Advanced Trauma Life Support® for Doctors

ATLS®

STUDENT COURSE MANUAL

EIGHTH EDITION

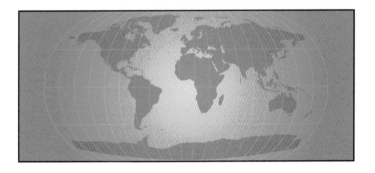

American College of Surgeons
Committee on Trauma

Chair of Committee on Trauma: John Fildes, MD, FACS
Medical Director of Trauma Program: J. Wayne Meredith, MD, FACS
ATLS Subcommittee Chairman: John Kortbeek, MD, FRCSC, FACS
ATLS Program Manager: Will Chapleau, EMT-P, RN, TNS
Project Manager: Claire Merrick
Development Editors: Nancy Peterson and Julie Scardiglia
Production Services: Laura Horowitz and Anne Seitz, Hearthside Publishing Services
Media Services: Steve Kidd and Angie Elliott, Delve Productions
Designer: Terri Wright Design
Artist: Dragonfly Media Group

EIGHTH EDITION
Second Impression

Copyright© 2008 American College of Surgeons
633 N. Saint Clair Street
Chicago, IL 60611-3211

Previous editions copyrighted 1980, 1982, 1984, 1993, 1997, and 2004 by the
American College of Surgeons.

Copyright enforceable internationally under the Bern Convention and the Uniform
Copyright Convention. All rights reserved. This manual is protected by copyright.
No part of it may be reproduced, stored in a retrieval system, or transmitted in any
form or by any means, electronic, mechanical, photocopying, recording, or
otherwise, without written permission from the American College of Surgeons.

The American College of Surgeons, its Committee on Trauma, and contributing
authors have taken care that the doses of drugs and recommendations for treatment
contained herein are correct and compatible with the standards generally accepted at
the time of publication. However, as new research and clinical experience broaden
our knowledge, changes in treatment and drug therapy may become necessary or
appropriate. Readers and participants of this course are advised to check the most
current product information provided by the manufacturer of each drug to be
administered to verify the recommended dose, the method and duration of
administration, and contraindications. It is the responsibility of the licensed
practitioner to be informed in all aspects of patient care and determine the best
treatment for each individual patient. The American College of Surgeons, its
Committee on Trauma, and contributing authors disclaim any liability, loss, or
damage incurred as a consequence, directly or indirectly, of the use and application
of any of the content of this 8th edition of the ATLS Program.

Advanced Trauma Life Support® and the acronym ATLS® are marks of the
American College of Surgeons.

Printed in the United States of America.

Advanced Trauma Life Support® Student Course Manual
Library of Congress Control Number: 2008905266
ISBN 978-1-880696-31-6

The 8th Edition of ATLS is dedicated to Irvene Hughes, RN. Ms. Hughes has served as a guiding light for ATLS from its inception in Nebraska, to its adoption by the American College of Surgeons, through seven editions published from her desk over 25 years. Irvene's commitment to quality, devotion to the program, and tireless efforts on behalf of the ATLS family were instrumental to the success of this international treasure. We, as her ATLS family, wish to thank Irvene for setting the example we attempt to follow.

FOREWORD

For more than a quarter century, the American College of Surgeons Committee on Trauma has taught the ATLS course to over 1 million doctors in more than 50 countries. ATLS has become the foundation of care for injured patients by teaching a common language and a common approach. The 8th edition was created using an international, multidisciplinary, and evidence-based approach. The result is an ATLS program that is contemporary and meaningful in the global community.

—*John Fildes,* MD, FACS
   Chair, AMERICAN COLLEGE OF SURGEONS COMMITTEE ON TRAUMA

PREFACE

Role of the American College of Surgeons Committee on Trauma

The American College of Surgeons (ACS) was founded to improve the care of surgical patients, and it has long been a leader in establishing and maintaining the high quality of surgical practice in North America. In accordance with that role, the ACS Committee on Trauma (COT) has worked to establish guidelines for the care of injured patients.

Accordingly, the COT sponsors and contributes to the continued development of the Advanced Trauma Life Support (ATLS) Program for Doctors. The ATLS Student Course does not present new concepts in the field of trauma care; rather, it teaches established treatment methods. A systematic, concise approach to the early care of trauma patients is the hallmark of the ATLS Program.

This eighth edition was developed for the ACS by members of the Subcommittee on ATLS and the ACS COT, other individual Fellows of the College, members of the international ATLS community, and nonsurgical consultants to the Subcommittee who were selected for their special competence in trauma care and their expertise in medical education. (Please see the listing at the end of the Preface and the Acknowledgements section for names and affiliations of these individuals.) The COT believes that those individuals who are responsible for caring for injured patients will find the information extremely valuable. The principles of patient care presented in this manual may also be beneficial for the care of patients with nontrauma-related diseases.

Injured patients present a wide range of complex problems. The ATLS Student Course presents a concise approach to assessing and managing multiply injured patients. The course presents doctors with knowledge and techniques that are comprehensive and easily adapted to fit their needs. The skills described in this manual represent one safe way to perform each technique. The ACS recognizes that there are other acceptable approaches. However, the knowledge and skills taught in the course are easily adapted to all venues for the care of these patients.

The ATLS Program is revised by the ATLS Subcommittee approximately every four years to respond to changes in available knowledge and incorporate newer and perhaps even safer skills. ATLS Committees in other countries and regions where the Program has been introduced

have participated in the revision process, and the ATLS Subcommittee appreciates their outstanding contributions. National and international educators review the educational materials to ensure that the course is conducted in a manner that facilitates learning. All of the course content is available in other resources, such as textbooks and journals. However, the ATLS Course is a specific entity, and the manuals, slides, skill procedures, and other resources are used for the entire course only and cannot be fragmented into separate, freestanding lectures or practical sessions. Members of the ACS COT and the ACS Regional and State/Provincial Committees, as well as the ACS ATLS Program Office staff members, are responsible for maintaining the high quality of the program. By introducing this course and maintaining its high quality, the COT hopes to provide another instrument by which to reduce the mortality and morbidity related to trauma. The COT recommends that doctors participating in the ATLS Student Course reverify their status every four years to maintain both their current status in the program and their knowledge of current ATLS core content.

New to this Edition

This eighth edition of the Advanced Trauma Life Support for Doctors Student Course Manual reflects several changes designed to enhance the educational content and its visual presentation.

CONTENT UPDATES

All chapters were rewritten and revised to ensure clear coverage of the most up-to-date technical content, which is also represented in updated references. New to this edition are:

▸▸ **New Sample Trauma Flow Sheet** (Appendix D)

▸▸ **Disaster Management and Emergency Preparedness** (Appendix H)

▸▸ **Skill X-B: Atlanto-occipital Joint Assessment**

▸▸ **Updated airway management algorithm**

▸▸ **Updated pelvic fracture management algorithm**

SKILLS VIDEO

You'll also note the inclusion of a DVD with this edition. This new course component includes video of critical skills that doctors should be familiar with before taking the course. Skill Stations during the course will allow doctors the opportunity to fine tune skill performance in preparation for the practical assessment. Review of the demonstrated skills prior to participating in the skills stations will enhance the learner's experience.

TEXTBOOK FEATURES

This edition features a new full-color design, along with new color photographs and medical illustrations. Content was presented in a narrative format rather than outline for ease of readability. In addition, an effort was made to augment the pedagogical features of the textbook to improve student comprehension and retention of knowledge. Look for the following features:

CHAPTER OUTLINE: This feature provides a "road map" to the chapter content

KEY QUESTIONS: ❓ These questions are aligned with the instructor's PowerPoint presentations to prepare students for key discussions during lectures

KEY POINTS: Sentences appear in red font to attract the reader's attention to key points of information.

LINKS ▪ Cross-references to other chapters, Skill Stations, and additional resources help to pull all of the information together

PITFALLS

PITFALL

These boxes highlight critical pitfalls to avoid while caring for trauma patients

SUMMARY

CHAPTER SUMMARY

Chapter summaries tie back to the Chapter Objectives to ensure understanding of the most pertinent chapter content

Editorial Notes

The ACS Committee on Trauma is referred to as the ACS COT or the Committee, and the State/Provincial Chair(s) is referred to as S/P Chair(s).

The international nature of this edition of the ATLS Student Manual may necessitate changes in commonly used terms to facilitate understanding by all students and teachers of the Program.

Advanced Trauma Life Support® and ATLS® are proprietary trademarks and service marks owned by the American College of Surgeons and cannot be used by individuals or entities outside the ACS COT organization for their goods and services without ACS approval. Accordingly, any reproduction of either or both marks in direct conjunction with the ACS ATLS Program within the ACS Committee on Trauma organization must be accompanied by the common law symbol of trademark ownership.

American College of Surgeons Committee on Trauma

John Fildes, MD, FACS
Committee on Trauma, Chair
Professor of Surgery, Vice Chair Department of Surgery, Program Director, General Surgery Residency Chief Division of Trauma & Critical Care
University of Nevada School of Medicine
Las Vegas, Nevada
United States

J. Wayne Meredith, MD, FACS
Trauma Program, Medical Director
Director of the Division of Surgical Sciences, Richard T. Myers Professor and Chairman
Wake Forest University
School of Medicine
Winston-Salem, North Carolina
United States

Subcommittee on Advanced Trauma Life Support of the American College of Surgeons Committee on Trauma

John B. Kortbeek, MD, FRCSC, FACS
ATLS Subcommittee, Chair
Professor Departments of Surgery and Critical Care
University of Calgary and Calgary Health Region
Calgary, Alberta
Canada

Christoph R. Kaufmann, MD, MPH, FACS
ATLS Subcommittee, International Course Director
Associate Medical Director
Trauma Services, Legacy Emanuel Hospital
Portland, Oregon
United States

Jameel Ali, MD, M.Med.Ed, FRCS, FACS
Professor of Surgery
University of Toronto
St. Michael's Hospital, Division of General Surgery/Trauma
Toronto, Ontario
Canada

Karen Brasel, MD, FACS
Associate Professor Trauma Surgery & Critical Care
Froedtert Hospital & Medical College of Wisconsin, Trauma
Surgery Division
Milwaukee, Wisconsin
United States

David G. Burris, MD, FACS
Professor & Chairman
USUHS, Norman M Rich Department of Surgery
Bethesda, Maryland
United States

William G. Cioffi, MD, FACS
Chief of Surgery
Rhode Island Hospital, Department of Surgery
Professor and Chairman
The Warren Alpert Medical School of Brown University,
Department of Surgery
Providence, Rhode Island
United States

Arthur Cooper, MD, MS, FACS, FAAP, FCCM
Professor of Surgery
Columbia University Medical Center
Affiliation at Harlem Hospital
New York, New York
United States

Michael Hollands, MB BS, FRACS, FACS
Head of Hepatobiliary and Gastro-oesophageal Surgery
Westmead Hospital
Sydney, New South Wales
Australia

Claus Falck Larsen, MD, dr.med., MPA, FACS
Medical Director
The Abdominal Centre, University of Copenhagen, Rigshopitalet
Denmark
Copenhagen
Denmark

West Livaudais, Jr, MD, FACS
Thoracic Surgeon
Southwest Wound Healing Center, Southwest Washington
Medical Center
Vancouver, Washington
United States

Fred A. Luchette, MD, FACS
Director, Division of Trauma, Critical Care, and Burns
Department of Surgery, Stritch School of Medicine, Loyola
University of Chicago
Maywood, Illinois
United States

John H. McVicker, MD, FACS
Neurosurgeon
Colorado Neurological Institute, Swedish Medical Center
Engelwood, Colorado
United States

Charles N. Mock, MD, PhD, MPH
*Professor of Surgery, Joint appointment, Professor of
Epidemiology*
Department of Surgery, Harborview Medical Center, University
of Washington
Seattle, Washington
United States

Frederick Moore, MD, FACS
Head, Division of Surgical Critical Care and Acute Care Surgery
Methodist Hospital
Houston, Texas
United States

Steven N. Parks, MD, FACS
Professor of Clinical Surgery
University of California, San Francisco, Department of Surgery,
Community Regional Medical Center
Fresno, California
United States

Renato Sergio Poggetti, MD, FACS
Director of Emergency Surgical Service
Hospital das Clinicas Universidad de São Paulo
Brazil

Thomas M. Scalea, MD, FACS
Physician in Chief
R Adams Cowley Shock Trauma Center
*Francis X Kelly Professor of Trauma Surgery, Director Program
in Trauma*
University of Maryland School of Medicine
Baltimore, Maryland
United States

R. Stephen Smith MD, RDMS, FACS
Vice Chair and Director of Surgical Education
Department of Surgery, The Virginia Tech - Carilion Medical
School
Roanoke, Virginia
United States

Richard Bell, MD, FACS (CON)
Professor and Chairman, Department of Surgery
University of South Carolina
Columbia, South Carolina
United States

Brent E. Krantz, MD, FACS (CON)
Professor of Surgery
University of South Carolina
Columbia, South Carolina
United States

Associate Members to the Subcommittee on Advanced Trauma Life Support of the American College of Surgeons Committee on Trauma

Reginald Burton, MD, FACS
Director, Trauma Program and Surgical Critical Care
Bryan LGH Medical Center, West
Lincoln, Nebraska
United States

Ronald Gross, MD, FACS
Associate Director of Trauma
Department of Emergency Medicine/Trauma, Hartford Hospital
Hartford, Connecticut
United States

Sharon M. Henry, MD, FACS
Associate Professor of Surgery
Director Wound Healing Service and Metabolism Service
University of Maryland, R. Adams Cowley Shock Trauma Center
Baltimore, Maryland
United States

Salvador Martín Mandujano, MD, FACS
General Surgeon
Medical Director
Cozumel Medical Center
Cozumel, Quintana Roo
Mexico

Charles E. Morrow, Jr, MD, FACS
Assistant Professor
Assistant Program Director, General Surgery
Medical Director, Trauma Surgery
Department of Trauma, Spartanburg Regional Medical Center
Spartanburg, South Carolina
United States

Frank Sacco, MD, FACS
Director of Trauma, Chief of Surgery
Alaska Native Medical Center, Department of Surgery
Anchorage, Alaska
United States

Martin A. Schreiber, MD, FACS
Associate Professor of Surgery
Chief of Trauma and Surgical Critical Care
Oregon Health & Science University, Trauma & Critical Care Section
Portland, Oregon
United States

Mary van Wijngaarden-Stephens, MD, FACS
Associate Clinical Professor Department of Surgery/Division Critical Care
Trauma Director
University of Alberta Hospitals
Edmonton, Alberta
Canada

Robert J. Winchell, MD, FACS
Head, Division of Trauma and Burn Surgery
Maine Medical Center
Associate Clinical Professor of Surgery
University of Vermont School of Medicine
Portland, Maine
United States

American Society of Anesthesiology Liasion to the Subcommittee on Advanced Trauma Life Support of the American College of Surgeons Committee on Trauma

Jill A. Antoine, MD
Associate Professor of Clinical Anesthesia
University of California, San Francisco, Department of Anesthesia and Perioperative Care
San Francisco, California
United States

American College of Emergency Physicians Liasion to the Subcommittee on Advanced Trauma Life Support of the American College of Surgeons Committee on Trauma

Richard C. Hunt, MD, FACEP
Director, Division of Injury Response
Centers for Disease Control and Prevention
Atlanta, Georgia
United States

Acknowledgments

CONTRIBUTORS

During development of this revision, we received a great deal of assistance from many individuals — whether reviewing information at meetings, submitting images, or evaluating research. ATLS® thanks the following contributors for their time and effort in the development of the 8th edition:

Melissa V. Abad
Regional Program Coordinator, CME Coordinator for Trauma Programs
American College of Surgeons ATLS Program Office
Chicago, Illinois
United States

Joe Acker, III, MS, MPH, EMT-P
Executive Director
Birmingham Regional EMS
Birmingham, Alabama
United States

Saud Al Turki, MD, FRCS, ODTS, FACA, FACS
Director
Trauma Courses Office, Postgraduate Education & Academic Affairs, King Abdulaziz Medical City
Riyadh
Kingdom of Saudi Arabia

Fatimah Albarracin, RN
Senior Officer
Life Support Training Center, Tawam Hospital, affiliate of Johns Hopkins Medicine
Al Ain, Abu Dhabi
United Arab Emirates

Celia Aldana
ATLS Coordinator
Committee on Trauma, Chile
Santiago
Chile

Jasmine Alkhatib
International Coordinator
American College of Surgeons
ATLS Program Office
Chicago, Illinois
United States

Donna Allerton, RN
Critical Care, Coordinator - ATLS Program
McMaster University Medical Centre
Hamilton, Ontario
Canada

Heri Aminuddin, MD
Neurosurgeon
Gatot Soebroto Central Army Hospital
Jakarta Timur, Jakarta
Indonesia

John A. Androulakis, MD, FACS
Emeritus Professor of Surgery
University Hospital of Patras
Patras
Greece

Guillermo Arana, MD, FACS
General Surgeon
National Hospital
Panama City
Panamá

Ivar Austlid
Department of Anaesthesia and Intensive Care
Haukeland University Hospital
Bergen
Norway

Margareta Behrbohm Fallsberg, PhD , BSc
Consultant
Consulting firm / small business
Linköping
Sweden

Renato Bessa de Melo, MD
Assistente Hospitalar
Serviço de Cirurgia Geral, Hospital de S.João
Porto
Portugal

Mike Betzner MD
Emergency Physician
Senior Medical Director STARS Air Ambulance
Calgary Health Region,
Calgary, Alberta
Canada
Clinical Lecturer, University of Calgary

Ken Boffard, MB BCh, FRCS, FRCS (Ed), FACS
Professor and Clinical Head
Department of Surgery, Johannesburg Hospital, University of the Witwatersrand
Johannesburg
South Africa

Raphael Bonvin, MD, PhD
Unite de pedagogie Medicale, Faculte de biologie et de medicine
Lausanne
Switzerland

Bertil Bouillon, MD
Professor
University of Witten Herdecke, Cologne, Merheim Medical Center, Department of Trauma and Orthopedic Surgery
Cologne
Germany

Mark W. Bowyer, MD, FACS, DMCC
Col (Ret), USAF, MC
Professor of Surgery
Chief, Division of Trauma and Combat Surgery
Director of Surgical Simulation
The Norman M. Rich Dept of Surgery
Uniformed Services University

Marianne Brandt
Special Education Teacher
Diabetes Educator
Caracas, Miranda
Venezuela

Fred Brenneman, MD, FRCSC, FACS
Chief, Trauma Program
Sunnybrook Health Sciences Center
Associate Professor
Department of Surgery, University of Toronto
Toronto, Ontario
Canada

Åse Brinchmann-Hansen, PhD
Managing Educational Consultant
The Norwegian Medical Association, Department of Professional Affairs
Oslo
Norway

Peter Brink, MD, PhD
Chief, Department of Traumatology
University Hospital Maastricht, Department of Traumatology
Maastricht
The Netherlands

Karim Brohi, MD
Consultant in Trauma, Vascular and Critical Care Surgery
The Royal London Hospital
London
United Kingdom

Laura Bruna, RN
Italian National Coordinator
Assitrauma
Torino
Italy

Jacqueline Bustraan, MSc
Educational Consultant and Researcher
PLATO, Centre for Research and Development of Education and Training, Leiden University
Leiden
Netherlands

Vilma Cabading
ATLS National Coordinator, Saudi Arabia
Academic Affairs Department
King Abdulaziz Medical City-NGHA
Riyadh
Kingdom of Saudi Arabia

Gerardo Cuauhtemoc Alvizo Cardenas
Assistant and Special Projects Coordinator
American College of Surgeons ATLS Program Office
Chicago, Illinois
United States

Carlos Carvajal Hafemann, MD, FACS
Professor of Surgery
Director of Surgery of the East Campus
Universidad de Chile
Santiago
Chile

Gustavo Castagneto, MD, FACS
Professor of Surgery
Buenos Aires British Hospital, Department of Surgery
Buenos Aires
Argentina

June Sau-Hung Chan
Skills Development Center, University of Hong
  Kong Medical Centre
Queen Mary Hospital, Department of Surgery
Hong Kong
China

Will Chapleau, EMT-P, RN, TNS
ATLS Program Manager
American College of Surgeons ATLS Program
  Office
Chicago, Illinois
United States

Zafarullah Chaudhry, MD, FRCS, FCPS, FACS
Professor of Surgery
National Hospital and Medical Center
President
College of Physicians and Surgeons Pakistan
Lahore
Pakistan

Peggy Chehardy, EdD, CHES
*Assistant Professor and Director of Surgical
  Education*
Tulane University School of Medicine,
  Department of Surgery
New Orleans, Louisiana
United States

Robert A. Cherry, MD, FACS
Trauma Program Medical Director
Penn State Milton S. Hershey Medical Center
  College of Medicine
Hershey, Pennsylvania
United States

Emmanuel Chrysos, MD, PhD, FACS
Associate Professor of Surgery
Department of General Surgery, University
  Hospital of Crete
Heraklion, Crete
Greece

Chin-Hung Chung, MB BS, FACS
Chief of Service
Department of Accident & Emergency, North
  District Hospital
Hong Kong
China

Francisco Collet e Silva, MD, FACS, PhD (med)
Medical Doctor
Emergency Surgical Services, Hospital das
  Clinicas of the University of São Paulo
São Paulo
Brazil

Jaime Cortes, MD
Chief, General Surgery
National Children's Hospital
Professor
University of Costa Rica
San Jose
Costa Rica

Scott D'Amours, MC.CM. FRCS(C), FRACS
ED Consultant
Royal Adelaide Hospital
Adelaide
Australia

Emily R.G. Delew
Regional Coordinator
American College of Surgeons
ATLS Program Office
Chicago, Illinois
United States

Laura Lee Demmons, RN, MBA
Manager
Critical Care Transport, University Hospital
Birmingham, Alabama
United States

Alejandro De Gracia, MD, FACS, MAAC
Chief, General Surgery
Agudos Parmenio Piñero General Hospital
Buenos Aires
Argentina

Mauricio Di Silvio-Lopez, MD, FACS
Clinical Residency and Research Program Director
20 de Noviembre National Medical Center,
  ISSSTE
Mexico City, Districto Federal
Mexico

Frank Doto, MS
Professor of Health Education
County College of Morris
Randolph, New Jersey
United States

Anne-Michéle Droux
ATLS National Coordinator, Switzerland
Swiss Society of Surgeons
Basel
Switzerland

Hermanus Jacobus Christoffel Du Plessis, MB,
ChB, MMed(Surg), FCS(SA), FACS
Chief Surgeon, Colonel
SAMHS (South African Military Health
  Services)
*Head of the Department of Surgery and
  Intensive Care*
1 Military Hospital
Adjunct Professor of Surgery
University of Pretoria
Pretoria
South Africa

Lesley Dunstall
EMST/ATLS National Coordinator, Australia
Royal Australasian College of Surgeons
North Adelaide, South Australia
Australia

Candida Durão
ATLS National Coordinator, Portugal
Portuguese Society of Surgeons
Lisbon
Portugal

Ruth Dyson, BA(hons)
ATLS Co-ordinator
The Royal College of Surgeons of England
London
United Kingdom

David Eduardo Eskenazi, MD, FACS
Chief, General and Thoracic Surgery
Htal. A. Oñativia

Buenos Aires
Argentina

Vagn Norgaard Eskesen, MD
Associate Professor
University Clinic of Neurosurgery, National
  Hospital - Copenhagen University Hospital
Copenhagen
Denmark

Denis Evoy, MCH, FRCSI
Consultant General Surgeon (Breast Endocrine)
St Vincents Private Hospital, Consultants Clinic
Dublin
Ireland

Froilan A. Fernandez, MD
Medical Director Emergency Service
Hospital del Trabajador
Santiago
Chile

Cornelia Rita Maria Getruda Fluit, MD,
MEdSci
Senior Consultant in Medical Education
University Medical Centre Nijmegen, Quality
  and Development of Medical Education
  Department
Nijmegen
The Netherlands

Jorge Esteban Foianini, MD, FACS
General Surgeon
Director
Foianini Clinic
Santa Cruz
Bolivia

Knut Fredriksen, MD, PhD
Consultant & Associate Professor
Department of Emergency Medical Services,
  University Hospital of North Norway
Faculty of Medicine,
University of Tromsø
Tromsø
Norway

Susanne Fristeen, RN
Former ATLS National Coordinator, Denmark
Danish Trauma Society
Copenhagen
Denmark

Christine Gaarder, MD
Head of Trauma Unit, General and GI surgeon
Emergency Division, Ullevaal University
  Hospital
Oslo
Norway

Subash Gautam, MD, MBBS, FRCS, FACS
*Senior Consultant and Head of Department of
  Surgery*
Fujairah Hospital
Fujairah
United Arab Emirates

Aggelos Geranios, MD
General Surgeon, Intensivist
Sur. Clinic of Livadeia Rural Hospital
Athens
Greece

Michael Gerazounis, MD
Greece

Javier González-Uriarte, MD, PhD, EBSQ,
FSpCS
General Surgeon
Hospital de Cruces, Bilbao, Liver Transplant
  Unit
Bilbao
Spain

John Greenwood
Director
Burns Unite, Royal Adelaide Hospital
Adelaide, South Australia
Australia

Russell L. Gruen, MBBS, PhD, FRACS
Associate Professor
University of Melbourne
Trauma Surgeon
The Royal Melbourne Hospital
Melbourne
Australia

Niels Gudmundsen-Vestre
Major
Danish Armed Forces Health Service
Hellerup
Denmark

Jeffrey S. Guy, MD, MSc, FACS
Director, Regional Burn Center
Associate Professor of Surgery
Vanderbilt University
Nashville, TN
United States

Enrique A. Guzman Cottallat, MD, FACS
Neurosurgeon
Diplomat in Public Health
Director, Neurosurgery Services
Guayaquil Hospital
Guayaquil
Ecuador

Arthur Hsieh, MA, NREMT-P
San Francisco Paramedic Association
San Francisco, California
United States

Richard Henn, RN, BSN, M.ED
Director, Education Department
Northern Arizona Healthcare
Flagstaff, Arizona
United States

Walter Henny, MD
Formerly of Erasmus Medical Center
Rotterdam
Netherlands

Grace Herrera-Fernandez
ATLS Coordinator
College of Physicians and Surgeons of Costa Rica
San Jose
Costa Rica

Fergal Hickey, FRCS, FRCS Ed.(A&E), DA(UK),
FCEM
Consultant in Emergency Medicine
Emergency Department, Sligo General Hospital

Sligo
Ireland

Scott Holmes
Duke University Lifeflight
Durham, North Carolina
United States

Jose María Jover Navalon, MD, FACS
Chief of Hepatopancreatic and Biliary Surgery
Hospital Universitario de Getafe, Department
  of General Surgery
Getafe
Spain

Aage W. Karlsen
ATLS Coordinator
Norwegian Air Ambulance
Drøbak
Norway

Darren Kilroy, FRCSEd, FCEM, M.Ed
Consultant in Emergency Medicine
Stockport NHS Foundation Trust
Cheshire
United Kingdom

Lena Klarin, RN
Former ATLS National Coordinator, Sweden
Sahlgrenska Universitetssjukhuset
Göteborg
Sweden

Peggy Knudson, MD, FACS
Professor of Surgery
University of California, San Francisco General
  Hospital, Department of Surgery
San Francisco, California
United States

Amy Koestner, RN, MSN
Trauma Program Manager
Borgess Medical Center
Kalamazoo, Michigan
United States

Radko Komadina , MD, PhD
*General Surgeon, Professor of Surgery, Head of
  Department for Medical Research*
General and Teaching Hospital Celje
Celje
Slovenia

Digna R. Kool, MD
Radiologist, Emergency Radiology
Department of Radiology, Radboud University
  Nijmegen Medical Centre
Nijmegen
The Netherlands

Roman Kosir, MD
Assistant of Surgery
University Clinical Center Maribor, Department
  of Traumatology
Maribor
Slovenia

Jon R. Krohmer, MD, FACEP
*Deputy Assistant Secretary for Health Affairs,
  Deputy Chief Medical Officer*
Department of Homeland Security
Washington, DC
United States

Ada Lai Yin Kwok
Skills Development Center, University of Hong
  Kong Medical Centre
Queen Mary Hospital, Department of Surgery
Hong Kong
China

LAM Suk-Ching, BN, MHM
Advanced Practice Nurse
Queen Mary Hospital
Hong Kong
China

Maria Lampi, BSc, RN
National ATLS Coordinator
Centre for Teaching & Research in Disaster
  Medicine and Traumatology, University Hospital
Linköping
Sweden

LEO Pien Ming MBBS, MRCS (Edin),
M.Med(Orthopaedics)
Changi General Hospital, General
  Orthopaedics, Department of Orthopaedics
Singapore
Republic of Singapore

Wilson Li, MD
Senior Medical Officer
Department of Orthopaedics & Traumatology,
  Queen Elizabeth Hospital
Hong Kong
China

Helen Livanios, RN
IC Unit Staff Nurse
Mediterraneo Hospital
Athens
Greece

Chong-Jeh Lo, MD, FACS
Associate Professor of Surgery
National Chen Kung University Medical Center
Tainan
Taiwan

Nur Rachmat Lubis, MD
Staff Department of Surgery
M. Hoesin General Hospital, Medical Faculty
  Sriwijaya University
Palembang, South Sumatra
Indonesia

J.S.K. Luitse, MD
Traumasurgeon
Medical Director Emergency Department
Trauma Coordinator
Academic Medical Center
Av Tilburg
Netherlands

Jaime Manzano, MD, FACS
General Surgeon
Hospital Metropolitano
Quito
Ecuador

Patrizio Mao, MD, FACS
Responsabile Urgenze Chirurgiche
Chirurgia Generale Universitaria, A.S.O. San
  Luigi Gonzaga di Orbassano
Torino
Italy

Emily Martens
Regional Program Coordinator, Surgical Skills Program Coordinator
American College of Surgeons ATLS Program Office
Chicago, Illinois
United States

Salvijus Milašius, MD
Chief of Primary Soldiers Health Care Center in Kaunas
Military Medical Services, Lithuanian Armed Forces
Kaunas
Lithuania

Soledad Monton, MD
General Surgeon
Department of General Surgery, Hospital García Orcoyen
Estella
Spain

Newton Djin Mori, MD
General Surgeon
Emergency Surgical Services,
Hospital das Clinicas Universidad de São Paulo
São Paulo
Brazil

Giorgio Olivero, MD, FACS
Professor of Surgery
University of Torino, Department of Medicine and Surgery, St. John the Baptist Hospital
Torino
Italy

Steve A. Olson, MD, FACS
Professor, Department of Surgery
Chief Orthopaedic Trauma
Chief Medical Officer
Duke University Hospital
Durham, North Carolina
United States

Gonzalo Ostria, MC, FACS
Director
Centro Medico Foianini
Santa Cruz
Bolivia

Fatima Pardo, MD
General Surgeon
ABC Medical Center
Mexico City, Districto Federal
Mexico

Andrew Pearce, BScHons MBBS, FACEM
Trauma Surgeon
Liverpool Hospital
Sydney
Australia

Nicolas Peloponissios, MD
General, Trauma, and Abdominal Surgeon
Department of Surgery, Daler Hospital
Fribourg
Switzerland

Pedro Moniz Pereira, MD, FACS
General Surgeon
Serviço de Cirurgia, Hospital Garcia de Orta
Almada
Portugal

Danielle Poretti, RN
Sanaxis, SA
Renens, Vaud
Switzerland

Jesper Ravn, MD
Consultant, Head of General Thoracic Department
Cardiothoracic Surgery, Rigshospitalet, Copenhagen University
Copenhagen
Denmark

Marcelo Recalde Hidrobo, MD, FACS
Professor of Oncological and General Surgeries
Loja University, International University, Ecuador;
Metropolitan Hospital
Quito
Ecuador

Peter Rhee, MD, MPH, FACS, FCCM, DMCC
Professor of Surgery
Chief, Section of Trauma, Critical Care, and Emergency Surgery
Arizona Health Sciences Center, Department of Surgery
Tucson, Arizona
United States

Martin Richardson
The Epworth Centre
Richmond, Victoria
Australia

Bo Richter
Major
Danish Armed Forces Health Services
Næstved
Denmark

Rosalind Roden, FFAEM
Consultant in Emergency Medicine
Leeds Teaching Hospitals NHS Trust
Yorkshire
United Kingdom

Diego Rodriguez, MD
Medical Director
Hospital Clinica San Agustin
San Agustin
Ecuador

Vicente Rodriguez, MD
Professor
Hospital Clinica San Agustin
San Agustin
Ecuador

Olav Røise, MD, PhD
Chairman of the Division of Neuroscience and Musculoskeletal Medicine
Ulleval University Hospital
Oslo
Norway

Daniel Ruiz, MD, FACS
Cardiovascular Surgeon
CMIC Clinic
Neuquén
Argentina

Octavio Ruiz, MD, FACS
Head of Transplant Services
American British Cowdray Medical Center
Mexico City, Districto Federal
Mexico

Jeffrey P. Salomone, MD, FACS
Associate Professor of Surgery
Emory University, Department of Surgery
Deputy Chief of Surgery
Grady Memorial Hospital
Atlanta, Georgia
United States

Rocio Sanchez-Aedo, RN
Former ATLS National Coordinator, Mexico
Committee on Trauma, Mexico
Mexico City, Districto Federal
Mexico

Mårtin Sandberg, MD, PhD
Senior Consultant in Anesthesiology
Air Ambulance Department, Ulleval University Hospital
Oslo
Norway

Nicole Schaapveld, RN
Managing Director / National Coordinator ATLS NL
Advanced Life Support Group - NL
Riel
The Netherlands

Domenic Scharplatz, MD, FACS
Head Surgeon
Hospital of Thusis
Thusis, Grisons
Switzerland

Inger B. Schipper, MD, PhD
Medical Director of the South West Netherlands Traumacenter
University Hospital Erasmus MC, Department of Trauma Surgery
Rotterdam
The Netherlands

Patrick Schoettker, MD, M.E.R.
Staff Specialist
Department of Anesthesiology, University Hospital Vaud
Lausanne
Switzerland

Kari Schrøder Hansen, MD
Consultant General Surgery
Department of Surgery, Haukeland University Hospital
Bergen
Norway

Bolivar Serrano, MD, FACS
General Surgeon
Hospital Latinoamericano
Cuenca
Ecuador

Juan Carlos Serrano, MD, FACS
Department of Trauma Director
Hospital Santa Inés
Cuenca
Ecuador

Mark Sheridan, MBBS, MMedSc, FRACS
Associate Professor
Director of Surgery and Director of
  Neurosurgery, Liverpool Hospital
Sydney, New South Wales
Australia

Richard K. Simons, MB, BChir, FRCS, FRCSC, FACS
Associate Professor, Medical Director, Trauma Services
Department of Surgery, UBC, Vancouver
  Coastal Health
Vancouver, British Columbia
Canada

Preecha Siritongtaworn, MD, FACS
Chief, Division of Trauma Surgery
Department of Surgery, Faculty of Medicine
  Siriraj Hospital, Mahidol University
Bangkok
Thailand

Nils Oddvar Skaga, MD
Chief Anaesthesiologist for Trauma
Ullevål University Hospital
Oslo
Norway

Peter Skippen, MBBS, FRCPC, FJFICM, MHA
Medical Director and Division Head
Clinical Associate Professor of Critical Care
BC Children's Hospital, Department of
  Pediatrics
Vancouver, British Columbia
Canada

Tone Slåke
ATLS National Coordinator, Norway
Norwegian Air Ambulance
Drøbak
Norway

Birgitte Soehus
ATLS National Coordinator, Denmark
Danish Trauma Society
Brønshøj
Denmark

Elizabeth de Solezio, MA, PhD
Advisor, Ecuadorian Secretary of State Culture Bureau
Committee on Trauma, Ecuador
Quito
Ecuador

Michael Stavropoulos, MD, FACS
Assistant Professor of Surgery
Surgery Department, Patras University Medical
  School
Patras
Greece

Spyridon Stergiopoulos, MD
Associate Professor of Surgery
Attikon University Hospital, 4th Surgical
  Department
Athens
Greece

Paul-Martin Sutter, MD
Department of Surgery, Spitalzentrum
Biel
Switzerland

Lars Bo Svendsen, MD, D M Sci
Associate Professor Surgery
Copenhagen University, Department of
  Abdominal Surgery and Transplantation,
  Rigshospitalet
Copenhagen
Denmark

Vasso Tagkalakis
ATLS National Coordinator, Greece
University of Patras
Patras
Greece

Wa'el S. Taha, MD
Assistant Professor of Surgery
Deputy Director of Trauma Courses Program
Department Orthopedic Surgery, King
  Abdulaziz Medical City
Riyadh
Kingdom of Saudi Arabia

Gustavo Tisminetzky, MD, FACS, MAAC
Professor of Surgery
Universidad de Buenos Aires, Escuela de
  Medicina Hospital Italiano de Buenos Aires,
  Jefe Unidad de Urgencia Hospital Fernández
Buenos Aires
Argentina

Philip Truskett , MB BS, FRACS
The Prince of Wales Hospital
Sydney, New South Wales
Australia

Wolfgang Ummenhofer, MD, DEAA
Professor of Anesthesiology and Intensive Care
University Hospital, Basel, Department of
  Anesthesia and Intensive Care
Basel
Switzerland

Yvonne van den Ende
Office Manager
Stichting Advanced Life Support Group
Riel
The Netherlands

Armand Robert van Kanten, MD
General Surgeon, Head of Trauma
University Hospital Paramaribo
Paramaribo
Suriname

Endre Varga, MD, PhD
Vice Chairman, Professor of Trauma Surgery
Department of Traumatology, Albert
  Szentgyörgyi Medical and Pharmaceutical
  Center, University of Szeged
Szeged
Hungary

Edina Várkonyi
Department of Traumatology, University of
  Szeged

Szeged
Hungary

Panteleimon Vassiliu, MD, PhD
Attending Surgeon
General Surgical Clinic
Attikon University Hospital
Athens
Greece

Eugenia Vassilopoulou, MD
Attending Anesthesiologist
General Hospital of Aigion
Aigion
Greece

Antigoni Vavarouta
ATLS Coordinator
University of Patras
Patras
Greece

Tore Vikström, MD, PhD
Director and Head, Consultant General Sugery
Professsor of Disaster Medicine & Traumatology
Centre for Teaching & Research in Disaster
  Medicine and Traumatology, University
  Hospital
Linköping
Sweden

Eric Voiglio, MD, PhD, FACS, FRCS
Senior Lecturer, Consultant Surgeon
Department of Emergency Surgery,
  University Hospitals of Lyon, Centre
  Hospitalier Lyon-Sud
Pierre-Bénite
France

Daryl Williams, MBBS, FANZCA, GDipBusAd, GdipCR
Associate Professor, University of Melbourne
Royal Melbourne Hospital, Department of
  Anaesthesia
Director Anaesthesia
Melbourne Hospital, University of Melbourne
Melbourne
Australia

Robert Winter, FRCP, FRCA, DM
Consultant in Critical Care Medicine
Mid Trent Critical Care Network and
  Nottingham University Hospitals
Nottingham
United Kingdom

Nopadol Wora-Urai, MD, FACS
President-Elect, Royal College of Surgeons
Royal College of Surgeons of Thailand
Bang

Wai-Key Yuen, MB BS, FRCS, FRACS, FACS
Consultant
Department of Surgery, Queen Mary
  Hospital
Hong Kong
China

HONOR ROLL

Over the past 30 years, ATLS has grown from a local course training Nebraska doctors to care for trauma patients to a family of trauma specialists from more than 50 countries who volunteer their time to ensure that our materials reflect the most current research and that our course is designed to improve patient outcomes. The 8th edition of ATLS reflects the efforts of the following individuals who contributed to the first seven editons, and we honor them here.

Sabas F. Abuabara, MD, FACS
Joe E. Acker, III, MS, MPH, EMT
Raymond H. Alexander, MD, FACS
Fareed Ali, MD, FRCS (C)
Jameel Ali, MD, MMed Ed, FRCS (C), FACS
Charles Aprahamian, MD, FACS
Guillermo Arana, MD, FACS
Ana Luisa Argomedo Manrique
Gonzalo Avilés
Richard Baillot, MD
Barbara A. Barlow, MA, MD, FACS
James Barone, MD, FACS
John Barrett, MD, FACS
Pierre Beaumont, MD
Richard M. Bell, MD, FACS
Eugene E. Berg, MD, FACS
Richard Bergeron, MD
François Bertrand, MD
Emidio Bianco, MD, JD
Don E. Boyle, MD, FACS
Rea Brown, MD, FACS
Allen F. Browne, MD, FACS
Gerry Bunting, MD
Andrew R. Burgess, MD, FACS
Richard E. Burney, MD, FACS
David Burris, MD, FACS
Sylvia Campbell, MD, FACS
C. James Carrico, MD, FACS
C. Gene Cayten, MD, FACS
David E. Clark, MD, FACS
Paul E. Collicott, MD, FACS
Arthur Cooper, MD, MS, FACS
Ronald D. Craig, MD
Doug Davey, MD
Elizabeth de Solezio, PhD
Subrato J. Deb, MD
Ronald Denis, MD
Jesus Díaz Portocarrero, MD, FACS
Frank X. Doto, MS
Marguerite Dupré, MD
Brent Eastman, MD, FACS
Frank E. Ehrlich, MD, FACS
Martin R. Eichelberger, MD, FACS
David Eduardo Eskenazi, MD, FACS
William F. Fallon, Jr, MD, FACS
David V. Feliciano, MD, FACS
Froilan Fernandez, MD
Carlos Fernandez-Bueno, MD
John J. Fildes, MD, FACS
Ronald P. Fischer, MD, FACS
Lewis M. Flint, Jr, MD, FACS
Stevenson Flanigan, MD, FACS
Esteban Foianini G., MD, FACS
Jorge E Foianini, MD, FACS
Richard Fruehling, MD
Sylvain Gagnon, MD
Richard Gamelli, MD, FACS
Thomas A. Gennarelli, MD, FACS
Paul Gebhard
James A. Geiling, MD, FCCP
John H. George, PhD
Roger Gilbertson, MD
Robert W. Gillespie, MD, FACS

Marc Giroux, MD
J. Alex Haller, Jr., MD, FACS
Burton H. Harris, MD, FACS
Michael L. Hawkins, MD, FACS
Ian Haywood, FRCS (Eng), MRCS, LRCP
James D. Heckman, MD, FACS
June E. Heilman, MD, FACS
David M. Heimbach, MD, FACS
David N. Herndon, MD, FACS
Erwin F. Hirsch, MD, FACS
Francisco Holguin, MD
David B. Hoyt, MD, FACS
Irvene K. Hughes, RN
Richard C. Hunt, MD, FACEP
John E. Hutton, Jr, MD, FACS
Miles H. Irving, FRCS (Ed), FRCS (Eng)
José María Jover Navalon, MD, FACS
Richard L. Judd, PhD
Gregory J. Jurkovich, MD, FACS
Christoph R. Kaufmann, MD, FACS
Howard B. Keith, MD, FACS
James F. Kellam, MD, FRCS, FACS
Steven J. Kilkenny, MD, FACS
John B. Kortbeek, MD, FACS
Brent Krantz, MD, FACS
Jon R. Krohmer, MD, FACEP
Katherine Lane, PhD
Francis G. Lapiana, MD, FACS
Pedro Larios Aznar
Anna M. Ledgerwood, MD, FACS
Dennis G. Leland, MD, FACS
Frank Lewis, MD, FACS
Edward B. Lucci, MD, FACEP
Eduardo Luck, MD, FACS
Thomas G. Luerssen, MD, FACS
Arnold Luterman, MD, FACS
Fernando Magallanes Negrete, MD
Donald W. Marion, MD, FACS
Michael R. Marohn, DO, FACS
Barry D. Martin, MD
Salvador Martín Mandujano, MD, FACS
Kimball I. Maull, MD, FACS
Mary C. McCarthy, MD, FACS
Gerald McCullough, MD, FACS
John E. McDermott, MD, FACS
James A. McGehee, DVM, MS
William F. McManus, MD, FACS
Norman E. McSwain, Jr., MD, FACS
Philip S. Metz, MD, FACS
Cynthia L. Meyer, MD
Frank B. Miller, MD, FACS
Sidney F. Miller, MD, FACS
Ernest E. Moore, MD, FACS
Johanne Morin, MD
David Mulder, MD, FACS
Raj K. Narayan, MD, FACS
James B. Nichols, DVM, MS
Martín Odriozola, MD, FACS
Franklin C. Olson, EdD
Gonzalo Ostria P, MD, FACS
Arthur Pagé, MD
José Paiz Tejada
Steven N. Parks, MD, FACS

Chester (Chet) Paul, MD
Mark D. Pearlman, MD
Andrew B. Peitzman, MD, FACS
Jean Péloquin, MD
Philip W. Perdue, MD, FACS
J.W. Rodney Peyton, FRCS (Ed), MRCP
Lawrence H. Pitts, MD FACS
Galen V. Poole, MD, FACS
Ernest Prégent, MD
Richard R. Price, MD, FACS
Herbert Proctor, MD, FACS
Jacques Provost, MD
Paul Pudimat, MD
Max L. Ramenofsky, MD, FACS
Marcelo Recalde, MD, FACS
John Reed, MD
Marleta Reynolds, MD, FACS
Stuart A. Reynolds, MD, FACS
Bernard Riley, FFARCS
Charles Rinker, MD, FACS
Avraham Rivkind, MD
Ronald E. Rosenthal, MD, FACS
Grace Rozycki, MD, FACS
J. Octavio Ruiz Speare, MD, MS, FACS
James M. Ryan, MCh, FRCS (Eng), RAMC
James M. Salander, MD, FACS
Gueider Salas, MD
Rocio Sánchez-Aedo Linares
Thomas G. Saul, MD, FACS
William P. Schecter, MD, FACS
Thomas E. Scott, MD, FACS
Stuart R. Seiff, MD, FACS
Steven R. Shackford, MD, FACS
Marc J. Shapiro, MD, FACS
Thomas E. Shaver, MD, FACS
Richard C. Simmonds, DVM, MS
David V. Skinner, FRCS (Ed), FRCS (Eng)
Arnold Sladen, MD, FACS
Ricardo Sonneborn, MD, FACS
Gerald O. Strauch, MD, FACS
Luther M. Strayer, III, MD
James K. Styner, MD
Joseph J. Tepas, III, MD, FACS
Stéphane Tétraeault, MD
Gregory A. Timberlake, MD, FACS
Peter G. Trafton, MD, FACS
Stanley Trooksin, MD, FACS
David Tuggle, MD, FACS
Jay Upright
Antonio Vera Bolea
Alan Verdant, MD
J. Leonel Villavicencio, MD, FACS
Franklin C. Wagner, MD, FACS
Raymond L. Warpeha, MD, FACS
Clark Watts, MD, FACS
John A. Weigelt, MD, FACS
John West, MD, FACS
Robert J. White, MD, FACS
Fremont P. Wirth, MD, FACS
Bradley D. Wong, MD, FACS
Peter H. Worlock, DM, FRCS (Ed), FRCS (Eng)

COURSE OVERVIEW: The Purpose, History, and Concepts of the ATLS Program

Program Goals

The Advanced Trauma Life Support (ATLS) course provides its participants with a safe and reliable method for the immediate treatment of injured patients and the basic knowledge necessary to:

1. Assess a patient's condition rapidly and accurately.

2. Resuscitate and stabilize patients according to priority.

3. Determine whether a patient's needs exceed a facility's resources and/or a doctor's capabilities.

4. Arrange appropriately for a patient's interhospital or intrahospital transfer (what, who, when, and how).

5. Ensure that optimal care is provided and that the level of care does not deteriorate at any point during the evaluation, resuscitation, or transfer processes.

Course Objectives

The content and skills presented in this course are designed to assist doctors in providing emergency care for trauma patients. The concept of the "golden hour" emphasizes the urgency necessary for successful treatment of injured patients and is not intended to represent a "fixed" time period of 60 minutes. Rather, it is the window of opportunity during which doctors can have a positive impact on the morbidity and mortality associated with injury. The ATLS course provides the essential information and skills for doctors to identify and treat life-threatening and potentially life-threatening injuries under the extreme pressures associated with the care of these patients in the fast-paced environment and anxiety of a trauma room. The ATLS course is applicable to all doctors in a variety of clinical situations. It is just as relevant to doctors in a large teaching facility in North America or Europe as it is in a developing nation with rudimentary facilities.

Upon completion of the ATLS student course, the doctor will be able to:

1. Demonstrate the concepts and principles of the primary and secondary patient assessments.

2. Establish management priorities in a trauma situation.

3. Initiate primary and secondary management necessary within the golden hour for the emergency management of acute life-threatening conditions.

4. In a given simulated clinical and surgical skills practicum, demonstrate the following skills, which are often required in the initial assessment and treatment of patients with multiple injuries:
   a. Primary and secondary assessment of a patient with simulated, multiple injuries
   b. Establishment of a patent airway and initiation of one- and two-person ventilation
   c. Orotracheal intubation on adult and infant manikins
   d. Pulse oximetry and carbon dioxide detection in exhaled gas
   e. Cricothyroidotomy
   f. Assessment and treatment of a patient in shock, particularly recognition of life-threatening hemorrhage
   g. Venous and intraosseous access
   h. Pleural decompression via needle thoracentesis and chest tube insertion
   i. Recognition of cardiac tamponade (and performance of pericardiocentesis)
   j. Clinical and radiographic identification of thoracic injuries
   k. Use of peritoneal lavage, ultrasound, and computed tomography (CT) in abdominal evaluation
   l. Evaluation and treatment of a patient with brain injury, including use of the Glasgow Coma Scale score and CT of the brain
   m. Assessment of head and facial trauma by physical examination
   n. Protection of the spinal cord, and radiographic and clinical evaluation of spine injuries
   o. Musculoskeletal trauma assessment and management
   p. Estimation of the size and depth of burn injury and volume resuscitation
   q. Recognition of the special problems of injuries in infants, the elderly, and pregnant women
   r. Understanding of the principles of disaster management

THE NEED

Injury deaths worldwide were estimated at more than 5 million in 2000 (Figure 1). The burden of injury is even more significant, accounting for 12% of the world's burden of disease. Motor vehicle crashes (road traffic injuries, in Figure 2) alone cause more than 1 million deaths annually and an estimated 20 million to 50 million significant injuries; they are the leading cause of death due to injury worldwide. Improvements in injury control efforts are having an impact in most developed countries, where trauma remains the leading cause of death in persons 1 through 44 years of age. Significantly, more than 90% of motor vehicle crashes occur in the developing world. Injury-related deaths are expected to rise dramatically by 2020, with deaths due to motor vehicle crashes projected to increase by 80% from current rates in low- and middle-income countries. By 2020 it is estimated that more than 1 in 10 people will die from injuries.

Global trauma-related costs are estimated to exceed $500 billion annually. These costs are much higher if one considers lost wages, medical expenses, insurance administration costs, property damage, fire loss, employer costs, and indirect loss from work-related injuries. Despite these staggering costs, less than 4 cents of each federal research dollar in the United States are spent on trauma research. As monumental as these data are, the true cost can be measured only when it is realized that trauma strikes down a society's youngest and potentially most productive members. Research dollars spent on communicable diseases such as polio and diphtheria have nearly eliminated the incidence of these diseases in the United States. Unfortunately the disease of trauma has not captured the public attention in the same way.

Injury is a disease. It has a host (the patient) and it has a vector of transmission (eg, motor vehicle, firearm, etc). Many significant changes have improved the care of the injured patient since the first edition of the ATLS Program appeared in 1980. The need for the program and for sustained, aggressive efforts to prevent injuries is as great now as it has ever been.

Trimodal Death Distribution

First described in 1982, the trimodal distribution of deaths implies that death due to injury occurs in one of three periods, or peaks (Figure 3). The *first peak* occurs within seconds to minutes of injury. During this early period, deaths generally result from apnea due to severe brain or high spinal cord injury or rupture of the heart,

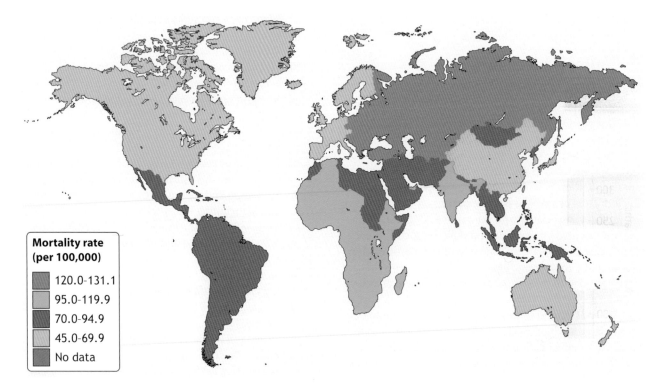

**Mortality rate
(per 100,000)**

120.0–131.1
95.0–119.9
70.0–94.9
45.0–69.9
No data

■ **Figure 1 Global Injury-Related Mortality.**

Reproduced with permission from *The Injury Chart Book: A Graphical Overview of the Global Burden of Injuries.* Geneva: World Health Organization Department of Injuries and Violence Prevention, Noncommunicable Diseases and Mental Health Cluster; 2002.

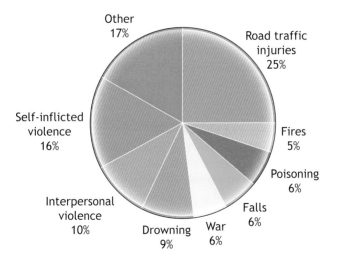

■ Figure 2 Distribution of Global Injury Mortality by Cause.

Reproduced with permission from *The Injury Chart Book: A Graphical Overview of the Global Burden of injuries.* Geneva: World Health Organization Department of Injuries and Violence Prevention, Noncommunicable Diseases and Mental Health Cluster; 2002.

aorta, or other large blood vessels. Very few of these patients can be saved because of the severity of their injuries. Only prevention can significantly reduce this peak of trauma-related deaths.

The *second peak* occurs within minutes to several hours following injury. Deaths that occur during this period are usually due to subdural and epidural

hematomas, hemopneumothorax, ruptured spleen, lacerations of the liver, pelvic fractures, and/or multiple other injuries associated with significant blood loss. The golden hour of care after injury is characterized by the need for rapid assessment and resuscitation, which are the fundamental principles of Advanced Trauma Life Support.

The *third peak,* which occurs several days to weeks after the initial injury, is most often due to sepsis and multiple organ system dysfunction. Care provided during each of the preceding periods impacts on outcomes during this stage. The first and every subsequent person to care for the injured patient has a direct effect on long-term outcome.

The temporal distribution of deaths reflects local advances and capabilities of trauma systems. The development of standardized trauma training for doctors, better prehospital care, and the development of trauma centers with dedicated trauma teams and established protocols to care for injured patients has altered the picture. A recent study in California demonstrated that approximately 50% of patients died at the scene or within the first hour, supporting continued emphasis on injury-prevention programs. Both the mechanism of injury and the body area injured were important determinants of the subsequent clinical course and the temporal risk of death. Eighty percent of deaths due to severe chest trauma occurred within the first 6 hours, whereas 90% of deaths from head injury occurred during the first week. The incidence of late deaths was much lower in this series (8%).

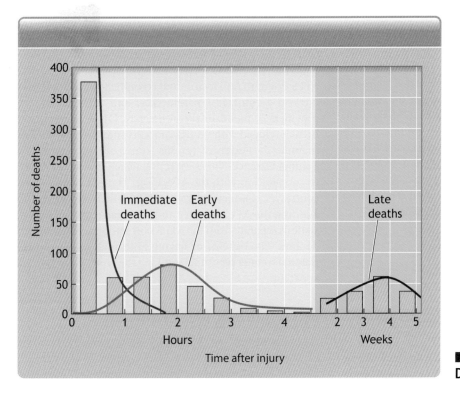

■ Figure 3 Trimodal Death Distribution.

History

The delivery of trauma care by doctors in the United States before 1980 was at best inconsistent. A tragedy occurred in February 1976 that changed trauma care in the "first hour" for injured patients in the United States and in much of the rest of the world. An orthopedic surgeon was piloting his plane and crashed in a rural Nebraska cornfield. The surgeon sustained serious injuries, three of his children sustained critical injuries, and one child sustained minor injuries. His wife was killed instantly. The care that he and his family subsequently received was inadequate by the day's standards. The surgeon, recognizing how inadequate their treatment was, stated: "When I can provide better care in the field with limited resources than what my children and I received at the primary care facility, there is something wrong with the system, and the system has to be changed."

A group of private-practice surgeons and doctors in Nebraska, the Lincoln Medical Education Foundation, and the Lincoln-area Mobile Heart Team Nurses, with the help of the University of Nebraska Medical Center, the Nebraska State Committee on Trauma (COT) of the American College of Surgeons (ACS), and the Southeast Nebraska Emergency Medical Services identified the need for training in advanced trauma life support. A combined educational format of lectures, lifesaving skill demonstrations, and practical laboratory experiences formed the first prototype ATLS course for doctors.

A new approach to the provision of care for individuals who suffer major, life-threatening injury premiered in 1978, the year of the first ATLS course. This prototype ATLS course was field-tested in conjunction with the Southeast Nebraska Emergency Medical Services. One year later, the ACS COT, recognizing trauma as a surgical disease, enthusiastically adopted the course under the imprimatur of the College and incorporated it as an educational program.

This course was based on the assumption that appropriate and timely care could significantly improve the outcome of injured patients. The original intent of the ATLS Program was to train doctors who do not manage major trauma on a daily basis, and the primary audience for the course has not changed. However, today the ATLS method is accepted as a standard for the "first hour" of trauma care by many who provide care for the injured, whether the patient is treated in an isolated rural area or a state-of the-art trauma center.

Course Development and Dissemination

THE 1980s AND 1990s

The ATLS course was conducted nationally for the first time under the auspices of the American College of Surgeons in January 1980. Canada became an active participant in the ATLS Program in 1981. Countries in Latin and South America joined the ACS COT in 1986 and implemented the ATLS Program. Under the auspices of the ACS Military Committee on Trauma, the program has been conducted for U.S. military doctors in other countries.

The program has grown each year in the number of both courses and participants. By 2007, the course had trained approximately 1 million doctors in more than 60,000 courses around the world. Currently, an average of 40,000 doctors are trained each year in approximately 2600 courses. The greatest growth in recent years has been in the international community, and this group currently represents approximately more than half of all ATLS activity.

The text for the course is revised approximately every 4 years and incorporates new methods of evaluation and treatment that have become accepted parts of the armamentarium of doctors who treat trauma patients. Course revisions incorporate suggestions from members of the Subcommittee on ATLS; members of the ACS COT; members of the international ATLS family; representatives to the ATLS Subcommittee from the American College of Emergency Physicians and the American College of Anesthesiologists; and course instructors, coordinators, educators, and participants. Changes that are made to the program reflect accepted, verified practice patterns, not "cutting edge" technology or experimental methods. The international nature of the program mandates that the course be adaptable to a variety of geographic, economic, social, and medical practice situations. To retain a current status in the ATLS Program, an individual must reverify with the latest edition of the materials.

A parallel course to the ATLS course is the Prehospital Trauma Life Support (PHTLS) course, which is sponsored by the National Association of Emergency Medical Technicians (NAEMT). The PHTLS course, developed in cooperation with the ACS COT, is based on the concepts of the ACS ATLS Program for Doctors and is conducted for emergency medical technicians, paramedics, and nurses who are providers of prehospital trauma care. Other courses have been developed with similar concepts and philosophies. For example, the Society of Trauma Nurses offers the Advanced Trauma Care for Nurses (ATCN), which is also developed in cooperation with the ACS COT. The ATCN and ATLS courses are conducted parallel to each other with the nurses auditing the ATLS lectures and then participating in skill stations separate from the ATLS skill stations conducted for doctors. The benefits of having both prehospital and in-hospital trauma personnel speaking the same "language" are apparent.

INTERNATIONAL DISSEMINATION

As a pilot project, the ATLS Program was exported outside of North America in 1986 to the Republic of Trinidad and Tobago. The ACS Board of Regents gave permission in 1987 for promulgation of the ATLS Program in other countries. The ATLS Program may be requested by a recognized surgical organization or ACS Chapter in another country by corresponding with the ATLS Subcommittee Chairperson, care of the ACS ATLS Program Office, Chicago, IL. At the time of publication, 47 countries were actively providing the ATLS course to their doctors. These countries include:

1. Argentina (ACS Chapter and Committee on Trauma)

2. Australia (Royal Australasian College of Surgeons)

3. Bahrain (Kingdom of Saudi Arabia ACS Chapter and Committee on Trauma)

4. Bolivia (Bolivian Surgeons Society)

5. Brazil (ACS Chapter and Committee on Trauma)

6. Canada (ACS Chapters and Provincial Committees on Trauma)

7. Chile (ACS Chapter and Committee on Trauma)

8. Colombia (ACS Chapter and Committee on Trauma)

9. Costa Rica (College of Physicians and Surgeons of Costa Rica)

10. Cyprus (ACS Chapter and Committee on Trauma, Greece)

11. Denmark (Danish Trauma Society)

12. Ecuador (ACS Chapter and Committee on Trauma)

13. Fiji and the nations of the Southwest Pacific (Royal Australasian College of Surgeons)

14. Germany (German Society for Trauma Surgery and Task Force for Early Trauma Care)

15. Greece (ACS Chapter and Committee on Trauma)

16. Grenada (Society of Surgeons of Trinidad and Tobago)

17. Hong Kong (ACS Chapter and Committee on Trauma)

18. Hungary (Hungarian Trauma Society)

19. Indonesia (Indonesian Surgeons Association)

20. Ireland (Royal College of Surgeons in Ireland)

21. Israel (Israel Surgical Society)

22. Italy (ACS Chapter and Committee on Trauma)

23. Jamaica (ACS Chapter and Committee on Trauma)

24. Kingdom of Saudi Arabia (ACS Chapter and Committee on Trauma)

25. Lithuania (Lithuanian Society of Traumatology and Orthopaedics)

26. Mexico (ACS Chapter and Committee on Trauma)

27. Netherlands, The (Dutch Trauma Society)

28. New Zealand (Royal Australasian College of Surgeons)

29. Norway (Norwegian Surgical Society)

30. Pakistan (College of Physicians and Surgeons Pakistan)

31. Panama (ACS Chapter and Committee on Trauma)

32. Papua New Guinea (Royal Australasian College of Surgeons)

33. Peru (ACS Chapter and Committee on Trauma)

34. Portugal (Portuguese Society of Surgeons)

35. Qatar (Kingdom of Saudi Arabia ACS Chapter and Committee on Trauma)

36. Republic of China, Taiwan (Surgical Association of the Republic of China, Taiwan)

37. Republic of Singapore (Chapter of Surgeons, Academy of Medicine)

38. Republic of South Africa (South African Trauma Society)

39. Spain (Spanish Society of Surgeons)

40. Sweden (Swedish Society of Surgeons)

41. Switzerland (Swiss Society of Surgeons)

42. Thailand (Royal College of Surgeons of Thailand)

43. Trinidad and Tobago (Society of Surgeons of Trinidad and Tobago)

44. United Arab Emirates (Surgical Advisory Committee)

45. United Kingdom (Royal College of Surgeons of England)

46. United States, U.S. territories (ACS Chapters and State Committees on Trauma)

47. Venezuela (ACS Chapter and Committee on Trauma)

The Concept

The concept behind the ATLS course has remained simple. Historically, the approach to treating injured patients, as taught in medical schools, was the same as that for patients with a previously undiagnosed medical condition: an extensive history including past medical history, a physical examination starting at the top of the head and progressing down the body, the development of a differential diagnosis, and a list of adjuncts to confirm the diagnosis. Although this approach was adequate for a patient with diabetes mellitus and many acute surgical illnesses, it did not satisfy the needs of patients suffering life-threatening injuries. The approach required change.

Three underlying concepts of the ATLS Program were initially difficult to accept:

1. Treat the greatest threat to life first.

2. The lack of a definitive diagnosis should never impede the application of an indicated treatment.

3. A detailed history is not essential to begin the evaluation of a patient with acute injuries.

The result was the development of the ABCDE approach to the evaluation and treatment of injured patients. These concepts are also in keeping with the observation that the care of injured patients in many circumstances is a team effort, allowing medical personnel with special skills and expertise to provide care simultaneously with surgical leadership of the process.

The ATLS course emphasizes that injury kills in certain reproducible time frames. For example, the loss of an airway kills more quickly than does the loss of the ability to breathe. The latter kills more quickly than loss of circulating blood volume. The presence of an expanding intracranial mass lesion is the next most lethal problem. Thus, the mnemonic ABCDE defines the specific, ordered evaluations and interventions that should be followed in all injured patients:

*A*irway with cervical spine protection

*B*reathing

*C*irculation, stop the bleeding

*D*isability or neurologic status

*E*xposure (undress) and *E*nvironment (temperature control)

Course Overview

The ATLS course emphasizes the rapid initial assessment and primary treatment of injured patients, starting at the time of injury and continuing through initial assessment, lifesaving intervention, reevaluation, stabilization, and, when needed, transfer to a trauma center. The course consists of precourse and postcourse tests, core content lectures, interactive case presentations, discussions, development of lifesaving skills, practical laboratory experiences, and a final performance proficiency evaluation. Upon completion of the course, doctors should feel confident in implementing the skills taught in the ATLS course.

The Impact

ATLS training for doctors in a developing country has resulted in a decrease in injury mortality. Lower per capita rates of deaths from injuries are observed in areas where doctors have ATLS training. In one study, a small trauma team led by a doctor with ATLS experience had equivalent patient survival when compared with a larger team with more doctors in an urban setting. In addition, there were more unexpected survivors than fatalities. There is abundant evidence that ATLS training improves the knowledge base, the psychomotor skills and their use in resuscitation, and the confidence and performance of doctors who have taken part in the program. The organization and procedural skills taught in the course are retained by course participants for at least 6 years, which may be the most significant impact of all.

Acknowledgments

The COT of the ACS and the ATLS Subcommittee gratefully acknowledge the following organizations for their time and efforts in developing and field testing the Advanced Trauma Life Support concept: The Lincoln Medical Education Foundation, Southeast Nebraska Emergency Medical Services, the University of Nebraska College of Medicine, and the Nebraska State Committee on Trauma of the ACS. The committee also is indebted to the Nebraska doctors who supported the development of this course and to the Lincoln Area Mobile Heart Team Nurses who shared their time and ideas to help build it. Appreciation is extended to the organizations identified previously in this overview for their support of the worldwide promulgation of the course. Special recognition is given to the spouses, significant others, children, and practice partners of the ATLS instructors and students. The time that doctors spend away from their homes and practices and effort afforded to this voluntary program are essential components for the existence and success of the ATLS Program.

Summary

The ATLS course provides an easily remembered approach to the evaluation and treatment of injured patients for any doctor, irrespective of practice specialty, even under the stress, anxiety, and intensity that accompanies the resuscitation process. In addition, the program provides a common language for all providers who care for injured patients. The ATLS course provides a foundation for evaluation, treatment, education, and quality assurance-in short, a system of trauma care that is measurable, reproducible, and comprehensive.

The ATLS Program has had a positive impact on the care provided to injured patients worldwide. This has resulted from the improved skills and knowledge of the doctors and other health care providers who have been course participants. The ATLS course establishes an organized and systematic approach for the evaluation and treatment of patients, promotes minimum standards of care, and recognizes injury as a world health care issue. Morbidity and mortality have been reduced, but the need to eradicate injury remains. The ATLS Program has changed and will continue to change as advances occur in medicine and the needs and expectations of our societies change.

Bibliography

1. Ali J, Adam R, Butler AK, et al, Trauma outcome improves following the Advanced Trauma Life Support program in a developing country. *J Trauma* 1993;34:890-899.

2. Ali J, Adam R, Josa D, et al. Comparison of interns completing the old (1993) and new interactive (1997) Advanced Trauma Life Support courses. *J Trauma* 1999;46:80-86.

3. Ali J, Adam R, Stedman M, et al. Advanced Trauma Life Support program increases emergency room application of trauma resuscitative procedures in a developing country. *J Trauma* 1994;36:391-394.

4. Ali J, Adam R, Stedman M, et al. Cognitive and attitudinal impact of the Advanced Trauma Life Support Course in a developing country. *J Trauma* 1994;36:695-702.

5. Ali J, Cohen R, Adam R, et al. Teaching effectiveness of the Advanced Trauma Life Support program as demonstrated by an objective structured clinical examination for practicing physicians. *World J Surg* 1996;20:1121-1125.

6. Ali J, Cohen R, Adams R, et al. Attrition of cognitive and trauma skills after the Advanced Trauma Life Support (ATLS) course. *J Trauma* 1996;40:860-866.

7. Ali J, Howard M. The Advanced Trauma Life Support Program in Manitoba: a 5-year review. *Can J Surg* 1993;36:181-183.

8. Anderson ID, Anderson IW, Clifford P, et al. Advanced Trauma Life Support in the UK: 8 years on. *Br J Hosp Med* 1997;57:272-273.

9. Aprahamian C, Nelson KT, Thompson BM, et al. The relationship of the level of training and area of medical specialization with registrant performance in the Advanced Trauma Life Support course. *J Emerg Med* 1984;2:137-140.

10. Ben Abraham R, Stein M, Kluger Y, et al. ATLS course in emergency medicine for physicians. *Harefuah* 1997;132:695-697, 743.

11. Ben Abraham R, Stein M, Kluger Y, et al. The impact of Advanced Trauma Life Support Course on graduates with non-surgical medical background. *Eur J Emerg Med* 1997;4:11-14.

12. Berger LR, Mohan D: *Injury Control: A Global View.* Delhi, India: Oxford University Press; 1996.

13. Blumenfield A, Ben Abraham R, Stein M, et al. Cognitive knowledge decline after Advanced Trauma Life Support courses. *J Trauma* 1998;44:513-516.

14. Burt CW. Injury-related visits to hospital emergency departments: United States, 1992. *Adv Data* 1995;261:1-20.

15. Demetriades D, Kimbrell B, Salim A, et al. Trauma deaths in a mature urban trauma system: is "trimodal" distribution a valid concept? *J Am Coll Surg* 2005;201:343-348.

16. Deo SD, Knottenbelt JD, Peden MM. Evaluation of a small trauma team for major resuscitation. *Injury* 1997;28:633-637.

17. Direccao Geral de Vicao, Lisboa, Portugal, data provided by Pedro Ferreira Moniz Pereira, MD, FACS.

18. Fingerhut LA, Cox CS, Warner M, et al. International comparative analysis of injury mortality: findings from the ICE on injury statistics. *Adv Data* 1998;303:1-20.

19. Firdley FM, Cohen DJ, Bienbaum ML, et al. Advanced Trauma Life Support: Assessment of cognitive achievement. *Milit Med* 1993;158:623-627.

20. Gautam V, Heyworth J. A method to measure the value of formal training in trauma management: comparison between ATLS and induction courses. *Injury* 1995;26:253-255.

21. Greenslade GL, Taylor RH. Advanced Trauma Life Support aboard RFA Argus. *J R Nav Med Serv* 1992;78:23-26.

22. Leibovici D, Fedman B, Gofrit ON, et al. Prehospital cricothyroidotomy by physicians. *Am J Emerg Med* 1997;15:91-93.

23. Mock CJ. International approaches to trauma care. *Trauma Q* 1998;14:191-348.

24. Murray CJ, Lopez A. The global burden of disease: I. A comprehensive assessment of mortality and disability from diseases, and injuries and risk factors in 1990 and projected to 2020. Cambridge, MA: Harvard University Press; 1996.

25. National Center for Health Statistics: Injury visits to emergency departments. please state so.

26. National Safety Council. *Injury Facts (1999).* Itasca, IL: National Safety Council.

27. Nourjah P. National hospital ambulatory medical care survey: 1997 emergency department summary. *Adv Data* 1999;304:1-24.

28. Olden van GDJ, Meeuwis JD, Bolhuis HW, et al. Clinical impact of advanced trauma life support. *Am J Emerg Med* 2004;22:522-525.

29. Rutledge R, Fakhry SM, Baker CC, et al. A population-based study of the association of medical manpower with county trauma death rates in the United States. *Ann Surg* 1994;219:547-563.

30. Walsh DP, Lammert GR, Devoll J. The effectiveness of the advanced trauma life support system in a mass casualty situation by non-trauma experienced physicians: Grenada 1983. *J Emerg Med* 1989;7:175-180.

31. Williams MJ, Lockey AS, Culshaw MC. Improved trauma management with Advanced Trauma Life Support (ATLS) training. *J Accident Emerg Med* 1997;14:81-83.

32. World Health Organization. *The Injury Chart Book: a Graphical Overview of the Global Burden of Injuries.* Geneva: World Health Organization Department of Injuries and Violence Prevention. Noncommunicable Diseases and Mental Health Cluster; 2002.

33. World Health Organization. *Violence and Injury Prevention and Disability (VIP).* http://www.who.int/violence_injury_prevention/publications/other_injury/chartb/en/index.html. Accessed January 9, 2008.

34. World Health Organization. *World Report on Road Traffic Injury Prevention.* Geneva: World Health Organization.

CONTENTS

3   Shock   55

7   Spine and Spinal Cord Trauma   157

8 Musculoskeletal Trauma   187

9 Thermal Injuries   211

10 Pediatric Trauma 225

11 Geriatric Trauma 247

Appendix H: Disaster Management and Emergency Preparedness
(Optional Lecture)   321

Appendix I: Triage Scenarios   337

Index   351

CHAPTER **1**

Initial Assessment and Management

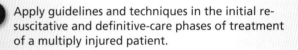

Upon completion of this topic, the student will demonstrate the ability to apply the principles of emergency medical care to multiply injured patients. Specifically, the doctor will be able to:

OBJECTIVES

1 Identify the correct sequence of priorities for assessment of a multiply injured patient.

2 Apply the principles outlined in the primary and secondary evaluation surveys to the assessment of a multiply injured patient.

3 Apply guidelines and techniques in the initial resuscitative and definitive-care phases of treatment of a multiply injured patient.

4 Explain how a patient's medical history and the mechanism of injury contribute to the identification of injuries.

5 Identify the pitfalls associated with the initial assessment and management of an injured patient and take steps to minimize their impact.

6 Conduct an initial assessment survey on a simulated multiply injured patient, using the correct sequence of priorities and explaining management techniques for primary treatment and stabilization.

Introduction

The treatment of seriously injured patients requires rapid assessment of the injuries and institution of life-preserving therapy. Because time is of the essence, a systematic approach that can be easily reviewed and practiced is most effective. This process is termed "initial assessment" and includes:

- Preparation
- Triage
- Primary survey (ABCDEs)
- Resuscitation
- Adjuncts to primary survey and resuscitation
- Consider need for patient transfer
- Secondary survey (head-to-toe evaluation and patient history)
- Adjuncts to the secondary survey
- Continued postresuscitation monitoring and reevaluation
- Definitive care

The primary and secondary surveys should be repeated frequently to identify any deterioration in the patient's status and to determine whether it is necessary to institute any treatment when adverse changes are identified.

The assessment sequence presented in this chapter reflects a linear, or longitudinal progression of events. In an actual clinical situation, many of these activities occur in parallel, or simultaneously. The longitudinal progression of the assessment process allows the doctor an opportunity to mentally review the progress of an actual trauma resuscitation.

ATLS® principles guide the assessment and resuscitation of injured patients. Judgment is required to determine which procedures are necessary, because not all patients require all of these procedures.

Preparation

❓ *How do I prepare for a smooth transition from the prehospital to the hospital environment?*

Preparation for the trauma patient occurs in two different clinical settings. First, during the *prehospital phase,* all events must be coordinated with the doctors at the receiving hospital. Second, during the *hospital phase,* preparations must be made to rapidly facilitate the trauma patient's resuscitation.

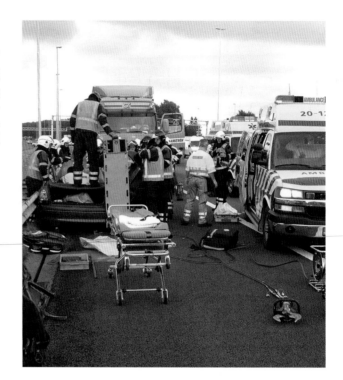

PREHOSPITAL PHASE

Coordination with the prehospital agency and personnel can greatly expedite treatment in the field. The prehospital system should be set up to notify the receiving hospital before personnel transport the patient from the scene. This allows for mobilization of the hospital's trauma team members so that all necessary personnel and resources are present in the emergency department (ED) at the time of the patient's arrival.

During the prehospital phase, emphasis should be placed on airway maintenance, control of external bleeding and shock, immobilization of the patient, and immediate transport to the closest appropriate facility, preferably a verified trauma center. Every effort should be made to minimize scene time (see Figure 1-1). Emphasis also should be placed on obtaining and reporting information needed for triage at the hospital, (eg, time of injury, events related to the injury, and patient history). The mechanisms of injury can suggest the degree of injury as well as specific injuries for which the patient must be evaluated.

The National Association of Emergency Medical Technicians' Prehospital Trauma Life Support Committee, in cooperation with the Committee on Trauma (COT) of the American College of Surgeons (ACS), has developed a course with a format similar to the ATLS Course that addresses prehospital care for injured patients.

HOSPITAL PHASE

Advance planning for the trauma patient's arrival is essential. Ideally, a resuscitation area is available for

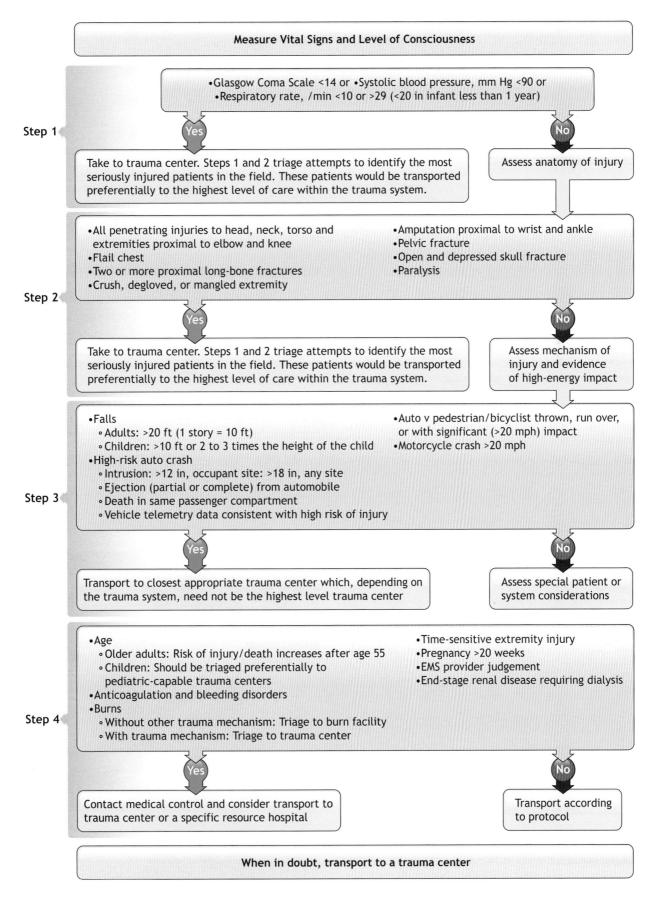

Measure Vital Signs and Level of Consciousness

Step 1

•Glasgow Coma Scale <14 or •Systolic blood pressure, mm Hg <90 or
•Respiratory rate, /min <10 or >29 (<20 in infant less than 1 year)

Yes → Take to trauma center. Steps 1 and 2 triage attempts to identify the most seriously injured patients in the field. These patients would be transported preferentially to the highest level of care within the trauma system.

No → Assess anatomy of injury

Step 2

•All penetrating injuries to head, neck, torso and extremities proximal to elbow and knee
•Flail chest
•Two or more proximal long-bone fractures
•Crush, degloved, or mangled extremity

•Amputation proximal to wrist and ankle
•Pelvic fracture
•Open and depressed skull fracture
•Paralysis

Yes → Take to trauma center. Steps 1 and 2 triage attempts to identify the most seriously injured patients in the field. These patients would be transported preferentially to the highest level of care within the trauma system.

No → Assess mechanism of injury and evidence of high-energy impact

Step 3

•Falls
  ◦Adults: >20 ft (1 story = 10 ft)
  ◦Children: >10 ft or 2 to 3 times the height of the child
•High-risk auto crash
  ◦Intrusion: >12 in, occupant site: >18 in, any site
  ◦Ejection (partial or complete) from automobile
  ◦Death in same passenger compartment
  ◦Vehicle telemetry data consistent with high risk of injury

•Auto v pedestrian/bicyclist thrown, run over, or with significant (>20 mph) impact
•Motorcycle crash >20 mph

Yes → Transport to closest appropriate trauma center which, depending on the trauma system, need not be the highest level trauma center

No → Assess special patient or system considerations

Step 4

•Age
  ◦Older adults: Risk of injury/death increases after age 55
  ◦Children: Should be triaged preferentially to pediatric-capable trauma centers
•Anticoagulation and bleeding disorders
•Burns
  ◦Without other trauma mechanism: Triage to burn facility
  ◦With trauma mechanism: Triage to trauma center

•Time-sensitive extremity injury
•Pregnancy >20 weeks
•EMS provider judgement
•End-stage renal disease requiring dialysis

Yes → Contact medical control and consider transport to trauma center or a specific resource hospital

No → Transport according to protocol

When in doubt, transport to a trauma center

■ Figure 1-1 Field Triage Decision Scheme.

trauma patients. Proper airway equipment (eg, laryngo-scopes and tubes) should be organized, tested, and placed where it is immediately accessible. Warmed in-travenous crystalloid solutions should be available and ready to infuse when the patient arrives. Appropriate monitoring capabilities should be immediately available. A method to summon additional medical assistance should be in place, as well as a means to ensure prompt responses by laboratory and radiology personnel. Trans-fer agreements with verified trauma centers should be established and operational. ◪ See American College of Surgeons Committee on Trauma (ACS COT), *Resources for Optimal Care of the Injured Patient, 2006.* Periodic re-view of patient care through the quality improvement process is an essential component of each hospital's trauma program.

All personnel who have contact with the patient must be protected from communicable diseases. Most promi-nent among these diseases are hepatitis and the acquired immunodeficiency syndrome (AIDS). The Centers for Dis-ease Control and Prevention (CDC) and other health agencies strongly recommend the use of standard precau-tions (eg, face mask, eye protection, water-impervious apron, leggings, and gloves) when coming into contact with body fluids. The ACS COT considers these to be *min-imum* precautions and protection for all health-care providers. Standard precautions are also an Occupational Safety and Health Administration (OSHA) requirement in the United States.

Triage

Triage involves the sorting of patients based on their need for treatment and the resources available to provide that treatment. Treatment is rendered based on the ABC priori-ties (**A**irway with cervical spine protection, **B**reathing, and **C**irculation with hemorrhage control), as outlined later in this chapter

Triage also pertains to the sorting of patients in the field and the decision regarding to which medical facil-ity they should be transported. It is the responsibility of the prehospital personnel and their medical director to ensure that appropriate patients arrive at appropriate hospitals. For example, it is inappropriate for prehospi-tal personnel to deliver a patient who has sustained se-vere trauma to a hospital that is not a trauma center if a trauma center is available at another hospital (see Fig-ure 1-1). Prehospital trauma scoring is helpful in identi-fying severely injured patients who should be transported to a trauma center. ◪ See Appendix I: Triage Scenarios and Appendix C: Trauma Scores: Revised and Pediatric.

Two types of triage situations usually exist: multiple ca-sualties and mass casualties.

MULTIPLE CASUALTIES

In multiple-casualty incidents, the number of patients and the severity of their injuries do not exceed the ability of the facility to render care. In such situations, patients with life-threatening problems and those sustaining multiple-system injuries are treated first. The use of prehospital care proto-cols and online medical direction can facilitate and improve care initiated in the field. Periodic multidisciplinary review of the care provided through quality improvement activi-ties is essential.

MASS CASUALTIES

In mass-casualty events, the number of patients and the severity of their injuries exceed the capability of the facility and staff. In such situations, the patients with the greatest chance of survival and requiring the least expenditure of time, equipment, supplies, and personnel, are treated first.

Primary Survey

❓ *What is a quick, simple way to assess the patient in 10 seconds?*

Patients are assessed, and their treatment priorities are established, based on their injuries, vital signs, and the

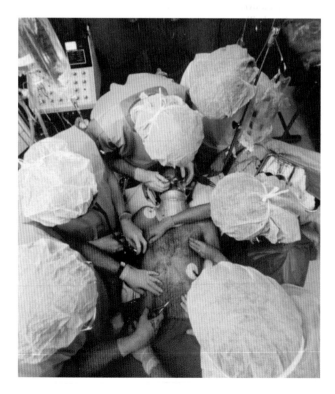

injury mechanisms. In severely injured patients, logical and sequential treatment priorities must be established based on overall patient assessment. The patient's vital functions must be assessed quickly and efficiently. Management consists of a rapid primary survey, resuscitation of vital functions, a more detailed secondary survey, and, finally, the initiation of definitive care. This process constitutes the ABCDEs of trauma care and identifies life-threatening conditions by adhering to the following sequence:

1. **A**irway maintenance with cervical spine protection

2. **B**reathing and ventilation

3. **C**irculation with hemorrhage control

4. **D**isability: Neurologic status

5. **E**xposure/Environmental control: Completely undress the patient, but prevent hypothermia

During the primary survey, life-threatening conditions are identified, and management is instituted simultaneously. The prioritized assessment and management procedures described in this chapter are presented as sequential steps in order of importance and for the purpose of clarity. However, these steps are frequently accomplished simultaneously.

Priorities for the care of *pediatric patients* are the same as those for adults. Although the quantities of blood, fluids, and medications; size of the child; degree and rapidity of heat loss; and injury patterns may differ, the assessment and management priorities are identical. ◢ Specific issues related to pediatric trauma patients are addressed in Chapter 10: Pediatric Trauma.

Priorities for the care of *pregnant females* are similar to those for nonpregnant females, but the anatomic and physiologic changes of pregnancy may modify the patient's response to injury. Early recognition of pregnancy by palpation of the abdomen for a gravid uterus and laboratory testing (human chorionic gonadotropin, or hCG) and early fetal assessment are important for maternal and fetal survival. ◢ Specific issues related to pregnant patients are addressed in Chapter 12: Trauma in Women.

Trauma is a common cause of death in the *elderly*. With increasing age, cardiovascular disease and cancer overtake the incidence of injury as the leading causes of death. Interestingly, the risk of death for any given injury at the lower and moderate Injury Severity Score (ISS) levels is greater for elderly males than for elderly females.

Resuscitation of elderly patients warrants special attention. The aging process diminishes the physiologic reserve of elderly trauma patients, and chronic cardiac, respiratory, and metabolic diseases can reduce the ability of these patients to respond to injury in the same manner in which younger patients are able to compensate for the physiologic stress caused by injury. Comorbidities such as diabetes, congestive heart failure, coronary artery disease, restrictive and obstructive pulmonary disease, coagulopathy, liver disease, and peripheral vascular disease are more common in older patients and adversely affect outcomes following injury. In addition, the long-term use of medications may alter the usual physiologic response to injury, and the narrow therapeutic window frequently leads to over-resuscitation or under-resuscitation in this patient population. As such, early, invasive monitoring is frequently a valuable adjunct to management. Despite these facts, most elderly trauma patients recover and return to their preinjury level of independent activity if appropriately treated. Prompt, aggressive resuscitation and the early recognition of preexisting medical conditions and medication use can improve survival in this patient group. ◢ See Chapter 11: Geriatric Trauma.

AIRWAY MAINTENANCE WITH CERVICAL SPINE PROTECTION

Upon initial evaluation of a trauma patient, the airway should be assessed first to ascertain patency. This rapid assessment for signs of airway obstruction should include inspection for foreign bodies and facial, mandibular, or tracheal/laryngeal fractures that may result in airway obstruction. Measures to establish a patent airway should be instituted while protecting the cervical spine. Initially, the chin-lift or jaw-thrust maneuver is recommended to achieve airway patency.

If the patient is able to communicate verbally, the airway is not likely to be in immediate jeopardy; however, repeated assessment of airway patency is prudent. In addition, patients with severe head injuries who have an altered level of consciousness or a Glasgow Coma Scale (GCS) score of 8 or less usually require the placement of a definitive airway. The finding of nonpurposeful motor responses strongly suggests the need for definitive airway management. Management of the airway in pediatric patients requires knowledge of the unique anatomic features of the position and size of the larynx in children, as well as special equipment. ◢ See Chapter 10: Pediatric Trauma.

While assessing and managing the patient's airway, great care should be taken to prevent excessive movement of the cervical spine. The patient's head and neck should not be hyperextended, hyperflexed, or rotated to establish and maintain the airway. Based on a history of a traumatic incident, loss of stability of the cervical spine should be suspected. Neurologic examination alone does not exclude a diagnosis of cervical spine injury. Protection of the patient's spinal cord with appropriate immobilization devices should be accomplished and maintained. If immobilization devices must be removed temporarily, one member of the trauma team should manually stabilize the patient's head and neck using inline immobilization techniques (Figure 1-2).

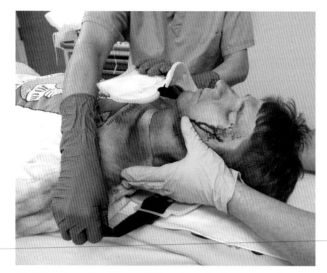

■ Figure 1-2 If immobilization devices must be removed temporarily, one member of the trauma team should manually stabilize the patient's head and neck using inline immobilization techniques.

The stabilization equipment used to protect the patient's spinal cord should be left in place until cervical spine injury has been excluded. **Protection of the spine and spinal cord is a critically important management principle.** Cervical spine radiographs may be obtained to confirm or exclude injury once immediate or potentially life-threatening conditions have been addressed. **Assume a cervical spine injury in any patient with multisystem trauma, especially those with an altered level of consciousness or a blunt injury above the clavicle.** ▪ See Chapter 7: Spine and Spinal Cord Trauma.

Every effort should be made to promptly identify airway compromise and secure a definitive airway. Equally important is the necessity to recognize the potential for progressive airway loss. Frequent reevaluation of airway patency is essential to identify and treat patients who are losing the ability to maintain an adequate airway.

BREATHING AND VENTILATION

Airway patency alone does not ensure adequate ventilation. Adequate gas exchange is required to maximize oxygenation and carbon dioxide elimination. Ventilation requires adequate function of the lungs, chest wall, and diaphragm. Each component must be examined and evaluated rapidly.

The patient's chest should be exposed to adequately assess chest wall excursion, and auscultation should be performed to ensure gas flow in the lungs. Visual inspection and palpation can detect injuries to the chest wall that might compromise ventilation. Percussion of the

---

PITFALLS

- Despite the efforts of even the most prudent and attentive doctor, there are circumstances in which airway management is exceptionally difficult and occasionally even impossible to achieve. Equipment failure often cannot be anticipated, for example, the light on the laryngoscope burns out or the cuff on the endotracheal tube that was placed with exceptional difficulty leaks because it was torn on the patient's teeth during intubation.
- Tragic pitfalls include patients in whom intubation cannot be performed after paralysis and patients in whom a surgical airway cannot be established expediently because of their obesity.
- Endotracheal intubation of a patient with an unknown laryngeal fracture or incomplete upper airway transection can precipitate total airway occlusion or complete airway transection. This may occur in the absence of clinical findings that suggest the potential for an airway problem, or when the urgency of the situation dictates the immediate need for a secure airway or ventilation.

These pitfalls cannot always be prevented. However, they should be anticipated, and preparations should be made to minimize their impact.

---

thorax during a noisy resuscitation may be difficult or produce unreliable results.

Injuries that can impair ventilation in the short term include tension pneumothorax, flail chest with pulmonary contusion, massive hemothorax, and open pneumothorax. These injuries should be identified during the primary survey. Simple pneumothorax or hemothorax, fractured ribs, and pulmonary contusion can compromise ventilation to a lesser degree and are usually identified during the secondary survey.

PITFALLS

Differentiating between ventilation problems and airway compromise can be difficult:

- A patient who has profound dyspnea and tachypnea gives the impression that his or her primary problem is related to an inadequate airway. However, if the ventilation problem is caused by a pneumothorax or tension pneumothorax, intubation with vigorous bag-valve ventilation can rapidly lead to further deterioration of the patient.
- When intubation and ventilation are necessary in an unconscious patient, the procedure itself can unmask or aggravate a pneumothorax, and the patient's chest must be reevaluated. Chest x-rays should be obtained as soon after intubation and initiation of ventilation as is practical.

CIRCULATION WITH HEMORRHAGE CONTROL

Circulation issues to consider include blood volume and cardiac output, and bleeding.

Blood Volume and Cardiac Output

Hemorrhage is the predominant cause of preventable deaths after injury. Hypotension following injury must be considered to be hypovolemic in origin until proved otherwise; therefore, rapid and accurate assessment of an injured patient's hemodynamic status is essential. The elements of clinical observation that yield important information within seconds are level of consciousness, skin color, and pulse.

Level of Consciousness   When circulating blood volume is reduced, cerebral perfusion may be critically impaired, resulting in altered levels of consciousness. However, a conscious patient also may have lost a significant amount of blood.

Skin Color   Skin color can be helpful in evaluating the injured patient who has hypovolemia. A patient with pink skin, especially in the face and extremities, rarely has critical hypovolemia after injury. Conversely, the patient with hypovolemia may have ashen, gray facial skin and white extremities.

Pulse   The pulse, typically an easily accessible central pulse (femoral or carotid artery), should be assessed bilaterally for quality, rate, and regularity. Full, slow, and regular peripheral pulses are usually signs of relative normovolemia in a patient who is not taking ß-adrenergic blocking medications. A rapid, thready pulse is typically a sign of hypovolemia, but the condition may have other causes. A normal pulse rate does not ensure that a patient has normovolemia, but an irregular pulse does warn of potential cardiac dysfunction. Absent central pulses that are not attributable to local factors signify the need for immediate resuscitative action to restore depleted blood volume and effective cardiac output.

Bleeding

External hemorrhage is identified and controlled during the primary survey. Rapid, external blood loss is managed by direct manual pressure on the wound. Pneumatic splinting devices also can help to control hemorrhage. These devices should be transparent to allow for monitoring of underlying bleeding. Tourniquets are infrequently used to control severe bleeding. The use of hemostats can damage nerves and veins. The major areas of occult blood loss are the chest, abdomen, retroperitoneum, pelvis, and long bones.

DISABILITY (NEUROLOGIC EVALUATION)

A rapid neurologic evaluation is performed at the end of the primary survey. This neurologic evaluation establishes the patient's level of consciousness, pupillary size and reaction, lateralizing signs, and spinal cord injury level.

PITFALLS

Trauma respects no patient population barrier. The elderly, children, athletes, and individuals with chronic medical conditions do not respond to volume loss in a similar or even in a "normal" manner.

- Elderly patients have a limited ability to increase their heart rate in response to blood loss, which obscures one of the earliest signs of volume depletion—tachycardia. Blood pressure has little correlation with cardiac output in older patients. Anticoagulation therapy for medical conditions such as atrial fibrillation, coronary artery disease, and transient ischemic attacks can increase blood loss.
- Children usually have abundant physiologic reserve and often have few signs of hypovolemia, even after severe volume depletion. When deterioration does occur, it is precipitous and catastrophic.
- Well-trained athletes have similar compensatory mechanisms, may have bradycardia, and may not have the usual level of tachycardia with blood loss.
- Often, the AMPLE history, described later in this chapter, is not available, so the health-care team is not aware of the patient's use of medications for chronic conditions.

Anticipation and an attitude of skepticism regarding the patient's "normal" hemodynamic status are appropriate.

The GCS is a quick, simple method for determining the level of consciousness that is predictive of patient outcome—particularly the best motor response. If it was not performed during the primary survey, the GCS should be performed as part of the more detailed, quantitative neurologic examination during the secondary survey. ■ See Chapter 6: Head Trauma and Appendix C: Trauma Scores: Revised and Pediatric.

A decrease in the level of consciousness may indicate decreased cerebral oxygenation and/or perfusion, or it may be caused by direct cerebral injury. An altered level of consciousness indicates the need for immediate reevaluation of the patient's oxygenation, ventilation, and perfusion status. Hypoglycemia and alcohol, narcotics, and other drugs also can alter the patient's level of consciousness. However, if these factors are excluded, changes in the level of consciousness should be considered to be of traumatic central nervous system origin until proven otherwise.

EXPOSURE/ENVIRONMENTAL CONTROL

The patient should be completely undressed, usually by cutting off his or her garments to facilitate a thorough examination and assessment. After the patient's clothing has been

PITFALL

Despite proper attention to all aspects of treating a patient with a closed head injury, neurologic deterioration can occur—often rapidly. The lucid interval classically associated with acute epidural hematoma is an example of a situation in which the patient will "talk and die." Frequent neurologic reevaluation can minimize this problem by allowing for early detection of changes. It may be necessary to return to the primary survey and to confirm that the patient has a secure airway, adequate ventilation and oxygenation, and adequate cerebral perfusion. Early consultation with a neurosurgeon also is necessary to guide additional management efforts.

removed and the assessment completed, cover the patient with warm blankets or an external warming device to prevent hypothermia in the ED. Intravenous fluids should be warmed before being infused, and a warm environment (room temperature) should be maintained. **The patient's body temperature is more important than the comfort of the health-care providers.**

Resuscitation

Aggressive resuscitation and the management of life-threatening injuries as they are identified are essential to maximize patient survival. Resusication also follows the ABC sequence.

AIRWAY

The airway should be protected in all patients and secured when there is a potential for airway compromise. The jaw-thrust or chin-lift maneuver may suffice as an initial intervention. If the patient is unconscious and has no gag reflex, the establishment of an oropharyngeal airway can be helpful temporarily. **A definitive airway (ie, intubation) should be established if there is any doubt about the patient's ability to maintain airway integrity.**

BREATHING/VENTILATION/OXYGENATION

Definitive control of the airway in patients who have compromised airways due to mechanical factors, have ventilatory problems, or are unconscious is achieved by endotracheal intubation. This procedure should be performed with continuous protection of the cervical spine. An airway should be established surgically if intubation is contraindicated or cannot be accomplished.

A tension pneumothorax compromises ventilation and circulation dramatically and acutely; if one is suspected, chest decompression should be started immediately. Every

injured patient should receive supplemental oxygen. If not intubated, the patient should have oxygen delivered by a mask-reservoir device to achieve optimal oxygenation. The use of the pulse oximeter is valuable in ensuring adequate hemoglobin saturation. See Chapter 2: Airway and Ventilatory Management.

CIRCULATION AND BLEEDING CONTROL

Definitive bleeding control is essential, and intravenous replacement of intravascular volume is important. A minimum of two large-caliber intravenous (IV) catheters should be introduced. The maximum rate of fluid administration is determined by the internal diameter of the catheter and inversely by its length—not by the size of the vein in which the catheter is placed. Establishment of upper-extremity peripheral IV access is preferred. Other peripheral lines, cutdowns, and central venous lines should be used as necessary in accordance with the skill level of the doctor who is caring for the patient. See Skill Station IV: Shock Assessment and Management, and Skill Station V: Venous Cutdown, in Chapter 3: Shock. At the time of IV insertion, draw blood for type and crossmatch and baseline hematologic studies, including a pregnancy test for all females of childbearing age.

Aggressive and continued volume resuscitation is not a substitute for definitive control of hemorrhage. Definitive control includes operation, angioembolization and pelvic stabilization. IV fluid therapy with crystalloids should be initiated. Such bolus IV therapy may require the administration of 1 to 2 L of an isotonic solution to achieve an appropriate response in the adult patient. All IV solutions should be warmed either by storage in a warm environment (37°C to 40°C, or 98.6° F to 104° F) or fluid-warming devices. Shock associated with injury is most often hypovolemic in origin. If the patient remains unresponsive to bolus IV therapy, blood transfusion may be required.

Hypothermia may be present when the patient arrives, or it may develop quickly in the ED if the patient is uncovered and undergoes rapid administration of room-temperature fluids or refrigerated blood. Hypothermia is a potentially lethal complication in injured patients, and aggressive mea-

PITFALL

Injured patients can arrive in the ED with hypothermia, and hypothermia may develop in some patients who require massive transfusions and crystalloid resuscitation despite aggressive efforts to maintain body heat. The problem is best minimized by early control of hemorrhage. This can require operative intervention or the application of an external compression device to reduce the pelvic volume for patients with certain types of pelvic fractures. Efforts to rewarm the patient and prevent hypothermia should be considered as important as any other component of the primary survey and resuscitation phase.

sures should be taken to prevent the loss of body heat and restore body temperature to normal. The temperature of the resuscitation area should be increased to minimize the loss of body heat. The use of a high-flow fluid warmer or microwave oven to heat crystalloid fluids to 39°C (102.2°F) is recommended. However blood products should not be warmed in a microwave oven. ◾ See Chapter 3: Shock.

Adjuncts to Primary Survey and Resuscitation

Adjuncts that are used during the primary survey and resuscitation phases include electrocardiographic monitoring; urinary and gastric catheters; other monitoring, such as of ventilatory rate, arterial blood gas (ABG) levels, pulse oximetry, and blood pressure; and x-ray examination and diagnostic studies.

ELECTROCARDIOGRAPHIC MONITORING

Electrocardiographic (ECG) monitoring of all trauma patients is important. Dysrhythmias—including unexplained tachycardia, atrial fibrillation, premature ventricular contractions, and ST segment changes—can indicate blunt cardiac injury. Pulseless electrical activity (PEA) can indicate cardiac tamponade, tension pneumothorax, and/or pro-

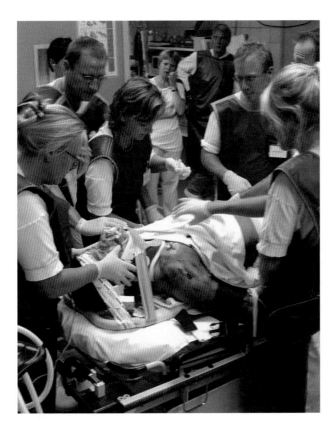

PITFALL

Sometimes anatomic abnormalities (eg, urethral stricture or prostatic hypertrophy) preclude placement of an indwelling bladder catheter, despite meticulous technique. Nonspecialists should avoid excessive manipulation of the urethra or use of specialized instrumentation. Consult a urologist early.

---

found hypovolemia. When bradycardia, aberrant conduction, and premature beats are present, hypoxia and hypoperfusion should be suspected immediately. Extreme hypothermia also produces these dysrhythmias. ◾ See Chapter 3: Shock.

URINARY AND GASTRIC CATHETERS

The placement of urinary and gastric catheters should be considered as part of the resuscitation phase. A urine specimen should be submitted for routine laboratory analysis.

Urinary Catheters

Urinary output is a sensitive indicator of the patient's volume status and reflects renal perfusion. Monitoring of urinary output is best accomplished by the insertion of an indwelling bladder catheter. Transurethral bladder catheterization is contraindicated in patients in whom urethral transection is suspected. Urethral injury should be suspected in the presence of one of the following:

- Blood at the urethral meatus
- Perineal ecchymosis
- Blood in the scrotum
- High-riding or nonpalpable prostate
- Pelvic fracture

Accordingly, a urinary catheter should not be inserted before the rectum and genitalia have been examined. If urethral injury is suspected, urethral integrity should be confirmed by a retrograde urethrogram before the catheter is inserted.

Gastric Catheters

A gastric tube is indicated to reduce stomach distention and decrease the risk of aspiration. Decompression of the stomach reduces the risk of aspiration, but does not prevent it entirely. Thick or semisolid gastric contents will not return through the tube, and actual passage of the tube can induce vomiting. For the tube to be effective, it must be positioned properly, be attached to appropriate suction, and be functional. Blood in the gastric aspirate can be indicative of oropharyngeal (swallowed) blood, traumatic insertion, or actual injury to the upper digestive tract. If the cribriform plate is known to be fractured or a fracture is suspected, the gastric tube should be inserted orally to prevent intracranial passage. In this situation, any nasopharyngeal instrumentation is potentially dangerous.

OTHER MONITORING

Adequate resuscitation is best assessed by improvement in physiologic parameters, such as pulse rate, blood pressure, pulse pressure, ventilatory rate, ABG levels, body temperature, and urinary output, rather than the qualitative assessment done during the primary survey. **Actual values for these parameters should be obtained as soon as is practical after completing the primary survey, and periodic reevaluation is prudent.**

Ventilatory Rate and Arterial Blood Gases

Ventilatory rate and ABG levels should be used to monitor the adequacy of respirations. Endotracheal tubes may be dislodged whenever the patient is moved. A colorimetric carbon dioxide detector is a device capable of detecting carbon dioxide in exhaled gas. Colorimetry, or capnography, is useful in confirming that the endotracheal tube is properly located in the respiratory tract of the patient on mechanical ventilation and not in the esophagus. However, it does not confirm proper placement of the tube in the trachea. ▪ See Chapter 2: Airway and Ventilatory Management.

Pulse Oximetry

Pulse oximetry is a valuable adjunct for monitoring oxygenation in injured patients. The pulse oximeter measures the oxygen saturation of hemoglobin colorimetrically, but it does *not* measure the partial pressure of oxygen. It also does not measure the partial pressure of carbon dioxide, which reflects the adequacy of ventilation. A small sensor is placed on the finger, toe, earlobe, or another convenient place. Most devices display pulse rate and oxygen saturation continuously.

Hemoglobin saturation from the pulse oximeter should be compared with the value obtained from the ABG analysis. Inconsistency indicates that at least one of the two determinations is in error.

Blood Pressure

The blood pressure should be measured. It should be kept in mind, though that it may be a poor measure of actual tissue perfusion.

X-RAY EXAMINATIONS AND DIAGNOSTIC STUDIES

X-ray examination should be used judiciously and should not delay patient resuscitation. Anteroposterior (AP) chest and AP pelvic films often provide information that can guide resuscitation efforts of patients with blunt trauma. Chest x-rays can show potentially life-threatening injuries that require

PITFALLS

- Placement of a gastric catheter may induce vomiting or gagging and produce the specific problem that its placement is intended to prevent—aspiration. Functional suction equipment should be immediately available.
- Combative trauma patients occasionally extubate themselves. They can also occlude their endotracheal tube or deflate the cuff by biting it. Frequent reevaluation of the airway is necessary.
- The pulse oximeter sensor should not be placed distal to the blood pressure cuff. Misleading information regarding hemoglobin saturation and pulse can be generated when the cuff is inflated and occludes blood flow.
- Normalization of hemodynamics in injured patients requires more than simply a normal blood pressure; a return to normal peripheral perfusion must be established. This can be problematic in the elderly, and consideration should be given to early invasive monitoring of cardiac function in these patients.

treatment, and pelvic films can show fractures of the pelvis that indicate the need for early blood transfusion. These films can be taken in the resuscitation area with a portable x-ray unit, but should not interrupt the resuscitation process.

During the secondary survey, complete cervical and thoracolumbar spine films may be obtained with a portable x-ray unit if the patient's care is not compromised and the mechanism of injury suggests the possibility of spinal injury. In a patient with obtundation who requires computed tomography (CT) of the brain, CT of the spine may be used as the method of radiographic assessment. Spinal cord protection that was established during the primary survey should be maintained. An AP chest film and additional films pertinent to the site(s) of suspected injury should be obtained. Essential diagnostic x-rays should be obtained even in pregnant patients.

Focused assessment sonography in trauma (FAST) and diagnostic peritoneal lavage (DPL) are useful tools for the quick detection of occult intraabdominal blood. Their use depends on the skill and experience of the doctor. Identification of the source of occult intraabdominal blood loss may indicate the need for operative control of hemorrhage.

Consider Need for Patient Transfer

During the primary survey and resuscitation phase, the evaluating doctor frequently has obtained enough information to indicate the need to transfer the patient to another facil-

PITFALL

Technical problems may be encountered when performing any diagnostic procedure, including those necessary to identify intraabdominal hemorrhage. Obesity and intraluminal bowel gas can compromise the images obtained by abdominal ultrasonography. Obesity, previous abdominal operations, and pregnancy also can make diagnostic peritoneal lavage difficult. Even in the hands of an experienced surgeon, the effluent volume from the lavage may be minimal or zero. In these circumstances, an alternative diagnostic tool should be chosen. A surgeon should be involved in the evaluation process and guide further diagnostic and therapeutic procedures.

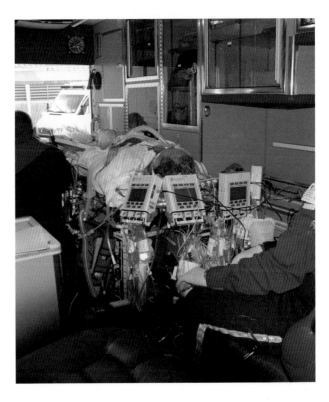

ity. This transfer process may be initiated immediately by administrative personnel at the direction of the examining doctor while additional evaluation and resuscitative measures are being performed. Once the decision to transfer the patient has been made, communication between the referring and receiving doctors is essential.

Secondary Survey

What is the secondary survey, and when does it start?

The secondary survey does not begin until the primary survey (ABCDEs) is completed, resuscitative efforts are underway, and the normalization of vital functions has been demonstrated.

The secondary survey is a head-to-toe evaluation of the trauma patient, that is, a complete history and physical examination, including reassessment of all vital signs. Each region of the body is completely examined. The potential for missing an injury or failure to appreciate the significance of an injury is great, especially in an unresponsive or unstable patient. ◾ See Table I-1: Secondary Survey, in Skill Station I: Initial Assessment and Management.

During the secondary survey, a complete neurologic examination is performed, including a GCS score determination, if it was not done during the primary survey, and x-rays are obtained, if indicated by the examination. Such examinations can be interspersed into the secondary survey at appropriate times. Special procedures, such as specific radiographic evaluations and laboratory studies, also are performed at this time. Complete patient evaluation requires repeated physical examinations.

HISTORY

Every complete medical assessment includes a history of the mechanism of injury. Often, such a history cannot be ob-

tained from a patient who has sustained trauma, and prehospital personnel and family must be consulted to obtain information that can enhance the understanding of the patient's physiologic state. The AMPLE history is a useful mnemonic for this purpose:

A —Allergies

M —Medications currently used

P —Past illnesses/Pregnancy

L —Last meal

E —Events/Environment related to the injury

The patient's condition is greatly influenced by the mechanism of injury. Prehospital personnel can provide valuable information on such mechanisms and should report pertinent data to the examining doctor. Some injuries can be predicted based on the direction and amount of energy behind the mechanism of injury. Injury usually is classified into two broad categories: blunt and penetrating trauma. ◾ See Appendix B: Biomechanics of Injury. Other types of injuries for which historical information is important include thermal injuries and those caused by a hazardous environment.

Blunt Trauma

Blunt trauma often results from automobile collisions, falls, and other injuries related to transportation, recreation, and occupations.

Important information to obtain about automobile collisions includes seat-belt use, steering wheel deformation,

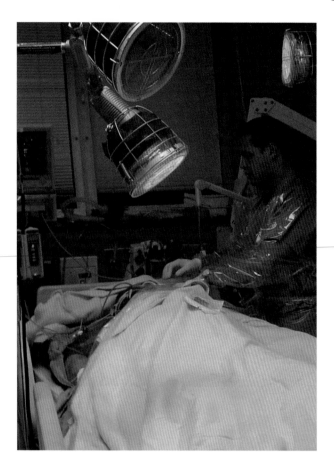

direction of impact, damage to the automobile in terms of major deformation or intrusion into the passenger compartment, and whether the patient was ejected from the vehicle. Ejection from the vehicle greatly increases the possibility of major injury.

Injury patterns can often be predicted by the mechanism of injury. Such injury patterns also are influenced by age groups and activities (see Table 1-1: Mechanisms of Injury and Related Suspected Injury Patterns).

Penetrating Trauma

The incidence of penetrating trauma (eg, injuries from firearms, stabbings, and impalement) has increased. Factors determining the type and extent of injury and subsequent management include the region of the body that was injured, the organs in the path of the penetrating object, and the velocity of the missile. Therefore, in gunshot victims, the velocity, caliber, presumed path of the bullet, and distance from the weapon to the wound can provide important clues as to the extent of injury. ▪ See Appendix B: Biomechanics of Injury.

Thermal Injury

Burns are a significant type of trauma that can occur alone or be coupled with blunt and penetrating trauma resulting from, for example, a burning automobile, explosion, falling

debris, the patient's attempt to escape a fire. Inhalation injury and carbon monoxide poisoning often complicate burn injuries. Therefore, it is important to know the circumstances of the burn injury. Specifically, knowledge of the environment in which the burn injury occurred (open or closed space), the substances consumed by the flames (eg, plastics and chemicals), and any possible associated injuries sustained, is critical for patient treatment.

Acute or chronic hypothermia without adequate protection against heat loss produces either local or generalized cold injuries. Significant heat loss can occur at moderate temperatures (15°C to 20°C or 59°F to 68°F) if wet clothes, decreased activity, and/or vasodilation caused by alcohol or drugs compromise the patient's ability to conserve heat. Such historical information can be obtained from prehospital personnel.

Hazardous Environment

A history of exposure to chemicals, toxins, and radiation is important to obtain for two main reasons: first, these agents can produce a variety of pulmonary, cardiac, and internal organ dysfunctions in injured patients. Second, these same agents may also present a hazard to healthcare providers. Frequently, the doctor's only means of preparation is to understand the general principles of management of such conditions and establish immediate contact with a Regional Poison Control Center.

PHYSICAL EXAMINATION

During the secondary survey, physical examination follows the sequence of head, maxillofacial structures, cervical spine and neck, chest, abdomen, perineum/rectum/vagina, musculoskeletal system, and neurologic system.

Head

The secondary survey begins with evaluating the head and identifying all related neurologic injuries and other significant injuries. The entire scalp and head should be examined for lacerations, contusions, and evidence of fractures. ▪ See Chapter 6: Head Trauma.

Because edema around the eyes can later preclude an in-depth examination, the eyes should be reevaluated for:

- Visual acuity
- Pupillary size
- Hemorrhage of the conjunctiva and/or fundi
- Penetrating injury
- Contact lenses (remove before edema occurs)
- Dislocation of the lens
- Ocular entrapment

TABLE 1-1 ■ Mechanisms of Injury and Related Suspected Injury Patterns

MECHANISM OF INJURY	SUSPECTED INJURY PATTERNS
Frontal impact automobile collision • Bent steering wheel • Knee imprint, dashboard • Bull's-eye fracture of the windshield	• Cervical spine fracture • Anterior flail chest • Myocardial contusion • Pneumothorax • Traumatic aortic disruption • Fractured spleen or liver • Posterior fracture/dislocation of hip and/or knee
Side impact automobile collision	• Contralateral neck sprain • Cervical spine fracture • Lateral flail chest • Pneumothorax • Traumatic aortic disruption • Diaphragmatic rupture • Fractured spleen/liver and/or kidney, depending on side of impact • Fractured pelvis or acetabulum
Rear impact automobile collision	• Cervical spine injury • Soft tissue injury to neck
Ejection from vehicle	• Ejection from the vehicle precludes meaningful prediction of injury patterns, but places patient at greater risk from virtually all injury mechanisms
Pedestrian struck by motor vehicle	• Head injury • Traumatic aortic disruption • Abdominal visceral injuries • Fractured lower extremities/pelvis

A quick visual-acuity examination of both eyes can be performed by asking the patient to read printed material, for example, a hand held Snellen chart, or words on an IV container or dressing package. Ocular mobility should be evaluated to exclude entrapment of extraocular muscles due to orbital fractures. These procedures frequently identify optic injuries that are not otherwise apparent. ■ See Appendix F: Ocular Trauma.

Maxillofacial Structures

Maxillofacial trauma that is not associated with airway obstruction or major bleeding should be treated only after the patient is stabilized completely and life-threatening injuries have been managed. At the discretion of appropriate specialists, definitive management may be safely delayed without compromising care. Patients with fractures of the midface can also have a fracture of the cribriform plate. For these patients, gastric intubation should be performed via the oral route. ■ See Chapter 6: Head Trauma, and Skill Station IX: Head and Neck Trauma: Assessment and Management.

Cervical Spine and Neck

Patients with maxillofacial or head trauma should be presumed to have an unstable cervical spine injury (eg, fracture and/or ligament injury), and the neck should be immobilized until all aspects of the cervical spine have been adequately studied and an injury has been excluded. The absence of neurologic deficit does not exclude injury to the cervical spine,

PITFALLS

- Facial edema in patients with massive facial injury or in comatose patients can preclude a complete eye examination. Such difficulties should not deter the doctor from performing the components of the ocular examination that are possible.
- Some maxillofacial fractures, such as nasal fracture, nondisplaced zygomatic fractures, and orbital rim fractures, can be difficult to identify early in the evaluation process. Therefore, frequent reassessment is crucial.

and such injury should be presumed until a complete cervical spine radiographic series and CT is reviewed by a doctor experienced in detecting cervical spine fractures radiographically.

Examination of the neck includes inspection, palpation, and auscultation. Cervical spine tenderness, subcutaneous emphysema, tracheal deviation, and laryngeal fracture can be discovered on a detailed examination. The carotid arteries should be palpated and auscultated for bruits. Evidence of blunt injury over these vessels should be noted and, if present, should arouse a high index of suspicion for carotid artery injury. Occlusion or dissection of the carotid artery can occur late in the injury process without antecedent signs or symptoms. Angiography or duplex ultrasonography may be required to exclude the possibility of major cervical vascular injury when the mechanism of injury suggests this possibility. Most major cervical vascular injuries are the result of penetrating injury; however, blunt force to the neck or a traction injury from a shoulder-harness restraint can result in intimal disruption, dissection, and thrombosis. ◾ See Chapter 7: Spine and Spinal Cord Trauma.

Protection of a potentially unstable cervical spine injury is imperative for patients who are wearing any type of protective helmet, and extreme care must be taken when removing the helmet. ◾ See Chapter 2: Airway and Ventilatory Management.

Penetrating injuries to the neck can potentially injure several organ systems. Wounds that extend through the platysma should not be explored manually, probed with instruments, or treated by individuals in the ED who are not trained to manage such injuries. The ED usually is not equipped to deal with the problems that can be encountered in such a situation. These injuries require evaluation by a surgeon operatively or with specialized diagnostic procedures under the direct supervision of a surgeon. The finding of active arterial bleeding, an expanding hematoma, arterial bruit, or airway compromise usually requires operative evaluation. Unexplained or isolated paralysis of an upper extremity should raise the suspicion of a cervical nerve root injury and should be accurately documented.

Chest

Visual evaluation of the chest, both anterior and posterior, can identify conditions such as open pneumothorax and large flail segments. A complete evaluation of the chest wall requires palpation of the entire chest cage, including the clavicles, ribs, and sternum. Sternal pressure can be painful if the sternum is fractured or costochondral separations exist. Contusions and hematomas of the chest wall should alert the doctor to the possibility of occult injury.

Significant chest injury can manifest with pain, dyspnea, and hypoxia. Evaluation includes auscultation of the chest and a chest x-ray examination. Breath sounds are auscultated high on the anterior chest wall for pneumothorax

PITFALLS

- Blunt injury to the neck can produce injuries in which the clinical signs and symptoms develop late and may not be present during the initial examination. Injury to the intima of the carotid arteries is an example.
- The identification of cervical nerve root or brachial plexus injury may not be possible in a comatose patient. Consideration of the mechanism of injury might be the doctor's only clue.
- In some patients, decubitus ulcers can develop quickly over the sacrum and other areas from immobilization on a rigid spine board and from the cervical collar. Efforts to exclude the possibility of spinal injury should be initiated as soon as is practical, and these devices should be removed. However, resuscitation and efforts to identify life-threatening or potentially life-threatening injuries should not be deferred.

and at the posterior bases for hemothorax. Although auscultatory findings can be difficult to evaluate in a noisy environment, they may be extremely helpful. Distant heart sounds and narrow pulse pressure can indicate cardiac tamponade. In addition, cardiac tamponade and tension pneumothorax are suggested by the presence of distended neck veins, although associated hypovolemia can minimize or eliminate this finding. Decreased breath sounds, hyperresonance to percussion, and shock may be the only indications of tension pneumothorax and the need for immediate chest decompression.

A chest x-ray may confirm the presence of a hemothorax or simple pneumothorax. Rib fractures may be present, but they may not be visible on the x-ray. A widened mediastinum or other radiographic signs can suggest an aortic rupture. ◾ See Chapter 4: Thoracic Trauma.

Abdomen

Abdominal injuries must be identified and treated aggressively. The specific diagnosis is not as important as recognizing that an injury exists and initiating surgical intervention, if necessary. A normal initial examination of the abdomen does not exclude a significant intraabdominal injury. Close observation and frequent reevaluation of the abdomen, preferably by the same observer, is important in managing blunt abdominal trauma, because over time, the patient's abdominal findings can change. Early involvement of a surgeon is essential.

Patients with unexplained hypotension, neurologic injury, impaired sensorium secondary to alcohol and/or other drugs, and equivocal abdominal findings should be considered candidates for peritoneal lavage, abdominal ultra-

PITFALLS

- Elderly patients may not tolerate even relatively minor chest injuries. Progression to acute respiratory insufficiency must be anticipated, and support should be instituted before collapse occurs.
- Children often sustain significant injury to the intrathoracic structures without evidence of thoracic skeletal trauma, so a high index of suspicion is essential.

sonography, or, if hemodynamic findings are normal, CT of the abdomen. Fractures of the pelvis or the lower rib cage also can hinder accurate diagnostic examination of the abdomen, because palpating the abdomen can elicit pain from these areas. See Chapter 5: Abdominal and Pelvic Trauma.

Perineum/Rectum/Vagina

The perineum should be examined for contusions, hematomas, lacerations, and urethral bleeding. See Chapter 5: Abdominal and Pelvic Trauma.

A rectal examination may be performed before placing a urinary catheter. If a rectal examination is required, the doctor should assess for the presence of blood within the bowel lumen, a high-riding prostate, the presence of pelvic fractures, the integrity of the rectal wall, and the quality of sphincter tone.

Vaginal examination should be performed in patients who are at risk of vaginal injury. The doctor should assess for the presence of blood in the vaginal vault and vaginal lacer-

PITFALLS

- Excessive manipulation of the pelvis should be avoided, because it may precipitate additional hemorrhage. The AP pelvic x-ray examination, performed as an adjunct to the primary survey and resuscitation, can provide valuable information regarding the presence of pelvic fractures, which are potentially associated with significant blood loss.
- Injury to the retroperitoneal organs may be difficult to identify, even with the use of CT. Classic examples include duodenal and pancreatic injuries.
- Knowledge of injury mechanism, identification of associated injuries, and a high index of suspicion are required. Despite the doctor's appropriate diligence, some of these injuries are not diagnosed initially.
- Female urethral injury, while uncommon, does occur in association with pelvic fractures and straddle injuries. When present, such injuries are difficult to detect.

ations. In addition, pregnancy tests should be performed on all females of childbearing age.

Musculoskeletal System

The extremities should be inspected for contusions and deformities. Palpation of the bones and examination for tenderness and abnormal movement aids in the identification of occult fractures.

Pelvic fractures can be suspected by the identification of ecchymosis over the iliac wings, pubis, labia, or scrotum. Pain on palpation of the pelvic ring is an important finding in alert patients. Mobility of the pelvis in response to gentle anterior-to-posterior pressure with the heels of the hands on both anterior iliac spines and the symphysis pubis can suggest pelvic ring disruption in unconscious patients. Because such manipulation can initiate unwanted bleeding, it should be done only once (if at all), and preferably by the orthopedic surgeon responsible for the patient's care. In addition, assessment of peripheral pulses can identify vascular injuries.

Significant extremity injuries can exist without fractures being evident on examination or x-rays. Ligament ruptures produce joint instability. Muscle-tendon unit injuries interfere with active motion of the affected structures. Impaired sensation and/or loss of voluntary muscle contraction strength can be caused by nerve injury or ischemia, including that due to compartment syndrome.

Thoracic and lumbar spinal fractures and/or neurologic injuries must be considered based on physical findings and mechanism of injury. Other injuries can mask the physical findings of spinal injuries, and they can remain undetected unless the doctor obtains the appropriate x-rays.

The musculoskeletal examination is not complete without an examination of the patient's back. Unless the patient's back is examined, significant injuries may be missed. See Chapter 7: Spine and Spinal Cord Trauma, and Chapter 8: Musculoskeletal Trauma.

Neurologic

A comprehensive neurologic examination includes not only motor and sensory evaluation of the extremities, but reevaluation of the patient's level of consciousness and pupillary size and response. The GCS score facilitates detection of early changes and trends in the neurologic status. See Appendix C: Trauma Scores: Revised and Pediatric.

Early consultation with a neurosurgeon is required for patients with neurologic injury. Patients should be frequently monitored for deterioration in level of consciousness and changes in the neurologic examination, as these findings can reflect progression of the intracranial injury. If a patient with a head injury deteriorates neurologically, oxygenation and perfusion of the brain and adequacy of ventilation (ie, the ABCDEs) must be reassessed. Intracranial surgical intervention or measures for reducing intracranial pressure may be necessary. The neurosurgeon will decide

PITFALLS

- Blood loss from pelvic fractures that increase pelvic volume can be difficult to control, and fatal hemorrhage can result. A sense of urgency should accompany the management of these injuries.
- Fractures involving the bones of the hands, wrists, and feet are often not diagnosed in the secondary survey performed in the ED. Sometimes, it is only after the patient has regained consciousness and/or other major injuries are resolved that pain in the area of an occult injury is noted.
- Injuries to the soft tissues around joints are frequently diagnosed after the patient begins to recover. Therefore, frequent reevaluation is essential.
- A high level of suspicion must be maintained to prevent the development of compartment syndrome.

whether conditions such as epidural and subdural hematomas require evacuation, and whether depressed skull fractures need operative intervention. See Chapter 6: Head Trauma, and Chapter 7: Spine and Spinal Cord Trauma.

Adjuncts to the Secondary Survey

❓ How can I minimize missed injuries?

Specialized diagnostic tests may be performed during the secondary survey to identify specific injuries. These include additional x-ray examinations of the spine and extremities; CT scans of the head, chest, abdomen, and spine; contrast urography and angiography; transesophageal ultrasound; bronchoscopy; esophagoscopy; and other diagnostic procedures. Often these procedures require transportation of the patient to other areas of the hospital, where equipment and personnel to manage life-threatening contingencies may not be immediately available. Therefore, these specialized tests should not be performed until the patient has been carefully examined and his or her hemodynamic status has been normalized.

Reevaluation

Trauma patients must be reevaluated constantly to ensure that new findings are not overlooked and to discover dete-

rioration in previously noted findings. As initial life-threatening injuries are managed, other equally life-threatening problems and less severe injuries can become apparent. Underlying medical problems that can significantly affect the ultimate prognosis of the patient can become evident. A high index of suspicion facilitates early diagnosis and management.

Continuous monitoring of vital signs and urinary output is essential. For adult patients, maintenance of urinary output at 0.5 mL/kg/hr is desirable. In pediatric patients who are older than 1 year, an output of 1 mL/kg/hr is typically adequate. ABG analyses and cardiac monitoring devices should be used. Pulse oximetry on critically injured patients and end-tidal carbon dioxide monitoring on intubated patients should be considered.

The relief of severe pain is an important part of the treatment of trauma patients. Many injuries, especially musculoskeletal injuries, produce pain and anxiety in conscious patients. Effective analgesia usually requires the administration of opiates or anxiolytics intravenously (intramuscular injections should be avoided). These agents should be used judiciously and in small doses to achieve the desired level of patient comfort and relief of anxiety, while avoiding respiratory depression, the masking of subtle injuries, and changes in the patient's status.

PITFALL

Any increase in intracranial pressure (ICP) can reduce cerebral perfusion pressure and lead to secondary brain injury. Most of the diagnostic and therapeutic maneuvers necessary for the evaluation and care of patients with brain injury will increase ICP. Tracheal intubation is a classic example; in patients with brain injury, it should be performed expeditiously and as smoothly as possible. Rapid neurologic deterioration of patients with brain injury can occur despite the application of all measures to control ICP and maintain appropriate support of the central nervous system.

Any evidence of loss of sensation, paralysis, or weakness suggests major injury to the spinal column or peripheral nervous system. Neurologic deficits should be documented when identified, even when transfer to another facility or doctor for specialty care is necessary. Immobilization of the entire patient, using a long spine board, semirigid cervical collar, and/or other cervical immobilization devices, must be maintained until spinal injury can be excluded. The common mistake of immobilizing the head but freeing the torso allows the cervical spine to flex with the body as a fulcrum. **Protection of the spinal cord is required at all times until a spine injury is excluded. Early consultation with a neurosurgeon or orthopedic surgeon is necessary if a spinal injury is detected.**

developed, reevaluated, and rehearsed frequently to enhance the possibility of saving the maximum number of injured patients. ATLS providers should understand their role in disaster management within their health-care institutions and remember the principles of ATLS relevant to patient care.

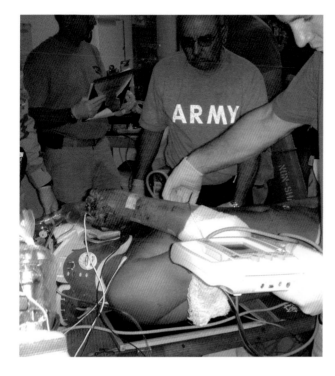

Records and Legal Considerations

Specific legal considerations, including records, consent for treatment, and forensic evidence, are relevant to ATLS providers.

RECORDS

Meticulous record keeping, including documenting the time for all events, is very important. Often more than one doctor cares for an individual patient. Precise records are essential to evaluate the patient's needs and clinical status. Accurate record keeping during resuscitation can be facilitated by a member of the nursing staff whose primary responsibility is to record and collate all patient care information.

Medicolegal problems arise frequently, and precise records are helpful for all individuals concerned. Chronologic reporting with flowsheets helps both the attending doctor and the consulting doctor to assess changes in the patient's condition quickly. See Appendix D: Sample Trauma Flow Sheet, Chapter 13: Transfer to Definitive Care, and Figure 13.1: Sample Transfer Form.

CONSENT FOR TREATMENT

Consent is sought before treatment, if possible. In life-threatening emergencies, it is often not possible to obtain such consent. In these cases, treatment should be provided first, with formal consent obtained later.

FORENSIC EVIDENCE

If criminal activity is suspected in conjunction with a patient's injury, the personnel caring for the patient must preserve the evidence. All items, such as clothing and bullets, must be saved for law enforcement personnel. Laboratory determinations of blood alcohol concentrations and other drugs may be particularly pertinent and have substantial legal implications. See Appendix B: Biomechanics of Injury.

Definitive Care

? Which patients do I transfer to a higher level of care? When should the transfer occur?

Interhospital triage criteria will help determine the level, pace, and intensity of initial treatment of the multiply injured patient. See ACS COT, *Resources for Optimal Care of the Injured Patient, 2006.* These criteria take into account the patient's physiologic status, obvious anatomic injury, mechanisms of injury, concurrent diseases, and other factors that can alter the patient's prognosis. ED and surgical personnel should use these criteria to determine whether the patient requires transfer to a trauma center or closest appropriate hospital capable of providing more specialized care. The closest appropriate local facility should be chosen based on its overall capabilities to care for the injured patient. See Chapter 13: Transfer to Definitive Care and Figure 1-1.

Disaster

Disasters frequently overwhelm local and regional resources. Plans for management of such conditions must be

CHAPTER SUMMARY

 1   The correct sequence of priorities for assessment of a multiply injured patient is preparation; triage; primary survey; resuscitation; adjuncts to primary survey and resuscitation; consider need for patient transfer; secondary survey, adjuncts to secondary survey; reevaluation; and definitive care.

2   The principles of the primary and secondary surveys are appropriate for the assessment of all multiply injured patients.

 3   The guidelines and techniques included in the initial resuscitative and definitive-care phases of treatment should be applied to all multiply injured patients.

 4   A patient's medical history and the mechanism of injury are critical to identifying injuries.

5   Pitfalls associated with the initial assessment and management of injured patients must be anticipated and managed to minimize their impact.

 6   The initial assessment of a multiply injured patient follows a sequence of priorities, as do the management techniques for primary treatment and stabilization.

BIBLIOGRAPHY

1. American College of Surgeons Committee on Trauma. *Resources for Optimal Care of the Injured Patient.* Chicago, IL: American College of Surgeons Committee on Trauma; 2006.

2. Battistella FD. Emergency department evaluation of the patient with multiple injuries. In: Wilmore DW, Cheung LY, Harken AH, et al., eds. *Scientific American Surgery.* New York, NY: Scientific American; 1988-2000.

3. Bhardwaj A, Ulatowski JA. Hypertonic saline solutions in brain injury. *Curr Opin Crit Care* 2004;10:126-131.

4. Doyle JA, Davis DP, Hoyt DB. The use of hypertonic saline in the treatment of traumatic brain injury. *J Trauma* 2001;50:367-383.

5. Enderson BL, Reath DB, Meadors J, et al. The tertiary trauma survey: a prospective study of missed injury. *J Trauma* 1990;30:666-670.

6. Esposito TJ, Ingraham A, Luchette FA, et al. Reasons to omit digital rectal exam in trauma patients: No fingers, no rectum, no useful additional information. *J Trauma* 2005;59(6):1314-1319.

7. Esposito TJ, Kuby A, Unfred C, et al. General surgeons and the Advanced Trauma Life Support course: Is it time to refocus? *J Trauma* 1995;39:929-934.

8. Kreimeier U, Messmer K. Small-volume resuscitation: from experimental evidence to clinical routine. Advantages and disadvantages of hypertonic solutions. *Acta Anaesthesiol Scand* 2002;46:625-638.

9. Mattox KL, Feliciano DV, Moore EE, eds. *Trauma.* 4th ed. New York, McGraw-Hill; 2000.

10. McSwain NE Jr., Salomone J, et al., eds. *Prehospital Trauma Life Support: Basic and Advanced.* 6th ed. St. Louis, MO: Mosby; 2007.

11. Morris JA, MacKinzie EJ, Daminso AM, et al. Mortality in trauma patients: interaction between host factors and severity. *J Trauma* 1990;30:1476-1482.

12. Murao Y, Hoyt DB, Loomis W, et al. Does the timing of hypertonic saline resuscitation affect its potential to prevent lung damage? *Shock* 2000;14:18-23.

13. Nahum AM, Melvin J, eds. *The Biomechanics of Trauma.* Norwalk, CT: Appleton-Century-Crofts; 1985.

14. Pope A, French G, Longnecker DE, eds. *Fluid Resuscitation: State of the Science for Treating Combat Casualties and Civilian Injuries.* Washington, DC: National Academies Press; 1999.

15. Rhodes M, Brader A, Lucke J, et al: Direct transport to the operating room for resuscitation of trauma patients. *J Trauma* 1989;29:907-915.

16. Rotstein OD. Novel strategies for immunomodulation after trauma: revisiting hypertonic saline as a resuscitation strategy for hemorrhagic shock. *J Trauma* 2000;49:580-583.

▶▶ **Interactive Skill Procedures**

THE FOLLOWING PROCEDURES ARE INCLUDED IN THIS SKILL STATION:

▶▶ **Skill I-A:** Primary Survey and Resuscitation

▶▶ **Skill I-B:** Secondary Survey and Management

▶▶ **Skill I-C:** Patient Reevaluation

▶▶ **Skill I-C:** Transfer to Definitive Care

Performance at this skill station will allow the participant to practice and demonstrate the following activities in a simulated clinical situation:

OBJECTIVES

1 Communicate and demonstrate to the instructor the systematic initial assessment and treatment of each patient.

2 Using the primary survey assessment techniques, determine and demonstrate:

  Airway patency and cervical spine control
  Breathing and ventilation
  Circulatory status with hemorrhage control
  Disability: neurologic status
  Exposure/environment: Undress the patient, but prevent hypothermia.

3 Establish resuscitation (management) priorities in a multiply injured patient based on findings from the primary survey.

4 Integrate appropriate history taking as an invaluable aid in patient assessment.

5 Identify the injury-producing mechanism and describe the injuries that may exist and/or may be anticipated as a result of the mechanism of injury.

6 Using secondary survey techniques, assess the patient from head to toe.

7 Using the primary and secondary survey techniques, reevaluate the patient's status and response to therapy instituted.

8 Given a series of x-rays:

  Diagnose fractures.
  Differentiate associated injuries.

9 Outline the definitive care necessary to stabilize each patient in preparation for possible transport to a trauma center or to the closest appropriate facility.

10 As referring doctor, communicate with the receiving doctor (instructor) in a logical, sequential manner:

  Patient's history, including mechanism of injury
  Physical findings
  Treatment instituted
  Patient's response to therapy
  Diagnostic tests performed and results
  Need for transport
  Method of transportation
  Anticipated time of arrival

▶ Skill I-A: Primary Survey and Resuscitation

The student should: (1) outline preparations that must be made to facilitate the rapid progression of assessment and resuscitation of the patient; (2) indicate the need to wear appropriate clothing to protect both the caregivers and the patient from communicable diseases; and (3) indicate that the patient is to be completely undressed, but that hypothermia should be prevented. *Note:* Standard precautions are required whenever caring for trauma patients.

▶▶ AIRWAY MAINTENANCE WITH CERVICAL SPINE PROTECTION

STEP 1. Assessment
  A. Ascertain patency.
  B. Rapidly assess for airway obstruction.

STEP 2. Management—Establish a patent airway
  A. Perform a chin-lift or jaw-thrust maneuver.
  B. Clear the airway of foreign bodies.
  C. Insert an oropharyngeal airway.
  D. Establish a definitive airway.
    1) Intubation
    2) Surgical cricothyroidotomy
  E. Describe jet insufflation of the airway, noting that it is only a temporary procedure.

STEP 3. Maintain the cervical spine in a neutral position with manual immobilization as necessary when establishing an airway.

STEP 4. Reinstate immobilization of the c-spine with appropriate devices after establishing an airway.

▶▶ BREATHING: VENTILATION AND OXYGENATION

STEP 1. Assessment
  A. Expose the neck and chest, and ensure immobilization of the head and neck.
  B. Determine the rate and depth of respirations.
  C. Inspect and palpate the neck and chest for tracheal deviation, unilateral and bilateral chest movement, use of accessory muscles, and any signs of injury.
  D. Percuss the chest for presence of dullness or hyperresonance.
  E. Auscultate the chest bilaterally.

STEP 2. Management
  A. Administer high-concentration oxygen.
  B. Ventilate with a bag-mask device.
  C. Alleviate tension pneumothorax.
  D. Seal open pneumothorax.

  E. Attach a CO_2 monitoring device to the endotracheal tube.
  F. Attach a pulse oximeter to the patient.

▶▶ CIRCULATION WITH HEMORRHAGE CONTROL

STEP 1. Assessment
  A. Identify source of external, exsanguinating hemorrhage.
  B. Identify potential source(s) of internal hemorrhage.
  C. Assess pulse: Quality, rate, regularity, and paradox.
  D. Evaluate skin color.
  E. Measure blood pressure, if time permits.

STEP 2. Management
  A. Apply direct pressure to external bleeding site(s).
  B. Consider presence of internal hemorrhage and potential need for operative intervention, and obtain surgical consult.
  C. Insert two large-caliber IV catheters.
  D. Simultaneously obtain blood for hematologic and chemical analyses; pregnancy test, when appropriate; type and crossmatch; and ABGs.
  E. Initiate IV fluid therapy with warmed crystalloid solution and blood replacement.
  F. Prevent hypothermia.

▶▶ DISABILITY: BRIEF NEUROLOGIC EXAMINATION

STEP 1. Determine the level of consciousness using the GCS.

STEP 2. Assess the pupils for size, equality, and reaction.

▶▶ EXPOSURE/ENVIRONMENTAL CONTROL

STEP 1. Completely undress the patient, but prevent hypothermia.

▶▶ ADJUNCTS TO PRIMARY SURVEY AND RESUSCITATION

STEP 1. Obtain ABG analysis and ventilatory rate.

STEP 2. Monitor the patient's exhaled CO_2 with an appropriate monitoring device.

STEP 3. Attach an ECG monitor to the patient.

STEP 4. Insert urinary and gastric catheters unless contraindicated, and monitor the patient's hourly output of urine.

STEP 5. Consider the need for and obtain AP chest and AP pelvic x-rays.

STEP 6. Consider the need for and perform FAST or DPL.

▶▶ **REASSESS PATIENT'S ABCDEs AND CONSIDER NEED FOR PATIENT TRANSFER**

▶ Skill I-B: Secondary Survey and Management

(Also See Table I-1: Secondary Survey)

▶▶ AMPLE HISTORY AND MECHANISM OF INJURY

STEP 1. Obtain AMPLE history from patient, family, or prehospital personnel.

STEP 2. Obtain history of injury-producing event and identify injury mechanisms.

▶▶ HEAD AND MAXILLOFACIAL

STEP 3. Assessment
   A. Inspect and palpate entire head and face for lacerations, contusions, fractures, and thermal injury.
   B. Reevaluate pupils.
   C. Reevaluate level of consciousness and GCS score.
   D. Assess eyes for hemorrhage, penetrating injury, visual acuity, dislocation of lens, and presence of contact lenses.
   E. Evaluate cranial-nerve function.
   F. Inspect ears and nose for cerebrospinal fluid leakage.
   G. Inspect mouth for evidence of bleeding and cerebrospinal fluid, soft-tissue lacerations, and loose teeth.

STEP 4. Management
   A. Maintain airway, and continue ventilation and oxygenation as indicated.
   B. Control hemorrhage.
   C. Prevent secondary brain injury.
   D. Remove contact lenses.

▶▶ CERVICAL SPINE AND NECK

STEP 5. Assessment
   A. Inspect for signs of blunt and penetrating injury, tracheal deviation, and use of accessory respiratory muscles.
   B. Palpate for tenderness, deformity, swelling, subcutaneous emphysema, tracheal deviation, and symmetry of pulses.
   C. Auscultate the carotid arteries for bruits.
   D. Obtain a CT of the cervical spine or a lateral, cross-table cervical spine x-ray.

STEP 6. Management: Maintain adequate in-line immobilization and protection of the cervical spine.

▶▶ CHEST

STEP 7. Assessment
   A. Inspect the anterior, lateral, and posterior chest wall for signs of blunt and penetrating injury, use of accessory breathing muscles, and bilateral respiratory excursions.
   B. Auscultate the anterior chest wall and posterior bases for bilateral breath sounds and heart sounds.
   C. Palpate the entire chest wall for evidence of blunt and penetrating injury, subcutaneous emphysema, tenderness, and crepitation.
   D. Percuss for evidence of hyperresonance or dullness.

STEP 8. Management
   A. Perform needle decompression of pleural space or tube thoracostomy, as indicated.
   B. Attach the chest tube to an underwater seal-drainage device.
   C. Correctly dress an open chest wound.
   D. Perform pericardiocentesis, as indicated.
   E. Transfer the patient to the operating room, if indicated.

▶▶ ABDOMEN

STEP 9. Assessment
   A. Inspect the anterior and posterior abdomen for signs of blunt and penetrating injury and internal bleeding.
   B. Auscultate for the presence of bowel sounds.
   C. Percuss the abdomen to elicit subtle rebound tenderness.

TABLE I-1   ■   Secondary Survey

ITEM TO ASSESS	ESTABLISHES/ IDENTIFIES	ASSESS	CONFIRM FINDING	BY
Level of Consciousness	• Severity of head injury	• GCS score	• 8, Severe head injury • 9–12, Moderate head injury • 13–15, Minor head injury	• CT scan • Repeat without paralyzing agents
Pupils	• Type of head injury • Presence of eye injury	• Size • Shape • Reactivity	• Mass effect • Diffuse brain injury • Ophthalmic injury	• CT scan
Head	• Scalp injury • Skull injury	• Inspect for lacerations and skull fractures • Palpable defects	• Scalp laceration • Depressed skull fracture • Basilar skull fracture	• CT scan
Maxillofacial	• Soft-tissue injury • Bone injury • Nerve injury • Teeth/mouth injury	• Visual deformity • Malocclusion • Palpation for crepitation	• Facial fracture • Soft-tissue injury	• Facial-bone x-ray • CT scan of facial bones
Neck	• Laryngeal injury • C-spine injury • Vascular injury • Esophageal injury • Neurologic deficit	• Visual inspection • Palpation • Auscultation	• Laryngeal deformity • Subcutaneous emphysema • Hematoma • Bruit • Platysmal penetration • Pain, tenderness of c-spine	• C-spine x-ray • Angiography/duplex exam • Esophagoscopy • Laryngoscopy
Thorax	• Thoracic-wall injury • Subcutaneous emphysema • Pneumothorax/ hemothorax • Bronchial injury • Pulmonary contusion • Thoracic aortic disruption	• Visual inspection • Palpation • Auscultation	• Bruising, deformity, or paradoxical motion • Chest-wall tenderness, crepitation • Diminished breath sounds • Muffled heart tones • Mediastinal crepitation • Severe back pain	• Chest x-ray • CT scan • Angiography • Bronchoscopy • Tube thoracostomy • Pericardiocentesis • TE ultrasound
Abdomen/Flank	• Abdominal-wall injury • Intraperitoneal injury • Retroperitoneal injury	• Visual inspection • Palpation • Auscultation • Determine path of penetration	• Abdominal-wall pain/tenderness • Peritoneal irritation • Visceral injury • Retroperitoneal organ injury	• DPL/ultrasound • CT scan • Laparotomy • Contrast GI x-ray studies • Angiography
Pelvis	• GU tract injuries • Pelvic fracture(s)	• Palpate symphysis pubis for widening • Palpate bony pelvis for tenderness • Determine pelvic stability only once • Inspect perineum • Rectal/vaginal exam	• GU tract injury (hematuria) • Pelvic fracture • Rectal, vaginal, and/or perineal injury	• Pelvic x-ray • GU contrast studies • Urethrogram • Cystogram • IVP • Contrast-enhanced CT

ITEM TO ASSESS	ESTABLISHES/ IDENTIFIES	ASSESS	CONFIRM FINDING	BY
Spinal Cord	• Cranial injury • Cord injury • Peripheral nerve(s) injury	• Motor response • Pain response	• Unilateral cranial mass effect • Quadriplegia • Paraplegia • Nerve root injury	• Plain spine x-rays • CT Scan • MRI
Vertebral Column	• Column injury • Vertebral instability • Nerve injury	• Verbal response to pain, lateralizing signs • Palpate for tenderness • Deformity	• Fracture versus dislocation	• Plain x-rays • CT scan • MRI
Extremities	• Soft-tissue injury • Bony deformities • Joint abnormalities • Neurovascular defects	• Visual inspection • Palpation	• Swelling, bruising, pallor • Malalignment • Pain, tenderness, crepitation • Absent/diminished pulses • Tense muscular compartments • Neurologic deficits	• Specific x-rays • Doppler examination • Compartment pressures • Angiography

D. Palpate the abdomen for tenderness, involuntary muscle guarding, unequivocal rebound tenderness, and a gravid uterus.

E. Obtain a pelvic x-ray film.

F. Perform DPL/abdominal ultrasound, if warranted.

G. Obtain CT of the abdomen if the patient is hemodynamically normal.

STEP 10. Management

A. Transfer the patient to the operating room, if indicated.

B. Wrap a sheet around the pelvis or apply a pelvic compression binder as indicated to reduce pelvic volume and control hemorrhage from a pelvic fracture.

▶▶ PERINEUM/RECTUM/VAGINA

STEP 11. Perineal assessment. Assess for:

A. Contusions and hematomas

B. Lacerations

C. Urethral bleeding

STEP 12. Rectal assessment in selected patients. Assess for:

A. Rectal blood

B. Anal sphincter tone

C. Bowel wall integrity

D. Bony fragments

E. Prostate position

STEP 13. Vaginal assessment in selected patients. Assess for:

A. Presence of blood in vaginal vault

B. Vaginal lacerations

▶▶ MUSCULOSKELETAL

STEP 14. Assessment

A. Inspect the upper and lower extremities for evidence of blunt and penetrating injury, including contusions, lacerations, and deformity.

B. Palpate the upper and lower extremities for tenderness, crepitation, abnormal movement, and sensation.

C. Palpate all peripheral pulses for presence, absence, and equality.

D. Assess the pelvis for evidence of fracture and associated hemorrhage.

E. Inspect and palpate the thoracic and lumbar spines for evidence of blunt and penetrating injury, including contusions, lacerations, tenderness, deformity, and sensation.

F. Evaluate the pelvic x-ray film for evidence of a fracture.

G. Obtain x-ray films of suspected fracture sites as indicated.

STEP 15. Management

A. Apply and/or readjust appropriate splinting devices for extremity fractures as indicated.

B. Maintain immobilization of the patient's thoracic and lumbar spines.

C. Wrap a sheet around the pelvis or apply a pelvic compression binder as indicated to reduce pelvic volume and control hemorrhage associated with a pelvic fracture.

D. Apply a splint to immobilize an extremity injury.

E. Administer tetanus immunization.

F. Administer medications as indicated or as directed by specialist.

G. Consider the possibility of compartment syndrome.

H. Perform a complete neurovascular examination of the extremities.

▶▶ NEUROLOGIC

STEP 16. Assessment

A. Reevaluate the pupils and level of consciousness.

B. Determine the GCS score.

C. Evaluate the upper and lower extremities for motor and sensory functions.

D. Observe for lateralizing signs.

STEP 17. Management

A. Continue ventilation and oxygenation.

B. Maintain adequate immobilization of the entire patient.

▶▶ ADJUNCTS TO SECONDARY SURVEY

STEP 18. Consider the need for and obtain these diagnostic tests as the patient's condition permits and warrants:

- Spinal x-rays
- CT of the head, chest, abdomen, and/or spine
- Contrast urography
- Angiography
- Extremity x-rays
- Transesophageal ultrasound
- Bronchoscopy
- Esophagoscopy

▶ Skill I-C: Patient Reevaluation

Reevaluate the patient, noting, reporting, and documenting any changes in the patient's condition and responses to resuscitative efforts. Judicious use of analgesics may be instituted. Continuous monitoring of vital signs, urinary output, and the patient's response to treatment is essential.

▶ Skill I-D: Transfer to Definitive Care

Outline rationale for patient transfer, transfer procedures, and patient's needs during transfer, and state the need for direct doctor-to-doctor communication.

CHAPTER **2**

Airway and Ventilatory Management

Upon completion of this topic, the student will identify actual or impending airway obstruction, explain the techniques of establishing and maintaining a patent airway, and confirm the adequacy of ventilation. Specifically, the doctor will be able to:

OBJECTIVES

1 Identify the clinical situations in which airway compromise is likely to occur.

2 Recognize the signs and symptoms of acute airway obstruction.

3 Describe the techniques for establishing and maintaining a patent airway.

4 Describe the techniques for confirming the adequacy of ventilation and oxygenation, including pulse oximetry and end-tidal CO_2 monitoring.

5 Define the term definitive airway.

6 Outline the steps necessary for maintaining oxygenation before, during, and after establishing a definitive airway.

Introduction

The inadequate delivery of oxygenated blood to the brain and other vital structures is the quickest killer of injured patients. Prevention of hypoxemia requires a protected, unobstructed airway and adequate ventilation, which take priority over management of all other conditions. An airway must be secured, oxygen delivered, and ventilatory support provided. **Supplemental oxygen must be administered to all trauma patients.**

Early preventable deaths from airway problems after trauma often result from:

- Failure to recognize the need for an airway intervention.
- Inability to establish an airway.
- Failure to recognize an incorrectly placed airway.
- Displacement of a previously established airway.
- Failure to recognize the need for ventilation.
- Aspiration of gastric contents.

Airway and ventilation are the first priorities.

Airway

❓ *How do I know the airway is adequate?*

The first steps toward identifying and managing potentially life-threatening airway compromise are to recognize problems involving maxillofacial, neck, and laryngeal trauma and to identify objective signs of airway obstruction.

PROBLEM RECOGNITION

Airway compromise can be sudden and complete, insidious and partial, and/or progressive and recurrent. Although it is often related to pain or anxiety or both, tachypnea can be a subtle but early sign of airway or ventilatory compromise. Therefore, assessment and frequent reassessment of airway patency and adequacy of ventilation are critical.

Patients with an altered level of consciousness are at particular risk for airway compromise and often require a definitive airway (a tube placed in the trachea with the cuff inflated, the tube connected to some form of oxygen-enriched assisted ventilation, and the airway secured in place with tape). Unconscious patients with head injuries, patients who are obtunded because of the use of alcohol

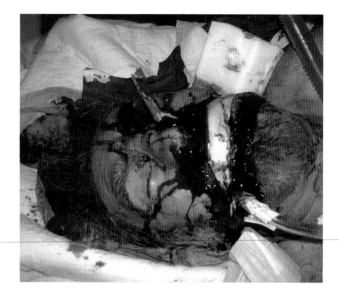

and/or other drugs, and patients with thoracic injuries all can have a compromised ventilatory effort. In these patients, the purpose of endotracheal intubation is to provide an airway, deliver supplementary oxygen, support ventilation, and prevent aspiration. **Maintaining oxygenation and preventing hypercarbia are critical in managing trauma patients, especially those who have sustained a head injury.**

Anticipating vomiting in all injured patients and being prepared to manage the situation are important. The presence of gastric contents in the oropharynx represents a significant risk of aspiration with the patient's next breath. Immediate suctioning and rotation of the entire patient to the lateral position are indicated.

Maxillofacial Trauma

Trauma to the face demands aggressive airway management. The mechanism for this injury is exemplified by an unbelted automobile passenger who is thrown into the windshield and dashboard. Trauma to the midface can produce fractures and dislocations that compromise the nasopharynx and oropharynx. Facial fractures can be associated with hemorrhage, increased secretions, and dislodged teeth, which cause additional difficulties in maintaining a patent airway. Fractures of the mandible, especially bilateral body fractures, can cause loss of normal airway support. Airway

---

PITFALL

Trauma patients can vomit and aspirate. Functional suction equipment must be immediately available to aid doctors in ensuring a secure, patent airway in all trauma patients.

obstruction can result if the patient is in a supine position. Patients who refuse to lie down may be experiencing difficulty in maintaining their airway or handling secretions.

Neck Trauma

Penetrating injury to the neck can cause vascular injury with significant hemorrhage, which can result in displacement and obstruction of the airway. Emergency placement of a surgical airway may be necessary if this displacement and obstruction make endotracheal intubation impossible. Hemorrhage from adjacent vascular injury can be massive, and operative control may be required.

Blunt or penetrating injury to the neck can cause disruption of the larynx or trachea, resulting in airway obstruction and/or severe bleeding into the tracheobronchial tree (Figure 2-1). A definitive airway is urgently required in this situation.

Neck injuries involving disruption of the larynx and trachea or compression of the airway from hemorrhage into the soft tissues of the neck can cause partial airway obstruction. Initially, a patient with this type of serious airway injury may be able to maintain airway patency and ventilation. However, if airway compromise is suspected, a definitive airway is required. To prevent extending an existing airway injury, an endotracheal tube must be inserted cautiously. Loss of airway patency can be precipitous, and an early surgical airway usually is indicated.

Laryngeal Trauma

Although fracture of the larynx is a rare injury, it can present with acute airway obstruction. It is indicated by the following triad of clinical signs:

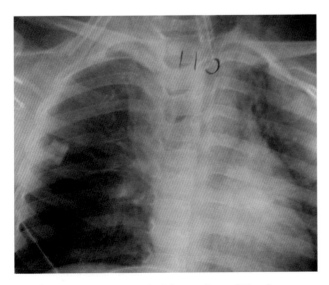

■ **Figure 2-1 Traumatic Disruption of Trachea,** as seen on radiograph. A definitive airway is urgently required in this situation.

1. Hoarseness

2. Subcutaneous emphysema

3. Palpable fracture

Complete obstruction of the airway or severe respiratory distress warrants an attempt at intubation. Flexible endoscopic intubation may be helpful in this situation, but only if it can be performed promptly. If intubation is unsuccessful, an emergency tracheostomy is indicated, followed by operative repair. However, a tracheostomy is difficult to perform under emergency conditions, it can be associated with profuse bleeding, and can be time-consuming. Surgical cricothyroidotomy, although not preferred for this situation, can be a lifesaving option.

Penetrating trauma to the larynx or trachea is overt and requires immediate management. Complete tracheal transection or occlusion of the airway with blood or soft tissue can cause acute airway compromise that requires immediate correction. These injuries are often associated with trauma to the esophagus, carotid artery, or jugular vein, as well as extensive tissue destruction. Noisy breathing indicates partial airway obstruction that can suddenly become complete, whereas absence of breathing suggests that complete obstruction already exists. When the level of consciousness is depressed, detection of significant airway obstruction is more subtle. Labored respiratory effort may be the only clue to airway obstruction and tracheobronchial injury.

If a fracture of the larynx is suspected, based on the mechanism of injury and subtle physical findings, computed tomography (CT) can help to identify this injury.

During initial assessment of the airway, the "talking patient" provides reassurance (at least for the moment) that the airway is patent and not compromised. Therefore, the most important early measure is to talk to the patient and stimulate a verbal response. A positive, appropriate verbal response indicates that the airway is patent, ventilation is intact, and brain perfusion is adequate. Failure to respond or an inappropriate response suggests an altered level of consciousness, airway and ventilatory compromise, or both.

OBJECTIVE SIGNS OF AIRWAY OBSTRUCTION

Several objective signs of airway obstruction can be identified by taking the following steps:

1. Observe the patient to determine whether he or she is agitated or obtunded. Agitation suggests hypoxia, and obtundation suggests hypercarbia. Cyanosis indicates hypoxemia due to inadequate oxygenation; it is identified by inspection of the nail beds and circumoral skin. Cyanosis is a late finding of hypoxia, and pulse oximetry is used early in the assessment of airway obstruction. Look for retractions and the use of accessory muscles of ventilation that, when present, provide additional evidence of airway compromise.

2. Listen for abnormal sounds. Noisy breathing is obstructed breathing. Snoring, gurgling, and crowing sounds (stridor) can be associated with partial occlusion of the pharynx or larynx. Hoarseness (dysphonia) implies functional, laryngeal obstruction. Abusive and belligerent patients may in fact have hypoxia and should not be presumed to be intoxicated.

3. Feel for the location of the trachea and quickly determine whether it is in the midline position.

Ventilation

Ensuring a patent airway is an important step in providing oxygen to the patient, but it is only the first step. An unobstructed airway is not likely to benefit the patient unless there is also adequate ventilation. The doctor must recognize problems with ventilation and look for objective signs of inadequate ventilation.

PROBLEM RECOGNITION

Ventilation can be compromised by airway obstruction, altered ventilatory mechanics, or central nervous system (CNS) depression. If a patient's breathing is not improved by clearing the airway, other causes of the problem must be identified and managed. Direct trauma to the chest, especially with rib fractures, causes pain with breathing and leads to rapid, shallow ventilation and hypoxemia. Elderly patients and those with preexisting pulmonary dysfunction are at significant risk for ventilatory failure under these circumstances. Intracranial injury can cause abnormal breathing patterns and compromise adequacy of ventilation. Cervical spinal cord injury can result in diaphragmatic breathing and interfere with the ability to meet increased oxygen demands. Complete cervical cord transection, which spares the phrenic nerves (C3 and C4), results in abdominal breathing and paralysis of the intercostal muscles; assisted ventilation may be required.

OBJECTIVE SIGNS OF INADEQUATE VENTILATION

? How do I know ventilation is adequate?

Several objective signs of inadequate ventilation can be identified by taking the following steps:

PITFALL

Patients who are breathing high concentrations of oxygen can maintain their oxygen saturation although breathing inadequately. Measure arterial or end-tidal carbon dioxide.

---

1. Look for symmetrical rise and fall of the chest and adequate chest wall excursion. Asymmetry suggests splinting of the rib cage or a flail chest. Labored breathing may indicate an imminent threat to the patient's ventilation.

2. Listen for movement of air on both sides of the chest. Decreased or absent breath sounds over one or both hemithoraces should alert the examiner to the presence of thoracic injury. ◾ See Chapter 4: Thoracic Trauma. Beware of a rapid respiratory rate—tachypnea can indicate respiratory distress.

3. Use a pulse oximeter. This device provides information regarding the patient's oxygen saturation and peripheral perfusion, but does not measure the adequacy of ventilation.

Airway Management

? How do I manage the airway of a trauma patient?

Airway patency and adequacy of ventilation must be assessed quickly and accurately. Pulse oximetry and end-tidal CO_2 measurement are essential. If problems are identified or suspected, measures should be instituted immediately to improve oxygenation and reduce the risk of further ventilatory compromise. These measures include airway maintenance techniques, definitive airway measures (including surgical airway), and methods of providing supplemental ventilation. Because all of these actions can require some neck motion, it is important to maintain cervical spine protection in all patients, especially those who are known to have an unstable cervical spine injury and those who have been incompletely evaluated and are at risk. The spinal cord must be protected until the possibility of a spinal injury has been excluded by clinical assessment and appropriate radiographic studies.

Patients who are wearing a helmet and require airway management need their head and neck held in a neutral position while the helmet is removed. This is a two-person procedure: One person provides in-line manual immobilization from below, while the second person expands the helmet laterally and removes it from above (Figure 2-2). Then, in-line manual immobilization is reestablished from above, and the patient's head and neck are secured during airway management. Removal of the helmet using a cast cutter while stabilizing the head and neck can minimize cervical spine motion in patients with known cervical spine injury.

High-flow oxygen is required both before and immediately after airway management measures are instituted. A rigid suction device is essential and should be readily available. Patients with facial injuries can have associated cribri-

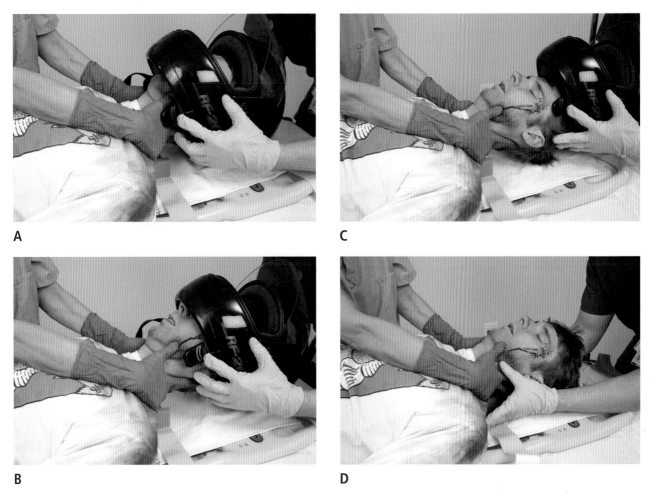

A

B

C

D

■ **Figure 2-2 Helmet Removal.** Removing a helmet properly is a two-person procedure. While one person provides manual in-line stabilization of the head and neck (**A**), the second person expands the helmet laterally. The second person then removes the helmet (**B**), with attention paid to the helmet clearing the nose and the occiput. Once removed, the first person supports the weight of the patient's head (**C**), and the second person takes over inline stabilization (**D**).

form plate fractures, and the insertion of any tube through the nose can result in passage into the cranial vault.

AIRWAY MAINTENANCE TECHNIQUES

In patients who have a decreased level of consciousness, the tongue can fall backward and obstruct the hypopharynx. This form of obstruction can be corrected readily by the chin-lift or jaw-thrust maneuver. The airway can then be maintained with an oropharyngeal or nasopharyngeal airway. Maneuvers used to establish an airway can produce or aggravate cervical spine injury, so in-line immobilization of the cervical spine is essential during these procedures.

Chin-Lift Maneuver

In the chin-lift maneuver, the fingers of one hand are placed under the mandible, which is then gently lifted upward to bring the chin anterior. The thumb of the same hand lightly depresses the lower lip to open the mouth (Figure 2-3). The thumb also may be placed behind the lower incisors and, simultaneously, the chin is gently lifted. The chin-lift maneuver should not hyperextend the neck. This maneuver is useful for trauma victims because it can prevent converting a cervical fracture without cord injury into one with cord injury.

Jaw-Thrust Maneuver

The jaw-thrust maneuver is performed by grasping the angles of the lower jaw, one hand on each side, and displacing the mandible forward (Figure 2-4). When this method is used with the face mask of a bag-mask device, a good seal and adequate ventilation can be achieved. Care must be taken to prevent neck extension.

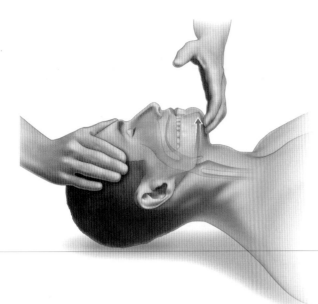

A

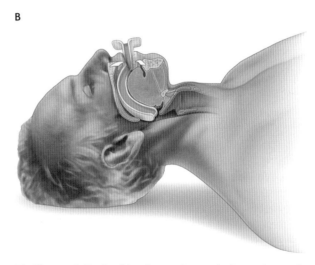

■ **Figure 2-3 Chin-Lift Maneuver to Establish an Airway.** This maneuver is useful for trauma victims because it can prevent converting a cervical fracture without cord injury into one with cord injury.

B

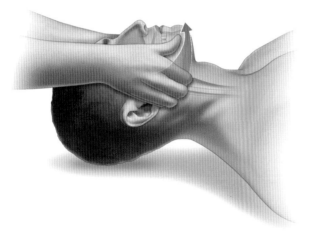

■ **Figure 2-4 Jaw-Thrust Maneuver to Establish an Airway.** Care must be taken to prevent neck extension.

■ **Figure 2-5**   In this alternative technique, the oral airway is inserted upside down **(A)** until the soft palate is encountered, at which point the device is rotated 180 degrees and slipped into place over the tongue. **(B)** This method should not be used in children.

Oropharyngeal Airway

Oral airways are inserted into the mouth behind the tongue. The preferred technique is to use a tongue blade to depress the tongue and then insert the airway posteriorly, taking care not to push the tongue backward, which would block—rather than clear—the airway. This device must not be used in conscious patients because it can induce gagging, vomiting, and aspiration. Patients who tolerate an oropharyngeal airway are highly likely to require intubation.

An alternative technique is to insert the oral airway upside down, so its concavity is directed upward, until the soft palate is encountered. At this point, with the device

rotated 180 degrees, the concavity is directed inferiorly, and the device is slipped into place over the tongue (Figure 2-5). This alternative method should not be used in children, because the rotation of the device can damage the mouth and pharynx. ▪▪ See Skill Station II: Airway and Ventilatory Management, Skill II-A: Oropharyngeal Airway Insertion.

Nasopharyngeal Airway

Nasopharyngeal airways are inserted in one nostril and passed gently into the posterior oropharynx. They should be well lubricated and inserted into the nostril that appears to be unobstructed. If obstruction is encountered during introduction of the airway, stop and try the other nostril. ▰ See Skill Station II: Airway and Ventilatory Management, Skill II-B: Nasopharyngeal Airway Insertion.

Laryngeal Mask Airway

There is an established role for the laryngeal mask airway (LMA) in the treatment of patients with difficult airways, particularly if attempts at endotracheal intubation or bag-mask ventilation have failed (Figure 2-6). However, the LMA does not provide a definitive airway, and proper placement of this device is difficult without appropriate training. When a patient has an LMA in place on arrival in the emergency department (ED), the doctor must plan for a definitive airway. ▰ See Skill Station II: Airway and Ventilatory Management, Skill II-E: Laryngeal Mask Airway Insertion.

Multilumen Esophageal Airway

Multilumen esophageal airway devices are used by some prehospital personnel to achieve an airway when a definitive airway is not feasible (Figure 2-7). One of the ports communicates with the esophagus and the other with the airway. The personnel who use this device are trained to observe which occludes the esophagus and which will provide air to the trachea. The esophageal port is then occluded with a balloon, and the other port is ventilated. A CO_2 detector improves the accuracy of this apparatus. The multilumen esophageal airway device must be removed and/or a definitive airway provided by the doctor after appropriate assessment.

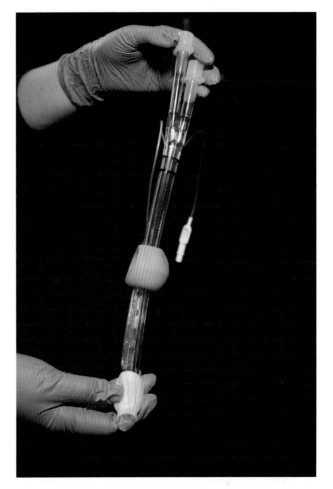

■ **Figure 2-7** Example of a multilumen esophageal airway.

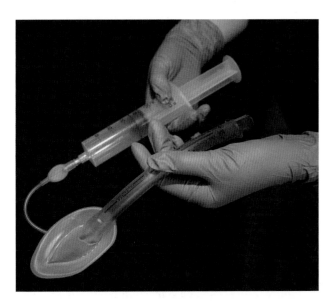

■ **Figure 2-6** Example of a laryngeal mask airway.

Laryngeal Tube Airway

The laryngeal tube airway (LTA) is an extraglottic airway device with capabilities similar to those of the LMA to provide successful patient ventilation (Figure 2-8). The LTA is not a definitive airway device, and plans to provide a definitive airway are necessary. Like the LMA, the LTA is placed without direct visualization of the glottis and does not require significant manipulation of the head and neck for placement. ▰ See Skill Station II: Airway and Ventilatory Management, Skill II-F: Laryngeal Tube Airway Insertion.

Gum Elastic Bougie

An excellent tool when faced with a difficult airway is the Eschmann Tracheal Tube Introducer (ETTI), also known as the gum elastic bougie (GEB) (Figure 2-9). First introduced as an aid to difficult intubations in 1949 by Macintosh, its use has been primarily in the operating room but has since been expanded to the ED and prehospital arena. It is a 60-cm-long, 15-French intubating stylette made from a woven polyester base with a resin coating, which is available in both disposable and reusable packaging. It has a Coude tip that is

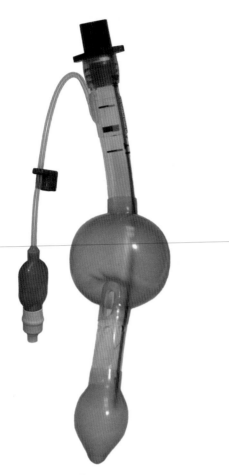

■ Figure 2-8 Example of a laryngeal tube airway.

angled at 40 degrees 3.5 cm from the distal end, with 10-cm gradations. No special preparation is required; it comes ready to use.

The GEB is used when vocal cords cannot be visualized on direct laryngoscopy. With the laryngoscope in place, the GEB is passed blindly beyond the epiglottis, with the angled tip positioned anteriorly. Tracheal position is confirmed by either feeling for clicks as the distal tip rubs along the cartilaginous tracheal rings (65%–90%), the tube rotates to the right or left when entering the bronchus, or when the tube is held up at the bronchial tree (10%–13%), which is usually at about the 50-cm mark. None of these indications occur if the GEB has entered the esophagus. The proximal end is lubricated, and a 6.0-mm internal diameter or larger endotracheal tube is passed over the GEB beyond the vocal cords. If the endotracheal tube is held up at the arytenoids or aryepiglottic folds, the tube is withdrawn slightly and turned 90 degrees to facilitate advancement beyond the obstruction. The GEB is then removed, and tube position is confirmed with auscultation of breath sounds and capnography.

In multiple operating room studies, successful intubation was achieved at rates greater than 95% with the GEB. In cases in which potential cervical spine injury was suspected,

GEB-aided intubation was successful in 100% of cases in less than 45 seconds. Although operating-room conditions are far superior to those of the ED and prehospital environments, the GEB has been successfully placed in these settings also. This simple device has allowed rapid intubation of nearly 80 percent of prehospital patients in whom direct laryngoscopy is difficult.

DEFINITIVE AIRWAY

A definitive airway requires a tube placed in the trachea with the cuff inflated, the tube connected to some form of oxygen-enriched assisted ventilation, and the airway secured in place with tape. There are three types of definitive airways: orotracheal tube, nasotracheal tube, and surgical airway (cricothyroidotomy or tracheostomy). The criteria for establishing a definitive airway are based on clinical findings and include (see Table 2-1):

- Presence of apnea

- Inability to maintain a patent airway by other means

- Need to protect the lower airway from aspiration of blood or vomitus

- Impending or potential compromise of the airway—for example, following inhalation injury, facial fractures, retropharyngeal hematoma, or sustained seizure activity

- Presence of a closed head injury requiring assisted ventilation (Glasgow Coma Scale score <8)

- Inability to maintain adequate oxygenation by facemask oxygen supplementation

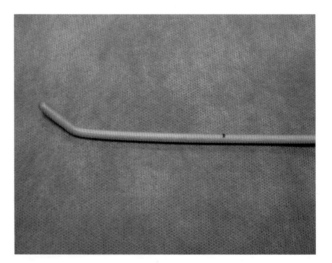

■ Figure 2-9 Eschmann Tracheal Tube Introducer (ETTI), also known as the gum elastic bougie.

TABLE 2-1 ■ Indications for Definitive Airway	
NEED FOR AIRWAY PROTECTION	**NEED FOR VENTILATION OR OXYGENATION**
Unconscious	Apnea • Neuromuscular paralysis • Unconscious
Severe maxillofacial fractures	Inadequate respiratory efforts • Tachypnea • Hypoxia • Hypercarbia • Cyanosis
Risk for aspiration • Bleeding • Vomiting	Severe, closed head injury with need for brief hyperventilation if acute neurologic deterioration occurs
Risk for obstruction • Neck hematoma • Laryngeal or tracheal injury • Stridor	Massive blood loss and need for volume resuscitation

The urgency of the situation and the circumstances indicating the need for airway intervention dictate the specific route and method to be used. Continued assisted ventilation is aided by supplemental sedation, analgesics, or muscle relaxants, as indicated. The use of a pulse oximeter can be helpful in determining the need for a definitive airway, the urgency of the need, and, by inference, the effectiveness of airway placement. The potential for concomitant cervical spine (c-spine) injury is of major concern in the patient requiring an airway. Figure 2-10 provides a scheme for deciding the appropriate route of airway management.

Endotracheal Intubation

Although it is important to establish the presence or absence of a cervical spine fracture, obtaining c-spine x-rays should not impede or delay placement of a definitive airway when one is clearly indicated. The patient who has a GCS score of 8 or less requires prompt intubation. If there is no immediate need for intubation, x-rays of the cervical spine may be obtained. **However, a normal lateral cervical spine film does not exclude the possibility of a c-spine injury.**

The most important determinant of whether to proceed with orotracheal or nasotracheal intubation is the experience of the doctor. Both techniques are safe and effective when performed properly. The orotracheal route is more commonly used. Esophageal occlusion by cricoid pressure is useful in preventing aspiration. Laryngeal manipulation by backward, upward, and rightward pressure (BURP) can aid in visualizing the vocal cords.

If the decision to perform orotracheal intubation is made, the two-person technique with in-line cervical spine immobilization is necessary (Figure 2-11). If the patient has apnea, orotracheal intubation is indicated. See Skill Station II: Airway and Ventilatory Management, Skill II-D: Adult Orotracheal Intubation (with and without Gum Elastic Bougie Device, and Skill II-G: Infant Endotracheal Intubation.

❓ How do I know the tube is in the right place?

Following direct laryngoscopy and insertion of the orotracheal tube, the cuff is inflated, and assisted ventilation instituted. Proper placement of the tube is suggested—but not confirmed—by hearing equal breath sounds bilaterally and detecting no borborygmi (ie, rumbling or gurgling noises) in the epigastrium. The presence of borborygmi in the epigastrium with inspiration suggests esophageal intubation and warrants repositioning of the tube. A carbon dioxide detector (ideally a capnograph, but, if that is not available, a colorimetric CO_2 monitoring device) is indicated to help confirm proper intubation of the airway. The presence of CO_2 in exhaled air indicates that the airway has been successfully intubated, but does not ensure the correct position of the endotracheal tube. If CO_2 is not detected, esophageal intubation has occurred. Proper position of the tube is best confirmed by chest x-ray, once the possibility of esophageal intubation is excluded. Colorimetric CO_2 indicators are not useful for physiologic monitoring or assessing the adequacy of ventilation, which requires arterial blood gas analysis or continual end-tidal carbon dioxide analysis. See Skill Station II: Airway and Ventilatory Management, Skill II-H: Pulse Oximetry Monitoring, and Skill II-I: Carbon Dioxide Detection.

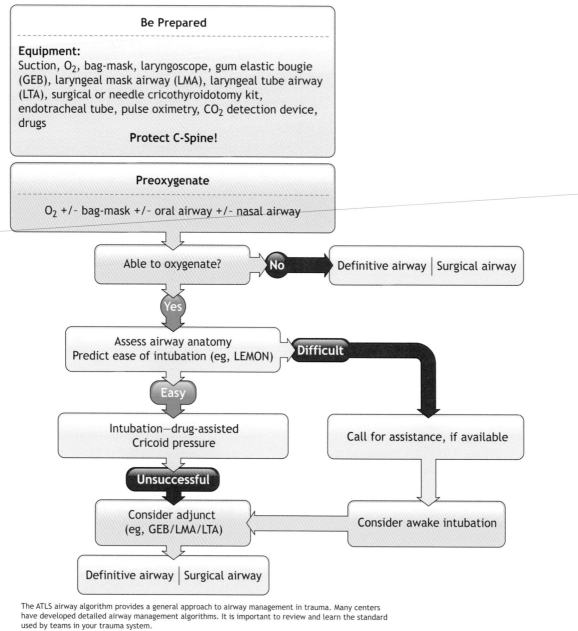

The ATLS airway algorithm provides a general approach to airway management in trauma. Many centers have developed detailed airway management algorithms. It is important to review and learn the standard used by teams in your trauma system.

■ **Figure 2-10 Airway Decision Scheme.** Used for deciding the appropriate route of airway management.

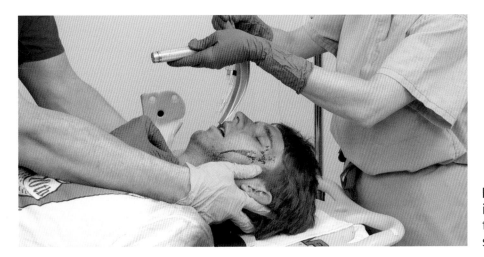

■ **Figure 2-11** Orotracheal intubation using two-person technique with inline cervical spine immobilization.

When the proper position of the tube is determined, it is secured in place. If the patient is moved, tube placement is reassessed by auscultation of both lateral lung fields for equality of breath sounds and by reassessment for exhaled CO_2.

If orotracheal intubation is unsuccessful on the first attempt or if the cords are difficult to visualize, a gum elastic bougie should be used.

Blind nasotracheal intubation requires spontaneous breathing. It is contraindicated in the patient with apnea. The deeper the patient breathes, the easier it is to follow the airflow through the larynx. Facial, frontal sinus, basilar skull, and cribriform plate fractures are relative contraindications to nasotracheal intubation. Evidence of nasal fracture, raccoon eyes (bilateral ecchymosis in the periorbital region), Battle sign (postauricular ecchymosis), and possible cerebrospinal fluid (CSF) leaks (rhinorrhea or otor-rhea) identify patients with these injuries. Precautions regarding cervical spine immobilization should be followed, as with orotracheal intubation.

A chest x-ray, CO_2 monitoring, oximetry, and physical exam are necessary to confirm correct position of the endotracheal tube. The tube may have been inserted into the esophagus or a mainstem bronchus, or dislodged during transport from the field or another hospital.

? How do I predict a potentially difficult airway?

It is important to assess the patient's airway prior to attempting intubation to predict the likely difficulty. Factors that may predict difficulties with airway maneuvers include cervical spine injury, severe arthritis of the cervical spine, significant maxillofacial or mandibular trauma, limited mouth opening, and anatomical variations such as receding chin, overbite, and a short, muscular neck. In such cases, skilled clinicians should assist in the event of difficulty. The mnemonic LEMON is helpful as a prompt when assessing the potential for difficulty (Box 2-1). Several components of LEMON are more useful in trauma. Look for evidence of a difficult airway (small mouth or jaw, large overbite, or facial trauma). Any obvious airway obstruction presents an immediate challenge. All blunt trauma patients will be in cervical spine immobilation, which increases the difficulty in establishing an airway. Clinical judgment and experience will determine whether to proceed immediately with drug-assisted intubation or to exercise caution.

The use of anesthetic, sedative, and neuromuscular blocking drugs for endotracheal intubation in trauma patients is potentially dangerous. In certain cases, the need for an airway justifies the risk of administering these drugs, but the doctor must understand their pharmacology, be skilled in the techniques of endotracheal intubation, and be able to obtain a surgical airway if necessary. In many cases in which an airway is acutely needed during the primary survey, the use of paralyzing or sedating drugs is not necessary.

The technique for rapid sequence intubation (RSI) is as follows:

1. Be prepared to perform a surgical airway in the event that airway control is lost.

2. Ensure that suction, as well as the ability to deliver positive pressure ventilation, is ready.

3. Preoxygenate the patient with 100% oxygen.

4. Apply pressure over the cricoid cartilage.

5. Administer an induction drug (eg, etomidate, 0.3 mg/kg, or 20 mg) or sedate, according to local practice.

6. Administer 1 to 2 mg/kg succinylcholine intravenously (usual dose, 100 mg).

7. After the patient relaxes, intubate the patient orotracheally.

8. Inflate the cuff and confirm tube placement (auscultate the patient's chest and determine presence of CO_2 in exhaled air).

9. Release cricoid pressure.

10. Ventilate the patient.

BOX 2-1
LEMON Assessment for Difficult Intubation

L = Look Externally: Look for characteristics that are known to cause difficult intubation or ventilation.

E = Evaluate the 3-3-2 Rule (see the figure on page 37): To allow for alignment of the pharyngeal, laryngeal, and oral axes, and therefore simple intubation, the following relationships should be observed:

- The distance between the patient's incisor teeth should be at least 3 finger breadths (3)
- The distance between the hyoid bone and the chin should be at least 3 finger breadths (3)
- The distance between the thyroid notch and floor of the mouth should be at least 2 finger breadths (2)

M = Mallampati (see below): The hypopharynx should be visualized adequately. This has been done traditionally by assessing the Mallampati classification. When possible, the patient is asked to sit upright, open the mouth fully, and protrude the tongue as far as possible. The examiner then looks into the mouth with a light to assess the degree of hypopharynx visible. In supine patients, the Mallampati score can be estimated by asking the patient to open the mouth fully and protrude the tongue; a laryngoscopy light is then shone into the hypopharynx from above.

O = Obstruction: Any condition that can cause obstruction of the airway will make laryngoscopy and ventilation difficult. Such conditions include epiglottitis, peritonsillar abscess, and trauma.

N = Neck Mobility: This is a vital requirement for successful intubation. It can be assessed easily by asking the patient to place his or her chin onto the chest and then extending the neck so that he or she is looking toward the ceiling. Patients in a hard collar neck immobilizer obviously have no neck movement and are therefore more difficult to intubate.

Modified with permission from: Reed, MJ, Dunn MJG, McKeown DW. Can an airway assessment score predict difficulty at intubation in the emergency department? *Emerg Med J* 2005;22:99-102.

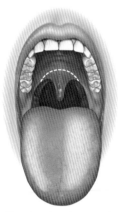 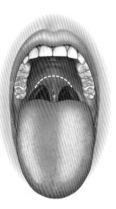 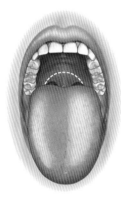

Class I: soft palate, uvula, fauces, pillars visible

Class II: soft palate, uvula, fauces visible

Class III: soft palate, base of uvula visible

Class IV: hard palate only visible

Mallampati Classifications. Used to visualize the hypopharynx. **Class I:** soft palate, uvula, fauces, pillars visible. **Class II:** soft palate, uvula, fauces visible. **Class III:** soft palate, base of uvula visible. **Class IV:** hard palate only visible.

(Continued)

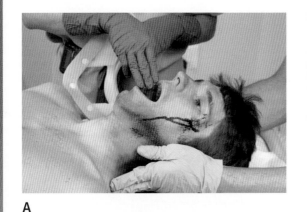

A

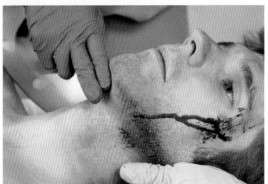

C

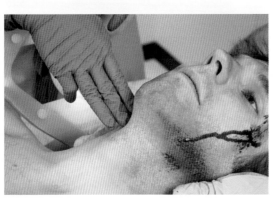

B

The 3-3-2 Rule. To allow for alignment of the pharyngeal, laryngeal, and oral axes and therefore simple intubation, the following relationships should be observed: The distance between the patient's incisor teeth should be at least 3 finger breadths **(A)**; the distance between the hyoid bone and the chin should be at least 3 finger breadths **(B)**; and the distance between the thyroid notch and floor of the mouth should be at least 2 finger breadths **(C)**.

Etomidate does not have a significant effect on blood pressure or intracranial pressure, but it can depress adrenal function and is not universally available. This drug does provide adequate sedation, which is advantageous in these patients. Etomidate and other sedatives must be used with great care to avoid loss of the airway as the patient becomes sedated. Then, succinylcholine, which is a short-acting drug, is administered. It has a rapid onset of paralysis (<1 minute) and a duration of 5 minutes or less. The most dangerous complication of using sedation and neuromuscular blocking agents is the inability to establish an airway. If endotracheal intubation is unsuccessful, the patient must be ventilated with a bag-mask device until the paralysis resolves; long-acting drugs are not routinely used for this reason. Because of

the potential for severe hyperkalemia, succinylcholine is not used in patients with severe crush injuries, major burns and electrical injuries, preexisting chronic renal failure, chronic paralysis, and chronic neuromuscular disease.

Induction agents, such as thiopental and sedatives, are potentially dangerous in trauma patients with hypovolemia. Small doses of diazepam or midazolam are appropriate to reduce anxiety in paralyzed patients. Flumazenil must be available to reverse the sedative effects after benzodiazepines have been administered. Practice patterns, drug preferences, and specific procedures for airway management vary among institutions. The principle that the individual using these techniques needs to be skilled in their use, knowledgeable of the inherent pitfalls associated with rapid sequence intu-

PITFALL

Equipment failure can occur at the most inopportune times and cannot always be anticipated. For example, the light on the laryngoscope burns out, the laryngoscope batteries are weak, the endotracheal tube cuff leaks, or the pulse oximeter does not function properly. Have spares available.

bation, and capable of managing the potential complications cannot be overstated.

Surgical Airway

The inability to intubate the trachea is a clear indication for creating a surgical airway. A surgical airway is established when edema of the glottis, fracture of the larynx, or severe oropharyngeal hemorrhage obstructs the airway or an endotracheal tube cannot be placed through the vocal cords. A surgical cricothyroidotomy is preferable to a tracheostomy for most patients who require establishment of an emergency surgical airway. A surgical cricothyroidotomy is easier to perform, is associated with less bleeding, and requires less time to perform than an emergency tracheostomy.

Needle Cricothyroidotomy.
Insertion of a needle through the cricothyroid membrane or into the trachea is a useful technique in emergency situations that provides oxygen on a short-term basis until a definitive airway can be placed. Needle cricothyroidotomy can provide temporary, supplemental oxygenation so that intubation can be accomplished on an urgent rather than an emergent basis.

The jet insufflation technique is performed by placing a large-caliber plastic cannula, 12- to 14-gauge for adults, and 16- to 18-gauge in children, through the cricothyroid membrane into the trachea below the level of the obstruction (Figure 2-12). The cannula is then connected to oxygen at 15 L/min (40 to 50 psi) with a Y-connector or a side hole cut in the tubing between the oxygen source and the plastic cannula. Intermittent insufflation, 1 second on and 4 seconds off, can then be achieved by placing the thumb over the open end of the Y-connector or the side hole.

The patient can be adequately oxygenated for only 30 to 45 minutes using this technique, and only patients with normal pulmonary function who do not have a significant chest injury may be oxygenated in this manner. During the 4 seconds that the oxygen is not being delivered under pressure, some exhalation occurs. Because of the inadequate exhalation, CO_2 slowly accumulates, limiting the use of this technique, especially in patients with head injuries.

See Skill Station III: Cricothyroidotomy, Skill III-A: Needle Cricothyroidotomy.

Jet insufflation must be used with caution when complete foreign-body obstruction of the glottic area is sus-

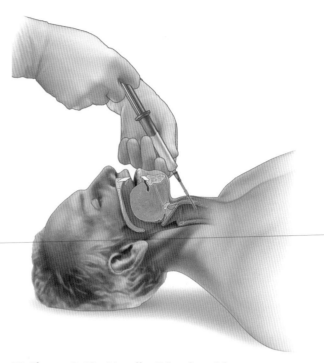

■ Figure 2-12 Needle Cricothyroidotomy. Performed by placing a large-caliber plastic cannula through the cricothyroid membrane into the trachea below the level of the obstruction.

pected. Although high pressure can expel the impacted material into the hypopharynx, where it can be removed readily, significant barotrauma can occur, including pulmonary rupture with tension pneumothorax. Low flow rates (5 to 7 L/min) should be used when persistent glottic obstruction is present.

Surgical Cricothyroidotomy.
Surgical cricothyroidotomy is performed by making a skin incision that extends through the cricothyroid membrane. A curved hemostat may be inserted to dilate the opening, and a small endotracheal tube or tracheostomy tube (preferably 5 to 7 mm OD) can be inserted. When an endotracheal tube is used, the cervical collar can be reapplied. It is possible for the endotracheal tube to become malpositioned and therefore easily advanced into a bronchus. Care must be taken, especially with children, to

PITFALL

The inability to intubate a patient expediently, to provide a temporary airway with a supraglottic device, or to establish a surgical airway results in hypoxia and patient deterioration. Remember that performing a needle cricothyroidotomy with jet insufflation can provide the time necessary to establish a definitive airway.

avoid damage to the cricoid cartilage, which is the only circumferential support for the upper trachea. Therefore, surgical cricothyroidotomy is not recommended for children under 12 years of age. ■ See Chapter 10: Pediatric Trauma.

In recent years, percutaneous tracheostomy has been reported as an alternative to open tracheostomy. This is not a safe procedure in the acute trauma situation, because the patient's neck must be hyperextended to properly position the head to perform the procedure safely. Percutaneous tracheostomy requires the use of a heavy guidewire and sharp dilator, or a guidewire and multiple or single large-bore dilators. This procedure can be dangerous and time-consuming, depending on the type of equipment used. ■ See Skill Station III: Cricothyroidotomy, Skill III-B: Surgical Cricothyroidotomy.

AIRWAY DECISION SCHEME

The airway decision scheme shown in Figure 2-10 applies only to patients who are in acute respiratory distress (or who have apnea), who are in need of an immediate airway, *and* in whom a cervical spine injury is suspected because of the mechanism of injury or suggested by the physical examination. The first priority is to ensure continued oxygenation with maintenance of cervical spine immobilization. This is accomplished initially by position (ie, chin-lift or jaw-thrust maneuver) and the preliminary airway techniques (ie, oropharyngeal airway or nasopharyngeal airway) previously described. An endotracheal tube is then passed while a second person provides in-line immobilization. If an endotracheal tube cannot be inserted and the patient's respiratory status is in jeopardy, ventilation via a laryngeal mask airway or other extraglottic airway device may be attempted as a bridge to a definitive airway. If this fails, a cricothyroidotomy should be performed.

Oxygenation and ventilation must be maintained before, during, and immediately upon completion of insertion of the definitive airway. Prolonged periods of inadequate or absent ventilation and oxygenation should be avoided.

Management of Oxygenation

? How do I know oxygenation is adequate?

Oxygenated inspired air is best provided via a tight-fitting oxygen reservoir face mask with a flow rate of at least 11 L/min. Other methods (eg, nasal catheter, nasal cannula, and nonrebreather mask) can improve inspired oxygen concentration.

Because changes in oxygenation occur rapidly and are impossible to detect clinically, pulse oximetry should be used when difficulties are anticipated in intubation or ventilation, including during transport of critically injured patients. Pulse oximetry is a noninvasive method to continuously

TABLE 2-2 ■ Approximate PaO_2 versus O_2 Hemoglobin Saturation Levels	
PaO_2 LEVELS	O_2 HEMOGLOBIN SATURATION LEVELS
90 mm Hg	100%
60 mm Hg	90%
30 mm Hg	60%
27 mm Hg	50%

measure the oxygen saturation (O_2 sat) of arterial blood. It does not measure the partial pressure of oxygen (PaO_2) and, depending on the position of the oxyhemoglobin dissociation curve, the PaO_2 can vary widely (see Table 2-2). However, a measured saturation of 95% or greater by pulse oximetry is strong corroborating evidence of adequate peripheral arterial oxygenation (PaO_2 >70 mm Hg, or 9.3 kPa).

Pulse oximetry requires intact peripheral perfusion and cannot distinguish oxyhemoglobin from carboxyhemoglobin or methemoglobin, which limits its usefulness in patients with severe vasoconstriction and those with carbon monoxide poisoning. Profound anemia (hemoglobin <5 g/dL) and hypothermia (<30° C, or <86° F) decrease the reliability of the technique. However, in most trauma patients pulse oximetry is useful, as the continuous monitoring of oxygen saturation provides an immediate assessment of therapeutic interventions.

Management of Ventilation

? How do I know ventilation is adequate?

Effective ventilation can be achieved by bag-mask techniques. However, one-person ventilation techniques using a bag-mask are less effective than two-person techniques in which both hands can be used to ensure a good seal. Bag-mask ventilation should be performed by two people whenever possible. ■ See Skill Station II: Airway and Ventilatory Management, Skill II-C: Bag-Mask Ventilation: Two-Person Technique.

PITFALL

Gastric distention can occur when ventilating the patient with a bag-mask device, which can result in the patient vomiting and aspirating. It also can cause distention of the stomach against the vena cava, resulting in hypotension and bradycardia.

Intubation of patients with hypoventilation and/or apnea patients may not be successful initially and may require multiple attempts. The patient must be ventilated periodically during prolonged efforts to intubate. The doctor should practice taking a deep breath and holding it when intubation is first attempted. When the doctor must breathe, the attempted intubation is aborted, and the patient ventilated.

With intubation of the trachea accomplished, assisted ventilation follows, using positive-pressure breathing techniques. A volume- or pressure-regulated respirator can be used, depending on availability of the equipment. The doctor should be alert to the complications of changes in intrathoracic pressure, which can convert a simple pneumothorax to a tension pneumothorax, or even create a pneumothorax secondary to barotrauma.

CHAPTER SUMMARY

1 Clinical situations in which airway compromise is likely to occur include maxillofacial trauma, neck trauma, laryngeal trauma, and airway obstruction.

2 Actual or impending airway obstruction should be suspected in all injured patients. Objective signs of airway obstruction include agitation, presentation with obtundation, cyanosis, abnormal sounds, and a displaced trachea.

3 Techniques for establishing and maintaining a patent airway include the chin-lift and jaw-thrust maneuvers, oropharyngeal and nasopharyngeal airways, laryngeal mask airway, multilumen esophageal airway, and the gum elastic bougie device. With all airway maneuvers, the cervical spine must be protected by in-line immobilization. The selection of orotracheal or nasotracheal routes for intubation is based on the experience and skill level of the doctor.

A surgical airway is indicated whenever an airway is needed and intubation is unsuccessful.

4 The assessment of airway patency and adequacy of ventilation must be performed quickly and accurately. Pulse oximetry and end-tidal CO_2 measurement are essential.

5 A definitive airway requires a tube placed in the trachea with the cuff inflated, the tube connected to some form of oxygen-enriched assisted ventilation, and the airway secured in place with tape. A definitive airway should be established if there is any doubt on the part of the doctor as to the integrity of the patient's airway. A definitive airway should be placed early after the patient has been ventilated with oxygen-enriched air, to prevent prolonged periods of apnea.

6 Oxygenated inspired air is best provided via a tight-fitting oxygen reservoir face mask with a flow rate of greater than 11 L/min. Other methods (eg, nasal catheter, nasal cannula, and nonrebreather mask) can improve inspired oxygen concentration.

Bibliography

1. Alexander R, Hodgson P, Lomax D, Bullen C. A comparison of the laryngeal mask airway and Guedel airway, bag and face-mask for manual ventilation following formal training. *Anaesthesia* 1993; 48(3):231-234.

2. Aprahamian C, Thompson BM, Finger WA, et al. Experimental cervical spine injury model: evaluation of airway management and splinting techniques. *Ann Emerg Med* 1984; 13(8):584-587.

3. Asai T, Shingu K. The laryngeal tube. *Br J Anaesth* 2005; 95(6):729-736.

4. Bergen JM, Smith DC. A review of etomidate for rapid sequence intubation in the emergency department. *J Emerg Med* 1997;15(2):221-230.

5. Brantigan CO, Grow JB Sr. Cricothyroidotomy: elective use in respiratory problems requiring tracheotomy. *J Thorac Cardiovasc Surg* 1976;71:72-81.

6. Combes X, Dumerat M, Dhonneur G. Emergency gum elastic bougie-assisted tracheal intubation in four patients with upper airway distortion. *Can J Anaesth* 2004; 51(10):1022-1024.

7. Crosby ET, Cooper RM, Douglas MJ, et al. The unanticipated difficult airway with recommendations for management. *Can J Anaesth* 1998; 45(8):757-776.

8. Danzl DF, Thomas DM. Nasotracheal intubation in the emergency department. *Crit Care Med* 1980;8(11):667-682.

9. Davies PR, Tighe SQ, Greenslade GL, Evans GH. Laryngeal mask airway and tracheal tube insertion by unskilled personnel. *Lancet* 1990; 336(8721):977-979.

10. Dogra S, Falconer R, Latto IP. Successful difficult intubation. Tracheal tube placement over a gum-elastic bougie. *Anaesthesia* 1990; 45(9):774-776.

11. Dorges V, Ocker H, Wenzel V, Sauer C, Schmucker P. Emergency airway management by non-anaesthesia house officers—a comparison of three strategies. *Emerg Med J* 2001; 18(2):90-94.

12. El-Orbany MI, Salem MR, Joseph NJ. The Eschmann tracheal tube introducer is not gum, elastic, or a bougie. *Anesthesiology* 2004;101(5);1240; author reply 1242-1240; author reply 1244.

13. Frame SB, Simon JM, Kerstein MD, et al. Percutaneous transtracheal catheter ventilation (PTCV) in complete airway obstructions canine model. *J Trauma* 1989;29(6):774-781.

14. Fremstad JD, Martin SH. Lethal complication from insertion of nasogastric tube after severe basilar skull fracture. *J Trauma* 1978;18:820-822.

15. Gataure PS, Vaughan RS, Latto IP. Simulated difficult intubation: comparison of the gum elastic bougie and the stylet. *Anaesthesia* 1996;1:935-938.

16. Greenberg RS, Brimacombe J, Berry A, Gouze V, Piantadosi S, Dake EM. A randomized controlled trial comparing the cuffed oropharyngeal airway and the laryngeal mask airway in spontaneously breathing anesthetized adults. *Anesthesiology* 1998; 88(4):970-977.

17. Grein AJ, Weiner GM. Laryngeal mask airway versus bag-mask ventilation or endotracheal intubation for neonatal resuscitation. *Cochrane Database Syst Rev* 2005;(2):CD003314.

18. Grmec S, Mally S. Prehospital determination of tracheal tube placement in severe head injury. *Emerg Med J* 2004; 21(4):518-520.

19. Guildner CV. Resuscitation—opening the airway: a comparative study of techniques for opening an airway obstructed by the tongue. *J Am Coll Emerg Physicians* 1976;5:588-590.

20. Hagberg C, Bogomolny Y, Gilmore C, Gibson V, Kaitner M, Khurana S. An evaluation of the insertion and function of a new supraglottic airway device, the King LT, during spontaneous ventilation. *Anesth Analg* 2006;102(2):621-625.

21. Iserson KV. Blind nasotracheal intubation. *Ann Emerg Med* 1981;10:468.

22. Jabre P, Combes X, Leroux B, Aaron E, Auger H, Margenet A, Dhonneur G. Use of the gum elastic bougie for prehospital difficult intubation. *Am J Emerg Med* 2005;23(4):552-555.

23. Jorden RC, Moore EE, Marx JA, et al. A comparison of PTV and endotracheal ventilation in an acute trauma model. *J Trauma* 1985;25(10):978-983.

24. Kidd JF, Dyson A, Latto IP. Successful difficult intubation. Use of the gum elastic bougie. *Anaesthesia* 1988;43:437-438.

25. Kress TD, et al. Cricothyroidotomy. *Ann Emerg Med* 1982;11:197.

26. Latto IP, Stacey M, Mecklenburgh J, Vaughan RS. Survey of the use of the gum elastic bougie in clinical practice. *Anaesthesia* 2002;57(4):379-384.

27. Levinson MM, Scuderi PE, Gibson RL, et al. Emergency percutaneous and transtracheal ventilation. *J Am Coll Emerg Physicians* 1979;8(10):396-400.

28. Levitan R, Ochroch EA. Airway management and direct laryngoscopy. A review and update. *Crit Care Clin* 2000;16(3):373-88, v.

29. Macintosh RR. An aid to oral intubation. *BMJ* 1949;1:28.

30. Majernick TG, Bieniek R, Houston JB, et al: Cervical spine movement during orotracheal intubation. *Ann Emerg Med* 1986;15(4):417-420.

31. Morton T, Brady S, Clancy M. Difficult airway equipment in English emergency departments. *Anaesthesia* 2000;55(5):485-488.

32. Nocera A. A flexible solution for emergency intubation difficulties. *Ann Emerg Med* 1996;27(5):665-667.

33. Noguchi T, Koga K, Shiga Y, Shigematsu A. The gum elastic bougie eases tracheal intubation while applying cricoid pressure compared to a stylet. *Can J Anaesth* 2003;50(7):712-717.

34. Nolan JP, Wilson ME. An evaluation of the gum elastic bougie. Intubation times and incidence of sore throat. *Anaesthesia* 1992;47(10):878-881.

35. Nolan JP, Wilson ME. Orotracheal intubation in patients with potential cervical spine injuries. An indication for the gum elastic bougie. *Anaesthesia* 1993;48(7):630-633.

36. Oczenski W, Krenn H, Dahaba AA, et al. Complications following the use of the Combitube, tracheal tube and laryngeal mask airway. *Anaesthesia* 1999;54(12):1161-1165.

37. Pennant JH, Pace NA, Gajraj NM. Role of the laryngeal mask airway in the immobile cervical spine. *J Clin Anesth* 1993;5(3):226-230.

38. Phelan MP. Use of the endotracheal bougie introducer for difficult intubations. *Am J Emerg Med* 2004;22(6):479-482.

39. Reed MJ, Dunn MJ, McKeown DW. Can an airway assessment score predict difficulty at intubation in the emergency department? *Emerg Med J* 2005;22(2):99-102.

40. Walls RM, Luten RC, Murphy MF and Schneider RE: The Manual of Emergency Airway Management, Philadelphia, Lippincott, Williams and Wilkins, 2000;34-36.

41. Russi C, Miller L. An Out-of-hospital Comparison of the King LT to Endotracheal Intubation and the Esophageal-Tracheal Combitube in a Simulated Difficult Airway Patient Encounter [In Process Citation]. *Acad Emerg Med* 2007;14(5 Suppl 1):S22.

42. Seshul MB Sr, Sinn DP, Gerlock AJ Jr. The Andy Gump fracture of the mandible: a cause of respiratory obstruction or distress. *J Trauma* 1978;18:611-612.

43. Silvestri S, Ralls GA, Krauss B, et al. The effectiveness of out-of-hospital use of continuous end-tidal carbon dioxide monitoring on the rate of unrecognized misplaced intubation within a regional emergency medical services system. *Ann Emerg Med* 2005;45(5):497-503.

44. Smith CE, Dejoy SJ. New equipment and techniques for airway management in trauma [In Process Citation]. *Curr Opin Anaesthesiol* 2001;14(2):197-209.

45. Walter J, Doris PE, Shaffer MA. Clinical presentation of patients with acute cervical spine injury. *Ann Emerg Med* 1984;13(7):512-515.

46. Yeston NS. Noninvasive measurement of blood gases. *Infect Surg* 1990;90:18-24.

▶▶ Interactive Skill Procedures

Note: Accompanying some of the skills procedures for this station is a series of scenarios, which are provided at the conclusion of the procedures for you to review and prepare for this station. **Standard precautions are required whenever caring for the trauma patient.**

THE FOLLOWING PROCEDURES ARE INCLUDED IN THIS SKILL STATION:

▶▶ **Skill II-A:** Oropharyngeal Airway Insertion

▶▶ **Skill II-B:** Nasopharyngeal Airway Insertion

▶▶ **Skill II-C:** Bag-Mask Ventilation: Two-Person Technique

▶▶ **Skill II-D:** Adult Orotracheal Intubation (with and without Gum Elastic Bougie Device)

▶▶ **Skill II-E:** Laryngeal Mask Airway (LMA) Insertion

▶▶ **Skill II-F:** Laryngeal Tube Airway (LTA) Insertion

▶▶ **Skill II-G:** Infant Endotracheal Intubation

▶▶ **Skill II-H:** Pulse Oximetry Monitoring

▶▶ **Skill II-I:** Carbon Dioxide Detection

Performance at this skill station will allow the participant to evaluate a series of clinical situations and acquire the cognitive skills for decision making in airway and ventilatory management. The student will practice and demonstrate the following skills on adult and infant intubation manikins:

OBJECTIVES

1 Insert oropharyngeal and nasopharyngeal airways.

2 Using both oral and nasal routes, intubate the trachea of an adult intubation manikin (within the guidelines listed), provide effective ventilation, and use capnography to determine proper placement of the endotracheal tube. Discuss and demonstrate methods to manage difficult or failed airways, including LMA/LTA and GEB.

3 Intubate the trachea of an infant intubation manikin with an endotracheal tube (within the guidelines listed) and provide effective ventilation.

4 Describe how trauma affects airway management when performing oral endotracheal intubation and nasotracheal intubation.

5 Using a pulse oximeter:

State the purpose of pulse oximetry monitoring.
Demonstrate the proper use of the device.
Describe the indications for its use, its functional limits of accuracy, and possible reasons for malfunction or inaccuracy.
Interpret accurately the pulse oximeter monitor readings and relate their significance to the care of trauma patients.

6 Discuss the indications for and use of end-tidal CO_2 detector devices.

▶ Skill II-A: Oropharyngeal Airway Insertion

Note: This procedure is for temporary ventilation while preparing to intubate an unconscious patient.

STEP 1. Select the proper-size airway. A correctly sized airway extends from the corner of the patient's mouth to the external auditory canal.

STEP 2. Open the patient's mouth with either the chin-lift maneuver or the crossed-finger technique (scissors technique).

STEP 3. Insert a tongue blade on top of the patient's tongue far enough back to depress the tongue

adequately. Be careful not cause the patient to gag.

STEP 4. Insert the airway posteriorly, gently sliding the airway over the curvature of the tongue until the device's flange rests on top of the patient's lips. The airway must not push the tongue backward and block the airway.

STEP 5. Remove the tongue blade.

STEP 6. Ventilate the patient with a bag-mask device.

▶ Skill II-B: Nasopharyngeal Airway Insertion

Note: This procedure is used when the patient would gag on an oropharyngeal airway.

STEP 1. Assess the nasal passages for any apparent obstruction (eg, polyps, fractures, or hemorrhage).

STEP 2. Select the proper-size airway, which will easily pass the selected nostril.

STEP 3. Lubricate the nasopharyngeal airway with a water-soluble lubricant or tap water.

STEP 4. Insert the tip of the airway into the nostril and direct it posteriorly and toward the ear.

STEP 5. Gently insert the nasopharyngeal airway through the nostril into the hypopharynx with a slight rotating motion until the flange rests against the nostril.

STEP 6. Apply ventilation with a bag-mask device.

▶ Skill II-C: Bag-Mask Ventilation: Two-Person Technique

STEP 1. Select the proper-size mask to fit the patient's face.

STEP 2. Connect the oxygen tubing to the bag-mask device and adjust the flow of oxygen to 12 L/min.

STEP 3. Ensure that the patient's airway is patent and secured according to previously described techniques.

STEP 4. The first person applies the mask to the patient's face, ascertaining a tight seal with both hands.

STEP 5. The second person applies ventilation by squeezing the bag with both hands.

STEP 6. Assess the adequacy of ventilation by observing the patient's chest movement.

STEP 7. Apply ventilation in this manner every 5 seconds.

▶ Skill II-D: Adult Orotracheal Intubation
(with and without Gum Elastic Bougie Device)

STEP 1. Ensure that adequate ventilation and oxygenation are in progress and that suctioning equipment is immediately available in the event that the patient vomits.

STEP 2. Inflate the cuff of the endotracheal tube to ascertain that the balloon does not leak, and then deflate the cuff.

STEP 3. Connect the laryngoscope blade to the handle, and check the bulb for brightness.

STEP 4. Assess the patient's airway for ease of intubation (LEMON mnemonic).

STEP 5. Direct an assistant to manually immobilize the head and neck. The patient's neck must not be hyperextended or hyperflexed during the procedure.

STEP 6. Hold the laryngoscope in the left hand.

STEP 7. Insert the laryngoscope into the right side of the patient's mouth, displacing the tongue to the left.

STEP 8. Visually identify the epiglottis and then the vocal cords.

STEP 9. Gently insert the endotracheal tube into the trachea without applying pressure on the teeth or oral tissues.

STEP 10. Inflate the cuff with enough air to provide an adequate seal. **Do not overinflate the cuff.**

STEP 11. Check the placement of the endotracheal tube by bag-mask-to-tube ventilation.

STEP 12. Visually observe chest excursions with ventilation.

STEP 13. Auscultate the chest and abdomen with a stethoscope to ascertain tube position.

STEP 14. Secure the tube. If the patient is moved, the tube placement should be reassessed.

STEP 15. If endotracheal intubation is not accomplished within seconds or in the same time required to hold your breath before exhaling, discontinue attempts, apply ventilation with a bag-mask device, and try again using the gum elastic bougie.

STEP 16. Placement of the tube must be checked carefully. A chest x-ray exam is helpful to assess the position of the tube, but it cannot exclude esophageal intubation.

STEP 17. Attach a CO_2 detector to the endotracheal tube between the adapter and the ventilating device to confirm the position of the endotracheal tube in the airway.

STEP 18. Attach a pulse oximeter to one of the patient's fingers (intact peripheral perfusion must exist) to measure and monitor the patient's oxygen saturation levels and provide an immediate assessment of therapeutic interventions.

▶ Skill II-E: Laryngeal Mask Airway (LMA) Insertion

STEP 1. Ensure that adequate ventilation and oxygenation are in progress and that suctioning equipment is immediately available in the event that the patient vomits.

STEP 2. Inflate the cuff of the LMA to ascertain that the balloon does not leak.

STEP 3. Direct an assistant to manually immobilize the head and neck. The patient's neck must not be hyperextended or hyperflexed during the procedure.

STEP 4. Before attempting insertion, completely deflate the LMA cuff by pressing it firmly onto a flat surface and lubricate it.

STEP 5. Choose the correct size LMA: 3 for a small woman, 4 for a large woman or small man, and 5 for a large man.

STEP 6. Hold the LMA with the dominant hand as you would a pen, with the index finger placed at the junction of the cuff and the shaft and the LMA opening oriented over the tongue.

STEP 7. Pass the LMA behind the upper incisors, with the shaft parallel to the patient's chest and the index finger pointing toward the intubator.

STEP 8. Push the lubricated LMA into position along the palatopharyngeal curve, with the index finger maintaining pressure on the tube and guiding the LMA into the final position.

STEP 9. Inflate the cuff with the correct volume of air (indicated on the shaft of the LMA).

STEP 10. Check the placement of the endotracheal tube by bag-mask-to-tube ventilation.

STEP 11. Visually observe chest excursions with ventilation.

▶ Skill II-F: Laryngeal Tube Airway (LTA) Insertion

STEP 1. Ensure proper sterilization.

STEP 2. Inspect all components for visible damage.

STEP 3. Examine the interior of the airway tube to ensure that it is free from blockage and loose particles.

STEP 4. Inflate the cuffs by injecting the maximum recommended volume of air into the cuffs.

STEP 5. Select the correct laryngeal tube size.

STEP 6. Apply a water-based lubricant to the beveled distal tip and posterior aspect of the tube, taking care to avoid introduction of lubricant into or near the ventilatory openings.

STEP 7. Preoxygenate the patient.

STEP 8. Achieve the appropriate depth of anesthesia.

STEP 9. Position the head. The ideal head position for LTA insertion is the "sniffing position." However, the angle and shortness of the tube also allow it to be inserted with the head in a neutral position.

STEP 10. Hold the LTA at the connector with the dominant hand. With the nondominant hand, hold the mouth open and apply the chin-lift maneuver.

STEP 11. With the LTA rotated laterally 45 to 90 degrees, introduce the tip into the mouth and advance it behind the base of the tongue.

STEP 12. Rotate the tube back to the midline as the tip reaches the posterior wall of the pharynx.

STEP 13. Without exerting excessive force, advance the LTA until the base of the connector is aligned with teeth or gums.

STEP 14. Inflate the LTA cuffs to the minimum volume necessary to seal the airway at the peak ventilatory pressure used (just seal volume).

STEP 15. While gently bagging the patient to assess ventilation, simultaneously withdraw the airway until ventilation is easy and free flowing (large tidal volume with minimal airway pressure).

STEP 16. Reference marks are provided at the proximal end of the LTA; when aligned with the upper teeth, these marks indicate the depth of insertion.

STEP 17. Confirm proper position by auscultation, chest movement, and verification of CO_2 by capnography.

STEP 18. Readjust cuff inflation to seal volume.

STEP 19. Secure LTA to patient using tape or other accepted means. A bite block can also be used, if desired.

▶ Skill II-G: Infant Endotracheal Intubation

STEP 1. Ensure that adequate ventilation and oxygenation are in progress.

STEP 2. Select the proper-size uncuffed tube, which should be the same size as the infant's nostril or little finger.

STEP 3. Connect the laryngoscope blade and handle; check the light bulb for brilliance.

STEP 4. Hold the laryngoscope in the left hand.

STEP 5. Insert the laryngoscope blade into the right side of the mouth, moving the tongue to the left.

STEP 6. Observe the epiglottis and then the vocal cords.

STEP 7. Insert the endotracheal tube not more than 2 cm past the cords.

STEP 8. Check the placement of the tube by bag-mask-to-tube ventilation.

STEP 9. Check the placement of the endotracheal tube by observing lung inflations and auscultating the chest and abdomen with a stethoscope.

STEP 10. Secure the tube. If the patient is moved, tube placement should be reassessed.

STEP 11. If endotracheal intubation is not accomplished within 30 seconds or in the same time required to hold your breath before exhaling, discontinue attempts, ventilate the patient with a bag-mask device, and try again.

STEP 12. Placement of the tube must be checked carefully. Chest x-ray examination may be helpful to assess the position of the tube, but it cannot exclude esophageal intubation.

STEP 13. Attach a CO_2 detector to the endotracheal tube between the adapter and the ventilating device to confirm the position of the endotracheal tube in the trachea.

STEP 14. Attach a pulse oximeter to one of the patient's fingers (intact peripheral perfusion must exist) to measure and monitor the patient's oxygen saturation levels and provide an immediate assessment of therapeutic interventions.

▶ Skill II-H: Pulse Oximetry Monitoring

The pulse oximeter is designed to measure oxygen saturation and pulse rate in peripheral circulation. This device is a microprocessor that calculates the percentage saturation of oxygen in each pulse of arterial blood that flows past a sensor. It simultaneously calculates the heart rate.

The pulse oximeter works by a low-intensity light beamed from a light-emitting diode (LED) to a light-receiving photodiode. Two thin beams of light, one red and the other infrared, are transmitted through blood and body tissue, and a portion is absorbed by the blood and body tissue. The photodiode measures the portion of the light that passes through the blood and body tissue. The relative amount of light absorbed by oxygenated hemoglobin differs from that absorbed by nonoxygenated hemoglobin. The microprocessor evaluates these differences in the arterial pulse and reports the values as calculated oxyhemoglobin saturation ($\%SaO_2$). Measurements are reliable and correlate well when compared with a cooximeter that directly measures SaO_2.

However, pulse oximetry is unreliable when the patient has poor peripheral perfusion, which can be caused by vasoconstriction, hypotension, a blood pressure cuff that is inflated above the sensor, hypothermia, and other causes of poor blood flow. Severe anemia can likewise influence the reading. Significantly high levels of carboxyhemoglobin or methemoglobin can cause abnormalities, and circulating dye (eg, indocyanine green and methylene blue) can interfere with the measurement. Excessive patient movement, other electrical devices, and intense ambient light can cause pulse oximeters to malfunction.

Using a pulse oximeter requires knowledge of the particular device being used. Different sensors are appropriate for different patients. The fingertip and earlobe are common sites for sensor application; however, both of these areas can be subject to vasoconstriction. The fingertip (or toe tip) of an injured extremity or below a blood pressure cuff should not be used.

When analyzing pulse oximetry results, evaluate the initial readings. Does the pulse rate correspond to the electrocardiographic monitor? Is the oxygen saturation appropriate? If the pulse oximeter is giving low readings or very poor readings, look for a physiologic cause, not a mechanical one.

The relationship between partial pressure of oxygen in arterial blood (PaO_2) and $\%SaO_2$ is shown in Figure II-1 (on page 48). The sigmoid shape of this curve indicates that the relationship between $\%SaO_2$ and PaO_2 is nonlinear. This is particularly important in the middle range of this curve, where small changes in PaO_2 will effect large changes in saturation. Remember, the pulse oximeter measures arterial oxygen saturation, *not* arterial oxygen partial pressure.

See Table 2-2: Approximate PaO_2 versus O_2 Hemoglobin Saturation Levels in Chapter 2: Airway and Ventilatory Management.

Standard blood gas measurements report both PaO_2 and $\%SaO_2$. When oxygen saturation is calculated from blood gas PaO_2, the calculated value can differ from the oxygen saturation measured by the pulse oximeter. This difference can occur because an oxygen saturation value that has been calculated from the blood gas PaO_2 has not necessarily been correctly adjusted for the effects of variables that shift the relationship between PaO_2 and saturation. These variables include temperature, pH, $PaCO_2$ (partial pressure of carbon dioxide), 2,3-DPG (diphosphoglycerates), and the concentration of fetal hemoglobin.

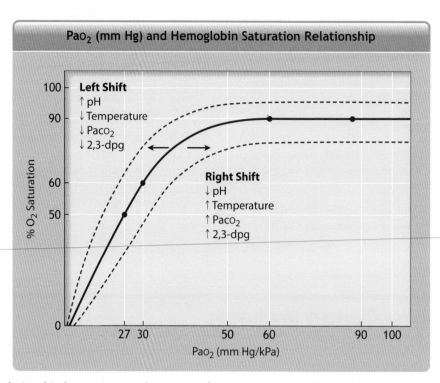

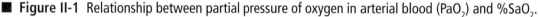

■ **Figure II-1** Relationship between partial pressure of oxygen in arterial blood (PaO_2) and $\%SaO_2$.

▶ Skill II-I: Carbon Dioxide Detection

When a patient is intubated, it is essential to check the position of the endotracheal tube. If carbon dioxide is detected in the exhaled air, the tube is in the airway. Methods of determining end-tidal CO_2 should be readily available in all EDs and any other locations where patients require intubation. The preferred method is quantitative, such as capnography, capnometry, or mass spectroscopy. Colorimetric devices use a chemically treated indicator strip that generally reflects the CO_2 level. At very low levels of CO_2, such as atmospheric air, the indicator turns purple. At higher CO_2 levels (eg, 2%–5%), the indicator turns yellow. A tan color indicates detection of CO_2 levels that are generally lower than those found in the exhaled tracheal gases.

It is important to note that, on rare occasion, patients with gastric distention can have elevated CO_2 levels in the esophagus. These elevated levels clear rapidly after several breaths, and the results of the colorimetric test should not be used until after at least six breaths. If the colorimetric device still shows an intermediate range, six additional breaths should be taken or given. If the patient sustains a cardiac arrest and has no cardiac output, CO_2 is not delivered to the lungs. In fact, with cardiac asystole, this can be a method of determining whether cardiopulmonary resuscitation is adequate.

The colorimetric device is not used for the detection of elevated CO_2 levels. Similarly, it is not used to detect a mainstem bronchial intubation. Physical and chest x-ray examinations are required to determine that the endotracheal tube is properly positioned in the airway. In a noisy ED or when the patient is transported several times, this device is extremely reliable in differentiating between tracheal and esophageal intubation.

▶ SCENARIOS

SCENARIO II-1

A 22-year-old male is an unrestrained passenger in a motor vehicle that collides head-on into a retaining wall. He has a strong odor of alcohol on his breath. At the time of the collision, he hits the windshield and sustains a scalp laceration. At the injury scene, he is combative, and his GCS score is 11. His blood pressure is 120/70 mm Hg, his heart rate is 100 beats/min, and his respirations are 20 breaths/min. A semi-rigid cervical collar is applied, and he is immobilized on a long backboard. He is receiving oxygen via a high-flow oxygen mask. Shortly after his arrival in the ED, he begins to vomit.

SCENARIO II-2

The patient described in the first Scenario II-1 is now unresponsive and has undergone endotracheal intubation. Ventilation with 100% oxygen is being applied. Part of his evaluation includes a CT scan of his brain. After he is transported to radiology for the scan, the pulse oximeter reveals 82% SaO_2.

SCENARIO II-3

A 3-year-old, unrestrained, front-seat passenger is injured when the car in which she is riding crashes into a stone wall. The child is unconscious at the injury scene. In the ED, bruises to her forehead, face, and chest wall are noted, and there is blood around her mouth. The blood pressure is 105/70 mm Hg, the heart rate is 120 beats/minute, and the respirations are rapid and shallow. The child's GCS score is 8.

SCENARIO II-4

A 35-year-old male sustains blunt chest trauma during a single-motor-vehicle collision. In the ED, he is alert and has evidence of a right-chest-wall contusion. He has point tenderness and fracture crepitation of several right ribs. His GCS score is 14. He is immobilized with a semi-rigid cervical spine collar and secured to a long backboard. High-flow oxygen is being administered via a face mask.

▶▶ Interactive Skill Procedures

Note: Standard precautions are required whenever caring for trauma patients.

THE FOLLOWING PROCEDURES ARE INCLUDED IN THIS SKILL STATION:

▶▶ **Skill III-A:** Needle Cricothyroidotomy

▶▶ **Skill III-B:** Surgical Cricothyroidotomy

Performance at this skill station will allow the student to practice and demonstrate the techniques of needle cricothyroidotomy and surgical cricothyroidotomy on a live, anesthetized animal, a fresh human cadaver, or an anatomic human body manikin. Specifically, the student will be able to:

OBJECTIVES

1 Identify the surface markings and structures to be noted when performing needle and surgical cricothyroidotomies.

2 State the indications and complications of needle and surgical cricothyroidotomies.

3 Perform needle and surgical cricothyroidotomies on a live, anesthetized animal, a fresh human cadaver, or an anatomic human body manikin, as outlined in this skill station.

▶ Skill III-A: Needle Cricothyroidotomy

STEP 1. Assemble and prepare oxygen tubing by cutting a hole toward one end of the tubing. Connect the other end of the oxygen tubing to an oxygen source capable of delivering 50 psi or greater at the nipple, and ensure the free flow of oxygen through the tubing.

STEP 2. Place the patient in a supine position.

STEP 3. Assemble a 12- or 14-gauge, 8.5-cm, over-the-needle catheter to a 6- to 12-mL syringe.

STEP 4. Surgically prepare the neck, using antiseptic swabs.

STEP 5. Palpate the cricothyroid membrane anteriorly between the thyroid cartilage and the cricoid cartilage. Stabilize the trachea with the thumb and forefinger of one hand to prevent lateral movement of the trachea during the procedure.

STEP 6. Puncture the skin in the midline with a 12- or 14-gauge needle attached to a syringe, directly over the cricothyroid membrane (ie, midsagittally). A small incision with a number 11 blade facilitates passage of the needle through the skin.

STEP 7. Direct the needle at a 45-degree angle caudally, while applying negative pressure to the syringe.

STEP 8. Carefully insert the needle through the lower half of the cricothyroid membrane, aspirating as the needle is advanced.

STEP 9. Note the aspiration of air, which signifies entry into the tracheal lumen.

STEP 10. Remove the syringe and withdraw the stylet, while gently advancing the catheter downward into position, taking care not to perforate the posterior wall of the trachea.

STEP 11. Attach the oxygen tubing over the catheter needle hub, and secure the catheter to the patient's neck.

STEP 12. Intermittent ventilation can be achieved by occluding the open hole cut into the oxygen tubing with your thumb for 1 second and releasing it for 4 seconds. After releasing your thumb from the hole in the tubing, passive exhalation occurs. *Note:* Adequate PaO_2 can be maintained for only 30 to 45 minutes, and CO_2 accumulation can occur more rapidly.

STEP 13. Continue to observe lung inflations and auscultate the chest for adequate ventilation.

▶▶ COMPLICATIONS OF NEEDLE CRICOTHYROIDOTOMY

- Inadequate ventilations, leading to hypoxia and death
- Aspiration (blood)
- Esophageal laceration
- Hematoma
- Perforation of the posterior tracheal wall
- Subcutaneous and/or mediastinal emphysema
- Thyroid perforation

▶ Skill III-B: Surgical Cricothyroidotomy
(See Figure III-1)

STEP 1. Place the patient in a supine position with the neck in a neutral position.

STEP 2. Palpate the thyroid notch, cricothyroid interval, and the sternal notch for orientation.

STEP 3. Assemble the necessary equipment.

STEP 4. Surgically prepare and anesthetize the area locally, if the patient is conscious.

STEP 5. Stabilize the thyroid cartilage with the left hand and maintain stabilization until the trachea is intubated.

STEP 6. Make a transverse skin incision over the cricothyroid membrane, and carefully incise through the membrane transversely.

STEP 7. Insert hemostat or tracheal spreader into the incision and rotate it 90 degrees to open the airway.

STEP 8. Insert a proper-size, cuffed endotracheal tube or tracheostomy tube (usually a number 5 or 6) into the cricothyroid membrane incision, directing the tube distally into the trachea.

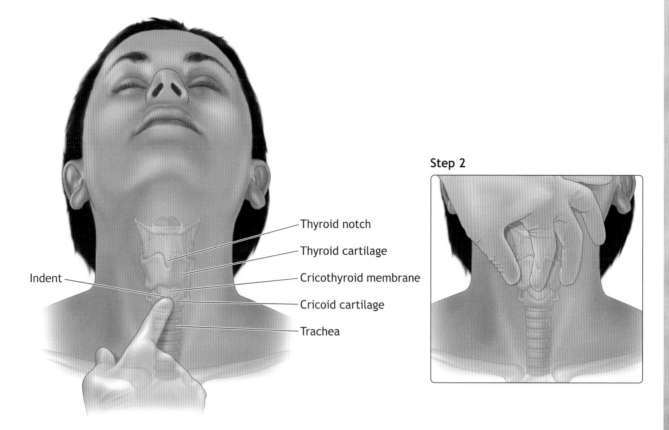

Indent

Thyroid notch
Thyroid cartilage
Cricothyroid membrane
Cricoid cartilage
Trachea

Step 2

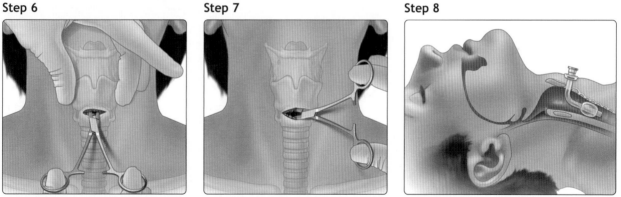

Step 6

Step 7

Step 8

■ **Figure III-1 Surgical Cricothyroidotomy.** (Illustrations correlate with selected steps in Skill III-B.)

STEP 9. Inflate the cuff and apply ventilation.

STEP 10. Observe lung inflations and auscultate the chest for adequate ventilation.

STEP 11. Secure the endotracheal or tracheostomy tube to the patient to prevent dislodging.

STEP 12. *Caution:* Do not cut or remove the cricoid and/or thyroid cartilages.

▶▶ **COMPLICATIONS OF SURGICAL CRICOTHYROIDOTOMY**

- Aspiration (eg, blood)
- Creation of a false passage into the tissues
- Subglottic stenosis/edema
- Laryngeal stenosis
- Hemorrhage or hematoma formation
- Laceration of the esophagus
- Laceration of the trachea
- Mediastinal emphysema
- Vocal cord paralysis, hoarseness

CHAPTER 3 Shock

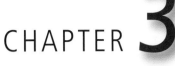

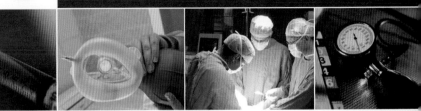

Upon completion of this topic, the student will identify and apply principles of management related to the initial diagnosis and treatment of shock in injured patients. Specifically, the doctor will be able to:

OBJECTIVES

1 Define shock and apply this definition to clinical practice.

2 Recognize the clinical shock syndrome and correlate a patient's acute clinical signs with the degree of volume deficit.

3 Explain the importance of early identification and control of the source of hemorrhage in trauma patients.

4 Compare and contrast the clinical presentation of patients with various causes of the shock state.

5 Describe the management and ongoing evaluation of hemorrhagic shock.

6 Recognize the physiologic responses to resuscitation in order to continually reassess patient response and avoid complications.

Introduction

The initial step in managing shock in injured patients is to recognize its presence. No laboratory test diagnoses shock; rather, the initial diagnosis is based on clinical appreciation of the presence of inadequate tissue perfusion and oxygenation. The definition of shock as an abnormality of the circulatory system that results in inadequate organ perfusion and tissue oxygenation also becomes an operative tool for diagnosis and treatment.

The second step in the initial management of shock is to identify the probable cause of the shock state. In trauma patients, this process is directly related to the mechanism of injury. Most injured patients in shock have hypovolemia, but they may suffer from cardiogenic, neurogenic, and even septic shock on occasion. In addition, tension pneumothorax can reduce venous return and produce shock; this diagnosis should be considered in patients who may have injuries above the diaphragm. Neurogenic shock results from extensive injury to the central nervous system (CNS) or spinal cord. For all practical purposes, shock does not result from isolated brain injuries. Patients with spinal cord injury may initially present in shock resulting from both vasodilation and relative hypovolemia. Septic shock is unusual, but must be considered in patients whose arrival at the emergency facility has been delayed by many hours.

The doctor's management responsibilities begin with recognizing the presence of the shock state, and treatment should be initiated simultaneously with the identification of a probable cause. The response to initial treatment, coupled with the findings during the primary and secondary patient surveys, usually provides sufficient information to determine the cause of the shock state. **Hemorrhage is the most common cause of shock in the injured patient.**

Shock Pathophysiology

❓ *What is shock?*

An overview of basic cardiac physiology and blood loss pathophysiology is essential to understanding the shock state.

BASIC CARDIAC PHYSIOLOGY

Cardiac output, which is defined as the volume of blood pumped by the heart per minute, is determined by multiplying the heart rate by the stroke volume. Stroke volume, the amount of blood pumped with each cardiac contraction, is classically determined by the following:

- Preload
- Myocardial contractility
- Afterload

Preload, the volume of venous return to the heart, is determined by venous capacitance, volume status, and the difference between mean venous systemic pressure and right atrial pressure (Figure 3-1). This pressure differential determines venous flow. The venous system can be considered a reservoir or capacitance system in which the volume of blood is divided into two components. One component does not contribute to the mean systemic venous pressure and represents the volume of blood that would remain in this capacitance circuit if the pressure in the system were zero.

The second, more important, component represents the venous volume that contributes to the mean systemic venous pressure. Nearly 70% of the body's total blood volume is estimated to be located in the venous circuit. The relationship between venous volume and venous pressure describes the compliance of the system. It is this pressure gradient that drives venous flow and therefore the volume of venous return to the heart. Blood loss depletes this component of venous volume and reduces the pressure gradient; as a consequence, venous return is reduced.

The volume of venous blood returned to the heart determines myocardial muscle fiber length after ventricular filling at the end of diastole. Muscle fiber length is related to the contractile properties of myocardial muscle according to Starling's law. *Myocardial contractility* is the pump that drives the system. *Afterload* is systemic (peripheral) vascular resistance or, simply stated, the resistance to the forward flow of blood.

BLOOD LOSS PATHOPHYSIOLOGY

Early circulatory responses to blood loss are compensatory—progressive vasoconstriction of cutaneous, muscle, and visceral circulation preserves blood flow to the kidneys, heart, and brain. The response to acute circulating volume depletion associated with injury is an increase in heart rate in an attempt to preserve cardiac output. In most cases, tachycardia is the earliest measurable circulatory sign of shock. The release of endogenous catecholamines increases peripheral vascular resistance, which in turn increases diastolic blood pressure and reduces pulse pressure, but does little to increase organ perfusion. Other hormones with vasoactive properties are released into the circulation during shock, including histamine, bradykinin, ß-endorphins, and a cascade of prostanoids and other cytokines. These substances have profound effects on the microcirculation and vascular permeability.

Venous return in early hemorrhagic shock is preserved to some degree by the compensatory mechanism of contraction of the volume of blood in the venous system, which

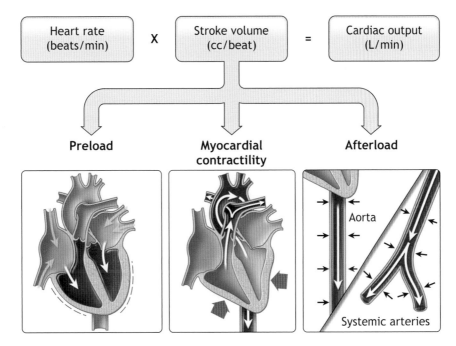

■ **Figure 3-1 Cardiac Output.**

does not contribute to mean systemic venous pressure. However, this compensatory mechanism is limited. The most effective method of restoring adequate cardiac output and end-organ perfusion is to restore venous return to normal by volume repletion.

At the cellular level, inadequately perfused and oxygenated cells are deprived of essential substrates for normal aerobic metabolism and energy production. Initially, compensation occurs by shifting to anaerobic metabolism, which results in the formation of lactic acid and the development of metabolic acidosis. If shock is prolonged and substrate delivery for the generation of adenosine triphosphate (ATP) is inadequate, the cellular membrane loses the ability to maintain its integrity, and the normal electrical gradient is lost.

Swelling of the endoplasmic reticulum is the first ultrastructural evidence of cellular hypoxia. Mitochondrial damage soon follows. Lysosomes rupture and release enzymes that digest other intracellular structural elements. Sodium and water enter the cell, and cellular swelling occurs. Intracellular calcium deposition also occurs. If the process is not reversed, progressive cellular damage, additional tissue swelling, and cellular death occur. This process compounds the impact of blood loss and hypoperfusion.

The administration of a sufficient quantity of isotonic electrolyte solutions helps combat this process. Patient treatment is directed toward reversing the shock state by providing adequate oxygenation, ventilation, and appropriate fluid resuscitation. Resuscitation may be accompanied by a marked increase in interstitial edema, which is caused by "reperfusion injury" to the capillary interstitial membrane. As a result, larger volumes of fluid may be required for resuscitation than initially anticipated.

The initial treatment of shock is directed toward restoring cellular and organ perfusion with adequately oxygenated blood. Control of hemorrhage and restoration of adequate circulating volume are the goals of treatment of hemorrhagic shock. With the possible exception of penetrating trauma to the torso without head injury, euvolemia should be maintained. Vasopressors are contraindicated for the treatment of hemorrhagic shock because they worsen tissue perfusion. Frequent monitoring of the patient's indices of perfusion is necessary to evaluate the response to therapy and detect deterioration in the patient's condition as early as possible.

Most injured patients who are in hypovolemic shock require early surgical intervention to reverse the shock state. **The presence of shock in an injured patient warrants the immediate involvement of a surgeon.**

Initial Patient Assessment

Optimally, doctors will recognize the shock state during the initial patient assessment. To do so, it is important to be familiar with the clinical differentiation of the causes of shock—chiefly, hemorrhagic and nonhemorrhagic.

RECOGNITION OF SHOCK

❓ *Is the patient in shock?*

Profound circulatory shock—evidenced by hemodynamic collapse with inadequate perfusion of the skin, kidneys, and central nervous system—is simple to recognize. However, after the airway and adequate ventilation have been ensured, careful evaluation of the patient's circulatory status is necessary to identify early manifestations of shock, including tachycardia and cutaneous vasoconstriction.

Reliance solely on systolic blood pressure as an indicator of shock may result in delayed recognition of the shock state. Compensatory mechanisms may preclude a measurable fall in systolic pressure until up to 30% of the patient's blood volume is lost. Specific attention should be directed to pulse rate, respiratory rate, skin circulation, and pulse pressure (the difference between systolic and diastolic pressure). Tachycardia and cutaneous vasoconstriction are the typical early physiologic responses to volume loss in most adults. **Any injured patient who is cool and has tachycardia is considered to be in shock until proven otherwise.** Occasionally, a normal heart rate or even bradycardia is associated with an acute reduction of blood volume. Other indices of perfusion must be monitored in these situations.

The normal heart rate varies with age. Tachycardia is present when the heart rate is greater than 160 in an infant, 140 in a preschool-age child, 120 in children from school age to puberty, and 100 in an adult. Elderly patients may not exhibit tachycardia because of their limited cardiac response to catecholamine stimulation or the concurrent use of medications, such as ß-adrenergic blocking agents. The ability of the body to increase the heart rate also may be limited by the presence of a pacemaker. A narrowed pulse pressure suggests significant blood loss and involvement of compensatory mechanisms.

Laboratory values for hematocrit or hemoglobin concentration are unreliable for estimating acute blood loss and inappropriate for diagnosing shock. Massive blood loss may produce only a minimal acute decrease in the hematocrit or hemoglobin concentration. Thus, a very low hematocrit value obtained shortly after injury suggests massive blood loss or a preexisting anemia, whereas a normal hematocrit does not exclude significant blood loss. Base deficit and/or lactate levels may be useful in determining the presence and severity of shock. Serial measurement of these parameters may be used to monitor a patient's response to therapy.

CLINICAL DIFFERENTIATION OF CAUSE OF SHOCK

❓ *What is the cause of the shock state?*

Shock in a trauma patient is classified as hemorrhagic or nonhemorrhagic. A patient with injuries above the diaphragm may have evidence of inadequate organ perfusion due to poor cardiac performance from blunt myocardial injury, cardiac tamponade, or a tension pneumothorax that produces inadequate venous return (preload). A high index of suspicion and careful observation of the patient's response to initial treatment will enable the doctor to recognize and manage all forms of shock.

Initial determination of the cause of shock depends on taking an appropriate history and performing a careful physical examination. Selected additional tests, such as monitoring central venous pressure (CVP) and obtaining data from a pulmonary artery catheter, chest and/or pelvic x-ray examinations, and ultrasonography, may provide confirmatory evidence for the cause of the shock state, but should not delay aggressive volume restoration.

Hemorrhagic Shock

Hemorrhage is the most common cause of shock after injury, and virtually all patients with multiple injuries have an element of hypovolemia. In addition, most nonhemorrhagic shock states respond partially or briefly to volume resuscitation. Therefore, if signs of shock are present, treatment usually is instituted as if the patient is hypovolemic. However, as treatment is instituted, it is important to identify the small number of patients whose shock has a different cause (eg, a secondary condition such as cardiac tamponade, tension pneumothorax, spinal cord injury, or blunt cardiac injury, which complicates hypovolemic/hemorrhagic shock). Specific information about the treatment of hemorrhagic shock is provided in the next section of this chapter. The primary focus in hemorrhagic shock is to identify and stop hemorrhage promptly.

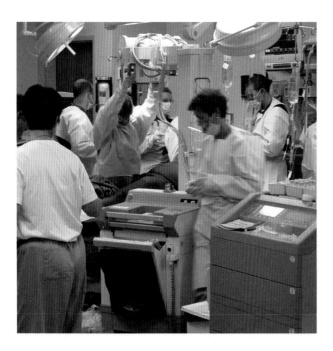

Nonhemorrhagic Shock

Nonhemorrhagic shock includes cardiogenic shock, cardiac tamponade, tension pneumothorax, neurogenic shock, and septic shock.

Cardiogenic Shock Myocardial dysfunction may be caused by blunt cardiac injury, cardiac tamponade, an air embolus, or, rarely, a myocardial infarction associated with the patient's injury. Blunt cardiac injury should be suspected when the mechanism of injury to the thorax is rapid deceleration. All patients with blunt thoracic trauma need constant electrocardiographic (ECG) monitoring to detect injury patterns and dysrhythmias. Blood creatine kinase (CK; formerly, creatine phosphokinase [CPK]) isoenzymes and specific isotope studies of the myocardium rarely assist the doctor in diagnosing or treating patients in the emergency department (ED). Echocardiography may be useful in the diagnosis of tamponade and valvular rupture, but it is often not practical or immediately available in the ED. Focused assessment sonography in trauma (FAST) in the ED can identify pericardial fluid and the likelihood of cardiac tamponade as the cause of shock. Blunt cardiac injury may be an indication for early CVP monitoring to guide fluid resuscitation in this situation.

Cardiac tamponade is most commonly identified in penetrating thoracic trauma, but it may occur as the result of blunt injury to the thorax. Tachycardia, muffled heart sounds, and dilated, engorged neck veins with hypotension resistant to fluid therapy suggest cardiac tamponade. However, the absence of these classic findings does not exclude the presence of this condition. Tension pneumothorax may mimic cardiac tamponade, but it is differentiated from the latter condition by the findings of absent breath sounds and a hyperresonant percussion note over the affected hemithorax. Appropriate placement of a needle into the pleural space in a case of tension pneumothorax temporarily relieves this life-threatening condition. Cardiac tamponade is best managed by thoracotomy. Pericardiocentesis may be used as a temporizing maneuver when thoracotomy is not an available option. ◾ See Skill Station VII: Chest Trauma Management, Skill VII-C: Pericardiocentesis.

Tension Pneumothorax Tension pneumothorax is a true surgical emergency that requires immediate diagnosis and treatment. It develops when air enters the pleural space, but a flap-valve mechanism prevents its escape. Intrapleural pressure rises, causing total lung collapse and a shift of the mediastinum to the opposite side with a subsequent impairment of venous return and fall in cardiac output. The presence of acute respiratory distress, subcutaneous emphysema, absent breath sounds, hyperresonance to percussion, and tracheal shift supports the diagnosis and warrants immediate thoracic decompression without waiting for x-ray confirmation of the diagnosis. ◾ See Skill Station VII: Chest Trauma Management, Skill VII-A: Needle Thoracentesis.

PITFALLS

- Missing tension pneumothorax.
- Assuming there is only one cause for shock.
- Young, healthy patients may have compensation for an extended period and then crash quickly.

Neurogenic Shock Isolated intracranial injuries do not cause shock. The presence of shock in a patient with a head injury necessitates a search for a cause other than an intracranial injury. Spinal cord injury may produce hypotension due to loss of sympathetic tone. Loss of sympathetic tone compounds the physiologic effects of hypovolemia, and hypovolemia compounds the physiologic effects of sympathetic denervation. The classic picture of neurogenic shock is hypotension without tachycardia or cutaneous vasoconstriction. A narrowed pulse pressure is not seen in neurogenic shock. Patients who have sustained a spinal injury often have concurrent torso trauma; therefore, patients with known or suspected neurogenic shock should be treated initially for hypovolemia. The failure of fluid resuscitation to restore organ perfusion suggests either continuing hemorrhage or neurogenic shock. CVP monitoring may be helpful in managing this sometimes complex problem. ◾ See Chapter 7: Spine and Spinal Cord Trauma.

Septic Shock Shock due to infection immediately after injury is uncommon; however, if a patient's arrival at an emergency facility is delayed for several hours, it could occur. Septic shock may occur in patients with penetrating abdominal injuries and contamination of the peritoneal cavity by intestinal contents. Patients with sepsis who also have hypotension and are afebrile are clinically difficult to distinguish from those in hypovolemic shock, as both groups may manifest tachycardia, cutaneous vasoconstriction, impaired urinary output, decreased systolic pressure, and narrow pulse pressure. Patients with early septic shock may have a normal circulating volume, modest tachycardia, warm, pink skin, systolic pressure near normal, and a wide pulse pressure.

Hemorrhagic Shock in Injured Patients

Hemorrhage is the most common cause of shock in trauma patients. The trauma patient's response to blood loss is made more complex by shifts of fluids among the fluid compartments in the body—particularly in the extracellular fluid compartment. The classic response to blood loss must be considered in the context of fluid shifts associated with soft tissue injury. In addition, the changes associated with severe, prolonged shock and the pathophysiologic results of resuscitation and reperfusion must also be considered, as previously discussed.

DEFINITION OF HEMORRHAGE

Hemorrhage is defined as an acute loss of circulating blood volume. Although there is considerable variability, the normal adult blood volume is approximately 7% of body weight. For example, a 70-kg male has a circulating blood volume of approximately 5 L. The blood volume of obese adults is estimated based on their ideal body weight, because calculation based on actual weight may result in significant overestimation. The blood volume for a child is calculated as 8% to 9% of body weight (80–90 mL/kg). ▪ See Chapter 10: Pediatric Trauma.

DIRECT EFFECTS OF HEMORRHAGE

The classification of hemorrhage into four classes based on clinical signs is a useful tool for estimating the percentage of acute blood loss. These changes represent a continuum of ongoing hemorrhage and guide initial therapy. **Volume replacement is guided by the patient's response to initial therapy, not solely by the initial classification.** This classification system is useful in emphasizing the early signs and pathophysiology of the shock state.

Class I hemorrhage is exemplified by the condition of an individual who has donated a unit of blood. *Class II* is uncomplicated hemorrhage for which crystalloid fluid resuscitation is required. *Class III* is a complicated hemorrhagic state in which at least crystalloid infusion is required and perhaps also blood replacement. *Class IV* hemorrhage is considered a preterminal event, and unless very aggressive measures are taken, the patient will die within minutes. Table 3-1 outlines the estimated blood loss and other critical measures for patients in each classification of shock.

Several confounding factors profoundly alter the classic hemodynamic response to an acute loss of circulating blood volume, and these must be promptly recognized by all individuals involved in the initial assessment and resuscitation of injured patients who are at risk for hemorrhagic shock. These factors include:

- Patient's age
- Severity of injury, with special attention to type and anatomic location of injury
- Time lapse between injury and initiation of treatment
- Prehospital fluid therapy and application of a pneumatic antishock garment (PASG)
- Medications used for chronic conditions

It is dangerous to wait until the trauma patient fits a precise physiologic classification of shock before initiating aggressive volume restoration. Fluid resuscitation must be initiated when early signs and symptoms of blood loss are apparent or suspected, not when the blood pressure is falling or absent.

Class I Hemorrhage—Up to 15% Blood Volume Loss

The clinical symptoms of volume loss with class I hemorrhage are minimal. In uncomplicated situations, minimal tachycardia occurs. No measurable changes occur in blood pressure, pulse pressure, or respiratory rate. For otherwise healthy patients, this amount of blood loss does not require replacement. Transcapillary refill and other compensatory mechanisms restore blood volume within 24 hours. However, in the presence of other fluid changes, this amount of blood loss may produce clinical symptoms, in which case replacement of the primary fluid losses corrects the circulatory state, usually without the need for blood transfusion.

Class II Hemorrhage—15% to 30% Blood Volume Loss

In a 70-kg male, volume loss with class II hemorrhage represents 750 to 1500 mL of blood. Clinical signs include tachycardia (heart rate above 100 in an adult), tachypnea, and decreased pulse pressure; the latter sign is related primarily to a rise in the diastolic component due to an increase in circulating catecholamines. These agents produce an increase in peripheral vascular tone and resistance. Systolic pressure changes minimally in early hemorrhagic shock; therefore, it is important to evaluate pulse pressure rather than systolic pressure. Other pertinent clinical findings with this amount of blood loss include subtle CNS changes, such as anxiety, fright, and hostility. Despite the significant blood loss and cardiovascular changes, urinary output is only mildly affected. The measured urine flow is usually 20 to 30 mL/hour in an adult.

Accompanying fluid losses can exaggerate the clinical manifestations of class II hemorrhage. Some of these patients may eventually require blood transfusion, but may be stabilized initially with crystalloid solutions.

Class III Hemorrhage—30% to 40% Blood Volume Loss

The blood loss with class III hemorrhage (approximately 2000 mL in an adult) may be devastating. Patients almost always present with the classic signs of inadequate perfusion, including marked tachycardia and tachypnea, significant changes in mental status, and a measurable fall in systolic pressure. In an uncomplicated case, this is the least amount of blood loss that consistently causes a drop in systolic pressure. Patients with this degree of blood loss almost always require transfusion. However, the priority of man-

TABLE 3-1 ■ Estimated Blood Loss[a] Based on Patient's Initial Presentation[b]				
	CLASS I	**CLASS II**	**CLASS III**	**CLASS IV**
Blood loss (mL)	Up to 750	750–1500	1500–2000	>2000
Blood loss (% blood volume)	Up to 15%	15%–30%	30%–40%	>40%
Pulse rate	<100	100–120	120–140	>140
Blood pressure	Normal	Normal	Decreased	Decreased
Pulse pressure (mm Hg)	Normal or increased	Decreased	Decreased	Decreased
Respiratory rate	14–20	20–30	30–40	>35
Urine output (mL/hr)	>30	20–30	5–15	Negligible
CNS/mental status	Slightly anxious	Mildly anxious	Anxious, confused	Confused, lethargic
Fluid replacement	Crystalloid	Crystalloid	Crystalloid and blood	Crystalloid and blood

[a]For a 70-kg male.

[b]The guidelines in this table are based on the 3-for-1 (3:1) rule, which derives from the empiric observation that most patients in hemorrhagic shock require as much as 300 mL of electrolyte solution for each 100 mL of blood loss. Applied blindly, these guidelines may result in excessive or inadequate fluid administration. For example, a patient with a crush injury to an extremity may have hypotension that is out of proportion to his or her blood loss and may require fluids in excess of the 3:1 guidelines. In contrast, a patient whose ongoing blood loss is being replaced by blood transfusion requires less than 3:1. The use of bolus therapy with careful monitoring of the patient's response may moderate these extremes.

agement is to stop the hemorrhage, by emergency operation if necessary, in order to decrease the need for transfusion. The decision to transfuse blood is based on the patient's response to initial fluid resuscitation and the adequacy of end-organ perfusion and oxygenation, as described later in this chapter.

Class IV Hemorrhage—More than 40% Blood Volume Loss

The degree of exsanguination with class IV hemorrhage is immediately life-threatening. Symptoms include marked tachycardia, a significant decrease in systolic blood pressure, and a very narrow pulse pressure (or an unobtainable diastolic pressure). Urinary output is negligible, and mental status is markedly depressed. The skin is cold and pale. Patients with class IV hemorrhage frequently require rapid transfusion and immediate surgical intervention. These decisions are based on the patient's response to the initial management techniques described in this chapter. Loss of more than 50% of blood volume results in loss of consciousness and decreased pulse and blood pressure.

The clinical usefulness of this classification scheme is illustrated by the following example: Because class III hemorrhage represents the smallest volume of blood loss that is consistently associated with a drop in systolic pressure, a 70-

kg patient with hypotension who arrives at an ED or trauma center has lost an estimated 1470 mL of blood (70 kg × 7% × 30% = 1.47 L, or 1470 mL). Nonresponse to fluid administration indicates persistent blood loss, unrecognized fluid losses, or nonhemorrhagic shock.

FLUID CHANGES SECONDARY TO SOFT TISSUE INJURY

Major soft tissue injuries and fractures compromise the hemodynamic status of injured patients in two ways. First, blood is lost into the site of injury, particularly in cases of major fractures. For example, a fractured tibia or humerus may be associated with the loss of as much as 1.5 units (750 mL) of blood. Twice that amount (up to 1500 mL) is commonly associated with femur fractures, and several liters of blood may accumulate in a retroperitoneal hematoma associated with a pelvic fracture.

The second factor to be considered is the edema that occurs in injured soft tissues. The degree of this additional volume loss is related to the magnitude of the soft tissue injury. Tissue injury results in activation of a systemic in-

PITFALL

Don't lose time focused on replacing fluid for blood. Find the source of bleeding.

flammatory response and production and release of multiple cytokines. Many of these locally active hormones have profound effects on the vascular endothelium, which increases permeability. Tissue edema is the result of shifts in fluid primarily from the plasma into the extravascular, extracellular space. Such shifts produce an additional depletion in intravascular volume.

Initial Management of Hemorrhagic Shock

What can I do about shock?

The diagnosis and treatment of shock must occur almost simultaneously. For most trauma patients, treatment is instituted as if the patient has hypovolemic shock, unless there is clear evidence that the shock state has a different cause. **The basic management principle is to stop the bleeding and replace the volume loss.**

PHYSICAL EXAMINATION

The physical examination is directed toward the immediate diagnosis of life-threatening injuries and includes assessment of the ABCDEs. Baseline recordings are important to monitor the patient's response to therapy. Vital signs, urinary output, and level of consciousness are essential. A more detailed examination of the patient follows as the situation permits. ◼ See Chapter 1: Initial Assessment and Management.

Airway and Breathing

Establishing a patent airway with adequate ventilation and oxygenation is the first priority. Supplementary oxygen is supplied to maintain oxygen saturation at greater than 95%. ◼ See Chapter 2: Airway and Ventilatory Management.

Circulation—Hemorrhage Control

Priorities for the circulation include controlling obvious hemorrhage, obtaining adequate intravenous access, and assessing tissue perfusion. Bleeding from external wounds usually can be controlled by direct pressure to the bleeding site. A PASG may be used to control bleeding from pelvic or lower extremity fractures, but its use should *not* interfere

with the rapid reestablishment of intravascular volume by intravenous fluid infusion. The adequacy of tissue perfusion dictates the amount of fluid resuscitation required. Surgery may be required to control internal hemorrhage.

Disability—Neurologic Examination

A brief neurologic examination will determine the level of consciousness, eye motion and pupillary response, best motor function, and degree of sensation. This information is useful in assessing cerebral perfusion, following the evolution of neurologic disability, and predicting future recovery. Alterations in CNS function in patients who have hypotension as a result of hypovolemic shock do not necessarily imply direct intracranial injury and may reflect inadequate brain perfusion. Restoration of cerebral perfusion and oxygenation must be achieved before ascribing these findings to intracranial injury. ◼ See Chapter 6: Head Trauma.

Exposure—Complete Examination

After lifesaving priorities are addressed, the patient must be completely undressed and carefully examined from head to toe to search for associated injuries. **When undressing the patient, it is essential to prevent hypothermia.** The use of fluid warmers as well as external passive and active warming techniques are essential to prevent hypothermia.

Gastric Dilation—Decompression

Gastric dilation often occurs in trauma patients, *especially in children,* and may cause unexplained hypotension or cardiac dysrhythmia, usually bradycardia from excessive vagal stimulation. **In unconscious patients, gastric distention increases the risk of aspiration of gastric contents, which is a potentially fatal complication.** Gastric decompression is accomplished by intubating the stomach with a tube passed nasally or orally and attaching it to suction to evacuate gastric contents. However, proper positioning of the tube does not completely obviate the risk of aspiration.

Urinary Catheterization

Bladder catheterization allows for assessment of the urine for hematuria and continuous evaluation of renal perfusion by monitoring urinary output. Blood at the urethral meatus or a high-riding, mobile, or nonpalpable prostate in males is an absolute contraindication to the insertion of a transurethral catheter prior to radiographic confirmation of an intact urethra. ◼ See Chapter 5: Abdominal and Pelvic Trauma.

VASCULAR ACCESS LINES

Access to the vascular system must be obtained promptly. This is best done by inserting two large-caliber (minimum of 16-gauge) peripheral intravenous catheters before placing a central venous line is considered. The rate of flow is proportional to the fourth power of the radius of the cannula and inversely related to its length (Poiseuille's law). Hence, short, large-caliber peripheral intravenous lines are preferred for the rapid infusion of large volumes of fluid. Fluid warmers and rapid infusion pumps are used in the presence of massive hemorrhage and severe hypotension.

The most desirable sites for peripheral, percutaneous intravenous lines in adults are the forearms and antecubital veins. If circumstances prevent the use of peripheral veins, large-caliber, central venous (femoral, jugular, or subclavian vein) access using the Seldinger technique or saphenous vein cutdown is indicated, depending on the skill and experience of the doctor. ■ See Skill Station IV: Shock Assessment and Management, and Skill Station V: Venous Cutdown.

Frequently in an emergency situation, central venous access is not accomplished under tightly controlled or completely sterile conditions. These lines should be changed in a more controlled environment as soon as the patient's condition permits. Consideration also must be given to the potential for serious complications related to attempted central venous catheter placement, such as pneumothorax or hemothorax, in patients who may already be unstable.

In children younger than 6 years, the placement of an intraosseous needle should be attempted before inserting a central line. The important determinant for selecting a procedure or route for establishing vascular access is the experience and skill of the doctor. Intraosseous access with specially designed equipment also is possible in adults.

As intravenous lines are started, blood samples are drawn for type and crossmatch, appropriate laboratory analyses, toxicology studies, and pregnancy testing for all females of childbearing age. Arterial blood gas (ABG) analysis is performed at this time. A chest x-ray must be obtained after attempts at inserting a subclavian or internal jugular CVP monitoring line to document the position of the line and to evaluate for a pneumothorax or hemothorax.

INITIAL FLUID THERAPY

Warmed isotonic electrolyte solutions, such as lactated Ringer's and normal saline, are used for initial resuscitation. This type of fluid provides transient intravascular expansion and further stabilizes the vascular volume by replacing accompanying fluid losses into the interstitial and intracellular spaces. An alternative initial fluid is hypertonic saline, although there is no evidence of survival advantage in the current literature.

An initial, warmed fluid bolus is given as rapidly as possible. The usual dose is 1 to 2 L for adults and 20 mL/kg for pediatric patients. This often requires application of pumping devices (mechanical or manual) to the fluid administration sets. The patient's response is observed during this initial fluid administration, and further therapeutic and diagnostic decisions are based on this response.

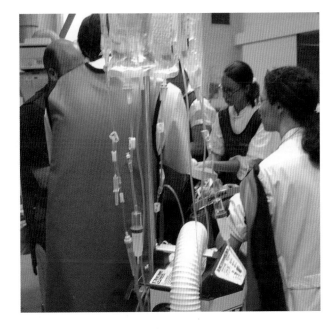

The amount of fluid and blood required for resuscitation is difficult to predict on initial evaluation of the patient. Table 3-1 provides general guidelines for establishing the amount of fluid and blood likely required. A rough guideline for the total amount of crystalloid volume required in the short term is to replace each 1 mL of blood loss with 3 mL of crystalloid fluid, thus allowing for restitution of plasma volume lost into the interstitial and intracellular spaces. This is known as the 3-for-1 rule. **It is most important to assess the patient's response to fluid resuscitation and evidence of adequate end-organ perfusion and oxygenation (ie, via urinary output, level of consciousness, and peripheral perfusion).** If, during resuscitation, the amount of fluid required to restore or maintain adequate organ perfusion greatly exceeds these estimates, a careful reassessment of the situation and a search for unrecognized injuries and other causes of shock are necessary.

The goal of resuscitation is to restore organ perfusion. This is accomplished by the use of resuscitation fluids to replace lost intravascular volume and guided by the goal of restoring a normal blood pressure. Note, however, that if blood pressure is raised rapidly before the hemorrhage has been definitively controlled, increased bleeding may occur. This can be seen in the small subset of patients in the transient or nonresponder category. **Persistent infusion of large volumes of fluids in an attempt to achieve a normal blood pressure is not a substitute for definitive control of bleeding.**

Fluid resuscitation and avoidance of hypotension are important principles in the initial management of blunt trauma patients, particularly those with traumatic brain injury (TBI). In penetrating trauma with hemorrhage, delaying aggressive fluid resuscitation until definitive control may prevent additional bleeding. Although complications associated with resuscitation injury are undesirable, the alterna-

PITFALL

Recognize the source of occult hemorrhage. Remember, "Blood on the floor × four more." Chest, pelvis, retroperitoneum, and long bones.

tive of exsanguination is even less so. A careful, balanced approach with frequent reevaluation is required.

Balancing the goal of organ perfusion with the risks of rebleeding by accepting a lower-than-normal blood pressure has been termed "controlled resuscitation," "balanced resuscitation," "hypotensive resuscitation," and "permissive hypotension." The goal is the balance, not the hypotension. Such a resuscitation strategy may be a bridge to, but is not a substitute for, definitive surgical control of bleeding.

Evaluation of Fluid Resuscitation and Organ Perfusion

? *What is the patient's response?*

The same signs and symptoms of inadequate perfusion that are used to diagnose shock are useful determinants of patient response. The return of normal blood pressure, pulse pressure, and pulse rate are signs that suggest perfusion is returning to normal. However, these observations give no information regarding organ perfusion. Improvements in the CVP status and skin circulation are important evidence of enhanced perfusion, but are difficult to quantitate. The volume of urinary output is a reasonably sensitive indicator of renal perfusion; normal urine volumes generally imply adequate renal blood flow, if not modified by the administration of diuretic agents. For this reason, urinary output is one of the prime monitors of resuscitation and patient response. Changes in CVP can provide useful information, and the risks incurred in the placement of a CVP line are justified for complex cases. Measurement of CVP is adequate for most cases.

URINARY OUTPUT

Within certain limits, urinary output is used to monitor renal blood flow. Adequate resuscitation volume replacement should produce a urinary output of approximately 0.5 mL/kg/hr in adults, whereas 1 mL/kg/hr is an adequate urinary output for pediatric patients. For children under 1 year of age, 2 mL/kg/hour should be maintained. The inability to obtain urinary output at these levels or a decreasing urinary output with an increasing specific gravity suggests in-

adequate resuscitation. This situation should stimulate further volume replacement and diagnostic endeavors.

ACID/BASE BALANCE

Patients in early hypovolemic shock have respiratory alkalosis due to tachypnea. Respiratory alkalosis is frequently followed by mild metabolic acidosis in the early phases of shock and does not require treatment. Severe metabolic acidosis may develop from long-standing or severe shock. Metabolic acidosis is caused by anaerobic metabolism, which results from inadequate tissue perfusion and the production of lactic acid. Persistent acidosis is usually caused by inadequate resuscitation or ongoing blood loss, and in the normothermic patient in shock it should be treated with fluids, blood, and consideration of operative intervention to control hemorrhage. Base deficit and/or lactate can be useful in determining the presence and severity of shock. Serial measurement of these parameters can be used to monitor the response to therapy. Sodium bicarbonate should *not* be used routinely to treat metabolic acidosis secondary to hypo-volemic shock.

Therapeutic Decisions Based on Response to Initial Fluid Resuscitation

The patient's response to initial fluid resuscitation is the key to determining subsequent therapy. Having established a preliminary diagnosis and treatment plan based on the initial evaluation, the doctor now modifies the plan based on the patient's response. Observing the response to the initial resuscitation identifies patients whose blood loss was greater than estimated and those with ongoing bleeding who require operative control of internal hemorrhage. Resuscitation in the operating room can accomplish simultaneously the direct control of bleeding by the surgeon and the restoration of intravascular volume. In addition, it limits the probability of overtransfusion or unnecessary transfusion of blood in patients whose initial status was disproportionate to the amount of blood loss.

It is particularly important to distinguish patients who are "hemodynamically stable" from those who are "hemodynamically normal." A hemodynamically stable patient may have persistent tachycardia, tachypnea, and oliguria—clearly underresuscitated and still in shock. In contrast, a hemodynamically normal patient is one who exhibits no signs of inadequate tissue perfusion. The potential patterns of response to initial fluid administration can be divided into three groups: rapid response, transient response, and minimal or no response. Vital signs and management guidelines for patients in each of these categories are outlined in Table 3-2.

TABLE 3-2 ■ Responses to Initial Fluid Resuscitation[a]			
	RAPID RESPONSE	**TRANSIENT RESPONSE**	**MINIMAL OR NO RESPONSE**
Vital signs	Return to normal	Transient improvement, recurrence of decreased blood pressure and increased heart rate	Remain abnormal
Estimated blood loss	Minimal (10%–20%)	Moderate and ongoing (20%–40%)	Severe (>40%)
Need for more crystalloid	Low	High	High
Need for blood	Low	Moderate to high	Immediate
Blood preparation	Type and crossmatch	Type-specific	Emergency blood release
Need for operative intervention	Possibly	Likely	Highly likely
Early presence of surgeon	Yes	Yes	Yes

[a]2000 mL of isotonic solution in adults; 20 mL/kg bolus of Ringer's lactate in children.

RAPID RESPONSE

Patients in this group, termed "rapid responders," respond rapidly to the initial fluid bolus and remain hemodynamically normal after the initial fluid bolus has been given and the fluids are slowed to maintenance rates. Such patients usually have lost minimal (less than 20%) blood volume. No further fluid bolus or immediate blood administration is indicated for this group. Typed and crossmatched blood should be kept available. **Surgical consultation and evaluation are necessary during initial assessment and treatment, as operative intervention may still be necessary.**

TRANSIENT RESPONSE

Patients in the second group, termed "transient responders" respond to the initial fluid bolus. However, they begin to show deterioration of perfusion indices as the initial fluids are slowed to maintenance levels, indicating either an ongoing blood loss or inadequate resuscitation. Most of these patients initially have lost an estimated 20% to 40% of their blood volume. Continued fluid administration and initiation of blood transfusion are indicated. A transient response to blood administration should identify patients who are still bleeding and require rapid surgical intervention.

MINIMAL OR NO RESPONSE

Failure to respond to crystalloid and blood administration in the ED dictates the need for immediate, definitive intervention (eg, operation or angioembolization) to control exsanguinating hemorrhage. On very rare occasions, failure to respond may be due to pump failure as a result of blunt cardiac injury, cardiac tamponade, or tension pneumothorax. Nonhemorrhagic shock always should be considered as a diagnosis in this group of patients. CVP monitoring or cardiac ultrasonography helps to differentiate between the various causes of shock.

PITFALLS

- Delay in definitive management can be lethal.
- Do not overlook a source of bleeding.

Blood Replacement

The decision to initiate blood transfusion is based on the patient's response, as described in the previous section.

CROSSMATCHED, TYPE-SPECIFIC, AND TYPE O BLOOD

The main purpose of blood transfusion is to restore the oxygen-carrying capacity of the intravascular volume. Volume resuscitation itself can be accomplished with crystalloids, with the added advantage that it contributes to interstitial and intracellular volume restitution.

Fully crossmatched blood is preferable. However, the complete crossmatching process requires approximately 1 hour in most blood banks. For patients who stabilize rapidly, crossmatched blood should be obtained and made available for transfusion when indicated.

Type-specific blood can be provided by most blood banks within 10 minutes. Such blood is compatible with ABO and Rh blood types, but incompatibilities of other antibodies may exist. Type-specific blood is preferred for patients who are transient responders, as described in the previous section. If type-specific blood is required, complete crossmatching should be performed by the blood bank.

If type-specific blood is unavailable, type O packed cells are indicated for patients with exsanguinating hemorrhage. To avoid sensitization and future complications, Rh-negative cells are preferred for females of childbearing age. For life-threatening blood loss, the use of unmatched, type-specific blood is preferred over type O blood. This is true unless multiple, unidentified casualties are being treated simultaneously and the risk of inadvertently administering the wrong unit of blood to a patient is great.

WARMING FLUIDS—PLASMA AND CRYSTALLOID

Hypothermia must be prevented and reversed if a patient has hypothermia on arrival at the hospital. The use of blood warmers in the ED is desirable, even if cumbersome. The most efficient way to prevent hypothermia in any patient receiving massive volumes of crystalloid is to heat the fluid to 39° C (102.2° F) before using it. This can be accomplished by storing crystalloids in a warmer or with the use of a microwave oven. Blood products cannot be warmed in a microwave oven, but they can be heated by passage through intravenous fluid warmers.

AUTOTRANSFUSION

Adaptations of standard tube thoracostomy collection devices are commercially available; these allow for sterile collection, anticoagulation (generally with sodium citrate solutions, not heparin), and retransfusion of shed blood. Collection of shed blood for autotransfusion should be considered for any patient with a major hemothorax.

COAGULOPATHY

Severe injury and hemorrhage result in the consumption of coagulation factors and early coagulopathy. Massive transfusion with the resultant dilution of platelets and clotting factors, along with the adverse effect of hypothermia on platelet aggregation and the clotting cascade, all contribute to coagulopathy in injured patients. Prothrombin time, partial thromboplastin time, and platelet count are valuable baseline studies to obtain in the first hour, especially if the patient has a history of coagulation disorders, takes medications that alter coagulation (eg, warfarin, aspirin, and nonsteroidal antiinflammatory agents [NSAIDs]), or a reliable bleeding history cannot be obtained. Transfusion of platelets, cryoprecipitate, and fresh-frozen plasma should be guided by these coagulation parameters, including fibrinogen levels. Routine use of such products is generally not warranted unless the patient has a known coagulation disorder or has undergone anticoagulation pharmacologically for management of a specific medical problem. In such cases, specific factor replacement therapy is immediately indicated when there is evidence of bleeding, or the potential for occult blood loss exists (eg, head, abdominal, or thoracic injury). However, consideration of early blood component therapy should be given to patients with class IV hemorrhage.

Patients with major brain injury are particularly prone to coagulation abnormalities as a result of substances, especially tissue thromboplastin, that are released by damaged neural tissue. These patients' coagulation parameters need to be closely monitored.

CALCIUM ADMINISTRATION

Most patients receiving blood transfusions do not need calcium supplements. Excessive, supplemental calcium may be harmful.

Special Considerations in the Diagnosis and Treatment of Shock

Special considerations in the diagnosis and treatment of shock include the mistaken equation of blood pressure with cardiac output; patient age; athletes in shock; pregnancy; patient medications; hypothermia; and the presence of pacemakers.

EQUATING BLOOD PRESSURE WITH CARDIAC OUTPUT

Treatment of hypovolemic (hemorrhagic) shock requires correction of inadequate organ perfusion by increasing organ blood flow and tissue oxygenation. Increasing blood flow requires an increase in cardiac output. Ohm's law ($V = I \times R$) applied to cardiovascular physiology states that blood pressure (V) is proportional to cardiac output (I) and systemic vascular resistance (R) (afterload). An increase in blood pressure should not be equated with a concomitant increase in cardiac output. An increase in peripheral resistance—for example, with vasopressor therapy—with no change in cardiac output results in increased blood pressure, but no improvement in tissue perfusion or oxygenation.

ADVANCED AGE

Elderly trauma patients require special consideration. The aging process produces a relative decrease in sympathetic activity with respect to the cardiovascular system. This is thought to result from a deficit in the receptor response to catecholamines, rather than from a reduction in catecholamine production. Cardiac compliance decreases with age, and older patients are unable to increase heart rate or the efficiency of myocardial contraction when stressed by blood volume loss, as are younger patients. Atherosclerotic vascular occlusive disease makes many vital organs extremely sensitive to even the slightest reduction in blood flow. Many elderly patients have preexisting volume depletion resulting from long-term diuretic use or subtle malnutrition. For these reasons, hypotension secondary to blood loss is poorly tolerated by elderly trauma patients. ß-adrenergic blockade may mask tachycardia as an early indicator of shock. Other medications may adversely affect the stress response to injury or block it completely. Because the therapeutic range for volume resuscitation is relatively narrow in elderly patients, it is prudent to consider early invasive monitoring as a means to avoid excessive or inadequate volume restoration.

The reduction in pulmonary compliance, decrease in diffusion capacity, and general weakness of the muscles of respiration limit the ability of elderly patients to meet the increased demands for gas exchange imposed by injury. This compounds the cellular hypoxia already produced by a reduction in local oxygen delivery. Glomerular and tubular senescence in the kidney reduces the ability of elderly patients to preserve volume in response to the release of stress hormones such as aldosterone, catecholamines, vasopressin, and cortisol. The kidney also is more susceptible to the effects of reduced blood flow and nephrotoxic agents such as drugs, contrast agents, and the toxic products of cellular destruction.

For all of these reasons, mortality and morbidity rates increase directly with age and long-term health status for mild and moderately severe injuries. Despite the adverse effects of the aging process, comorbidities from preexisting disease, and a general reduction in the "physiologic reserve" of geriatric patients, the majority of these patients may recover and return to their preinjury status. Treatment begins with prompt, aggressive resuscitation and careful monitoring. ◾ See Chapter 11: Geriatric Trauma.

ATHLETES

Rigorous athletic training routines change the cardiovascular dynamics of this group of patients. Blood volume may increase 15% to 20%, cardiac output sixfold, and stroke volume 50%, and the resting pulse can average 50. The ability of athletes' bodies to compensate for blood loss is truly remarkable. The usual responses to hypovolemia may not be manifested in athletes, even when significant blood loss has occurred.

PREGNANCY

Physiologic maternal hypervolemia requires a greater blood loss to manifest perfusion abnormalities in the mother, which also may be reflected in decreased fetal perfusion. ◾ See Chapter 12: Trauma in Women.

MEDICATIONS

ß-adrenergic receptor blockers and calcium-channel blockers can significantly alter a patient's hemodynamic response to hemorrhage. Insulin overdosing may be responsible for hypoglycemia and may have contributed to the injury-producing event. Long-term diuretic therapy may explain unexpected hypokalemia, and NSAIDs may adversely affect platelet function.

HYPOTHERMIA

Patients suffering from hypothermia and hemorrhagic shock do not respond normally to the administration of blood and fluid resuscitation, and coagulopathy often develops. Body temperature is an important vital sign to monitor during the initial assessment phase. Esophageal or bladder temperature is an accurate clinical measurement of the core temperature. A trauma victim under the influence of alcohol and exposed to cold temperature extremes is more likely to have hypothermia as a result of vasodilation. Rapid rewarming in a environment with appropriate external warming devices, heat lamps, thermal caps, heated respiratory gases, and warmed intravenous fluids and blood will generally correct hypotension and hypothermia. Core rewarming (irrigation of the peritoneal or thoracic cavity with crystalloid solutions warmed to 39° C [102.2° F] or extracorporeal bypass) may occasionally be indicated. Hypothermia is best treated by prevention. ◾ See Chapter 9: Thermal Injuries.

PACEMAKER

Patients with pacemakers are unable to respond to blood loss in the expected fashion, because cardiac output is di-

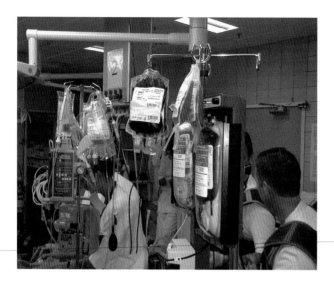

rectly related to heart rate. In the significant number of patients with myocardial conduction defects who have such devices in place, CVP monitoring is invaluable to guide fluid therapy.

Reassessing Patient Response and Avoiding Complications

Inadequate volume replacement is the most common complication of hemorrhagic shock. Immediate, appropriate, and aggressive therapy that restores organ perfusion minimizes these problematic events.

CONTINUED HEMORRHAGE

Obscure hemorrhage is the most common cause of poor response to fluid therapy. Patients with this condition are generally included in the transient response category as defined previously. Immediate surgical intervention may be necessary.

FLUID OVERLOAD AND CVP MONITORING

After a patient's initial assessment and treatment have been completed, the risk of fluid overload is minimized by careful monitoring. Remember, the goal of therapy is restoration of organ perfusion and adequate tissue oxygenation, confirmed by appropriate urinary output, CNS function, skin color, and return of pulse and blood pressure toward normal.

Monitoring the response to resuscitation is best accomplished for some patients in an environment in which

sophisticated techniques are used. Early transfer of the patient to an intensive care unit should be considered for elderly patients and patients with nonhemorrhagic causes of shock.

CVP monitoring is a relatively simple procedure used as a standard guide for assessing the ability of the right side of the heart to accept a fluid load. Properly interpreted, the response of the CVP to fluid administration helps evaluate volume replacement. Several points to remember are:

1. The precise measure of cardiac function is the relationship between ventricular end diastolic volume and stroke volume. Right atrial pressure (CVP) and cardiac output (as reflected by evidence of perfusion or blood pressure, or even by direct measurement) are indirect and, at best, insensitive estimates of this relationship. Remembering these facts is important to avoid overdependency on CVP monitoring.

2. The initial CVP level and actual blood volume are not necessarily related. The initial CVP is sometimes high, even with a significant volume deficit, especially in patients with chronic obstructive pulmonary disease, generalized vasoconstriction, and rapid fluid replacement. The initial venous pressure also may be high because of the application of PASG or the inappropriate use of exogenous vasopressors.

3. A minimal rise in the initially low CVP with fluid therapy suggests the need for further volume expansion (minimal or no response to fluid resuscitation category).

4. A declining CVP suggests ongoing fluid loss and the need for additional fluid or blood replacement (transient response to fluid resuscitation category).

5. An abrupt or persistent elevation in CVP suggests that volume replacement is adequate or too rapid or that cardiac function is compromised.

6. Pronounced elevations of CVP may be caused by hypervolemia as a result of overtransfusion, cardiac dysfunction, cardiac tamponade, or increased intrathoracic pressure from a tension pneumothorax. Catheter malposition may produce erroneously high CVP measurements.

Aseptic techniques must be used when central venous lines are placed. Multiple sites provide access to the central circulation, and the decision regarding which route to use is determined by the skill and experience of the doctor. The ideal position for the tip of the catheter is in the superior vena cava, just proximal to the right atrium. ◾ Techniques for catheter placement are discussed in detail in Skill Station IV: Shock Assessment and Management.

The placement of central venous lines carries the risk of potentially life-threatening complications. Infections, vascular injury, nerve injury, embolization, thrombosis, and pneumothorax may result. CVP monitoring reflects right heart function. It may not be representative of left heart function in patients with primary myocardial dysfunction or abnormal pulmonary circulation.

RECOGNITION OF OTHER PROBLEMS

When a patient fails to respond to therapy, consider cardiac tamponade, tension pneumothorax, ventilatory problems, unrecognized fluid loss, acute gastric distention, myocardial infarction, diabetic acidosis, hypoadrenalism, and neurogenic shock. Constant reevaluation, especially when patients' conditions deviate from expected patterns, is the key to recognizing such problems as early as possible.

CHAPTER SUMMARY

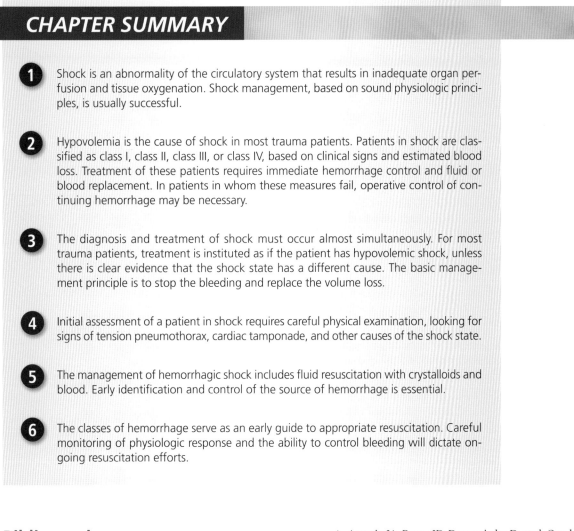

1. Shock is an abnormality of the circulatory system that results in inadequate organ perfusion and tissue oxygenation. Shock management, based on sound physiologic principles, is usually successful.

2. Hypovolemia is the cause of shock in most trauma patients. Patients in shock are classified as class I, class II, class III, or class IV, based on clinical signs and estimated blood loss. Treatment of these patients requires immediate hemorrhage control and fluid or blood replacement. In patients in whom these measures fail, operative control of continuing hemorrhage may be necessary.

3. The diagnosis and treatment of shock must occur almost simultaneously. For most trauma patients, treatment is instituted as if the patient has hypovolemic shock, unless there is clear evidence that the shock state has a different cause. The basic management principle is to stop the bleeding and replace the volume loss.

4. Initial assessment of a patient in shock requires careful physical examination, looking for signs of tension pneumothorax, cardiac tamponade, and other causes of the shock state.

5. The management of hemorrhagic shock includes fluid resuscitation with crystalloids and blood. Early identification and control of the source of hemorrhage is essential.

6. The classes of hemorrhage serve as an early guide to appropriate resuscitation. Careful monitoring of physiologic response and the ability to control bleeding will dictate ongoing resuscitation efforts.

Bibliography

1. Abou-Khalil B, Scalea TM, Trooskin SZ, et al. Hemodynamic responses to shock in young trauma patients: need for invasive monitoring. *Crit Care Med* 1994;22(4):633-639.

2. Alam HB, Rhee P. New developments in fluid resuscitation. *Surg Clin North Am* 2007; 87(1):55-72, vi.

3. Alam HB. An update on fluid resuscitation. *Scand J Surg* 2006; 95(3):136-145.

4. Asensio JA, Berne JD, Demetriades D, et al. One hundred five penetrating cardiac injuries: a 2-year prospective evaluation. *J Trauma* 1998; 44(6):1073-1082.

5. Asensio JA, Murray J, Demetriades D, et al. Penetrating cardiac injuries: a prospective study of variables predicting outcomes. *J Am Coll Surg* 1998; 186(1):24-34.

6. Bickell WH, Wall MJ, Pepe PE, et al. Immediate versus delayed fluid resuscitation for hypotensive patients with penetrating torso injuries. *N Engl J Med* 1994; 331(17):1105-1109.

7. Brown MD. Evidence-based emergency medicine. Hypertonic versus isotonic crystalloid for fluid resuscitation in critically ill patients. *Ann Emerg Med* 2002; 40(1):113-114.

8. Bunn F, Roberts I, Tasker R, Akpa E. Hypertonic versus near isotonic crystalloid for fluid resuscitation in critically ill patients. *Cochrane Database Syst Rev* 2004; (3):CD002045.

9. Burris D, Rhee P, Kaufmann C, et al. Controlled resuscitation for uncontrolled hemorrhagic shock. *J Trauma* 1999; 46(2):216-223.

10. Carrico CJ, Canizaro PC, Shires GT. Fluid resuscitation following injury: rationale for the use of balanced salt solutions. *Crit Care Med* 1976;4(2):46-54.

11. Chernow B, Rainey TG, Lake CR. Endogenous and exogenous catecholamines. *Crit Care Med* 1982;10:409.

12. Cogbill TH, Blintz M, Johnson JA, et al. Acute gastric dilatation after trauma. *J Trauma* 1987;27(10):1113-1117.

13. Cook RE, Keating JF, Gillespie I. The role of angiography in the management of haemorrhage from major fractures of the pelvis. *J Bone Joint Surg Br* 2002; 84(2):178-182.

14. Cooney R, Ku J, Cherry R, et al. Limitations of splenic angioembolization in treating blunt splenic injury. *J Trauma* 2005; 59(4), 926-932; discussion 932.

15. Cooper DJ, Walley KR, Wiggs RB, et al. Bicarbonate does not improve hemodynamics in critically ill patients who have lactic acidosis. *Ann Intern Med* 1990;112:492.

16. Counts RB, Haisch C, Simon TL, et al. Hemostasis in massively transfused trauma patients. *Ann Surg* 1979;190(l):91-99.

17. Davis JW, Kaups KL, Parks SN. Base deficit is superior to pH in evaluating clearance of acidosis after traumatic shock. *J Trauma* 1998 Jan;44(1):114-118.

18. Davis JW, Parks SN, Kaups KL et al. *J Trauma* Admission base deficit predicts transfusion requirements and risk of complications. 1997 Mar;42(3):571-573.

19. Dent D, Alsabrook G, Erickson BA, et al. Blunt splenic injuries: high nonoperative management rate can be achieved with selective embolization. *J Trauma* 2004; 56(5):1063-1067.

20. Dutton RP, Mackenzie CF, Scalea TM. Hypotensive resuscitation during active hemorrhage: impact on in-hospital mortality. *J Trauma* 2002; 52(6):1141-1146.

21. Fangio P, Asehnoune K, Edouard A, Smail N, Benhamou D. Early embolization and vasopressor administration for management of life-threatening hemorrhage from pelvic fracture. *J Trauma* 2005; 58(5), 978-984; discussion 984.

22. Ferrara A, MacArthur JD, Wright HK, et al. Hypothermia and acidosis worsen coagulopathy in patients requiring massive transfusion. *Am J Surg* 1990;160:515.

23. Gaarder C, Dormagen JB, Eken T, et al. Nonoperative management of splenic injuries: improved results with angioembolization. *J Trauma* 2006; 61(1):192-198.

24. Glover JL, Broadie TA. Intraoperative autotransfusion. *World J Surg* 1987;11:60-64.

25. Gould SA, Moore EE, Hoyt DB, et al. The first randomized trial of human polymerized hemoglobin as a blood substitute in acute trauma and emergent surgery. *J Am Coll Surg* 1998;187(2):113-122.

26. Granger DN. Role of xanthine oxidase and granulocytes in ischemia-reperfusion injury. *Am J Physiol* 1988;255:H1269-H1275.

27. Greaves I, Porter KM, Revell MP. Fluid resuscitation in prehospital trauma care: a consensus view. *J R Coll Surg Edinb* 2002; 47(2):451-457.

28. Greco L, Francioso G, Pratichizzo A, Testini M, Impedovo G, Ettorre GC. Arterial embolization in the treatment of severe blunt hepatic trauma. *Hepatogastroenterology* 2003; 50(51):746-749.

29. Guyton AC, Lindsey AW, Kaufman BN. Effect of mean circulatory filling pressure and other peripheral circulatory factors on cardiac output. *Am J Physiol* 1955;180:463-468.

30. Haan J, Scott J, Boyd-Kranis RL, Ho S, Kramer M, Scalea TM. Admission angiography for blunt splenic injury: advantages and pitfalls. *J Trauma* 2001; 51(6):1161-1165.

31. Hagiwara A, Yukioka T, Ohta S, Nitatori T, Matsuda H, Shimazaki S. Nonsurgical management of patients with blunt splenic injury: efficacy of transcatheter arterial embolization. *AJR Am J Roentgenol* 1996; 167(1):159-166.

32. Hak DJ. The role of pelvic angiography in evaluation and management of pelvic trauma. *Orthop Clin North Am* 2004; 35(4):439-443, v.

33. Harrigan C, Lucas CE, Ledgerwood AM, et al. Serial changes in primary hemostasis after massive transfusion. *Surgery* 1985;98:836-840.

34. Hoyt DB. Fluid resuscitation: the target from an analysis of trauma systems and patient survival. *J Trauma* 2003; 54(5 Suppl):S31-35.

35. Jurkovich QJ. Hypothermia in the trauma patient. In: Maull KI, ed. *Advances in Trauma.* Chicago: Yearbook; 1989:111-140.

36. Kaplan LJ, Kellum JA. Initial pH, base deficit, lactate, anion gap, strong ion difference, and strong ion gap predict outcome from major vascular injury. *Crit Care Med* 2004;32(5):1120-1124.

37. Karmy-Jones R, Nathens A, Jurkovich GJ, et al. Urgent and emergent thoracotomy for penetrating chest trauma. *J Trauma* 2004; 56(3), 664-668; discussion 668-669.

38. Knudson MM, Maull KI. Nonoperative management of solid organ injuries. Past, present, and future. *Surg Clin North Am* 1999;79(6):1357-1371.

39. Krausz MM. Fluid resuscitation strategies in the Israeli army. *J Trauma* 2003; 54(5 Suppl):S39-42.

40. Kruse JA, Vyskocil JJ, Haupt MT. Intraosseous: a flexible option for the adult or child with delayed, difficult, or impossible conventional vascular access. *Crit Care Med* 1994;22:728-735.

41. Lowry SF, Fong Y. Cytokines and the cellular response to injury and infection. In: Wilmore DW, Brennan MF, Harken AH, et

al., eds. *Care of the Surgical Patient.* New York: Scientific American; 1990.

42. Lucas CE, Ledgerwood AM. Cardiovascular and renal response to hemorrhagic and septic shock. In: Clowes GHA Jr, ed. *Trauma, Sepsis and Shock: The Physiological Basis of Therapy.* New York: Marcel Dekker; 1988:87-215.

43. Mandal AK, Sanusi M. Penetrating chest wounds: 24 years experience. *World J Surg* 2001;25(9):1145-1149.

44. Mansour MA, Moore EE, Moore FA, Read RR. Exigent postinjury thoracotomy analysis of blunt versus penetrating trauma. *Surg Gynecol Obstet* 1992;175(2):97-101.

45. Martin DJ, Lucas CE, Ledgerwood AM, et al. Fresh frozen plasma supplement to massive red blood cell transfusion. *Ann Surg* 1985;202:505.

46. Martin, MJ, Fitz, Sullivan E, Salim, A, et al. Discordance between lactate and base deficit in the surgical intensive care unit: which one do you trust? *Am J Surg* 2006;191(5): 625-630.

47. Mizushima Y, Tohira H, Mizobata Y, Matsuoka T, Yokota J. Fluid resuscitation of trauma patients: how fast is the optimal rate? *Am J Emerg Med* 2005;23(7):833-837.

48. Novak L, Shackford SR, Bourguignon P, et al. Comparison of standard and alternative prehospital resuscitation in uncontrolled hemorrhagic shock and head injury. *J Trauma* 1999;47(5):834-844.

49. O'Neill PA, Riina J, Sclafani S, Tornetta P. Angiographic findings in pelvic fractures. *Clin Orthop Relat Res* 1996;(329):60-67.

50. Pappas P, Brathwaite CE, Ross SE. Emergency central venous catheterization during resuscitation of trauma patients. *Am Surg* 1992;58:108-111.

51. Peck KR, Altieri M. Intraosseous infusions: an old technique with modern applications. *Pediatr Nurs* 1988;14(4):296-298.

52. Poole GV, Meredith JW, Pennell T, et al. Comparison of colloids and crystalloids in resuscitation from hemorrhagic shock. *Surg Gynecol Obstet* 1982;154:577-586.

53. Revell M, Greaves I, Porter K. Endpoints for fluid resuscitation in hemorrhagic shock. *J Trauma* 2003;54(5 Suppl):S63-S67.

54. Rhodes M, Brader A, Lucke J, et al. A direct transport to the operating room for resuscitation of trauma patients. *J Trauma* 1989;29:907-915.

55. Rohrer MJ, Natale AM. Effect of hypothermia on the coagulation cascade. *Crit Care Med* 1992;20:490.

56. Rotondo MF, Schwab CW, McGonigal MD, et al. "Damage control": an approach for improved survival in exsanguinating penetrating abdominal injury. *J Trauma* 1993;35:375-382.

57. Sadri H, Nguyen-Tang T, Stern R, Hoffmeyer P, Peter R. Control of severe hemorrhage using C-clamp and arterial embolization in hemodynamically unstable patients with pelvic ring disruption. *Arch Orthop Trauma Surg* 2005;125(7):443-447.

58. Sarnoff SJ. Myocardial contractility as described by ventricular function curves: observations on Starling's law of the heart. *Physiol Rev* 1988;35:107-122.

59. Sawyer RW, Bodai BI. The current status of intraosseous infusion. *J Am Coll Surg* 1994;179:353-361.

60. Scalea TM, Hartnett RW, Duncan AO, et al. Central venous oxygen saturation: a useful clinical tool in trauma patients. *J Trauma* 1990;30(12):1539-1543.

61. Scalea TM, Simon HM, Duncan AO, et al. Geriatric blunt multiple trauma: improved survival with early invasive monitoring. *J Trauma* 1990;30:129-136.

62. Schierhout G, Roberts I. Fluid resuscitation with colloid or crystalloid solutions in critically ill patients: a systematic review of randomised trials. *Br J Med* 1998;316:961-964.

63. Shapiro M, McDonald AA, Knight D, Johannigman JA, Cuschieri J. The role of repeat angiography in the management of pelvic fractures. *J Trauma* 2005;58(2):227-231.

64. Smith HE, Biffl WL, Majercik SD, Jednacz J, Lambiase R, Cioffi WG. Splenic artery embolization: Have we gone too far? *J Trauma* 2006; 61(3):541-544; discussion 545-546.

65. Thourani VH, Feliciano DV, Cooper WA, et al. Penetrating cardiac trauma at an urban trauma center: a 22-year perspective. *Am Surg* 1999; 65(9):811-816; discussion 817-818.

66. Tyburski JG, Astra L, Wilson RF, Dente C, Steffes C. Factors affecting prognosis with penetrating wounds of the heart. *J Trauma* 2000;48(4):587-590; discussion 590-591.

67. Velanovich V. Crystalloid versus colloid fluid resuscitation: a meta-analysis of mortality. *Surgery* 1990;105:65-71.

68. Velmahos GC, Toutouzas KG, Vassiliu P, et al. A prospective study on the safety and efficacy of angiographic embolization for pelvic and visceral injuries. *J Trauma* 2002;53(2):303-308; discussion 308.

69. Virgilio RW, Rice CL, Smith DE, et al. Crystalloid vs colloid resuscitation: is one better? A randomized clinical study. *Surgery* 1979;85(2):129-139.

70. von OUO, Bautz P, De GM. Penetrating thoracic injuries: what we have learnt. *Thorac Cardiovasc Surg* 2000;48(1):55-61.

71. Wahl WL, Ahrns KS, Chen S, Hemmila MR, Rowe SA, Arbabi S. Blunt splenic injury: operation versus angiographic embolization. *Surgery* 2004;136(4):891-899.

72. Werwath DL, Schwab CW, Scholter JR, et al. Microwave oven: a safe new method of warming crystalloids. *Am J Surg* 1984;12:656-659.

73. Williams JF, Seneff MG, Friedman BC, et al. Use of femoral venous catheters in critically ill adults: prospective study. *Crit Care Med* 1991;19:550-553.

74. York J, Arrilaga A, Graham R, et al. Fluid resuscitation of patients with multiple injuries and severe closed head injury: experience with an aggressive fluid resuscitation strategy. *J Trauma* 2000;48(3):376-379.

▶▶ Interactive Skill Procedures

Note: Accompanying some of the skills procedures for this station is a series of scenarios, which are provided at the conclusion of the procedures for you to review and prepare for this station. Tables pertaining to the initial assessment and management of the patient in shock also are provided for your review after the scenarios. *Note:* **Standard precautions are required when caring for trauma patients.**

THE FOLLOWING PROCEDURES ARE INCLUDED IN THIS SKILL STATION:

▶▶ **Skill IV-A:** Peripheral Venous Access

▶▶ **Skill IV-B:** Femoral Venipuncture: Seldinger Technique

▶▶ **Skill IV-C:** Subclavian Venipuncture: Infraclavicular Approach

▶▶ **Skill IV-D:** Internal Jugular Venipuncture: Middle or Central Route

▶▶ **Skill IV-E:** Intraosseous Puncture/Infusion: Proximal Tibial Route

▶▶ **Skill IV-F:** Broselow™ Pediatric Emergency Tape

Performance at this skill station will allow the participant to practice the assessment of a patient in shock, determine the cause of the shock state, institute the initial management of shock, and evaluate the patient's response to treatment. Specifically, the student will be able to:

OBJECTIVES

1 Recognize the shock state.

2 Evaluate a patient to determine the extent of organ perfusion, including performing a physical examination and the relevant adjuncts to the primary survey.

3 Identify the causes of the shock state.

4 Initiate the resuscitation of a patient in shock by identifying and controlling hemorrhage and promptly initiating volume replacement.

5 Identify the surface markings and demonstrate the techniques of vascular access for the following:

Peripheral venous system
Femoral vein
Internal jugular vein
Subclavian vein
Intraosseous infusion in children

6 Use adjuncts in the assessment and management of the shock state, including:

X-ray examination (chest and pelvic film)
Diagnostic peritoneal lavage (DPL)
Abdominal ultrasound
Computed tomography (CT)
Broselow™ Pediatric Emergency Tape

7 Identify patients who require definitive hemorrhage control or transfer to the intensive care unit, where extended monitoring capabilities are available.

8 Identify which additional therapeutic measures are necessary based on the patient's response to treatment and the clinical significance of the responses of patients as classified by:

Rapid response
Transient response
Nonresponse

▶ Skill IV-A: Peripheral Venous Access

STEP 1. Select an appropriate site on an extremity (antecubital, forearm, or saphenous vein).

STEP 2. Apply an elastic tourniquet above the proposed puncture site.

STEP 3. Clean the site with antiseptic solution.

STEP 4. Puncture the vein with a large-caliber, plastic, over-the-needle catheter. Observe for blood return.

STEP 5. Thread the catheter into the vein over the needle.

STEP 6. Remove the needle and tourniquet.

STEP 7. If appropriate, obtain blood samples for laboratory tests.

STEP 8. Connect the catheter to the intravenous infusion tubing and begin the infusion of warmed crystalloid solution.

STEP 9. Observe for possible infiltration of the fluids into the tissues.

STEP 10. Secure the catheter and tubing to the skin of the extremity.

▶ Skill IV-B: Femoral Venipuncture: Seldinger Technique
(See Figure IV-1)

Note: Sterile technique should be used when performing this procedure.

STEP 1. Place the patient in the supine position.

STEP 2. Cleanse the skin around the venipuncture site well and drape the area.

STEP 3. Locate the femoral vein by palpating the femoral artery. The vein lies directly medial to the femoral artery (nerve, artery, vein, empty space). A finger should remain on the artery to facilitate anatomical location and avoid insertion of the catheter into the artery. Ultrasound can be used as an adjunct for placement of central venous lines.

STEP 4. If the patient is awake, use a local anesthetic at the venipuncture site.

STEP 5. Introduce a large-caliber needle attached to a 12-mL syringe with 0.5 to 1 mL of saline. The needle, directed toward the patient's head, should enter the skin directly over the femoral vein. Hold the needle and syringe parallel to the frontal plane.

STEP 6. Directing the needle cephalad and posteriorly, slowly advance the needle while gently withdrawing the plunger of the syringe.

STEP 7. When a free flow of blood appears in the syringe, remove the syringe and occlude the needle with a finger to prevent air embolism.

STEP 8. Insert the guidewire and remove the needle. Use an introducer if required.

STEP 9. Insert the catheter over the guidewire.

STEP 10. Remove the guidewire and connect the catheter to the intravenous tubing.

STEP 11. Affix the catheter in place (with a suture), apply antibiotic ointment, and dress the area.

STEP 12. Tape the intravenous tubing in place.

STEP 13. Obtain chest and abdominal x-ray films to confirm the position and placement of the intravenous catheter.

STEP 14. The catheter should be changed as soon as is practical.

▶▶ MAJOR COMPLICATIONS OF FEMORAL VENOUS ACCESS

- Deep-vein thrombosis
- Arterial or neurologic injury
- Infection
- Arteriovenous fistula

Step 5

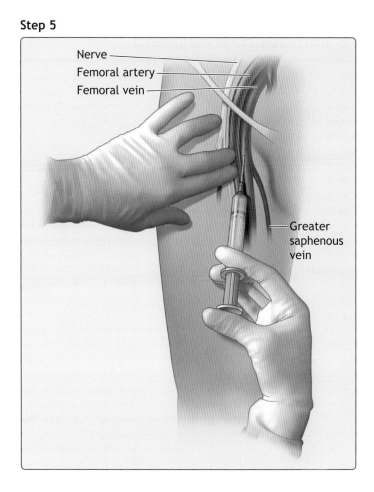

Nerve
Femoral artery
Femoral vein

Greater
saphenous
vein

Step 8

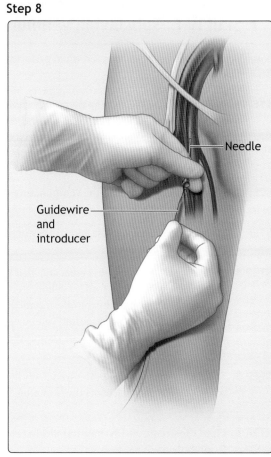

Needle

Guidewire
and
introducer

Step 9

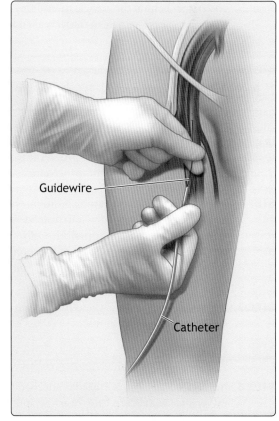

Guidewire

Catheter

■ **Figure IV-1 Femoral Venipuncture: Seldinger Technique.**
(Illustrations correlate with selected steps in Skill IV-B.)

▶ Skill IV-C: Subclavian Venipuncture: Infraclavicular Approach

Note: Sterile technique should be used when performing this procedure.

STEP 1. Place the patient in the supine position, with the head at least 15 degrees down to distend the neck veins and prevent air embolism. Only if a cervical spine injury has been excluded can the patient's head be turned away from the venipuncture site.

STEP 2. Cleanse the skin around the venipuncture site well and drape the area.

STEP 3. If the patient is awake, use a local anesthetic at the venipuncture site.

STEP 4. Introduce a large-caliber needle, attached to a 12-mL syringe with 0.5 to 1 mL of saline, 1 cm below the junction of the middle and medial thirds of the clavicle. Ultrasound can be used as an adjunct for the placement of central venous lines

STEP 5. After the skin has been punctured, with the bevel of the needle upward, expel the skin plug that can occlude the needle.

STEP 6. Hold the needle and syringe parallel to the frontal plane.

STEP 7. Direct the needle medially, slightly cephalad, and posteriorly behind the clavicle toward the posterior, superior angle to the sternal end of the clavicle (toward the finger placed in the suprasternal notch).

STEP 8. Slowly advance the needle while gently withdrawing the plunger of the syringe.

STEP 9. When a free flow of blood appears in the syringe, rotate the bevel of the needle caudally, remove the syringe, and occlude the needle with a finger to prevent air embolism.

STEP 10. Insert the guidewire while monitoring the electrocardiogram for rhythm abnormalities.

STEP 11. Remove the needle while holding the guidewire in place.

STEP 12. Insert the catheter over the guidewire to a predetermined depth (the tip of the catheter should be above the right atrium for fluid administration).

STEP 13. Connect the catheter to the intravenous tubing.

STEP 14. Affix the catheter securely to the skin (with a suture), apply antibiotic ointment, and dress the area.

STEP 15. Tape the intravenous tubing in place.

STEP 16. Obtain a chest x-ray film to confirm the position of the intravenous line and identify a possible pneumothorax.

▶ Skill IV-D: Internal Jugular Venipuncture: Middle or Central Route

Note: Internal jugular catheterization is frequently difficult in injured patients because of the immobilization necessary to protect the patient's cervical spinal cord. Sterile technique should be used when performing this procedure.

STEP 1. Place the patient in the supine position, with the head at least 15 degrees down to distend the neck veins and prevent an air embolism. Only if the cervical spine has been cleared radiographically can the patient's head be turned away from the venipuncture site.

STEP 2. Cleanse the skin around the venipuncture site well and drape the area.

STEP 3. If the patient is awake, use a local anesthetic at the venipuncture site.

STEP 4. Introduce a large-caliber needle, attached to a 12-mL syringe with 0.5 to 1 mL of saline, into the center of the triangle formed by the two lower heads of the sternomastoid and the clavicle. Ultrasound can be used as an adjunct for the placement of central venous lines.

STEP 5. After the skin has been punctured, with the bevel of the needle upward, expel the skin plug that can occlude the needle.

STEP 6. Direct the needle caudally, parallel to the sagittal plane, at an angle 30 degrees posterior to the frontal plane.

STEP 7. Slowly advance the needle while gently withdrawing the plunger of the syringe.

STEP 8. When a free flow of blood appears in the syringe, remove the syringe and occlude the needle with a finger to prevent air embolism. If the vein is not entered, withdraw the needle and redirect it 5 to 10 degrees laterally.

STEP 9. Insert the guidewire while monitoring the ECG for rhythm abnormalities.

STEP 10. Remove the needle while securing the guidewire and advance the catheter over the wire. Connect the catheter to the intravenous tubing.

STEP 11. Affix the catheter in place to the skin (with suture), apply antibiotic ointment, and dress the area.

STEP 12. Tape the intravenous tubing in place.

STEP 13. Obtain a chest film to confirm the position of the intravenous line and identify a possible pneumothorax.

▶▶ **COMPLICATIONS OF CENTRAL VENOUS PUNCTURE**

- Pneumothorax or hemothorax
- Venous thrombosis
- Arterial or neurologic injury
- Arteriovenous fistula
- Chylothorax
- Infection
- Air embolism

▶ Skill IV-E: Intraosseous Puncture/Infusion: Proximal Tibial Route
(See Figure IV-2)

Note: Sterile technique should be used when performing this procedure.

The procedure described here is appropriate for children 6 years of age or younger for whom venous access is impossible because of circulatory collapse or for whom percutaneous peripheral venous cannulation has failed on two attempts. Intraosseous infusions should be limited to emergency resuscitation of the child and discontinued as soon as other venous access has been obtained. (Techniques for intraosseous infusion in adults are not discussed here. See references in the bibliography for Chapter 3: Shock for further information.)

Methylene blue dye can be mixed with the saline or water for demonstration purposes on chicken or turkey bones only. When the needle is properly placed within the medullary canal, the methylene blue dye/saline solution seeps from the upper end of the chicken or turkey bone when the solution is injected (see Step 8).

STEP 1. Place the patient in the supine position. Select an uninjured lower extremity, place sufficient padding under the knee to effect an approximate 30-degree flexion of the knee, and allow the patient's heel to rest comfortably on the gurney (stretcher).

STEP 2. Identify the puncture site—the anteromedial surface of the proximal tibia, approximately one fingerbreadth (1 to 3 cm) below the tubercle.

STEP 3. Cleanse the skin around the puncture site well and drape the area.

STEP 4. If the patient is awake, use a local anesthetic at the puncture site.

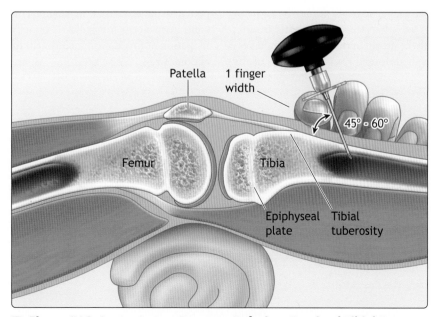

■ **Figure IV-2 Intraosseous Puncture/Infusion: Proximal Tibial Route.**

STEP 5. Initially at a 90-degree angle, introduce a short (threaded or smooth), large-caliber, bone-marrow aspiration needle (or a short, 18-gauge spinal needle with stylet) into the skin and periosteum with the needle bevel directed toward the foot and away from the epiphyseal plate.

STEP 6. After gaining purchase in the bone, direct the needle 45 to 60 degrees away from the epiphyseal plate. Using a gentle twisting or boring motion, advance the needle through the bone cortex and into the bone marrow.

STEP 7. Remove the stylet and attach to the needle a 12-mL syringe with approximately 6 mL of sterile saline. Gently draw on the plunger of the syringe. Aspiration of bone marrow into the syringe signifies entrance into the medullary cavity.

STEP 8. Inject the saline into the needle to expel any clot that can occlude the needle. If the saline flushes through the needle easily and there is no evidence of swelling, the needle is likely in the appropriate place. If bone marrow was not aspirated as outlined in Step 7, but the needle flushes easily when injecting the saline and there is no evidence of swelling, the needle is likely in the appropriate place. In addition, proper placement of the needle is indicated if the needle remains upright without support and intravenous solution flows freely without evidence of subcutaneous infiltration.

STEP 9. Connect the needle to the large-caliber intravenous tubing and begin fluid infusion. Carefully screw the needle further into the medullary cavity until the needle hub rests on the patient's skin and free flow continues. If a smooth needle is used, it should be stabilized at a 45- to 60-degree angle to the anteromedial surface of the child's leg.

STEP 10. Apply antibiotic ointment and a 3-×-3 sterile dressing. Secure the needle and tubing in place.

STEP 11. Routinely reevaluate the placement of the intraosseous needle, ensuring that it remains through the bone cortex and in the medullary canal. Remember, intraosseous infusion should be limited to emergency resuscitation of the child and discontinued as soon as other venous access has been obtained.

▸▸ COMPLICATIONS OF INTRAOSSEOUS PUNCTURE

- Infection
- Through-and-through penetration of the bone
- Subcutaneous or subperiosteal infiltration
- Pressure necrosis of the skin
- Physeal plate injury
- Hematoma

▸ Skill IV-F: Broselow™ Pediatric Emergency Tape

A specific skill is not outlined for the Broselow™ Emergency Tape. However, participants need to be aware of its availability and its use when treating pediatric trauma patients. By measuring the height of the child, the child's estimated weight can be determined readily. One side of the tape provides drugs and their recommended doses for the pediatric patient based on weight. The other side stipulates equipment needs for pediatric patients based on size. Participation at this station includes an orientation to the tape and its use.

▶ SCENARIOS

SCENARIO IV-1

A 42-year-old woman was ejected from a vehicle during an automobile collision. En route to the ED, prehospital personnel report that her heart rate is 110 beats/min, her blood pressure is 88/46 mm Hg, and her respiratory rate is 30 breaths/min. The patient is confused, and her peripheral capillary refill is reduced. (See Table IV-1.) Her airway is patent. She is in respiratory distress with neck vein distention, absent breath sounds on the right and tracheal deviation to the left.

SCENARIO IV-2 (continuation of previous scenario)

After needle decompression and chest-tube insertion, the patient's heart rate is 120 beats/min, the blood pressure is 80/46 mm Hg, and the respiratory rate is 30 breaths/min. Her skin is pale, cool, and moist to touch. She moans when stimulated. (See Table IV-2.)

SCENARIO IV-3 (continuation of previous scenario)

After the initiation of vascular access and infusion of 2000 mL of warmed crystalloid solution, the patient's heart rate has decreased to 90 beats/min; the blood pressure is 110/80 mm Hg and the respiratory rate is 22 breaths/min. The patient is now able to speak, her breathing is less labored, and her peripheral perfusion has improved. (See Table IV-2.)

SCENARIO IV-4 (continuation of previous scenario)

The patient responds initially to the rapid infusion of 1500 mL of warmed crystalloid solution by a transient increase in blood pressure to 110/80 mm Hg, a decrease in the heart rate to 96 beats/min, and improvements in level of consciousness and peripheral perfusion. Fluid infusion is slowed to maintenance levels. Five minutes later, the assistant reports a deterioration in the blood pressure to 88/60 mm Hg, an

TABLE IV-1 ■ **Initial Assessment and Shock Management**

CONDITION	ASSESSMENT (PHYSICAL EXAMINATION)	MANAGEMENT
Tension pneumothorax	• Tracheal deviation • Distended neck veins • Tympany • Absent breath sounds	• Needle decompression • Tube thoracostomy
Massive hemothorax	• Tracheal deviation • Flat neck veins • Percussion dullness • Absent breath sounds	• Venous access • Volume replacement • Surgical consultation/thoracotomy • Tube thoracostomy
Cardiac tamponade	• Distended neck veins • Muffled heart tones • Ultrasound	• Venous access • Volume replacement • Pericardiotomy • Thoracotomy • Pericardiocentesis
Intraabdominal hemorrhage	• Distended abdomen • Uterine lift, if pregnant • DPL/ultrasonography • Vaginal examination	• Venous access • Volume replacement • Surgical consultation • Displace uterus from vena cava
Obvious external bleeding	• Identify source of obvious external bleeding	• Direct pressure • Splints • Closure of actively bleeding scalp wounds

TABLE IV-2 ■ Pelvic Fractures

CONDITION	IMAGE FINDINGS	SIGNIFICANCE	INTERVENTION
Pelvic fracture	**Pelvic x-ray** • Pubic ramus fracture • Open book • Vertical shear	• Less blood loss than other types • Lateral compression mechanism • Pelvic volume increased • Major source of blood loss • Major source of blood loss	• Volume replacement • Probable transfusion • Decreased pelvic volume • Internal hip rotation • PASG • External fixator • Angiography • Skeletal traction • Orthopedic consultation
Visceral organ injury	**CT scan** • Intraabdominal hemorrhage	• Potential for continuing blood loss • Performed only in hemodynamically normal patients	• Volume replacement • Possible transfusion • Surgical consultation

increase in the heart rate to 115 beats/min, and a return in the delay of the peripheral capillary refill. (See Table IV-3.)

Alternative Scenario: The rapid infusion of 2000 mL of warmed crystalloid solution produces only a modest increase in the patient's blood pressure to 90/60 mm Hg, and her heart rate remains at 110 beats/min. Her urinary output since the insertion of the urinary catheter has been only 5 mL of very dark urine.

SCENARIO IV-5

A 42-year-old woman, ejected from her vehicle during a crash, arrives in the ED unconscious with a heart rate of 140 beats/min, a blood pressure of 60 mm Hg by palpation, and pale, cool, and pulseless extremities. Endotracheal intubation and assisted ventilation are initiated. The rapid volume infusion of 2000 mL of warmed crystalloid solution does not improve her vital signs, and she does not demonstrate evidence of improved organ perfusion. (See Table IV-4.)

SCENARIO IV-6

An 18-month-old boy is brought to the ED by his mother, who apparently experiences spousal abuse. The child has evidence of multiple soft-tissue injuries about the chest, abdomen, and extremities. His skin color is pale, he has a weak, thready pulse rate of 160 beats/min, and he responds only to painful stimuli with a weak cry.

TABLE IV-3 ■ Transient Responder

CAUSE	PHYSICAL EXAM	ADDITIONAL DIAGNOSTIC STEPS	INTERVENTION
Underestimation of blood loss or continuing blood loss	• Abdominal distention • Pelvic fracture • Extremity fracture • Obvious external bleeding	• DPL or ultrasonography	• Surgical consultation • Volume infusion • Blood transfusion • Apply appropriate splints
Nonhemorrhagic • Cardiac tamponade • Recurrent/persistent tension pneumothorax	• Distended neck veins • Decreased heart sounds • Normal breath sounds • Distended neck veins • Tracheal shift • Absent breath sounds • Hyperresonant chest percussion	• Echocardiogram • FAST • Pericardiocentesis • Clinical diagnosis	• Thoracotomy • Reevaluate chest • Needle decompression • Tube thoracostomy

TABLE IV-4 ■ Nonresponder

CAUSE	PHYSICAL EXAM	ADDITIONAL DIAGNOSTIC STEPS	INTERVENTION
Massive blood loss (Class III or IV) • Intraabdominal bleeding	• Abdominal distention	• DPL or ultrasonography	• Immediate intervention by surgeon • Volume restoration • Operative resuscitation
Nonhemorrhagic • Tension pneumothorax	• Distended neck veins • Tracheal shift • Absent breath sounds • Hyperresonant chest percussion	• Clinical diagnosis	• Reevaluate chest • Needle decompression • Tube thoracotomy
• Cardiac tamponade	• Distended neck veins • Decreased heart sounds • Normal breath sounds	• Echocardiogram • FAST • Pericardiocentesis	• Thoracotomy
• Blunt cardiac injury	• Irregular heart rate • Inadequate perfusion	• Ischemic ECG changes • Echocardiogram	• Prepare for OR • Invasive monitoring • Inotropic support • Consider operative intervention • Invasive monitoring may be required

Venous Cutdown (Optional Station)

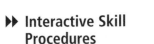

▶▶ **Interactive Skill Procedures**

Note: **Standard precautions are required when caring for trauma patients.**

THE FOLLOWING PROCEDURE IS INCLUDED IN THIS SKILL STATION:

▶▶ **Skill V-A: Venous Cutdown**

Performance at this skill station will allow the participant to practice and demonstrate on a live, anesthetized animal or a fresh, human cadaver the technique of peripheral venous cutdown. Specifically, the student will be able to:

OBJECTIVES

1 Identify and describe the surface markings and structures to be noted in performing a peripheral venous cutdown.

2 Describe the indications and contraindications for a peripheral venous cutdown.

ANATOMIC CONSIDERATIONS FOR VENOUS CUTDOWN

3 The primary site for a peripheral venous cutdown is the greater saphenous vein at the ankle, which is located at a point approximately 2 cm anterior and superior to the medial malleolus. (See Figure V-1.)

4 A secondary site is the antecubital medial basilic vein, located 2.5 cm lateral to the medial epicondyle of the humerus at the flexion crease of the elbow.

▶ Skill V-A: Venous Cutdown
(See Figure V-1)

STEP 1. Prepare the skin of the ankle with antiseptic solution and drape the area.

STEP 2. Infiltrate the skin over the vein with 0.5% lidocaine.

STEP 3. Make a full-thickness, transverse skin incision through the anesthetized area to a length of 2.5 cm.

STEP 4. By blunt dissection, using a curved hemostat, identify the vein and dissect it free from any accompanying structures.

STEP 5. Elevate and dissect the vein for a distance of approximately 2 cm to free it from its bed.

STEP 6. Ligate the distal mobilized vein, leaving the suture in place for traction.

STEP 7. Pass a tie around the vein in a cephalad direction.

STEP 8. Make a small, transverse venotomy and gently dilate the venotomy with the tip of a closed hemostat.

STEP 9. Introduce a plastic cannula through the venotomy and secure it in place by tying the upper ligature around the vein and cannula. The cannula should be inserted an adequate distance to prevent dislodging.

STEP 10. Attach the intravenous tubing to the cannula and close the incision with interrupted sutures.

STEP 11. Apply a sterile dressing with a topical antibiotic ointment.

▶▶ COMPLICATIONS OF PERIPHERAL VENOUS CUTDOWN

- Cellulitis
- Hematoma
- Phlebitis
- Perforation of the posterior wall of the vein
- Venous thrombosis
- Nerve transaction
- Arterial transaction

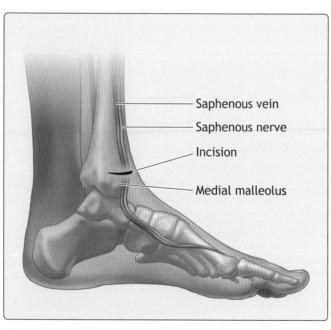
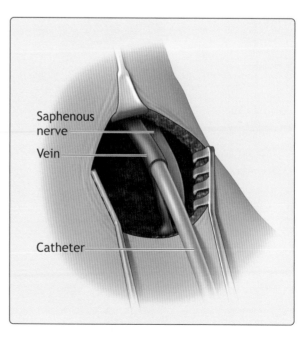

■ Figure V-1 Venous Cutdown

CHAPTER **4** **Thoracic Trauma**

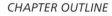

CHAPTER OUTLINE

Objectives

Introduction

Primary Survey: Life-Threatening Injuries
Airway
Breathing
Circulation

Resuscitative Thoracotomy

Secondary Survey: Potentially Life-Threatening Chest Injuries
Simple Pneumothorax
Hemothorax
Pulmonary Contusion
Tracheobronchial Tree Injury
Blunt Cardiac Injury
Traumatic Aortic Disruption
Traumatic Diaphragmatic Injury
Blunt Esophageal Rupture

Other Manifestations of Chest Injuries
Subcutaneous Emphysema
Crushing Injury to the Chest (Traumatic Asphyxia)
Rib, Sternum, and Scapular Fractures

Other Indications for Chest Tube Insertion

Chapter Summary

Bibliography

Upon completion of this topic, the student will identify and initiate treatment of common and life-threatening thoracic injuries. Specifically, the doctor will be able to:

OBJECTIVES

1 Identify and initiate treatment of the following injuries during the primary survey:

Airway obstruction

Tension pneumothorax

Open pneumothorax

Flail chest and pulmonary contusion

Massive hemothorax

Cardiac tamponade

2 Identify and initiate treatment of the following potentially life-threatening injuries during the secondary survey:

Simple pneumothorax

Hemothorax

Pulmonary contusion

Tracheobronchial tree injury

Blunt cardiac injury

Traumatic aortic disruption

Traumatic diaphragmatic injury

Blunt esophageal rupture

3 Describe the significance and treatment of subcutaneous emphysema, thoracic crush injuries, and sternal, rib, and clavicular fractures.

Introduction

? What life-threatening chest injuries should I recognize as causing major pathophysiologic events?

Thoracic trauma is a significant cause of mortality. Many patients with thoracic trauma die after reaching the hospital, yet many of these deaths could be prevented with prompt diagnosis and treatment. Less than 10% of blunt chest injuries and only 15% to 30% of penetrating chest injuries require thoracotomy. Most patients who sustain thoracic trauma can be treated by technical procedures within the capabilities of doctors who take this course. It is important to remember that iatrogenic thoracic injuries are common (eg, hemothorax or pneumothorax with central line placement and esophageal injury during endoscopy).

Hypoxia, hypercarbia, and acidosis often result from chest injuries. Tissue hypoxia results from inadequate delivery of oxygen to the tissues because of hypovolemia (blood loss), pulmonary ventilation/perfusion mismatch (eg, contusion, hematoma, and alveolar collapse), and changes in intrathoracic pressure relationships (eg, tension pneumothorax and open pneumothorax). Hypercarbia most often results from inadequate ventilation caused by changes in intrathoracic pressure relationships and depressed level of consciousness. Metabolic acidosis is caused by hypoperfusion of the tissues (shock).

Initial assessment and treatment of patients with thoracic trauma consists of the primary survey, resuscitation of vital functions, detailed secondary survey, and definitive care. Because hypoxia is the most serious feature of chest injury, the goal of early intervention is to prevent or correct hypoxia. Injuries that are an immediate threat to life are treated as quickly and simply as is possible. Most life-threatening thoracic injuries are treated by airway control or an appropriately placed chest tube or needle. The secondary survey is influenced by the history of the injury and a high index of suspicion for specific injuries.

Primary Survey: Life-Threatening Injuries

? What are the significant patho-physiologic effects of chest injury that I should identify in the primary survey, and when and how do I correct them?

The primary survey of patients with thoracic injuries begins with the airway. **Major problems should be corrected as they are identified.**

AIRWAY

It is necessary to recognize and address major injuries affecting the airway during the primary survey. Airway patency and air exchange should be assessed by listening for air movement at the patient's nose, mouth, and lung fields; inspecting the oropharynx for foreign-body obstruction; and observing for intercostal and supraclavicular muscle retractions.

Laryngeal injury can accompany major thoracic trauma. Although the clinical presentation is occasionally subtle, acute airway obstruction from laryngeal trauma is a life-threatening injury. ▪ See Chapter 2: Airway and Ventilatory Management.

Injury to the upper chest can create a palpable defect in the region of the sternoclavicular joint with posterior dislocation of the clavicular head, causing upper airway obstruction. Identification of this injury is made by observation of upper airway obstruction (stridor) or a marked change in the expected voice quality (if the patient is able to talk). Management consists of a closed reduction of the injury, which can be performed by extending the shoulders or grasping the clavicle with a pointed clamp, such as a towel clip, and manually reducing the fracture. This injury, once reduced, usually is stable if the patient is in the supine position.

▪ Other injuries affecting the airway are addressed in Chapter 2: Airway and Ventilatory Management.

BREATHING

The patient's chest and neck should be completely exposed to allow for assessment of breathing and the neck veins. Respiratory movement and quality of respirations are assessed by observing, palpating, and listening.

Important, yet often subtle, signs of chest injury or hypoxia include an increased respiratory rate and change in the breathing pattern, especially progressively more shallow respirations. Cyanosis is a late sign of hypoxia in trauma patients. However, the absence of cyanosis does not necessarily indicate adequate tissue oxygenation or an adequate airway. The major thoracic injuries that affect breathing and that must be recognized and addressed during the primary survey include tension pneumothorax, open pneumothorax (sucking chest wound), flail chest and pulmonary contusion, and massive hemothorax.

PITFALL

After intubation, one of the common reasons for loss of breath sounds in the left thorax is a right mainstem intubation. During the reassessment, be sure to check the position of the endotracheal tube before assuming that the change in physical examination results is due to a pneumothorax or hemothorax.

Tension Pneumothorax

A tension pneumothorax develops when a "one-way valve" air leak occurs from the lung or through the chest wall (Figure 4-1). Air is forced into the thoracic cavity without any means of escape, completely collapsing the affected lung. The mediastinum is displaced to the opposite side, decreasing venous return and compressing the opposite lung.

The most common cause of tension pneumothorax is mechanical ventilation with positive-pressure ventilation in patients with visceral pleural injury. However, a tension pneumothorax may complicate a simple pneumothorax following penetrating or blunt chest trauma in which a parenchymal lung injury fails to seal, or after a misguided attempt at subclavian or internal jugular venous catheter insertion. Occasionally, traumatic defects in the chest wall also may cause a tension pneumothorax if incorrectly covered with occlusive dressings or if the defect itself constitutes a flap-valve mechanism. Tension pneumothorax also may occur from markedly displaced thoracic spine fractures.

Tension pneumothorax is a clinical diagnosis reflecting air under pressure in the pleural space. Treatment should not be delayed to wait for radiologic confirmation. Tension pneumothorax is characterized by some or all of the following signs and symptoms: chest pain, air hunger, respiratory distress, tachycardia, hypotension, tracheal deviation, unilateral absence of breath sounds, neck vein distention, and cyanosis (late manifestation). Because of the similarity in their signs, tension pneumothorax may be confused initially with cardiac tamponade. Differentiation can be made by a hyperresonant note on percussion and absent breath sounds over the affected hemithorax.

Tension pneumothorax requires immediate decompression and is managed initially by rapidly inserting a large-caliber needle into the second intercostal space in the midclavicular line of the affected hemithorax (Figure 4-2). ▟ See Skill Station VII: Chest Trauma Management, Skill VII-A: Needle Thoracentesis. This maneuver converts the injury to a simple pneumothorax; however, the possibility of subsequent pneumothorax as a result of the needle stick now exists. Repeated reassessment of the patient is necessary. Definitive treatment usually requires only the insertion of a chest tube into the fifth intercostal space (usually the nipple level), just anterior to the midaxillary line.

Open Pneumothorax (Sucking Chest Wound)

Large defects of the chest wall that remain open may result in an open pneumothorax, or sucking chest wound (Figure 4-3). Equilibration between intrathoracic pressure and atmospheric pressure is immediate. If the opening in the chest wall is approximately two-thirds the diameter of the trachea, air passes preferentially through the chest wall defect with each respiratory effort, because air tends to follow the path of least resistance. Effective ventilation is thereby impaired, leading to hypoxia and hypercarbia.

Initial management of an open pneumothorax is accomplished by promptly closing the defect with a sterile occlusive dressing. The dressing should be large enough to overlap the wound's edges and then taped securely on three sides in order to provide a flutter-type valve effect (Figure 4-4). As the patient breathes in, the dressing occludes the wound, preventing air from entering. During exhalation, the open end of the dressing allows air to escape from the pleural space. A chest tube remote from the wound should be placed as soon as possible. Securely taping all edges of

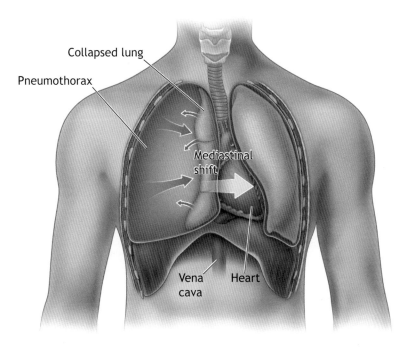

Collapsed lung

Pneumothorax

Mediastinal shift

Vena cava   Heart

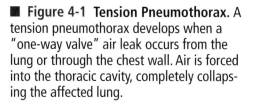

■ **Figure 4-1 Tension Pneumothorax.** A tension pneumothorax develops when a "one-way valve" air leak occurs from the lung or through the chest wall. Air is forced into the thoracic cavity, completely collapsing the affected lung.

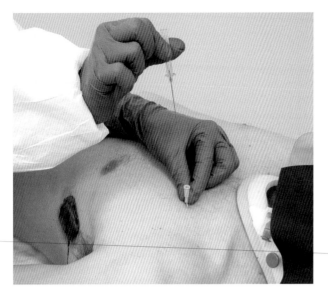

■ **Figure 4-2 Needle Decompression.** Tension pneumothorax is managed initially by rapidly inserting a large-caliber needle into the second intercostal space in the midclavicular line of the affected hemithorax.

the dressing may cause air to accumulate in the thoracic cavity, resulting in a tension pneumothorax unless a chest tube is in place. Any occlusive dressing (eg, plastic wrap or petrolatum gauze) may be used as a temporary measure so that rapid assessment can continue. Definitive surgical clo-

sure of the defect is frequently required. See Skill Station VII: Chest Trauma Management, Skill VII-B: Chest Tube Insertion.

Flail Chest and Pulmonary Contusion

A flail chest occurs when a segment of the chest wall does not have bony continuity with the rest of the thoracic cage (Figure 4-5). This condition usually results from trauma associated with multiple rib fractures—that is, two or more ribs fractured in two or more places. The presence of a flail chest segment results in severe disruption of normal chest wall movement. If the injury to the underlying lung is significant, serious hypoxia may result. The major difficulty in flail chest stems from the injury to the underlying lung (pulmonary contusion). Although chest wall instability leads to paradoxical motion of the chest wall during inspiration and expiration, this defect alone does not cause hypoxia. Restricted chest wall movement associated with pain and underlying lung injury are important causes of hypoxia.

Flail chest may not be apparent initially because of splinting of the chest wall. The patient moves air poorly, and movement of the thorax is asymmetrical and uncoordinated. Palpation of abnormal respiratory motion and crepitation of rib or cartilage fractures aid the diagnosis. A satisfactory chest x-ray film may suggest multiple rib fractures, but may not show costochondral separation. Arterial blood gas (ABG) analyses that suggest respiratory failure with hypoxia also may aid in diagnosing a flail chest.

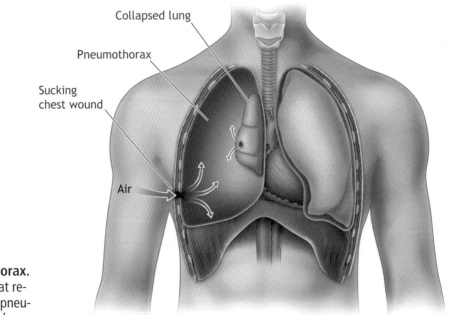

■ **Figure 4-3 Open Pneumothorax.** Large defects of the chest wall that remain open may result in an open pneumothorax, or sucking chest wound.

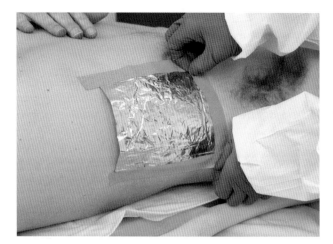

■ **Figure 4-4 Dressing for Treatment of Open Pneumothorax.** Promptly close the defect with a sterile occlusive dressing that is large enough to overlap the wound's edges. Tape it securely on three sides to provide a flutter-type valve effect.

achieved by using intravenous narcotics or various methods of local anesthetic administration that avoid the potential respiratory depression seen with systemic narcotics. The choices for administration of local anesthetics include intermittent intercostal nerve block(s) and intrapleural, extrapleural, or epidural anesthesia. When used properly, local anesthetic agents may provide excellent analgesia and avoid the need for intubation. However, prevention of hypoxia is of paramount importance for trauma patients, and a short period of intubation and ventilation may be necessary until diagnosis of the entire injury pattern is complete. A careful assessment of the respiratory rate, arterial oxygen tension, and the work of breathing will indicate appropriate timing for intubation and ventilation.

Massive Hemothorax

Accumulation of blood and fluid in a hemithorax may significantly compromise respiratory efforts by compressing the lung and preventing adequate ventilation. Such massive

Initial therapy includes adequate ventilation, administration of humidified oxygen, and fluid resuscitation. In the absence of systemic hypotension, the administration of crystalloid intravenous solutions should be carefully controlled to prevent overhydration.

The definitive treatment is to ensure oxygenation as completely as possible, administer fluids judiciously, and provide analgesia to improve ventilation. This can be

PITFALL

Both tension pneumothorax and massive hemothorax are associated with decreased breath sounds on auscultation. Differentiation on physical examination is made by percussion; hyperresonance confirms a pneumothorax, whereas dullness confirms a massive hemothorax.

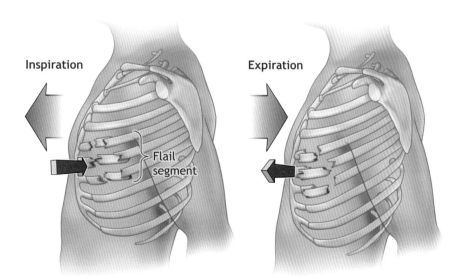

■ **Figure 4-5 Flail Chest.** The presence of a flail chest segment results in severe disruption of normal chest wall movement. If the injury to the underlying lung is significant, serious hypoxia may result.

acute accumulations of blood more dramatically present as hypotension and shock, and are discussed further below.

CIRCULATION

The patient's pulse should be assessed for quality, rate, and regularity. In patients with hypovolemia, the radial and dorsalis pedis pulses may be absent because of volume depletion. Blood pressure and pulse pressure is measured and the peripheral circulation assessed by observing and palpating the skin for color and temperature. Neck veins should be assessed for distention, remembering that neck veins may not be distended in patients with hypovolemia and cardiac tamponade, tension pneumothorax, or traumatic diaphragmatic injury.

A cardiac monitor and pulse oximeter should be attached to the patient. Patients who sustain thoracic trauma—especially in the area of the sternum or from a rapid deceleration injury—are susceptible to myocardial injury, which may lead to dysrhythmias. Hypoxia and acidosis enhance this possibility. Dysrhythmias should be managed according to standard protocols. Pulseless electric activity (PEA) is manifested by an ECG that shows a rhythm while the patient has no identifiable pulse. PEA may be present in cardiac tamponade, tension pneumothorax, profound hypovolemia, and cardiac rupture.

The major thoracic injuries that affect circulation and should be recognized and addressed during the primary survey include massive hemothorax and cardiac tamponade.

Massive Hemothorax

Massive hemothorax results from the rapid accumulation of more than 1500 mL of blood or one-third or more of the patient's blood volume in the chest cavity (Figure 4-6). It is most commonly caused by a penetrating wound that disrupts the systemic or hilar vessels. Massive hemothorax also may result from blunt trauma.

Blood loss is complicated by hypoxia. The neck veins may be flat as a result of severe hypovolemia, or they may be distended if there is an associated tension pneumothorax. However, rarely will the mechanical effects of massive intrathoracic blood shift the mediastinum enough to cause distended neck veins. A massive hemothorax is discovered when shock is associated with the absence of breath sounds or dullness to percussion on one side of the chest.

Massive hemothorax is initially managed by the simultaneous restoration of blood volume and decompression of the chest cavity. Large-caliber intravenous lines and a rapid crystalloid infusion are begun, and type-specific blood is administered as soon as possible. Blood from the chest tube should be collected in a device suitable for autotransfusion. A single chest tube (#38 French) is inserted, usually at the nipple level, just anterior to the midaxillary line, and rapid restoration of volume continues as decompression of the chest cavity is completed. When massive hemothorax is suspected, prepare for autotransfusion. If 1500 mL is immediately evacuated, it is highly likely that an early thoracotomy will be required.

Some patients who have an initial volume output of less than 1500 mL but continue to bleed may require a thoracotomy. This decision is based not on the rate of continuing blood loss (200 mL/hr for 2 to 4 hr), but on the patient's physiologic status. A persistent need for blood transfusions is an indication for thoracotomy. During patient resuscitation, the volume of blood initially drained from the chest

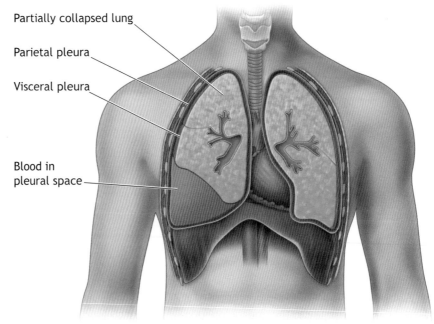

Partially collapsed lung

Parietal pleura

Visceral pleura

Blood in pleural space

■ **Figure 4-6 Massive Hemothorax.** This condition results from the rapid accumulation of more than 1500 mL of blood or one-third or more of the patient's blood volume in the chest cavity.

tube and the rate of continuing blood loss must be factored into the amount of intravenous fluid required for replacement. The color of the blood (indicating an arterial or venous source) is a poor indicator of the necessity for thoracotomy.

Penetrating anterior chest wounds medial to the nipple line and posterior wounds medial to the scapula should alert the doctor to the possible need for thoracotomy, because of the likelihood of damage to the great vessels, hilar structures, and the heart, with the associated potential for cardiac tamponade. **Thoracotomy is not indicated unless a surgeon, qualified by training and experience, is present.**

Cardiac Tamponade

Cardiac tamponade most commonly results from penetrating injuries. However, blunt injury also may cause the pericardium to fill with blood from the heart, great vessels, or pericardial vessels (Figure 4-7). The human pericardial sac is a fixed fibrous structure; only a relatively small amount of blood is required to restrict cardiac activity and interfere with cardiac filling. Cardiac tamponade may develop slowly, allowing for a more leisurely evaluation, or may occur rapidly, requiring rapid diagnosis and treatment. The diagnosis of cardiac tamponade can be difficult.

The classic diagnostic Beck's triad consists of venous pressure elevation, decline in arterial pressure, and muffled heart tones. However, muffled heart tones are difficult to assess in the noisy emergency department, and distended neck veins may be absent due to hypovolemia. Additionally, tension pneumothorax, particularly on the left side, may mimic cardiac tamponade. Kussmaul's sign (a rise in venous pressure with inspiration when breathing spontaneously) is a true paradoxical venous pressure abnormality associated with tamponade. PEA is suggestive of cardiac tamponade, but has other causes, as listed above. Insertion of a central venous line with measurement of central venous pressure (CVP) may aid diagnosis, but CVP can be elevated for a variety of reasons.

Diagnostic methods include echocardiogram, focused assessment sonogram in trauma (FAST), or pericardial window. Prompt transthoracic ultrasound (echocardiogram) may be a valuable noninvasive method of assessing the pericardium, but reports suggest it has a significant false-negative rate of about 5% to 10%. In hemodynamically abnormal patients with blunt trauma, provided it does **not** delay patient resuscitation, an examination of the pericardial sac for the presence of fluid may be obtained as part of a focused abdominal ultrasound examination performed by properly trained and credentialed surgical team in the emergency department. FAST is a rapid and accurate method of imaging the heart and pericardium. It may be 90% accurate for the presence of pericardial fluid for the experienced operator. ◾ See Chapter 5: Abdominal and Pelvic Trauma.

Prompt diagnosis and evacuation of pericardial blood is indicated for patients who do not respond to the usual

Normal   Pericardial tamponade

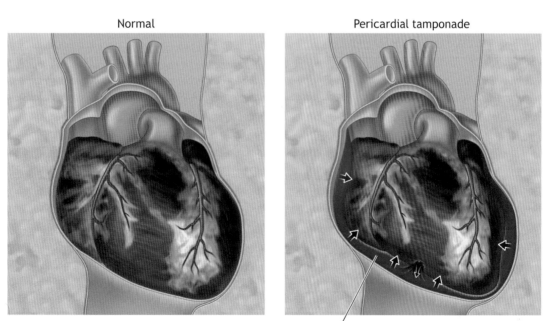

Pericardial sac

■ **Figure 4-7 Cardiac Tamponade.** Cardiac tamponade results from penetrating or blunt injuries that cause the pericardium to fill with blood from the heart, great vessels, or pericardial vessels.

measures of resuscitation for hemorrhagic shock and have the potential for cardiac tamponade. If a qualified surgeon is present, surgery should be performed to relieve the tamponade. This is best performed in the operating room if the patient's condition allows. **If surgical intervention is not available, pericardiocentesis can be diagnostic as well as therapeutic, but is not definitive treatment for cardiac tamponade.** ◾ For further information regarding FAST, see Chapter 5: Abdominal and Pelvic Trauma.

Although cardiac tamponade may be strongly suspected, the initial administration of intravenous fluid raises the venous pressure and improves cardiac output transiently while preparations are made for surgery. If subxyphoid pericardiocentesis is used as a temporizing maneuver the use of a plastic-sheathed needle or the Seldinger technique for insertion of a flexible catheter is ideal, but the urgent priority is to aspirate blood from the pericardial sac. If ultrasound imaging is available, it can facilitate accurate insertion of the needle into the pericardial space. Because of the self-sealing qualities of the injured myocardium, aspiration of pericardial blood alone may relieve symptoms temporarily. However, all patients with acute tamponade and positive pericardiocentesis will require surgery for examination of the heart and repair of the injury. Pericardiocentesis may not be diagnostic or therapeutic when the blood in the pericardial sac has clotted. Preparations for transfer of these patients to an appropriate facility for definitive care are necessary. Pericardiotomy via thoracotomy is indicated *only* when a qualified surgeon is available.

Resuscitative Thoracotomy

Closed heart massage for cardiac arrest or PEA is ineffective in patients with hypovolemia. Patients with *penetrating* thoracic injuries who arrive pulseless, but with myocardial electrical activity, may be candidates for immediate resuscitative thoracotomy. **A qualified surgeon must be present at the time of the patient's arrival to determine the need and potential for success of a resuscitative thoracotomy in the ED.** Restoration of intravascular volume is continued, and endotracheal intubation and mechanical ventilation are essential.

A patient who has sustained a penetrating wound and required CPR in the prehospital setting should be evaluated for any signs of life. If there are none, and no cardiac electrical activity is present, no further resuscitative effort should be made. Patients who sustain blunt injuries and arrive pulseless but with myocardial electrical activity (PEA) are not candidates for emergency department resuscitative thoracotomy. Signs of life include reactive pupils, spontaneous movement, or organized ECG activity.

The therapeutic maneuvers that can be effectively accomplished with a resuscitative thoracotomy are:

- evacuation of pericardial blood causing tamponade
- direct control of exsanguinating intrathoracic hemorrhage
- open cardiac massage
- cross-clamping of the descending aorta to slow blood loss below the diaphragm and increase perfusion to the brain and heart

Despite the value of these maneuvers, multiple reports confirm that thoracotomy in the ED for patients with blunt trauma and cardiac arrest is rarely effective.

Once these and other immediately life-threatening injuries have been treated, attention may be directed to the secondary survey.

Secondary Survey: Potentially Life-Threatening Chest Injuries

What adjunctive tests are used during the secondary survey to allow complete evaluation for potentially life-threatening thoracic injuries?

The secondary survey involves further, in-depth, physical examination, an upright chest x-ray examination if the patient's condition permits, ABG measurements, and pulse oximetry and ECG monitoring. In addition to lung expansion and the presence of fluid, the chest film should be examined for widening of the mediastinum, a shift of the midline, and loss of anatomic detail. Multiple rib fractures and fractures of the first or second rib(s) suggest that a severe force has been delivered to the chest and underlying tissues. ◾ See Skill Station VI: X-Ray Identification of Thoracic Injuries.

The following eight lethal injuries are described below:

- Simple pneumothorax
- Hemothorax
- Pulmonary contusion
- Tracheobronchial tree injury
- Blunt cardiac injury
- Traumatic aortic disruption
- Traumatic diaphragmatic injury
- Blunt esophageal rupture

Unlike immediately life-threatening conditions that are recognized during the primary survey, the injuries listed here usually are not obvious on physical examination. Diagnosis requires a high index of suspicion and appropriate use of adjunctive studies. These injuries are more often missed than diagnosed during the initial posttraumatic period; however, if overlooked, lives can be lost.

SIMPLE PNEUMOTHORAX

Pneumothorax results from air entering the potential space between the visceral and parietal pleura (Figure 4-8). Both penetrating and nonpenetrating trauma can cause this injury. Thoracic spine fracture dislocations also can be associated with a pneumothorax. Lung laceration with air leakage is the most common cause of pneumothorax resulting from blunt trauma.

The thorax is normally completely filled by the lung, being held to the chest wall by surface tension between the pleural surfaces. Air in the pleural space disrupts the cohesive forces between the visceral and parietal pleura, which allows the lung to collapse. A ventilation/perfusion defect occurs because the blood that perfuses the nonventilated area is not oxygenated.

When a pneumothorax is present, breath sounds are decreased on the affected side, and percussion demonstrates hyperresonance. An upright, expiratory x-ray film of the chest aids in the diagnosis.

Any pneumothorax is best treated with a chest tube placed in the fourth or fifth intercostal space, just anterior to the midaxillary line. Observation and aspiration of an asymptomatic pneumothorax may be appropriate, but the choice should be made by a qualified doctor; otherwise, placement of a chest tube should be performed. Once a chest tube is inserted and connected to an underwater seal apparatus with or without suction, a chest x-ray examination is necessary to confirm reexpansion of the lung. Neither general anesthesia nor positive-pressure ventilation should be administered in a patient who has sustained a traumatic pneumothorax or who is at risk for unexpected intraoperative pneumothorax until a chest tube has been inserted. A simple pneumothorax can readily convert to a life-threatening tension pneumothorax, particularly if it is initially unrecognized and positive-pressure ventilation is applied. The patient with a pneumothorax should also undergo chest decompression before he or she is transported via air ambulance.

HEMOTHORAX

The primary cause of hemothorax (<1500 mL blood) is lung laceration or laceration of an intercostal vessel or internal mammary artery due to either penetrating or blunt trauma. Thoracic spine fracture dislocations also may be associated with a hemothorax. Bleeding is usually self-limited and does not require operative intervention.

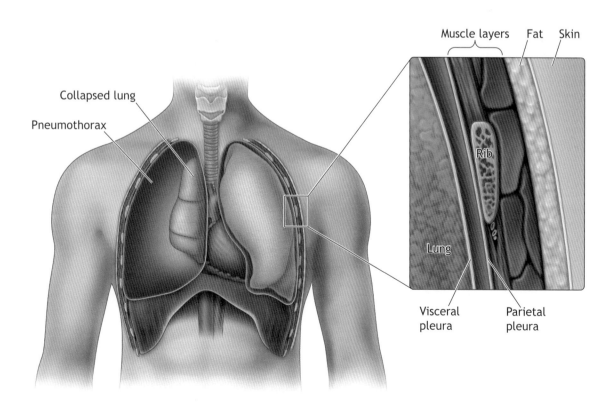

■ **Figure 4-8 Simple Pneumothorax.** Pneumothorax results from air entering the potential space between the visceral and parietal pleura.

PITFALL

A simple pneumothorax in a trauma patient should not be ignored or overlooked. It may progress to a tension pneumothorax.

PITFALL

A simple hemothorax, not fully evacuated, may result in a retained, clotted hemothorax with lung entrapment or, if infected, develop into an empyema.

An acute hemothorax large enough to appear on a chest x-ray film is best treated with a large-caliber (36 French) chest tube. The chest tube evacuates blood, reduces the risk of a clotted hemothorax, and, importantly, provides a method for continuous monitoring of blood loss. Evacuation of blood and fluid also facilitates a more complete assessment of potential diaphragmatic injury. Although many factors are involved in the decision to operate on a patient with a hemothorax, the patient's physiologic status and the volume of blood drainage from the chest tube are major factors. As a guideline, if 1500 mL of blood is obtained immediately through the chest tube, if drainage of more than 200 mL/hr for 2 to 4 hr occurs, or if blood transfusion is required, operative exploration should be considered.

PULMONARY CONTUSION

Pulmonary contusion may occur without rib fractures or flail chest, particularly in young patients without completely ossified ribs. However, pulmonary contusion is the most common potentially lethal chest injury. The resultant respiratory failure can be subtle, and it develops over time, rather than occurring instantaneously. The plan for definitive management may change with time, warranting careful monitoring and reevaluation of the patient.

Patients with significant hypoxia (ie, PaO_2 <65 mm Hg [8.6 kPa] or SaO_2 <90%) on room air *may* require intubation and ventilation within the first hour after injury. Associated medical conditions, such as chronic pulmonary disease and renal failure, increase the necessity of early intubation and mechanical ventilation. Some patients with stable conditions may be treated selectively without endotracheal intubation or mechanical ventilation.

Pulse oximetry monitoring, ABG determinations, ECG monitoring, and appropriate ventilatory equipment are necessary for optimal treatment. Any patient with the aforementioned preexisting conditions who is to be transferred should undergo intubation and ventilation.

TRACHEOBRONCHIAL TREE INJURY

Injury to the trachea or major bronchus is an unusual and potentially fatal condition that is often overlooked on initial assessment. In blunt trauma the majority of such injuries occur within 1 in. (2.54 cm) of the carina. Most patients with this injury die at the scene. Those who reach the hospital alive have a high mortality rate from associated injuries.

If tracheobronchial injury is suspected, immediate surgical consultation is warranted. Such patients typically present with hemoptysis, subcutaneous emphysema, or tension pneumothorax with a mediastinal shift. A pneumothorax associated with a persistent large air leak after tube thoracostomy suggests a tracheobronchial injury. Bronchoscopy confirms the diagnosis of the injury. Placement of more than one chest tube often is necessary to overcome a very large leak and expand the lung. Temporary intubation of the opposite mainstem bronchus may be required to provide adequate oxygenation.

Intubation of patients with tracheobronchial injuries is frequently difficult because of anatomic distortion from paratracheal hematoma, associated oropharyngeal injuries, and/or the tracheobronchial injury itself. For such patients, immediate operative intervention is indicated. In more stable patients, operative treatment of tracheobronchial injuries may be delayed until the acute inflammation and edema resolve.

BLUNT CARDIAC INJURY

Blunt cardiac injury can result in myocardial muscle contusion, cardiac chamber rupture, coronary artery dissection and/or thrombosis, or valvular disruption. Cardiac rupture typically presents with cardiac injury tamponade and should be recognized during the primary survey. However, occasionally the signs and symptoms of tamponade are slow to develop with an atrial rupture. Early use of FAST can facilitate diagnosis.

Patients with myocardial contusion may report chest discomfort, but this symptom is often attributed to chest wall contusion or fractures of the sternum and/or ribs. The true diagnosis of myocardial contusion can be established only by direct inspection of the injured myocardium. The clinically important sequelae of myocardial contusion are

PITFALL

Avoid underestimating the severity of blunt pulmonary injury. Pulmonary contusion may present as a wide spectrum of clinical signs that are often not well correlated with chest x-ray findings. Careful monitoring of ventilation, oxygenation, and fluid status is required, often for several days. With proper management, mechanical ventilation can be avoided.

hypotension, dysrhythmias, or wall-motion abnormality on two-dimensional echocardiography. The electrocardiographic changes are variable and may even indicate frank myocardial infarction. Multiple premature ventricular contractions, unexplained sinus tachycardia, atrial fibrillation, bundle-branch block (usually right), and ST-segment changes are the most common ECG findings. Elevated central venous pressure in the absence of an obvious cause may indicate right ventricular dysfunction secondary to contusion. It also is important to remember that the traumatic event may have been precipitated by a myocardial ischemic episode.

The presence of cardiac troponins may be diagnostic of myocardial infarction. However, their use in diagnosing blunt cardiac injury is inconclusive and offers no additional information beyond that available from ECG. Therefore, they have no role in the evaluation and treatment of patients with blunt cardiac injury.

Patients with a blunt injury to the heart diagnosed by conduction abnormalities are at risk for sudden dysrhythmias and should be monitored for the first 24 hours. After this interval, the risk of a dysrhythmia appears to decrease substantially.

TRAUMATIC AORTIC DISRUPTION

Traumatic aortic rupture is a common cause of sudden death after an automobile collision or fall from a great height (Figure 4-9). For survivors, recovery is frequently possible if aortic rupture is identified and treated immediately.

Patients with aortic rupture, who may potentially survive, tend to have an incomplete laceration near the ligamentum arteriosum of the aorta. Continuity maintained by an intact adventitial layer or contained mediastinal hematoma prevents immediate death. Many surviving patients die in the hospital if left untreated. Some blood can escape into the mediastinum, but one characteristic shared by all survivors is that they have a contained hematoma. Per-

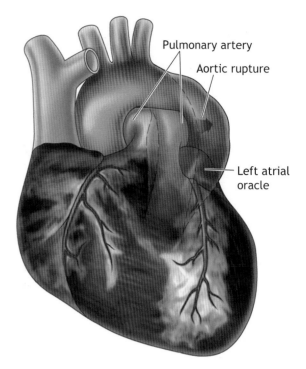

■ Figure 4-9 Aortic Rupture. Traumatic aortic rupture is a common cause of sudden death after an automobile collision or fall from a great height.

sistent or recurrent hypotension is usually due to a separate, unidentified bleeding site. Although free rupture of a transected aorta into the left chest does occur and may cause hypotension, it usually is fatal unless the patient is operated on within a few minutes.

Specific signs and symptoms of traumatic aortic disruption are frequently absent. A high index of suspicion prompted by a history of decelerating force and characteristic findings on chest x-ray films should be maintained, and the patient should be further evaluated. Adjunctive radiologic signs on chest x-ray films, which may or may not be present, indicate the likelihood of major vascular injury in the chest. They include:

- Widened mediastinum

- Obliteration of the aortic knob

- Deviation of the trachea to the right

- Depression of the left mainstem bronchus

- Elevation of the right mainstem bronchus

- Obliteration of the space between the pulmonary artery and the aorta (obscuration of the aortopulmonary window)

- Deviation of the esophagus (nasogastric tube) to the right

- Widened paratracheal stripe

PITFALL

Penetrating objects that traverse the mediastinum may injure the major mediastinal structures, such as the heart, great vessels, tracheobronchial tree, and esophagus. The diagnosis is made when careful examination and a chest x-ray film reveal an entrance wound in one hemithorax and an exit wound or a missile lodged in the contralateral hemithorax. Wounds in which metallic fragments from the missile are in proximity to mediastinal structures also should raise suspicion of a mediastinal traversing injury. Such wounds warrant careful consideration, and surgical consultation is mandatory.

- Widened paraspinal interfaces

- Presence of a pleural or apical cap

- Left hemothorax

- Fractures of the first or second rib or scapula

False positive and false negative findings may occur with each x-ray sign, and, rarely (1%–2%), no mediastinal or initial chest x-ray abnormality is present in patients with great-vessel injury. If there is even a slight suspicion of aortic injury, the patient should be evaluated at a facility capable of repairing a diagnosed injury.

Helical contrast-enhanced computed tomography (CT) of the chest has been shown to be an accurate screening method for patients with suspected blunt aortic injury. CT scanning should be performed liberally, because the findings on chest x-ray, especially the supine view, are unreliable. If the results are equivocal, aortography should be performed. In general, patients who are hemodynamically abnormal should not be placed in a CT scanner. The sensitivity and specificity of helical contrast-enhanced CT have been shown to be 100% each, but this result is very technology-dependent. If enhanced helical CT of the chest is negative for mediastinal hematoma and aortic rupture, no further diagnostic imaging of the aorta is necessary. When the CT is positive for blunt aortic rupture, the extent of the injury may need to be further defined with aortography. Transesophageal echocardiography (TEE) also appears to be a useful, less invasive diagnostic tool. The trauma surgeon caring for the patient is in the best position to determine which, if any, other diagnostic tests are warranted.

In hospitals that lack the capability to care for cardiothoracic injuries, the decision to transfer patients with potential aortic injury may be difficult. A properly performed and interpreted helical CT that is normal may obviate the need for transfer to a higher level of care to exclude thoracic aortic injury.

A qualified surgeon should treat patients with blunt traumatic aortic injury and assist in the diagnosis. The treatment is either primary repair or resection of the torn segment and replacement with an interposition graft.

Techniques of endovascular repair are rapidly evolving as an alternative approach for surgical repair of blunt traumatic aortic injury.

TRAUMATIC DIAPHRAGMATIC INJURY

Traumatic diaphragmatic ruptures are more commonly diagnosed on the left side, perhaps because the liver obliterates the defect or protects it on the right side of the diaphragm, whereas the appearance of the bowel, stomach, and nasogastric (NG) tube is more easily detected in the left chest. However, this fact may not represent the true incidence of laterality. Blunt trauma produces large radial tears that lead to herniation (Figure 4-10), whereas penetrating trauma produces small perforations that often take some time, even years, to develop into diaphragmatic hernias.

Diaphragmatic injuries are frequently missed initially when the chest film is misinterpreted as showing an elevated diaphragm, acute gastric dilatation, loculated hemopneumothorax, or subpulmonary hematoma. If a laceration of the left diaphragm is suspected, a gastric tube should be inserted. When the gastric tube appears in the thoracic cavity on the chest film, the need for special contrast studies is eliminated. Occasionally, the condition is not identified on the initial x-ray film or until after chest tube evacuation of the left thorax. An upper gastrointestinal contrast study should be performed if the diagnosis is not clear. The appearance of peritoneal lavage fluid in the chest tube drainage also confirms the diagnosis. Minimally invasive endoscopic procedures (eg, laparoscopy or thoracoscopy) may be helpful in evaluating the diaphragm in indeterminate cases.

Right diaphragmatic ruptures are rarely diagnosed in the early postinjury period. The liver often prevents herniation of other abdominal organs into the chest. The appearance of an elevated right diaphragm on chest x-ray may be the only finding.

Operation for other abdominal injuries often reveals a diaphragmatic tear. Treatment is by direct repair.

BLUNT ESOPHAGEAL RUPTURE

Esophageal trauma is most commonly penetrating in nature. Blunt esophageal trauma, although very rare, can be lethal if unrecognized. Blunt injury of the esophagus is caused by the forceful expulsion of gastric contents into the

---

PITFALL

Delayed or extensive evaluation of the wide mediastinum without cardiothoracic surgery capabilities may result in an early in-hospital rupture of the contained hematoma and rapid death from exsanguination. All patients with a mechanism of injury and simple chest x-ray findings suggestive of aortic disruption should be transferred to a facility capable of rapid definitive diagnosis and treatment of this injury.

PITFALL

Diaphragm injuries are notorious for not being diagnosed during the initial trauma evaluation. An undiagnosed diaphragm injury can result in pulmonary compromise or entrapment and strangulation of peritoneal contents.

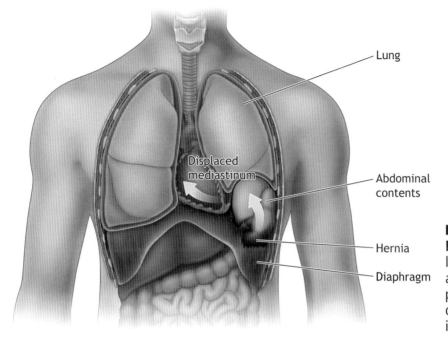

■ **Figure 4-10 Diaphragmatic Rupture.** Blunt trauma produces large radial tears that lead to herniation, whereas penetrating trauma produces small perforations that often take some time to develop into diaphragmatic hernias.

esophagus from a severe blow to the upper abdomen. This forceful ejection produces a linear tear in the lower esophagus, allowing leakage into the mediastinum (Figure 4-11). The resulting mediastinitis and immediate or delayed rupture into the pleural space cause empyema.

The clinical picture of patients with blunt esophageal rupture is identical to that of postemetic esophageal rupture. Esophageal injury should be considered in any patient who: (1) has a left pneumothorax or hemothorax without a rib fracture; (2) has received a severe blow to the lower sternum or epigastrium and is in pain or shock out of proportion to the apparent injury; and (3) has particulate matter in the chest tube after the blood begins to clear. Presence of mediastinal air also suggests the diagnosis, which often can be confirmed by contrast studies and/or esophagoscopy.

Treatment consists of wide drainage of the pleural space and mediastinum with direct repair of the injury via thoracotomy, if feasible. Repairs performed within a few hours of injury lead to a much better prognosis.

Other Manifestations of Chest Injuries

Other significant thoracic injuries—including subcutaneous emphysema; crushing injury (traumatic asphyxia); and rib, sternum, and scapular fractures—should be detected during the secondary survey. Although these injuries may not be immediately life-threatening, they have the potential to do significant harm.

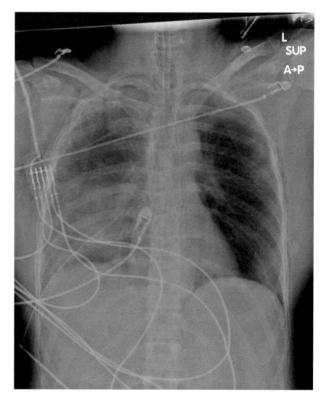

■ **Figure 4-11** Radiograph showing rib fractures. Fractures of the scapula, first or second rib, or the sternum suggest a magnitude of injury that places the head, neck, spinal cord, lungs, and great vessels at risk for serious associated injury.

SUBCUTANEOUS EMPHYSEMA

Subcutaneous emphysema can result from airway injury, lung injury, or, rarely, blast injury. Although it does not require treatment, the underlying injury must be addressed. If positive-pressure ventilation is required, tube thoracostomy should be considered on the side of the subcutaneous emphysema in anticipation of a tension pneumothorax developing.

CRUSHING INJURY TO THE CHEST (TRAUMATIC ASPHYXIA)

Findings associated with a crush injury to the chest include upper torso, facial, and arm plethora with petechiae secondary to acute, temporary compression of the superior vena cava. Massive swelling and even cerebral edema may be present. Associated injuries must be treated.

RIB, STERNUM, AND SCAPULAR FRACTURES

The ribs are the most commonly injured component of the thoracic cage, and injuries to the ribs are often significant. Pain on motion typically results in splinting of the thorax, which impairs ventilation, oxygenation, and effective coughing. The incidence of atelectasis and pneumonia rises significantly with preexisting lung disease.

The upper ribs (1 to 3) are protected by the bony framework of the upper limb. The scapula, humerus, and clavicle, along with their muscular attachments, provide a barrier to rib injury. Fractures of the scapula, first or second rib, or the sternum suggest a magnitude of injury that places the head, neck, spinal cord, lungs, and great vessels at risk for serious associated injury. Because of the severity of the associated injuries, mortality may be as high as 35%. Surgical consultation is warranted.

Sternal and scapular fractures are generally the result of a direct blow. Pulmonary contusion may accompany sternal fractures, and blunt cardiac injury should be considered with all such fractures. Operative repair of sternal and scapular fractures occasionally is indicated. Rarely, posterior sternoclavicular dislocation results in mediastinal displacement of the clavicular heads with accompanying superior vena caval obstruction. Immediate reduction is required.

The middle ribs (4 to 9) sustain the majority of blunt trauma. Anteroposterior compression of the thoracic cage will bow the ribs outward with a fracture in the midshaft. Direct force applied to the ribs tends to fracture them and drive the ends of the bones into the thorax, raising the potential for more intrathoracic injury, such as a pneumothorax or hemothorax. As a general rule, a young patient with a more flexible chest wall is less likely to sustain rib fractures. Therefore, the presence of multiple rib fractures in young patients implies a greater transfer of force than in older patients. Fractures of the lower ribs (10 to 12) should increase suspicion for hepatosplenic injury.

Localized pain, tenderness on palpation, and crepitation are present in patients with rib injury. A palpable or visible deformity suggests rib fractures. A chest x-ray film should be obtained primarily to exclude other intrathoracic injuries and not just to identify rib fractures. Fractures of anterior cartilages or separation of costochondral junctions have the same significance as rib fractures, but will not be seen on the x-ray examinations. Special rib-technique x-ray films are expensive, may not detect all rib injuries, add nothing to treatment, require painful positioning of the patient, and are not useful. ⌐ See Skill Station VI: X-Ray Identification of Thoracic Injuries.

Taping, rib belts, and external splints are contraindicated. Relief of pain is important to enable adequate ventilation. Intercostal block, epidural anesthesia, and systemic analgesics are effective and may be necessary.

PITFALL

Underestimating the severe pathophysiology of rib fractures is a common pitfall, particularly in patients at the extremes of age. Aggressive pain control without respiratory depression is the key management principle.

Other Indications for Chest Tube Insertion

Other indications for chest tube insertion include:

- Selected patients with suspected severe lung injury, especially those being transferred by air or ground vehicle

- Individuals undergoing general anesthesia for treatment of other injuries (eg, cranial or extremity), who have suspected significant lung injury

- Individuals requiring positive-pressure ventilation in whom substantial chest injury is suspected

CHAPTER SUMMARY

1 Thoracic trauma is common in the multiply injured patient and may be associated with life-threatening problems. These patients can usually be treated or their conditions temporarily relieved by relatively simple measures such as intubation, ventilation, tube thoracostomy, fluid resuscitation. The ability to recognize these important injuries and the skill to perform the necessary procedures can be lifesaving. The primary survey includes management of the following conditions:

- Airway obstruction—Early assessment and recognition of the need for establishing a controlled airway while maintaining in-line immobilization of the cervical spine at all times.

- Tension pneumothorax—Clinical diagnosis (decreased breath sounds and hyperresonance) with immediate decompression of the pleural space.

- Open pneumothorax—Obvious chest wall deformity with sucking chest wound is initially managed with flutter-valve dressing.

- Flail chest and pulmonary contusion—Unstable segment of chest wall with paradoxical motion requires judicious fluid resuscitation and adequate analgesia with selective intubation for pulmonary support.

- Massive hemothorax—Diagnosed by finding decreased breath sounds and dullness to percussion on physical examination. Initial management requires evacuation with insertion of a large (#36 French) chest tube. A qualified surgeon must be involved in the decision for thoracotomy.

- Cardiac tamponade—Diagnosis by clinical examination, with ultrasound examination to confirm. Initial management includes fluid resuscitation and surgery. Pericardiocentesis may be used as a temporizing maneuver if surgical intervention is not immediately available.

2 The secondary survey includes identification and initial treatment of the following potentially life-threatening injuries, utilizing adjunctive studies (x-rays, laboratory test, ECG):

- Simple pneumothorax—Typically diagnosed by chest x-ray or CT scan and treated with tube thoracostomy.

- Hemothorax—Typically diagnosed by chest x-ray or CT scan and treated with tube thoracostomy.

- Pulmonary contusion—Typically diagnosed by chest x-ray or CT scan. Management includes judicious fluid resuscitation and selective intubation for pulmonary support.

- Tracheobronchial tree injury—Associated with hemoptysis, pneumomediastinum, pneumopericardium, persistent air leak from chest tube, or persistent pneumothorax after insertion of a chest tube. Requires operative repair.

- Blunt cardiac injury—Most common complication is arrhythmias, which are managed according to standard protocols. Less common complications include acute myocardial infarction and valvular disruption.

- Traumatic aortic disruption—Early diagnosis requires a high index of suspicion. Most common radiographic sign is widened mediastinum seen on anteroposterior chest x-ray. Diagnosis is confirmed by dynamic helical CT scanning or aortography. Qualified surgeon must be involved in management.

- Traumatic diaphragmatic injury—Early diagnosis requires a high index of suspicion. Most common radiographic sign is elevation of diaphragm on involved side. Requires early laparotomy for repair and to address associated injuries.

- Blunt esophageal rupture—Physical examination reveals pain out of proportion for injuries. Associated with left pleural effusion and/or pneumomediastinum. Early operative intervention by a qualified surgeon reduces morbidity and mortality.

3 Several manifestations of thoracic trauma are indicative of a greater risk of associated injuries.

- Subcutaneous emphysema is associated with airway or lung injury. Tube thoracostomy should be considered for patients requiring positive pressure ventilation.

- Crush injuries of the chest present with petechiae and plethora of the head, neck, and upper torso. Brain injury with progressive cerebral edema should be suspected.

Injuries to the upper ribs (1–3), scapula, and sternum are associated with significant mechanisms of injury. Underlying head, spine, and cardiothoracic injury should be suspected.

Bibliography

1. Ball CG, Kirkpatrick AW, Laupland KB, et al. Incidence, risk factors, and outcomes for occult pneumothoraces in victims of major trauma. *J Trauma* 2005; 59(4), 917-924; discussion 924-925.

2. Bertinchant JP, Robert E, Polge A, et al. Release kinetics of cardiac troponin I and cardiac troponin T in effluents from isolated perfused rabbit hearts after graded experimental myocardial contusion. *J Trauma* 1999;47(3):474-480.

3. Boyd M, Vanek VW, Bourguet CC. Emergency room resuscitative thoracotomy: when is it indicated? *J Trauma* 1992;33(5):714-721.

4. Brasel KJ, Stafford RE, Weigelt JA, Tenquist JE, Borgstrom DC. Treatment of occult pneumothoraces from blunt trauma. *J Trauma* 1999; 46(6), 987-990; discussion 990-991.

5. Brooks AP, Olson LK, Shackford SR. Computed tomography in the diagnosis of traumatic rupture of the thoracic aorta. *Clin Radiol* 1989;40:133-138.

6. Bulger EM, Edwards T, Klotz P, Jurkovich GJ. Epidural analgesia improves outcome after multiple rib fractures. *Surgery* 2004;136(2):426-430.

7. Callaham M. Pericardiocentesis in traumatic and nontraumatic cardiac tamponade. *Ann Emerg Med* 1984;13(10):924-945.

8. Cook J, Salerno C, Krishnadasan B, Nicholls S, Meissner M, Karmy-Jones R. The effect of changing presentation and management on the outcome of blunt rupture of the thoracic aorta. *J Thorac Cardiovasc Surg* 2006; 131(3), 594-600.

9. Dunham CM, Barraco RD, Clark DE, et al. Guidelines for emergency tracheal intubation immediately following traumatic injury: an EAST Practice Management Guidelines Workgroup. *J Trauma Infect Crit Care Burns* 2003;55:162-179.

10. Dyer DS, Moore EE, Mestek MF, et al. Can chest CT be used to exclude aortic injury? *Radiology* 1999;213(1):195-202.

11. Esposito TJ, Jurkovich GJ, Rice CL, et al. Reappraisal of emergency room thoracotomy in a changing environment. *J Trauma* 1991;31(7):881-887.

12. Fabian TC, Richardson JD, Croce MA, et al. Prospective study of blunt aortic injury: multicenter trial of the American Association for the Surgery of Trauma. *J Trauma* 1997;42:374-383.

13. Flagel B, Luchette FA, Reed RL, et al. Half a dozen ribs: the breakpoint for mortality. *Surgery* 2005;138:717-725.

14. Gavant ML, Menke PG, Fabian TC, et al. Blunt traumatic aortic rupture: detection with helical CT of the chest. *Radiology* 1995;197:125-133.

15. Goldberg SP, Karalis DG, Ross JJ, et al. Severe right ventricular contusion mimicking cardiac tamponade: the value of transesophageal echocardiography in blunt chest trauma. *Ann Emerg Med* 1993;22(4):745-747.

16. Graham JG, Mattox KL, Beall AC Jr. Penetrating trauma of the lung. *J Trauma* 1979;19:665.

17. Heniford BT, Carrillo EG, Spain DA, et al. The role of thoracoscopy in the management of retained thoracic collections after trauma. *Ann Thorac Surg* 1997;63(4):940-943.

18. Hopson LR, Hirsh E, Delgado J, Domeier RM, McSwain NE, Krohmer J. Guidelines for withholding or termination of resuscitation in prehospital traumatic cardiopulmonary arrest: a joint position paper from the National Association of EMS Physicians Standards and Clinical Practice Committee and the American College of Surgeons Committee on Trauma. *Prehosp Emerg Care* 2003; 7(1), 141-146.

19. Hopson LR, Hirsh E, Delgado J, et al. Guidelines for withholding or termination of resuscitation in prehospital traumatic cardiopulmonary arrest. *J Am Coll Surg* 2003; 196(3), 475-481.

20. Hunt PA, Greaves I, Owens WA. Emergency thoracotomy in thoracic trauma-a review. *Injury* 2006; 37(1), 1-19.

21. Karalis DG, Victor MF, Davis GA, et al. The role of echocardiography in blunt chest trauma: a transthoracic and transesophageal echocardiography study. *J Trauma* 1994;36 (l):53-58.

22. Lang-Lazdunski L, Mourox J, Pons F, et al. Role of videothoracoscopy in chest trauma. *Ann Thorac Surg* 1997; 63(2):327-333.

23. Lee JT, White RA. Current status of thoracic aortic endograft repair. *Surg Clin North Am* 2004;84(5):1295-1318.

24. Lockey D, Crewdson K, Davies G. Traumatic cardiac arrest: who are the survivors? *Ann Emerg Med* 2006; 48(3), 240-244.

25. Marnocha KE, Maglinte DDT, Woods J, et al. Blunt chest trauma and suspected aortic rupture: reliability of chest radiograph findings. *Ann Emerg Med* 1985;14(7):644-649.

26. Mattox KL, Flint LM, Carrico CJ, et al. Blunt cardiac injury. *J Trauma* 1994;33(5):649-650.

27. Mattox KL, Wall MJ. Newer diagnostic measures and emergency management. *Chest Surg Clin North Am* 1997;2:213-226.

28. McPhee JT, Asham EH, Rohrer MJ, et al. The midterm results of stent graft treatment of thoracic aortic injuries. *J Surg Res* 2007;138(2):181-188.

29. Meyer DM, Jessen ME, Wait MA. Early evacuation of traumatic retained hemothoraces using thoracoscopy: A prospective randomized trial. *Ann Thorac Surg* 1997;64(5):1396-1400.

30. Mirvis SE, Shanmugantham K, Buell J, et al. Use of spiral computed tomography for the assessment of blunt trauma patients with potential aortic injury. *J Trauma* 1999;45:922-930.

31. Moon MR, Luchette FA, Gibson SW, et al. Prospective, randomized comparison of epidural versus parenteral opioid analgesia in thoracic trauma. *Ann Surg* 1999;229:684-692.

32. Peterson BG, Matsumura JS, Morasch MD, West MA, Eskandari MK. Percutaneous endovascular repair of blunt thoracic aortic transection. *J Trauma* 2005 Nov;59(5):1062-1065.

33. Pezzella AT, Silva WE, Lancey RA. Cardiothoracic trauma. *Curr Probl Surg* 1998;35(8):649-650.

34. Poole G, Myers RT. Morbidity and mortality rates in major blunt trauma to the upper chest. *Ann Surg* 1980;193(1):70-75.

35. Powell DW, Moore EE, Cothren CC, et al. Is emergency department resuscitative thoracotomy futile care for the critically injured patient requiring prehospital cardiopulmonary resuscitation? *J Am Coll Surg* 2004;199(2):211-215.

36. Ramzy AI, Rodriguez A, Turney SZ. Management of major tracheobronchial ruptures in patients with multiple system trauma. *J Trauma* 1988;28:914-920.

37. Reed AB, Thompson JK, Crafton CJ, et al. Timing of endovascular repair of blunt traumatic thoracic aortic transections. *J Vasc Surg* 2006;43(4):684-688.

38. Rhee PM, Acosta J, Bridgeman A, Wang D, Jordan M, Rich N. Survival after emergency department thoracotomy: review of published data from the past 25 years. *J Am Coll Surg* 2000; 190(3), 288-298.

39. Richardson JD, Adams L, Flint LM. Selective management of flail chest and pulmonary contusion. *Ann Surg* 1982;196(4):481-487.

40. Richardson JD, Flint LM, Snow NJ, et al. Management of transmediastinal gunshot wounds. *Surgery* 1981;90(4):671-676.

41. Rosato RM, Shapiro MJ, Keegan MJ, et al. Cardiac injury complicating traumatic asphyxia. *J Trauma* 1991;31(10):1387-1389.

42. Rozycki GS, Feliciano DV, Oschner MG, et al. The role of ultrasound in patients with possible penetrating cardiac wounds: a prospective multicenter study. *J Trauma* 1999;46(4):542-551.

43. Rozycki GS, Feliciano DV, Schmidt JA. The role of surgeon-performed ultrasound in patients with possible cardiac wounds. *Ann Surg* 1996;223(6):737-744.

44. Simeone A, Freitas M, Frankel HL. Management options in blunt aortic injury: a case series and literature review. *Am Surg* 2006; 72(1), 25-30.

45. Simon B, Cushman J, Barraco R, et al. Pain management in blunt thoracic trauma: an EAST Practice Management Guidelines Workgroup. *J Trauma Infect Crit Care Burns* 2005;59:1256-1267.

46. Smith MD, Cassidy JM, Souther S, et al. Transesophageal echocardiography in the diagnosis of traumatic rupture of the aorta. *N Engl J Med* 1995;332:356-362.

47. Søreide K, Søiland H, Lossius HM, et al. Resuscitative emergency thoracotomy in a Scandinavian trauma hospital—Is it justified? *Injury* 2007;38(1):34-42.

48. Søreide K, Søiland H, Lossius HM, Vetrhus M, Soreide JA, Soreide E. Resuscitative emergency thoracotomy in a Scandinavian trauma hospital—is it justified? *Injury* 2007; 38(1), 34-42.

49. Stafford RE, Linn J, Washington L. Incidence and management of occult hemothoraces. *Am J Surg* 2006; 192(6), 722-726.

50. Swaaenburg JC, Klaase JM, DeJongste MJ, et al. Troponin I, troponin T, CKMB-activity and CKMG-mass as markers for the detection of myocardial contusion in patients who experienced blunt trauma. *Clin Chim Acta* 1998;272(2):171-181.

51. Symbas PN. Cardiothoracic trauma. *Curr Probl Surg* 1991;28(11):741-797.

52. Tehrani HY, Peterson BG, Katariya K, et al. Endovascular repair of thoracic aortic tears. *Ann Thorac Surg* 2006;82(3):873-877.

53. Weiss RL, Brier JA, O'Connor W, et al. The usefulness of transesophageal echocardiography in diagnosing cardiac contusions. *Chest* 1996;109(1):73-77.

54. Woodring D. Radiographic manifestations of mediastinal hemorrhage from blunt chest trauma. *Ann Thorac Surg* 1984;37(2):171-178.

55. Woodring JH. A normal mediastinum in blunt trauma rupture of the thoracic aorta and brachiocephalic arteries. *J Emerg Med* 1990;8:467-476.

▶▶ Interactive Skill Procedures

Note: This Skill Station includes a systematic method for evaluating chest x-ray films. A series of x-rays with related scenarios is then shown to students for their evaluation and management decisions based on the findings.

THE FOLLOWING PROCEDURE IS INCLUDED IN THIS SKILL STATION:

▶▶ **Skill VI-A:** Process for Initial Review of Chest X-Rays

Performance at this skill station will allow the participant to:

OBJECTIVES

1 Describe the process for viewing a chest x-ray film for the purpose of identifying life-threatening and potentially life-threatening thoracic injuries.

2 Identify various thoracic injuries by using the following seven specific anatomic guidelines for examining a series of chest x-rays:

> Trachea and bronchi
> Pleural spaces and lung parenchyma
> Mediastinum
> Diaphragm
> Bony thorax
> Soft tissues
> Tubes and lines

3 Given a series of x-rays:

> Diagnose fractures.
> Diagnose a pneumothorax and a hemothorax.
> Identify a widened mediastinum.
> Delineate associated injuries.
> Identify other areas of possible injury.

▶ Skill VI-A: Process for Initial Review of Chest X-Rays

▶▶ I. OVERVIEW

STEP 1. Confirm that the film being viewed is of your patient.

STEP 2. Quickly assess for suspected pathology.

STEP 3. Use the patient's clinical findings to focus the review of the chest x-ray film, and use the x-ray findings to guide further physical evaluation.

▶▶ II. TRACHEA AND BRONCHI

STEP 1. Assess the position of the tube in cases of endotracheal intubation.

STEP 2. Assess for the presence of interstitial or pleural air that can represent tracheobronchial injury.

STEP 3. Assess for tracheal lacerations that can present as pneumomediastinum, pneumothorax, subcutaneous and interstitial emphysema of the neck, or pneumoperitoneum.

STEP 4. Assess for bronchial disruption that can present as a free pleural communication and produce a massive pneumothorax with a persistent air leak that is unresponsive to tube thoracostomy.

▶▶ III. PLEURAL SPACES AND LUNG PARENCHYMA

STEP 1. Assess the pleural space for abnormal collections of fluid that can represent a hemothorax.

STEP 2. Assess the pleural space for abnormal collections of air that can represent a pneumothorax—usually seen as an apical lucent area without bronchial or vascular markings.

STEP 3. Assess the lung fields for infiltrates that can suggest pulmonary contusion, hematoma, aspiration, etc. Pulmonary contusion appears as air-space consolidation that can be irregular and patchy, homogeneous, diffuse, or extensive.

STEP 4. Assess the parenchyma for evidence of laceration. Lacerations appear as a hematoma, vary according to the magnitude of injury, and appear as areas of consolidation.

▶▶ IV. MEDIASTINUM

STEP 1. Assess for air or blood that can displace mediastinal structures or blur the demarcation between tissue planes or outline them with radiolucency.

STEP 2. Assess for radiologic signs associated with cardiac or major vascular injury.

a. Air or blood in the pericardium can result in an enlarged cardiac silhouette. Progressive changes in cardiac size can represent an expanding pneumopericardium or hemopericardium.

b. Aortic rupture can be suggested by:
- A widened mediastinum—most reliable finding
- Fractures of the first and second ribs
- Obliteration of the aortic knob
- Deviation of the trachea to the right
- Presence of a pleural cap
- Elevation and rightward shift of the right mainstem bronchus
- Depression of the left mainstem bronchus
- Obliteration of the space between the pulmonary artery and aorta
- Deviation of the esophagus (NG tube) to the right

▶▶ V. DIAPHRAGM

Note: Diaphragmatic rupture requires a high index of suspicion, based on the mechanism of injury, signs and symptoms, and x-ray findings. Initial chest x-ray examination may not clearly identify a diaphragmatic injury. Sequential films or additional studies may be required.

STEP 1. Carefully evaluate the diaphragm for:

a. Elevation (may rise to fourth intercostal space with full expiration)

b. Disruption (stomach, bowel gas, or NG tube above the diaphragm)

c. Poor identification (irregular or obscure) due to overlying fluid or soft-tissue masses

STEP 2. X-ray changes suggesting injury include:

a. Elevation, irregularity, or obliteration of the diaphragm—segmental or total

b. A mass-like density above the diaphragm that can be due to a fluid-filled bowel, omentum, liver, kidney, spleen, or pancreas (may appear as a "loculated pneumothorax")

c. Air or contrast-containing stomach or bowel above the diaphragm

d. Contralateral mediastinal shift

e. Widening of the cardiac silhouette if the peritoneal contents herniate into the pericardial sac

f. Pleural effusion

STEP 3. Assess for associated injuries, such as splenic, pancreatic, renal, and liver.

▶▶ VI. BONY THORAX

STEP 1. Assess the clavicle for evidence of:

    a. Fracture

    b. Associated injury, such as great-vessel injury

STEP 2. Assess the scapula for evidence of:

    a. Fracture

    b. Associated injury, such as airway or great-vessel injury, pulmonary contusion

STEP 3. Assess ribs 1 through 3 for evidence of:

    a. Fracture

    b. Associated injury, such as pneumothorax, major airway, or great-vessel injury

STEP 4. Assess ribs 4 through 9 for evidence of:

    a. Fracture, especially in two or more contiguous ribs in two places (flail chest)

    b. Associated injury, such as pneumothorax, hemothorax, pulmonary contusion

STEP 5. Assess ribs 9 through 12 for evidence of:

    a. Fracture, especially in two or more places (flail chest)

    b. Associated injury, such as pneumothorax, pulmonary contusion, spleen, liver, and/or kidney

STEP 6. Assess the sternomanubrial junction and sternal body for evidence of fracture or dislocation. (Sternal fractures can be mistaken on the AP film for a mediastinal hematoma. After the patient is stabilized, a coned-down view, overpenetrated film, lateral view, or CT may be obtained to better identify suspected sternal fracture.)

STEP 7. Assess the sternum for associated injuries, such as myocardial contusion and great-vessel injury (widened mediastinum), although these combinations are relatively infrequent.

▶▶ VII. SOFT TISSUES

STEP 1. Assess for:

    a. Displacement or disruption of tissue planes

    b. Evidence of subcutaneous air

TABLE VI-1 ■ Chest X-Ray Suggestions

FINDINGS	DIAGNOSES TO CONSIDER
Respiratory distress without x-ray findings	CNS injury, aspiration, traumatic asphyxia
Any rib fracture	Pneumothorax, pulmonary contusion
Fracture of first three ribs or sternoclavicular fracture–dislocation	Airway or great-vessel injury
Fracture of lower ribs 9 to 12	Abdominal injury
Two or more rib fractures in two or more places	Flail chest, pulmonary contusion
Scapular fracture	Great-vessel injury, pulmonary contusion, brachial plexus injury
Mediastinal widening	Great-vessel injury, sternal fracture, thoracic spine injury
Persistent large pneumothorax or air leak after chest tube insertion	Bronchial tear
Mediastinal air	Esophageal disruption, tracheal injury, pneumoperitoneum
GI gas pattern in the chest (loculated air)	Diaphragmatic rupture
NG tube in the chest	Diaphragmatic rupture or ruptured esophagus
Air fluid level in the chest	Hemopneumothorax or diaphragmatic rupture
Disrupted diaphragm	Abdominal visceral injury
Free air under the diaphragm	Ruptured hollow abdominal viscus

▸▸ VIII. TUBES AND LINES

STEP 1. Assess for placement and positioning of:

    a. Endotracheal tube

    b. Chest tubes

    c. Central access lines

    d. Nasogastric tube

    e. Other monitoring devices

▸▸ IX. X-RAY REASSESSMENT

The patient's clinical findings should be correlated with the x-ray findings, and vice versa. After careful, systematic eval- uation of the initial chest film, additional x-rays or ra- diographic and/or imaging studies may be necessary as his- torical facts and physical findings dictate. Remember, nei- ther the physical examination nor the chest x-ray film should be viewed in isolation. Findings on the physical examination should be used to focus the review of the chest x-ray film, and findings on the chest x-ray film should be used to guide the physical examination and direct the use of ancillary di- agnostic procedures. For example, review of the previous x- ray film and repeat chest films may be indicated if significant changes occur in the patient's status. Thoracic CT, thoracic arteriography, or pericardial ultrasonography/echocardiog- raphy may be indicated for specificity of diagnosis.

▸ THORAX X-RAY SCENARIOS

PATIENT VI-1

X-ray film of a 33-year-old bicyclist who was hit by a car.

PATIENT VI-2

X-ray film of a young female with a small stab wound above the nipple on the right side with ipsilateral diminished breath sounds.

PATIENT VI-3

X-ray film of a 56-year-old truck driver who hit an abut- ment and reported left-sided chest pain and respiratory dis- tress.

PATIENT VI-4

X-ray film of a 22-year-old male in distress after a fight in a bar (stab wound in the back, fourth intercostal space on left).

PATIENT VI-5

X-ray film of a 42-year-old male in respiratory distress after sustaining a gunshot wound in a jewelry shop robbery.

PATIENT VI-6

X-ray film of a motorcyclist with severe head trauma on ad- mission.

PATIENT VI-7

X-ray film of a 36-year-old male after treatment of an obvi- ous pneumothorax on the right side, still desaturated.

PATIENT VI-8

X-ray film of a 45-year-old male motorcyclist who hit a tree at high speed. He was intubated by EMS and presents as he- modynamically normal.

PATIENT VI-9

X-ray film of a 56-year-old motorcyclist who sustained a collision with a truck. He was intubated and received a tho- rax drain in the prehospital setting.

PATIENT VI-10

X-ray film of an 18-year-old gang leader who was assaulted. He has multiple contusions, an altered level of conscious- ness, and a small entrance wound on the right hemithorax. He has received initial resuscitation.

PATIENT VI-11

X-ray film of a 56-year-old male who fell off a ladder (6 m) with severe head injury.

VII Chest Trauma Management

▶▶ Interactive Skill Procedures

Note: **Standard precautions are required when caring for trauma patients.**

THE FOLLOWING PROCEDURES ARE INCLUDED IN THIS SKILL STATION:

▶▶ **Skill VII-A:** Needle Thoracentesis

▶▶ **Skill VII-B:** Chest Tube Insertion

▶▶ **Skill VII-C:** Pericardiocentesis

Performance at this skill station will allow the student to practice and demonstrate on a live, anesthetized animal; a fresh, human cadaver; or an anatomic human body manikin the techniques of needle thoracic decompression of a tension pneumothorax, chest tube insertion for the emergency management of hemopneumothorax, and pericardiocentesis. Specifically, the student also will be able to:

OBJECTIVES

1 Identify the surface markings and techniques for pleural decompression with needle thoracentesis, chest tube insertion, and needle pericardiocentesis.

2 Describe the underlying pathophysiology of tension pneumothorax and cardiac tamponade as a result of trauma.

3 Describe the complications of needle thoracentesis, chest tube insertion, and pericardiocentesis.

▶ Skill VII-A : Needle Thoracentesis

Note: This procedure is appropriate for patients in critical condition with rapid deterioration who have a life-threatening tension pneumothorax. If this technique is used and the patient does not have a tension pneumothorax, a pneumothorax and/or damage to the lung may occur.

STEP 1. Assess the patient's chest and respiratory status.

STEP 2. Administer high-flow oxygen and apply ventilation as necessary.

STEP 3. Identify the second intercostal space, in the midclavicular line on the side of the tension pneumothorax.

STEP 4. Surgically prepare the chest.

STEP 5. Locally anesthetize the area if the patient is conscious and if time permits.

STEP 6. Place the patient in an upright position if a cervical spine injury has been excluded.

STEP 7. Keeping the Luer-Lok in the distal end of the catheter, insert an over-the-needle catheter (2 in. [5 cm] long) into the skin and direct the needle just over (ie, superior to) the rib into the intercostal space.

STEP 8. Puncture the parietal pleura.

STEP 9. Remove the Luer-Lok from the catheter and listen for the sudden escape of air when the needle enters the parietal pleura, indicating that the tension pneumothorax has been relieved.

STEP 10. Remove the needle. Leave the plastic catheter in place and apply a bandage or small dressing over the insertion site.

STEP 11. Prepare for a chest tube insertion, if necessary. The chest tube is typically inserted at the nipple level just anterior to the midaxillary line of the affected hemithorax.

STEP 12. Connect the chest tube to an underwater-seal device or a flutter-type valve apparatus and remove the catheter used to relieve the tension pneumothorax initially.

STEP 13. Obtain a chest x-ray film.

▶▶ COMPLICATIONS OF NEEDLE THORACENTESIS

- Local hematoma
- Pneumothorax
- Lung laceration

▶ Skill VII-B: Chest Tube Insertion

STEP 1. Determine the insertion site, usually at the nipple level (fifth intercostal space), just anterior to the midaxillary line on the affected side. A second chest tube may be used for a hemothorax.

STEP 2. Surgically prepare and drape the chest at the predetermined site of the tube insertion.

STEP 3. Locally anesthetize the skin and rib periosteum.

STEP 4. Make a 2- to 3-cm transverse (horizontal) incision at the predetermined site and bluntly dissect through the subcutaneous tissues, just over the top of the rib.

STEP 5. Puncture the parietal pleura with the tip of a clamp and put a gloved finger into the incision to avoid injury to other organs and to clear any adhesions, clots, etc.

STEP 6. Clamp the proximal end of the thoracostomy tube and advance it into the pleural space to the desired length. The tube should be directed posteriorly along the inside of the chest wall.

STEP 7. Look for "fogging" of the chest tube with expiration or listen for air movement.

STEP 8. Connect the end of the thoracostomy tube to an underwater-seal apparatus.

STEP 9. Suture the tube in place.

STEP 10. Apply a dressing, and tape the tube to the chest.

STEP 11. Obtain a chest x-ray film.

STEP 12. Obtain arterial blood gas values and/or institute pulse oximetry monitoring as necessary.

▶▶ COMPLICATIONS OF CHEST TUBE INSERTION

- Laceration or puncture of intrathoracic and/or abdominal organs, which can be prevented by using the finger technique before inserting the chest tube

- Introduction of pleural infection—eg, thoracic empyema
- Damage to the intercostal nerve, artery, or vein
  - Converting a pneumothorax to a hemopneumothorax
  - Resulting in intercostal neuritis/neuralgia
- Incorrect tube position, extrathoracic or intrathoracic
- Chest tube kinking, clogging, or dislodging from the chest wall, or disconnection from the underwater-seal apparatus
- Persistent pneumothorax

- Large primary leak
- Leak at the skin around the chest tube; suction on tube too strong
  - Leaky underwater-seal apparatus
- Subcutaneous emphysema, usually at tube site
- Recurrence of pneumothorax upon removal of chest tube; seal of thoracostomy wound not immediate
- Lung fails to expand because of plugged bronchus; bronchoscopy required
- Anaphylactic or allergic reaction to surgical preparation or anesthetic

▶ Skill VII-C: Pericardiocentesis

STEP 1. Monitor the patient's vital signs and ECG before, during, and after the procedure.

STEP 2. Surgically prepare the xiphoid and subxiphoid areas, if time allows.

STEP 3. Locally anesthetize the puncture site, if necessary.

STEP 4. Using a 16- to 18-gauge, 6-in. (15-cm) or longer over-the-needle catheter, attach a 35-mL empty syringe with a three-way stopcock.

STEP 5. Assess the patient for any mediastinal shift that may have caused the heart to shift significantly.

STEP 6. Puncture the skin 1 to 2 cm inferior to the left of the xiphochondral junction, at a 45-degree angle to the skin.

STEP 7. Carefully advance the needle cephalad and aim toward the tip of the left scapula.

STEP 8. If the needle is advanced too far (ie, into the ventricular muscle), an injury pattern known as the "current of injury" appears on the ECG monitor (eg, extreme ST-T wave changes or widened and enlarged QRS complex). This pattern indicates that the pericardiocentesis needle should be withdrawn until the previous baseline ECG tracing reappears. Premature ventricular contractions also can occur, secondary to irritation of the ventricular myocardium.

STEP 9. When the needle tip enters the blood-filled pericardial sac, withdraw as much nonclotted blood as possible.

STEP 10. During the aspiration, the epicardium approaches the inner pericardial surface again, as does the needle tip. Subsequently, an ECG current of injury pattern may reappear. This indicates that the pericardiocentesis needle should be withdrawn slightly. Should this

injury pattern persist, withdraw the needle completely.

STEP 11. After aspiration is completed, remove the syringe, and attach a three-way stopcock, leaving the stopcock closed. Secure the catheter in place.

STEP 12. Option: Applying the Seldinger technique, pass a flexible guidewire through the needle into the pericardial sac, remove the needle, and pass a 14-gauge flexible catheter over the guidewire. Remove the guidewire and attach a three-way stopcock.

STEP 13. Should the cardiac tamponade symptoms persist, the stopcock may be opened and the pericardial sac reaspirated. The plastic pericardiocentesis catheter can be sutured or taped in place and covered with a small dressing to allow for continued decompression en route to surgery or transfer to another care facility.

▶▶ COMPLICATIONS OF PERICARDIOCENTESIS

- Aspiration of ventricular blood instead of pericardial blood
- Laceration of ventricular epicardium/myocardium
- Laceration of coronary artery or vein
- New hemopericardium, secondary to lacerations of the coronary artery or vein, and/or ventricular epicardium/myocardium
- Ventricular fibrillation
- Pneumothorax, secondary to lung puncture
- Puncture of great vessels with worsening of pericardial tamponade
- Puncture of esophagus with subsequent mediastinitis
- Puncture of peritoneum with subsequent peritonitis or false positive aspirate

CHAPTER 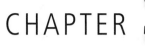 5 **Abdominal and Pelvic Trauma**

Upon completion of this topic, the student will identify common patterns of abdominal trauma based on mechanism of injury and establish management priorities accordingly. Specifically, the doctor will be able to:

OBJECTIVES

1 Identify the key anatomic regions of the abdomen.

2 Identify the patient at risk for abdominal and pelvic injuries based on the mechanism of injury.

3 Apply the appropriate diagnostic procedures to identify ongoing hemorrhage and injuries that can cause delayed morbidity and mortality

Describe the short-term management of abdominal and pelvic injuries.

Introduction

When should the abdomen be assessed in the treatment of multiply injured patients?

Evaluation of the abdomen is a challenging component of the initial assessment of injured patients. **The assessment of circulation during the primary survey includes early evaluation of the possibility of occult hemorrhage in the abdomen and pelvis in any patient who has sustained blunt trauma.** Penetrating torso wounds between the nipple and perineum also must be considered as potential causes of intraabdominal injury. The mechanism of injury, the force with which the injury was sustained, the location of injury, and the hemodynamic status of the patient determine the best method of abdominal assessment.

Unrecognized abdominal injury continues to be a cause of preventable death after truncal trauma. Rupture of a hollow viscus and bleeding from a solid organ are not easily recognized, and patient assessment is often compromised by alcohol intoxication, use of illicit drugs, injury to the brain or spinal cord, and injury to adjacent structures such as the ribs, spine, or pelvis. *Significant* amounts of blood may be present in the abdominal cavity with no dramatic change in appearance or dimensions and with no obvious signs of peritoneal irritation. Any patient who has sustained significant blunt torso injury from a direct blow, deceleration, or a penetrating torso injury must be considered to have an abdominal visceral or vascular injury until proven otherwise.

External Anatomy of the Abdomen

The abdomen is partially enclosed by the lower thorax; the anterior abdomen is defined as the area between the transnipple line superiorly, the inguinal ligaments and symphysis pubis inferiorly, and the anterior axillary lines laterally.

The flank is the area between the anterior and posterior axillary lines from the sixth intercostal space to the iliac crest. The thick musculature of the abdominal wall in this location, rather than the much thinner aponeurotic sheaths

PITFALL

Delay in recognizing intraabdominal or pelvic injury leads to early death from hemorrhage or delayed death from visceral injury.

of the anterior abdomen, acts as a partial barrier to penetrating wounds, particularly stab wounds.

The back is the area located posterior to the posterior axillary lines from the tip of the scapulae to the iliac crests. Similar to the abdominal-wall muscles in the flank, the thick back and paraspinal muscles act as a partial barrier to penetrating wounds.

Internal Anatomy of the Abdomen

The three distinct regions of the abdomen are the peritoneal cavity, the retroperitoneal space, and the pelvic cavity. The pelvic cavity, in fact, contains components of both the peritoneal cavity and retroperitoneal spaces (Figure 5-1).

PERITONEAL CAVITY

It is convenient to divide the peritoneal cavity into two parts—upper and lower. The upper peritoneal cavity, which is covered by the lower aspect of the bony thorax, includes the diaphragm, liver, spleen, stomach, and transverse colon.

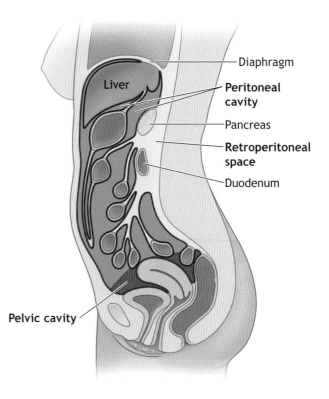

■ **Figure 5-1 Regions of Abdomen.** The three distinct regions of the abdomen are the peritoneal cavity, retroperitoneal space, and pelvic cavity.

PITFALL

Injuries to hidden areas of the abdomen such as the retroperitoneum must be suspected and evaluated.

This area is also referred to as the "thoracoabdominal component" of the abdomen. As the diaphragm rises to the fourth intercostal space during full expiration, fractures of the lower ribs or penetrating wounds below the nipple line may injure abdominal viscera. The lower peritoneal cavity contains the small bowel, parts of the ascending and descending colons, the sigmoid colon, and, in females, the internal reproductive organs.

RETROPERITONEAL SPACE

This potential space is the area posterior to the peritoneal lining of the abdomen. It contains the abdominal aorta; the inferior vena cava; most of the duodenum, pancreas, kidneys and ureters; the posterior aspects of the ascending and descending colons; and the retroperitoneal components of the pelvic cavity. **Injuries to the retroperitoneal visceral structures are difficult to recognize because the area is remote from physical examination, and injuries do not initially present with signs or symptoms of peritonitis.** In addition, this space is not sampled by diagnostic peritoneal lavage (DPL). ◾ See Skill Station VIII: Diagnostic Peritoneal Lavage.

PELVIC CAVITY

The pelvic cavity, surrounded by the pelvic bones, is essentially the lower part of the retroperitoneal and intraperitoneal spaces. It contains the rectum, bladder, iliac vessels, and, in females, internal reproductive organs. As with the thoracoabdominal area, examination of pelvic structures is compromised by overlying bones.

Mechanism of Injury

Why is the mechanism of injury important?

Information provided by prehospital personnel or witnesses can be very helpful in predicting injury patterns. This information should always be considered and evaluated when assessing trauma patients. ◾ See Appendix B: Biomechanics of Injury.

BLUNT TRAUMA

A direct blow, such as contact with the lower rim of the steering wheel or a door intruding into the passenger space as the result of a motor vehicle crash, can cause compression and crushing injuries to abdominal viscera. Such forces deform solid and hollow organs and may cause rupture, with secondary hemorrhage, contamination by visceral contents, and peritonitis. Shearing injuries are a form of crushing injury that may result when a restraint device, such as a lap-type seat belt or shoulder harness component, is worn improperly (Figure 5-2). Patients injured in motor vehicle crashes also may sustain deceleration injuries, in which there is a differential movement of fixed and nonfixed parts of the body. Examples include the frequent lacerations of the liver and spleen, both movable organs, at the sites of their fixed supporting ligaments.

Air-bag deployment does not preclude abdominal injury. In patients who sustain blunt trauma, the organs most frequently injured include the spleen (40%–55%), liver (35%–45%), and small bowel (5%–10%). In addition, there is a 15% incidence of retroperitoneal hematoma in patients who undergo laparotomy for blunt trauma. Although restraint devices prevent more major injuries, they may produce specific patterns of injury, as shown in Table 5-1.

PENETRATING TRAUMA

Stab wounds and low-velocity gunshot wounds cause tissue damage by lacerating and cutting. High-velocity gunshot wounds transfer more kinetic energy to abdominal viscera. High-velocity wounds may cause increased damage lateral to the track of the missile due to temporary cavitation.

Stab wounds traverse adjacent abdominal structures and most commonly involve the liver (40%), small bowel

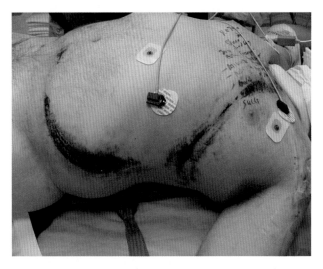

◾ **Figure 5-2 Lap Belt Injury.** Injuries can result when a restraint device, such as a lap-type seat belt or shoulder harness component, is worn improperly.

TABLE 5-1 ■ **Truncal and Cervical Injuries from Restraint Devices**

RESTRAINT DEVICE	INJURY
Lap Seat Belt • Compression • Hyperflexion	• Tear or avulsion of mesentery • Rupture of small bowel or colon • Thrombosis of iliac artery or abdominal aorta • Chance fracture of lumbar vertebrae • Pancreatic or duodenal injury
Shoulder Harness • Sliding under the seat belt ("submarining") • Compression	• Intimal tear or thrombosis in innominate, carotid, subclavian, or vertebral arteries • Fracture or dislocation of cervical spine • Rib fractures • Pulmonary contusion • Rupture of upper abdominal viscera
Air Bag • Contact • Contact/deceleration • Flexion (unrestrained) • Hyperextension (unrestrained)	• Corneal abrasions • Abrasions of face, neck, and chest • Cardiac rupture • Cervical or thoracic spine fracture

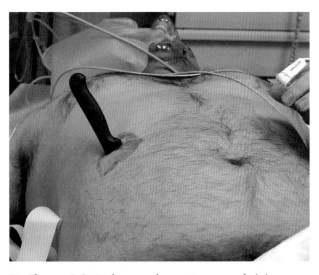

■ **Figure 5-3** Stab wounds most commonly injure the liver, small bowel, diaphragm, and colon.

(30%), diaphragm (20%), and colon (15%) (Figure 5-3). Gunshot wounds may cause additional intraabdominal injuries based on the length of the missile's path through the body, the greater kinetic energy, the possibility of ricochet off of bony structures, and the possibility of fragmentation, creating secondary missiles. Gunshot wounds most commonly involve the small bowel (50%), colon (40%), liver (30%), and abdominal vascular structures (25%).

Explosive devices cause injuries through several mechanisms, including penetrating fragment wounds and blunt injuries caused by the patient being thrown or struck. Combined penetrating and blunt mechanisms must be considered. Patients close to the source of the explosion may have additional pulmonary injuries and injuries to the hollow viscera related to blast pressure. **The potential for blast overpressure injury should not distract the doctor from a systematic, ABC approach to identification and treatment of the common blunt and penetrating injuries.**

PITFALLS

Failure to understand the mechanism leads to a lowered index of suspicion and missed injuries, such as:

• Underestimation of energy delivered to the abdomen in blunt trauma

• Visceral and vascular injuries caused by small external low-velocity wounds, especially stab and fragment wounds

• Underestimation of the amount of energy delivered in high-velocity wounds, leading to missed injuries tangential to the path of the missile

Assessment

❓ *How do I know if shock is the result of an intraabdominal injury?*

In patients with hypotension, the doctor's goal is to rapidly determine whether an abdominal injury is present and whether it is the cause of the hypotension. The history may predict, and the physical exam, along with rapidly available diagnostic tools, may confirm the presence of abdominal and pelvic injuries that require urgent control of hemorrhage. **Hemodynamically normal patients without signs of peritonitis may undergo a more detailed evaluation to determine whether specific injuries that can cause delayed morbidity and mortality are present.** This may include repeated examination to determine whether signs of bleeding or peritonitis develop over time.

HISTORY

When assessing a patient injured in a motor vehicle crash, pertinent historical information includes speed of the vehicle, type of collision (eg, frontal impact, lateral impact, sideswipe, rear impact, or rollover), vehicle intrusion into the passenger compartment, types of restraints used, deployment of air bags, patient's position in the vehicle, and status of passengers, if any. This information may be provided by the patient, other passengers, the police, or emergency medical personnel. Information about vital signs, obvious injuries, and response to prehospital treatment also should be provided by the prehospital care providers.

When assessing a patient who has sustained penetrating trauma, pertinent information includes the time of injury, type of weapon (eg, knife, handgun, rifle, or shotgun), distance from the assailant (particularly important with shotgun wounds, as the likelihood of major visceral injuries decreases beyond the 10-foot, or 3-meter, range), number of stab or gunshot wounds sustained, and the amount of external bleeding noted at the scene. If possible to obtain it, important additional information includes the magnitude and location of abdominal pain and whether this pain is referred to the shoulder.

When injuries are caused by an explosive device, the likelihood of visceral high pressure injuries is increased if the explosion occurred in an enclosed space and with decreasing distance of the patient from the explosion.

PHYSICAL EXAMINATION

❓ *How do I determine whether there is an abdominal injury?*

The abdominal examination should be conducted in a meticulous, systematic fashion in the standard sequence: inspection, auscultation, percussion, and palpation. This is followed by assessment of pelvic stability; urethral, perineal, and rectal exam; vaginal exam; and gluteal exam. The find-

> **PITFALL**
>
> Hypothermia contributes to coagulopathy and ongoing bleeding.

ings, whether positive or negative, should be documented carefully in the patient's medical record.

Inspection

In most circumstances, the patient must be fully undressed. The anterior and posterior abdomen, as well as the lower chest and perineum, is inspected for abrasions, contusions from restraint devices, lacerations, penetrating wounds, impaled foreign bodies, evisceration of omentum or small bowel, and pregnancy. The patient should be cautiously logrolled to facilitate a complete examination. At the conclusion of the rapid physical exam, the patient should be covered with warmed blankets to help prevent hypothermia.

Auscultation

Auscultation of the abdomen may be difficult in a noisy emergency department, but it may be used to confirm the presence or absence of bowel sounds. Free intraperitoneal blood or gastrointestinal contents may produce an ileus, resulting in the loss of bowel sounds; however, this finding is nonspecific, as ileus may also be caused by extraabdominal injuries. **These findings are most useful when they are normal initially and then change over time.**

Percussion and Palpation

Percussion causes slight movement of the peritoneum and may elicit signs of peritoneal irritation. **When present, no additional evidence of rebound tenderness need or should be sought as such an examination may cause the patient unnecessary further pain.**

Voluntary guarding by the patient may make the abdominal examination unreliable. In contrast, involuntary muscle guarding is a reliable sign of peritoneal irritation. Palpation may also elicit and distinguish superficial (abdominal wall) and deep tenderness. The presence of a pregnant uterus, as well as estimation of fetal age, also can be determined.

Assessment of Pelvic Stability

Major hemorrhage may occur from a pelvic fracture in patients who sustain blunt truncal trauma. An early assessment

> **PITFALL**
>
> Repeated manipulation of a fractured pelvis can aggravate hemorrhage.

of the likelihood of hemorrhage from this source can be made during the physical exam by evaluating pelvic stability. This begins with manual compression of the anterosuperior iliac spines or iliac crests. Abnormal movement or bony pain suggests fracture, and the exam may stop with this maneuver. If the pelvis seems stable to compression, a maneuver to distract the anterosuperior iliac spines is accomplished, also evaluating for bony movement or pain. **Caution should be exercised, as this maneuver can cause or aggravate bleeding.** When rapidly available, some doctors substitute x-ray examination of the pelvis to avoid pain and the potential for aggravating hemorrhage.

Urethral, Perineal, and Rectal Examination

The presence of blood at the urethral meatus strongly suggests a urethral tear. Inspection of the scrotum and perineum should be performed to look for ecchymoses or hematoma, suggestive of the same injury. In patients who have sustained blunt trauma, goals of the rectal examination are to assess sphincter tone, determine the position of the prostate (a high-riding prostate indicates urethral disruption), and identify any fractures of the pelvic bones. In patients with penetrating wounds, the rectal examination is used to assess sphincter tone and look for gross blood from a bowel perforation.

Vaginal Examination

Laceration of the vagina may occur from bony fragments from pelvic fracture(s) or from penetrating wounds. Vaginal exam should be performed when injury is suspected (eg, in the presence of complex perineal laceration). Also see Chapter 12: Trauma in Women.

Gluteal Examination

The gluteal region extends from the iliac crests to the gluteal folds. Penetrating injuries to this area are associated with an incidence of up to a 50% of significant intraabdominal injuries, including rectal injuries below the peritoneal reflection. Gunshot and stab wounds are associated with intraabdominal injuries; these wounds mandate a search for such injuries.

ADJUNCTS TO PHYSICAL EXAMINATION

Gastric and urinary catheters are frequently inserted as part of the resuscitation phase, once problems with the airway, breathing, and circulation are diagnosed and treated.

Gastric Tube

The therapeutic goals of inserting gastric tubes early in the resuscitation process are to relieve acute gastric dilation, decompress the stomach before performing a DPL, and remove gastric contents, thereby reducing the risk of aspiration. The presence of blood in the gastric secretions suggests an injury to the esophagus or upper gastrointestinal tract if nasopharyngeal and/or oropharyngeal sources are excluded. **If severe facial fractures exist or basilar skull fracture is suspected, the gastric tube should be inserted through the mouth to prevent passage of the tube through the cribriform plate into the brain.**

Urinary Catheter

The goals of inserting urinary catheters early in the resuscitation process are to relieve retention, decompress the bladder before performing DPL, and allow for monitoring of urinary output as an index of tissue perfusion. Hematuria is a sign of trauma to the genitourinary tract and nonrenal intraabdominal organs. **The inability to void, unstable pelvic fracture, blood at the meatus, scrotal hematoma, or perineal ecchymoses and a high-riding prostate on rectal examination mandate retrograde urethrography to confirm an intact urethra before inserting a urinary catheter. A disrupted urethra detected during the primary or secondary survey may require the insertion of a suprapubic tube by an experienced doctor and may be performed more safely with ultrasound guidance.**

Other Studies

With preparation and an organized team approach, the preceding evaluation can be performed very quickly. The following additional studies are chosen based on the hemodynamic status of the patient and the suspected injuries. When intraabdominal injury is suspected, a number of studies can provide useful information; however, these studies should not delay the transfer of a patient to definitive care.

X-Ray Examination for Abdominal Trauma Anteroposterior (AP) chest and pelvic x-ray examinations are recommended in the assessment of patients with multisystem blunt trauma. Patients with hemodynamic abnormalities who have penetrating abdominal wounds do not require screening x-ray examination in the emergency department (ED). If the patient has no hemodynamic abnormalities and has penetrating trauma above the umbilicus or a suspected thoracoabdominal injury, an upright chest x-ray examination is useful to exclude an associated hemothorax or pneumothorax or to document the presence of intraperitoneal air. With marker rings or clips applied to all entrance and exit wound sites, a supine abdominal x-ray may be obtained in patients with no hemodynamic abnormalities to determine the track of the missile or presence of retroperitoneal air.

PITFALL

Avoid nasal gastric tube in midface injury. Use oral gastric route.

Focused Assessment Sonography in Trauma   Focused assessment sonography in trauma (FAST) is one of the two most rapid studies for the identification of hemorrhage or the potential for hollow viscus injury. In FAST, ultrasound technology is used by properly trained individuals to detect the presence of hemoperitoneum (Figure 5-4). With specific equipment and in experienced hands, ultrasound has a sensitivity, specificity, and accuracy in detecting intraabdominal fluid comparable to DPL and abdominal computed tomography. Thus, ultrasound provides a rapid, noninvasive, accurate, and inexpensive means of diagnosing hemoperitoneum that can be repeated frequently. Ultrasound scanning can be done at the bedside in the resuscitation room while simultaneously performing other diagnostic or therapeutic procedures. The indications for the procedure are the same as for DPL. Factors that compromise the utility of ultrasound are obesity, the presence of subcutaneous air, and previous abdominal operations.

Ultrasound scanning to detect hemoperitoneum can be accomplished rapidly. Furthermore, it can detect one of the nonhypovolemic reasons for hypotension: pericardial tamponade. Scans are obtained of the pericardial sac, hepatorenal fossa, splenorenal fossa, and pelvis or pouch of Douglas. **After the initial scan is completed, a second or "control" scan should ideally be performed after an interval of 30 minutes.** The control scan can detect progressive hemoperitoneum in patients with a low rate of bleeding and short intervals from injury to the initial scan.

Diagnostic Peritoneal Lavage   Diagnostic peritoneal lavage (DPL) is the second of the two most rapid studies for the identification of hemorrhage or the potential for hollow viscus injury. DPL is an invasive procedure that significantly alters subsequent examinations of the patient and is considered 98% sensitive for intraperitoneal bleeding (Figure 5-5). It should be performed by a surgical team caring for a patient with hemodynamic abnormalities and multiple blunt injuries, especially when any of the following situations exists:

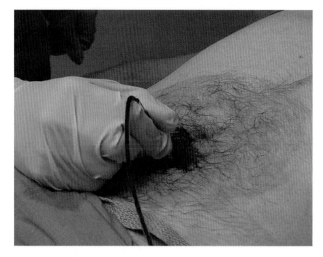

■ **Figure 5-5 Diagnostic Peritoneal Lavage (DPL).** DPL is a rapidly performed, invasive procedure that is considered 98% sensitive for intraperitoneal bleeding.

- Change in sensorium—brain injury, alcohol intoxication, and use of illicit drugs
- Change in sensation—injury to spinal cord
- Injury to adjacent structures—lower ribs, pelvis, lumbar spine
- Equivocal results on physical examination
- Prolonged loss of contact with patient anticipated—general anesthesia for extraabdominal injuries, lengthy x-ray studies (eg, angiography in a patient with or without hemodynamic abnormalities)
- Lap-belt sign (abdominal wall contusion) with suspicion of bowel injury

DPL also is indicated in patients with no hemodynamic abnormalities when the same situations are present, but ultrasound and computed tomography (CT) are not available. The only absolute contraindication to DPL is an existing indication for laparotomy. Relative contraindications include previous abdominal operations, morbid obesity, advanced cirrhosis, and preexisting coagulopathy. Either an open or closed (Seldinger) infraumbilical technique is acceptable in the hands of trained doctors. In patients with pelvic fractures or advanced pregnancy, an open supraumbilical approach is preferred to avoid entering a pelvic hematoma or

PITFALL

A single physical exam or adjunct should not allay clinical suspicion based on the mechanism of injury. Repeated exams and complementary adjuncts may be necessary.

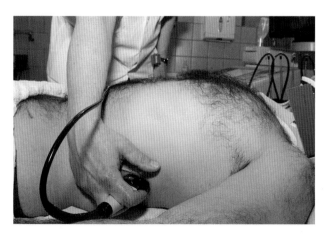

■ **Figure 5-4 Focused Assessment Sonography in Trauma (FAST).** In FAST, ultrasound technology is used to detect the presence of hemoperitoneum.

damaging the enlarged uterus. **Free aspiration of blood, gastrointestinal contents, vegetable fibers, or bile through the lavage catheter in patients with hemodynamic abnormalities mandates the use of laparotomy.**

If gross blood (>10 mL) or gastrointestinal contents are not aspirated, lavage is performed with 1000 mL of warmed isotonic crystalloid solution (10 mL/kg in a child). After ensuring adequate mixing of peritoneal contents with the lavage fluid by compressing the abdomen and moving the patient by logrolling or tilting him or her into head-down and head-up positions, the effluent is sent to the laboratory for quantitative analysis if gastrointestinal contents, vegetable fibers, or bile are not obviously present. A positive test for blunt trauma is indicated by >100,000 red cells per cubic millimeter, 500 white cells per cubic millimeter, or the presence of bacteria shown on Gram staining. ◾ See Skill Station VIII: Diagnostic Peritoneal Lavage.

Computed Tomography   Computed tomography (CT) is a diagnostic procedure that requires transport of the patient to the scanner, administration of contrast, and scanning of the upper and lower abdomen, as well as the pelvis. **It is a time-consuming procedure that should be used only in patients with no hemodynamic abnormalities in whom there is no apparent indication for an emergency laparotomy.** The CT scan provides information relative to specific organ injury and its extent, and can diagnose retroperitoneal and pelvic organ injuries that are difficult to assess by a physical examination, FAST, and peritoneal lavage. Relative contraindications to the use of CT include delay until the scanner is available, an uncooperative patient who cannot be safely sedated, and allergy to the contrast agent when nonionic contrast is not available. **Some gastrointestinal, diaphragmatic, and pancreatic injuries may be missed on CT. In the absence of hepatic or splenic injuries, the presence of free fluid in the abdominal cavity suggests an injury to the gastrointestinal tract and/or its mesentery, and many trauma surgeons find this to be an indication for early operative intervention.**

Contrast Studies   A number of contrast studies can aid in the diagnosis of specifically suspected injuries, but they should not delay the care of patients with hemodynamic abnormalities. These include:

- Urethrography
- Cystography
- Intravenous pyelography
- Gastrointestinal contrast studies

Urethrography should be performed before inserting an indwelling urinary catheter when a urethral tear is suspected. It is performed with an #8 French urinary catheter secured in the meatal fossa by balloon inflation to 1.5 to 2 mL. Approximately 15 to 20 mL of undiluted contrast material is instilled with gentle pressure. A radiograph is taken with an oblique projection and with slight stretching of the penis.

An intraperitoneal or extraperitoneal bladder rupture is best diagnosed by a cystogram. A syringe barrel is attached to the indwelling bladder catheter, held 40 cm above the patient, and 300 mL of water-soluble contrast is allowed to flow into the bladder or until: (1) flow stops, (2) the patient voids spontaneously, or (3) the patient is in discomfort. AP, oblique, and postdrainage views are essential to definitively exclude injury. CT evaluation of the bladder and pelvis (CT cystography) is an alternative study that is particularly useful in providing additional information about the kidneys and pelvic bones.

Suspected urinary system injuries are best evaluated by contrast-enhanced CT scan. If CT is not available, intravenous pyelography (IVP) provides an alternative. A high-dose, rapid injection of renal contrast ("screening IVP") is best performed using the recommended dosage of 200 mg of iodine/kg body weight. This involves a bolus injection of 100 mL (standard, 1.5 mL/kg for a 70-kg individual) of a 60% iodine solution performed through two 50-mL syringes over 30 to 60 seconds. If only 30% iodine solution is available, the ideal dose is 3.0 mL/kg. The calyces of the kidneys should be visualized on a flat-plate x-ray of the abdomen 2 minutes after the injection is completed. Unilateral nonfunctioning indicates an absent kidney, thrombosis, avulsion of the renal artery, or massive parenchymal disruption. Nonfunctioning warrants further radiologic evaluation with contrast-enhanced CT or renal arteriography, or surgical exploration, depending on the mechanism of injury and local availability or expertise.

Isolated injuries to retroperitoneal gastrointestinal structures (ie, duodenum, ascending or descending colon, rectum, biliary tract, and pancreas) may not cause peritonitis and may not be detected on DPL. When injury to one of these structures is suspected, CT with contrast, specific upper and lower gastrointestinal contrast studies, and pancreaticobiliary imaging studies may be useful. **These studies should be guided by the surgeon who will ultimately care for the patient.**

EVALUATION OF BLUNT TRAUMA

If there is early or obvious evidence that the patient will be transferred to another facility, time-consuming tests, such as contrast urologic and gastrointestinal studies, DPL, and CT,

PITFALL

Evaluations should not delay the transfer of the patient to a more appropriate level of care for severe injuries that have already been identified.

should _not_ be performed. Table 5-2 compares the use of DPL, FAST, and CT, including their advantages and disadvantages, in the evaluation of blunt trauma.

EVALUATION OF PENETRATING TRAUMA

The evaluation of penetrating trauma involves special consideration to address penetrating wounds to the abdomen and thoracoabdominal region. Options include local wound exploration and serial physical examination. DPL, or CT in anterior abdominal stab wounds. Double or triple contrast CT are useful in flank and back injuries. Surgery may be required for immediate diagnosis and treatment.

Penetrating Wounds

Most gunshot wounds to the abdomen are managed by exploratory laparotomy, as the incidence of significant intraperitoneal injury approaches 90%. Tangential gunshot wounds often are not truly tangential, and concussive and blast injuries can cause intraperitoneal injury without peritoneal penetration. Stab wounds to the abdomen may be managed more selectively, but approximately 30% do cause intraperitoneal injury. Thus, indications for laparotomy in patients with penetrating abdominal wounds include:

- Any patient with hemodynamic abnormalities
- Gunshot wound
- Signs of peritoneal irritation
- Signs of fascial penetration

When there is suspicion that a penetrating wound is superficial and does not appear to travel below the abdominal musculoaponeurotic layer, an experienced surgeon may elect to explore the wound locally to determine the depth of penetration. This procedure is not used with wounds overlying the ribs because of the risk of causing a pneumothorax, and it is not indicated in patients with peritonitis or hypotension from suspected abdominal injury.

Because 25% to 33% of stab wounds to the anterior abdomen do not penetrate the peritoneum, laparotomy for such patients is often nonproductive. Under sterile conditions, local anesthesia is injected, and the wound track is followed through the layers of the abdominal wall or until its termination. Confirmation of penetration through the anterior fascia places the patient at higher risk for intraperitoneal injury, and many trauma surgeons view this as an indication for laparotomy. Any patient in whom the track cannot be followed because of obesity, lack of cooperation, or soft-tissue hemorrhage or distortion should be admitted for continued evaluation or surgical exploration (laparotomy).

Thoracoabdominal Lower Chest Wounds

Diagnostic options in asymptomatic patients with possible injuries to the diaphragm and upper abdominal structures include serial physical and chest x-ray examinations, thoracoscopy, laparoscopy, and CT (for right thoracoabdominal wounds). Despite all these options, late posttraumatic left-sided diaphragmatic hernias continue to occur after thoracoabdominal stab wounds; thus early or immediate surgical exploration (laparotomy) for such wounds also is an option. For left-sided thoracoabdominal gunshot wounds, the safest alternative is laparotomy.

Local Wound Exploration and Serial Physical Examinations versus DPL in Anterior Abdominal Stab Wounds

Approximately 55% to 60% of patients with stab wounds that penetrate the anterior peritoneum have hypotension, peritonitis, or evisceration of omentum or small bowel. These patients require emergency laparotomy. In the remaining patients, in whom anterior peritoneal penetration can be confirmed or is strongly suspected after local wound exploration, approximately 50% eventually require operation. Laparotomy remains a reasonable option for all such

TABLE 5-2 ■ Comparison of DPL, FAST, and CT in Blunt Abdominal Trauma			
	DPL	**FAST**	**CT SCAN**
Advantages	• Early diagnosis • Performed rapidly • 98% sensitive • Detects bowel injury	• Early diagnosis • Noninvasive • Performed rapidly • Repeatable	• Most specific for injury • Sensitive: 92%–98% accurate
Disadvantages	• Invasive • Low specificity • Misses injuries to diaphragm and retroperitoneum	• Operator-dependent • Bowel gas and subcutaneous air distortion • Misses diaphragm, bowel, pancreatic, and solid organ injuries	• Cost and time • Misses diaphragm, bowel, and some pancreatic injuries • Transport required

PITFALL

These evaluations are seeking to prove that there is no injury in the patients with no hemodynamic abnormalities. They should not delay laparotomy in patients with hemodynamic abnormalities that likely have an abdominal source.

patients. Less invasive diagnostic options for relatively asymptomatic patients (who may have pain at the site of the stab wound) include serial physical examinations over a 24-hour period, DPL, or diagnostic laparoscopy. **Although a positive FAST may be helpful in this situation, a negative FAST does not exclude the possibility of significant intraabdominal injury producing small volumes of fluid.** Serial physical examinations are labor-intensive, but have an overall accuracy rate of 94%. DPL may allow for earlier diagnosis of injury in relatively asymptomatic patients. The accuracy rate is greater than 90% when specific cell counts, rather than gross inspection of the fluid, are used. Use of lower thresholds for penetrating trauma increases sensitivity and decreases specificity. Diagnostic laparoscopy can confirm or exclude peritoneal penetration, but it is less useful in identifying specific injuries.

Serial Physical Examinations versus Double- or Triple-Contrast CT in Flank and Back Injuries

The thickness of the flank and back muscles protects the underlying viscera from injury from many stab wounds and some gunshot wounds to these areas. Although laparotomy is a reasonable option for all such patients, less invasive diagnostic options in patients who are initially asymptomatic include serial physical examinations, double- or triple-contrast CT, and DPL. Serial physical examination in patients who are initially asymptomatic and then become symptomatic is very accurate in detecting retroperitoneal and intraperitoneal injuries with wounds posterior to the anterior axillary line.

Double- (intravenous and oral) or triple- (intravenous, oral, and rectal) contrast-enhanced CT assesses the retroperitoneal colon on the side of the wound. The accuracy is comparable to that of serial physical examinations, but should allow for earlier diagnosis of injury in relatively asymptomatic patients when CT is performed properly.

On rare occasions, these retroperitoneal injuries may be missed by serial examinations and contrast CT. Early outpatient follow-up is mandatory after the 24-hour period of in-hospital observation because of the subtle presentation of certain colonic injuries.

DPL can also be used as an early screening test in such patients. A positive DPL is an indication for an urgent laparotomy.

Indications for Laparotomy in Adults

In which patients is a laparotomy warranted?

In individual patients, surgical judgment is required to determine the timing and need for laparotomy. The following indications are commonly used to facilitate the surgeon's decision-making process.

- Blunt abdominal trauma with hypotension with a positive FAST or clinical evidence of intraperitoneal bleeding

- Blunt abdominal trauma with positive DPL

- Hypotension with penetrating abdominal wound

- Gunshot wounds traversing the peritoneal cavity or visceral/vascular retroperitoneum

- Evisceration

- Bleeding from the stomach, rectum, or genitourinary tract from penetrating trauma

- Peritonitis

- Free air, retroperitoneal air, or rupture of the hemidiaphragm after blunt trauma

- Ruptured gastrointestinal tract, intraperitoneal bladder injury, renal pedicle injury, or severe visceral parenchymal injury after blunt or penetrating trauma, as demonstrated on contrast-enhanced CT

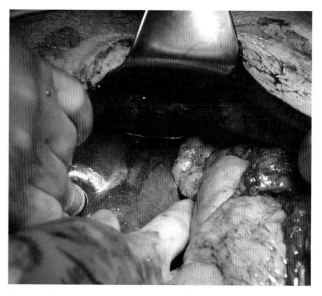

Surgical judgment is required to determine the timing and need for laparotomy.

Specific Diagnoses

The liver, spleen, and kidney are the organs predominantly involved after blunt trauma, although the relative incidence of hollow visceral perforation, lumbar spinal injuries, and uterine rupture increases with incorrect seat-belt usage (see Table 5-1). Difficulties in diagnosis may occur with injuries to the diaphragm, duodenum, pancreas, genitourinary system, or small bowel.

DIAPHRAGM INJURIES

Blunt tears may occur in any portion of either diaphragm; however, the left hemidiaphragm is more commonly injured. The most common injury is 5 to 10 cm in length and involves the posterolateral left hemidiaphragm. Abnormalities on the initial chest x-ray include elevation or "blurring" of the hemidiaphragm, hemothorax, an abnormal gas shadow that obscures the hemidiaphragm, or the gastric tube being positioned in the chest. However, the initial chest x-ray may be normal in a small percentage of patients.

DUODENAL INJURIES

Duodenal rupture is classically encountered in unrestrained drivers involved in frontal-impact motor vehicle collisions and patients who sustain direct blows to the abdomen, such as from bicycle handlebars. Bloody gastric aspirate or retroperitoneal air seen on a flat-plate x-ray film of the abdomen or abdominal CT should raise suspicion for this injury. An upper gastrointestinal x-ray series or double-contrast CT is indicated for high-risk patients.

PANCREATIC INJURIES

Pancreatic injuries most often result from a direct epigastric blow that compresses the organ against the vertebral column. **An early normal serum amylase level does not exclude major pancreatic trauma.** Conversely, the amylase level may be elevated from nonpancreatic sources. However, persistently elevated or rising serum amylase levels should prompt further evaluation of the pancreas and other abdominal viscera. **Double-contrast CT may not identify significant pancreatic trauma in the immediate postinjury period (up to 8 hours); it should be repeated later if pancreatic injury is suspected.** Should there be concern after equivocal results on CT, surgical exploration of the pancreas is warranted.

GENITOURINARY INJURIES

Direct blows to the back or flank that result in contusions, hematomas, or ecchymoses are markers of potential underlying renal injury and warrant an evaluation (CT or IVP) of the urinary tract. Additional indications for evaluating the urinary tract include gross hematuria or microscopic hematuria in patients with: (1) a penetrating abdominal wound, (2) an episode of hypotension (systolic blood pressure less than 90 mm Hg) in conjunction with blunt abdominal trauma, and (3) intraabdominal injuries associated with blunt trauma. Gross hematuria and microscopic hematuria in patients with an episode of shock indicate that they are at risk for nonrenal abdominal injuries. An abdominal CT scan with IV contrast can document the presence and extent of a blunt renal injury, 95% of which can be treated nonoperatively. Thrombosis of the renal artery or disruption of the renal pedicle secondary to deceleration is a rare upper tract injury in which hematuria may be absent, although the patient may have severe abdominal pain. With either injury, IVP, CT, or renal arteriography may be useful in diagnosis.

An anterior pelvic fracture usually is present in patients with urethral injuries. Urethral disruptions are divided into those above (posterior) or below (anterior) the urogenital diaphragm. A posterior urethral injury usually occurs in patients with multisystem injuries and pelvic fractures. In contrast, an anterior urethral injury results from a straddle impact and may be an isolated injury.

SMALL BOWEL INJURIES

Blunt injury to the intestines generally results from sudden deceleration with subsequent tearing near a fixed point of attachment, especially if the patient's seat belt was used incorrectly. The appearance of transverse, linear ecchymoses on the abdominal wall (seat-belt sign) or the presence of a lumbar distraction fracture (Chance fracture) on x-ray examination should alert the doctor to the possibility of intestinal injury. **Although some patients have early abdominal pain and tenderness, diagnosis may be difficult in others, especially because only minimal bleeding may result from torn intestinal organs.** Early ultrasound and CT are often not diagnostic for these subtle injuries, and DPL is a better choice when abdominal wall ecchymoses are present.

SOLID ORGAN INJURIES

Injuries to the liver, spleen, and kidney that result in shock, hemodynamic instability, or evidence of continuing bleeding are indications for urgent laparotomy. Solid organ injury in patients with no hemodynamic abnormalities can often be treated nonoperatively. Such patients must be admitted to the hospital for careful observation, and evaluation by a surgeon is essential. Concomitant hollow viscus injury occurs in less than 5% of patients initially thought to have isolated solid organ injuries.

PELVIC FRACTURES AND ASSOCIATED INJURIES

❓ *How do I treat patients with pelvic fractures?*

The sacrum and innominate bones (ilium, ischium, and pubis), along with many ligamentous complexes, comprise the pelvis. Fractures and ligamentous disruptions of the pelvis suggest that major forces were applied to the patient. Such injuries usually result from auto–pedestrian, motor vehicle, and motorcycle crashes. Pelvic fractures have a significant association with injuries to intraperitoneal and retroperitoneal visceral and vascular structures. The incidence of tears of the thoracic aorta also appears to be significantly increased in patients with pelvic fractures, especially anteroposterior fractures. Therefore, hypotension may or may not be related to the pelvic fracture itself when blunt trauma is the mechanism of injury.

Patients with hemorrhagic shock and unstable pelvic fractures have four potential sources of blood loss: (1) fractured bone surfaces, (2) pelvic venous plexus, (3) pelvic arterial injury, and (4) extrapelvic sources. **The pelvis should be temporarily stabilized or "closed" using an available commercial compression device or sheet to decrease bleeding.** Intraabdominal sources of hemorrhage must be excluded or treated operatively. Further decisions to control ongoing pelvic bleeding include angiographic embolization, surgical stabilization, and direct surgical control (see Figure 5-6).

Mechanism of Injury/Classification

The four patterns of force leading to pelvic fractures are the following: (1) AP compression, (2) lateral compression, (3) vertical shear, and (4) complex (combination) pattern.

An AP compression injury may be caused by an auto–pedestrian collision or motorcycle crash, a direct crushing injury to the pelvis, or a fall from a height greater than 12 feet (3.6 meters). With disruption of the symphysis pubis, there often is tearing of the posterior osseous liga-

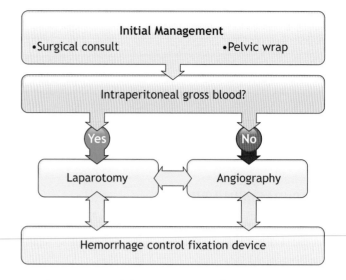

■ **Figure 5-6 Pelvic Fractures and Hemorrhagic Shock—Management Algorithm.**

mentous complex (sacroiliac, sacrospinous, sacrotuberous, and fibromuscular pelvic floor) represented by a sacroiliac fracture and/or dislocation or sacral fracture. With opening of the pelvic ring, there may be hemorrhage from the posterior pelvic venous complex and, occasionally, branches of the internal iliac artery. Figure 5-8 shows an "open book" fracture.

Lateral compression injuries often result from motor vehicle crashes and lead to internal rotation of the involved hemipelvis. This rotation drives the pubis into the lower genitourinary system, injuring the bladder and/or urethra. The pelvic volume is actually compressed in such an injury, so life-threatening hemorrhage is not common. Figure 5-7 shows a "closed" fracture.

A high-energy shear force applied in a vertical plane across the anterior and posterior aspects of the ring disrupts

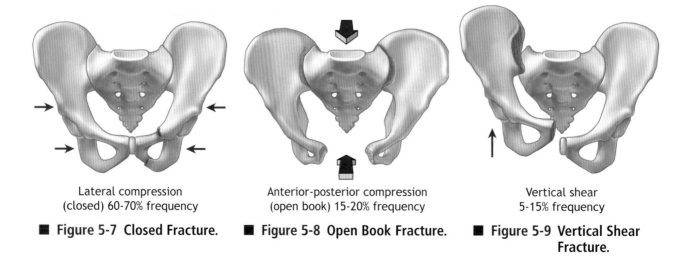

Lateral compression (closed) 60-70% frequency

Anterior-posterior compression (open book) 15-20% frequency

Vertical shear 5-15% frequency

■ **Figure 5-7 Closed Fracture.**   ■ **Figure 5-8 Open Book Fracture.**   ■ **Figure 5-9 Vertical Shear Fracture.**

PITFALL

Delay in stabilization of the pelvis allows continued hemorrhage.

the sacrospinous and sacrotuberous ligaments and leads to a major pelvic instability. Figure 5-9 shows a vertical shear fracture.

In some cases of severe injury, combinations of compression and shear forces result in complex combination patterns. These injuries are associated with major bleeding.

Assessment

The flank, scrotum, and perianal area should be inspected quickly for blood at the urethral meatus; swelling or bruising; or laceration in the perineum, vagina, rectum, or buttocks, which is suggestive of an open pelvic fracture. Palpation of a high-riding prostate gland also is a sign of a significant pelvic fracture.

Mechanical instability of the pelvic ring can be quickly ascertained during physical examination of the pelvis. Once instability has been verified, a source of hemorrhage has been suggested; no further maneuvers to demonstrate instability are necessary. A rapidly available x-ray may avoid the pain and potential hemmorrhage associated with manipulating the pelvis.

The first indication of mechanical instability is seen on inspection for leg-length discrepancy or rotational deformity (usually external) without a fracture of that extremity. Because the unstable pelvis is able to rotate externally, the pelvis can be closed by pushing on the iliac crests at the level of the anterior superior iliac spine. Motion can be felt if the iliac crests are grasped and the unstable hemipelvis is pushed inward and then outward (compression distraction maneuver). With posterior disruption, the involved hemipelvis can be pushed cephalad as well as pulled caudally. This translational motion can be felt by palpating the posterior iliac spine and tubercle while pushing or pulling the unstable hemipelvis. When appropriate, an AP x-ray film of the pelvis confirms the clinical examination. When time, availability, and patient condition permit, the x-ray may be used in lieu of manipulation to make the diagnosis. See Chapter 3: Shock; and Skill Station IV: Shock Assessment and Management.

Management

Simple techniques may be used to splint unstable pelvic fractures and close the increased pelvic volume prior to patient transfer and during the resuscitation with crystalloid fluids and blood. These techniques include: (1) a sheet wrapped around the pelvis as a sling, causing internal rotation of the lower limbs, (2) commercially available pelvic splints, and (3) other pelvis-stabilizing devices (Figure 5-10).

Reduction of an acetabular fracture by longitudinal traction of the lower extremity also can be useful. Although definitive management of pelvic fractures varies, one treatment algorithm based on the hemodynamic status for patients in emergency situations in shown in Figure 5-6: Management of Pelvic Fractures. **Since significant resources are required to care for patients with severe pelvic fractures, early consideration of transfer to a trauma center is essential.**

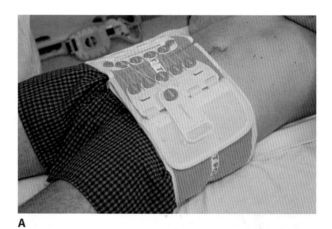

A

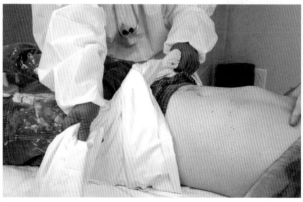

B

■ **Figure 5-10 Pelvic Stabilization.** Pelvic binder **(A)** and pelvic stabilization using a sheet **(B)**.

CHAPTER SUMMARY

1 The three distinct regions of the abdomen are the peritoneal cavity, the retroperitoneal space, and the pelvic cavity. The pelvic cavity contains components of both the peritoneal cavity and retroperitoneal spaces.

2 Early consultation with a surgeon is necessary whenever a patient with possible intraabdominal injuries is brought to the emergency department. Once the patient's vital functions have been restored, evaluation and management vary depending on the mechanism of injury as described herein.

3 Patients with hemodynamic abnormalities and multiple blunt injuries should be rapidly assessed for intraabdominal bleeding or contamination from the gastrointestinal tract by performing a FAST or diagnostic peritoneal lavage. Patients with no hemodynamic abnormalities and no peritonitis should be evaluated by contrast-enhanced CT, with the decision to operate based on the specific organ(s) involved and the magnitude of injury. All patients with penetrating wounds in proximity to the abdomen and associated hypotension, peritonitis, or evisceration require emergency laparotomy. Patients with gunshot wounds that obviously traverse the peritoneal cavity or visceral/vascular area of the retroperitoneum on physical or routine x-ray examination also require emergency laparotomy. Asymptomatic patients with anterior abdominal stab wounds that are shown on local wound exploration to penetrate the fascia or peritoneum are evaluated by serial physical examinations or DPL. However, laparoscopy or laparotomy remains an acceptable option. Asymptomatic patients with flank or back stab wounds that are not obviously superficial are evaluated by serial physical examinations or contrast-enhanced CT. Exploratory laparotomy is an acceptable option with these patients as well. It is safer to perform a laparotomy in patients with gunshot wounds to the flank and back.

4 Management of blunt and penetrating trauma to the abdomen and pelvis includes:
- Reestablishing vital functions and optimizing oxygenation and tissue perfusion
- Prompt recognition of sources of hemorrhage with efforts at hemorrhage control (such as pelvic stabilization)
- Delineating the injury mechanism
- Meticulous initial physical examination, repeated at regular intervals
- Selecting special diagnostic maneuvers as needed, performed with a minimal loss of time
- Maintaining a high index of suspicion related to occult vascular and retroperitoneal injuries
- Early recognition for surgical intervention and prompt laparotomy

Bibliography

1. Agolini SF, Shah K, Jaffe J, et al. Arterial embolization is a rapid and effective technique for controlling pelvic fracture hemorrhage. *J Trauma* 1997;43(3):395-399.

2. Almogy G, Mintz Y, Zamir G, et al. Suicide bombing attacks: Can external signs predict internal injuries? *Ann Surg* 2006;243(4):541-546.

3. Anderson PA, Rivara FP, Maier RV, et al. The epidemiology of seat belt-associated injuries. *J Trauma* 1991;31:60-67.

4. Appenzeller GN. Injury patterns in peacekeeping missions: the Kosovo experience. *Mil Med* 2004;169(3):187-191.

5. Aquilera PA, Choi T, Durham BH. Ultrasound-aided suprapubic cystostomy catheter placement in the emergency department. *J Emerg Med* 2004;26(3):319-321.

6. Ballard RB, Rozycki GS, Newman PG, et al. An algorithm to reduce the incidence of false-negative FAST examinations in

patients at high risk for occult injury. *J Am Coll Surg* 1999;189(2):145-150.

7. Beekley AC, Starnes BW, Sebesta JA. Lessons learned from modern military surgery. *Surg Clin North Am* 2007;87(1):157-84, vii.

8. Born CT. Blast trauma: the fourth weapon of mass destruction. *Scand J Surg* 2005;94(4):279-285.

9. Boyle EM, Maier RV, Salazar JD, et al: Diagnosis of injuries after stab wounds to the back and flank. *J Trauma* 1997;42(2):260-265.

10. Cook RE, Keating JF, Gillespie I. The role of angiography in the management of haemorrhage from major fractures of the pelvis. *J Bone Joint Surg Br* 2002;84(2):178-182.

11. Cryer HM, Miller FB, Evers BM, et al. Pelvic fracture classification: correlation with hemorrhage. *J Trauma* 1988;28:973-980.

12. Dalal SA, Burgess AR, Siegel JH, et al. Pelvic fracture in multiple trauma: classification by mechanism is key to pattern of organ injury, resuscitative requirements, and outcome. *J Trauma* 1989;29:981-1002.

13. De PRG, Burris DG, Champion HR, Hodgson MJ. Blast injuries. *N Engl J Med* 2005;352(13):1335-1342.

14. Demetriades D, Rabinowitz B, Sofianos C, et al. The management of penetrating injuries of the back: a prospective study of 230 patients. *Ann Surg* 1988;207:72-74.

15. Dischinger PC, Cushing BM, Kerns TJ. Injury patterns associated with direction of impact: drivers admitted to trauma centers. *J Trauma* 1993;35:454-459.

16. Donohue JH, Federle MP, Griffiths BG, et al. Computed tomography in the diagnosis of blunt intestinal and mesenteric injuries. *J Trauma* 1987;27:11-17.

17. Durkin A, Sagi HC, Durham R, Flint L. Contemporary management of pelvic fractures. *Am J Surg* 2006;192(2): 211-223.

18. Dyer GS, Vrahas MS. Review of the pathophysiology and acute management of haemorrhage in pelvic fracture. *Injury* 2006;37(7):602-613.

19. Fallon WF Jr, Reyna TM, Brunner RG, et al. Penetrating trauma to the buttock. *South Med J* 1988;81(10):1236-1238.

20. Fangio P, Asehnoune K, Edouard A, Smail N, Benhamou D. Early embolization and vasopressor administration for management of life-threatening hemorrhage from pelvic fracture. *J Trauma* 2005;58(5):978-984; discussion 984.

21. Feliciano DV, Bitondo CG, Steed G, et al. Five hundred open taps or lavages in patients with abdominal stab wounds. *Am J Surg* 1984;146:772-777.

22. Giannoudis PV, Pape HC. Damage control orthopaedics in unstable pelvic ring injuries. *Injury* 2004;35(7):671-677.

23. Grotz MR, Allami MK, Harwood P, Pape HC, Krettek C, Giannoudis PV. Open pelvic fractures: epidemiology, current concepts of management and outcome. *Injury* 2005;36(1):1-13.

24. Gylling SF, Ward RE, Holcroft JW, et al. Immediate external fixation of unstable pelvic fractures. *Am J Surg* 1985;150:721-724.

25. Hak DJ. The role of pelvic angiography in evaluation and management of pelvic trauma. *Orthop Clin North Am* 2004;35(4):439-443, v.

26. Hare SS, Goddard I, Ward P, Naraghi A, Dick EA. The radiological management of bomb blast injury. *Clin Radiol* 2007; 62(1):1-9.

27. Heetveld MJ, Harris I, Schlaphoff G, Balogh Z, D'Amours SK, Sugrue M. Hemodynamically unstable pelvic fractures: recent care and new guidelines. *World J Surg* 2004;28(9):904-909.

28. Heetveld MJ, Harris I, Schlaphoff G, Sugrue M. Guidelines for the management of haemodynamically unstable pelvic fracture patients. *ANZ J Surg* 2004;74(7):520-529.

29. Holmes JF, Harris D, Battistella FD. Performance of abdominal ultrasonography in blunt trauma patients with out-of-hospital or emergency department hypotension. *Ann Emerg Med* 2004;43(3):354-361.

30. Huizinga WK, Baker LW, Mtshali ZW. Selective management of abdominal and thoracic stab wounds with established peritoneal penetration: the eviscerated omentum. *Am J Surg* 1987;153:564-568.

31. Ivatury RR, Rao RM, Nallathambi M, et al. Penetrating gluteal injury. *J Trauma* 1982;23(8):706-709.

32. Kluger Y, Peleg K, Daniel-Aharonson L, Mayo A. The special injury pattern in terrorist bombings. *J Am Coll Surg* 2004; 199(6):875-879.

33. Knudson MM, McAninch JW, Gomez R, Hematuria as a predictor of abdominal injury after blunt trauma. *Am J Surg* 1992;164(5):482-486.

34. Koraitim MM. Pelvic fracture urethral injuries: the unresolved controversy. *J Urol* 1999;161(5):1433-1441.

35. Kregor PJ, Routt ML. Unstable pelvic ring disruptions in unstable patients. *Injury* 1999; 30 Suppl 2:B19-28.

36. Lee C, Porter K. The prehospital management of pelvic fractures. *Emerg Med J* 2007;24(2):130-133.

37. Liu M, Lee C, Veng F. Prospective comparison of diagnostic peritoneal lavage, computed tomographic scanning, and ultrasonography for the diagnosis of blunt abdominal trauma. *J Trauma* 1993;35:267-270.

38. Marti M, Parron M, Baudraxler F, Royo A, Gomez LN, Alvarez-Sala R. Blast injuries from Madrid terrorist bombing attacks on March 11, 2004. *Emerg Radiol* 2006; 13(3):113-122.

39. McCarthy MC, Lowdermilk GA, Canal DF, et al. Prediction of injury caused by penetrating wounds to the abdomen, flank, and back. *Arch Surg* 1991;26:962-966.

40. Mendez C, Gubler KD, Maier RV. Diagnostic accuracy of peritoneal lavage in patients with pelvic fractures. *Arch Surg* 1994;129(5):477-481.

41. Metz CM, Hak DJ, Goulet JA, Williams D. Pelvic fracture patterns and their corresponding angiographic sources of hemorrhage. *Orthop Clin North Am* 2004; 35(4):431-437, v.

42. Meyer DM, Thal ER, Weigelt JA, et al. The role of abdominal CT in the evaluation of stab wounds to the back. *J Trauma* 1989;29:1226-1230.

43. Miller KS, McAnnich JW. Radiographic assessment of renal trauma: our 15-year experience. *J Urol* 1995;154(2 Pt 1):352-355.

44. Mirza A, Ellis T. Initial management of pelvic and femoral fractures in the multiply injured patient. *Crit Care Clin* 2004; 20(1):159-170.

45. Mohanty K, Musso D, Powell JN, Kortbeek JB, Kirkpatrick AW. Emergent management of pelvic ring injuries: an update. *Can J Surg* 2005; 48(1):49-56.

46. Montgomery SP, Swiecki CW, Shriver CD. The evaluation of casualties from Operation Iraqi Freedom on return to the continental United States from March to June 2003. *J Am Coll Surg* 2005; 201(1):7-12; discussion 12-13.

47. Nance FC, Wennar MH, Johnson LW, et al. Surgical judgement in the management of penetrating wounds to the abdomen: experience with 2,212 patients. *Ann Surg* 1974;179(5):639-646.

48. Nelson TJ, Wall DB, Stedje-Larsen ET, Clark RT, Chambers LW, Bohman HR. Predictors of mortality in close proximity blast injuries during Operation Iraqi Freedom. *J Am Coll Surg* 2006; 202(3):418-422.

49. Niwa T, Takebayashi S, Igari H, et al. The value of plain radiographs in the prediction of outcome in pelvic fractures treated with embolisation therapy. *Br J Radiol* 2000; 73(873):945-950.

50. Nordenholz KE, Rubin MA, Gularte GG, et al. Ultrasound in the evaluation and management of blunt abdominal trauma. *Ann Emerg Med* 1997;29(3):357-366.

51. O'Neill PA, Riina J, Sclafani S, Tornetta P. Angiographic findings in pelvic fractures. *Clin Orthop Relat Res* 1996; (329):60-67.

52. Phillips T, Sclafani SJA, Goldstein A, et al. Use of the contrast-enhanced CT enema in the management of penetrating trauma to the flank and back. *J Trauma* 1986;26:593-601.

53. Reid AB, Letts RM, Black GB. Pediatric Chance fractures: association with intraabdominal injuries and seat belt use. *J Trauma* 1990;30:384-391.

54. Robin AP, Andrews JR, Lange DA, et al. Selective management of anterior abdominal stab wounds. *J Trauma* 1989;29:1684-1689.

55. Rommens PM. Pelvic ring injuries: a challenge for the trauma surgeon. *Acta Chir Belg* 1996; 96(2):78-84.

56. Root HD. Abdominal trauma and diagnostic peritoneal lavage revisited. *Am J Surg* 1990;159:363-364.

57. Routt ML Jr, Simonian PT, Swiontkowski MF. Stabilization of pelvic ring disruptions. *Orthop Clin North Am* 1997;28(3):369-388.

58. Rozycki GS. Abdominal ultrasonography in trauma. *Surg Clin North Am* 1995;75:175-191.

59. Rozycki GS, Ballard RB, Feliciano DV, et al. Surgeon-performed ultrasound for the assessment of truncal injuries: lessons learned from 1540 patients. *Ann Surg* 1998;228(4):557-565.

60. Ruchholtz S, Waydhas C, Lewan U, et al. Free abdominal fluid on ultrasound in unstable pelvic ring fracture: is laparotomy always necessary? *J Trauma* 2004; 57(2):278-285; discussion 285-287.

61. Sadri H, Nguyen-Tang T, Stern R, Hoffmeyer P, Peter R. Control of severe hemorrhage using C-clamp and arterial embolization in hemodynamically unstable patients with pelvic ring disruption. *Arch Orthop Trauma Surg* 2005; 125(7):443-447.

62. Schreiber M, Gentilello L, Rhee P, et al. Limiting computed tomography to patients with peritoneal lavage—positive results reduces cost and unnecessary celiotomies in blunt trauma. *Arch Surg* 1996;13:954-959.

63. Shackford SR, Rogers FB, Osler TM, et al. Focused abdominal sonography for trauma: the learning curve of nonradiologist clinicians in detecting hemoperitoneum. *J Trauma* 1999;46(4):553-562.

64. Shapiro M, McDonald AA, Knight D, Johannigman JA, Cuschieri J. The role of repeat angiography in the management of pelvic fractures. *J Trauma* 2005; 58(2):227-231.

65. Sharma OP, Oswanski MF, White PW. Injuries to the colon from blast effect of penetrating extra-peritoneal thoraco-abdominal trauma. *Injury* 2004; 35(3):320-324.

66. Takishima T, Sugimota K, Hirata M, et al. Serum amylase level on admission in the diagnosis of blunt injury to the pancreas: its significance and limitations. *Ann Surg* 1997;226(1):70-76.

67. Thal ER. Evolution of peritoneal lavage and local exploration in lower chest and abdominal stab wounds. *J Trauma* 1977;17:642-648.

68. Udobi KF, Roderiques A, Chiu WC, Scalea TM. Role of ultrasonography in penetrating abdominal trauma: a prospective clinical study. *J Trauma* 2001;50(3):475-479.

69. Velmahos GC, Chahwan S, Falabella A, Hanks SE, Demetriades D. Angiographic embolization for intraperitoneal and retroperitoneal injuries. *World J Surg* 2000; 24(5):539-545.

70. Velmahos GC, Toutouzas KG, Vassiliu P, et al. A prospective study on the safety and efficacy of angiographic embolization for pelvic and visceral injuries. *J Trauma* 2002; 53(2):303-308; discussion 308.

71. Wightman JM, Gladish SL. Explosions and blast injuries. *Ann Emerg Med* 2001;37(6):664-678.

72. Zantut LF, Ivatury RR, Smith RS, et al. Diagnostic and therapeutic laparoscopy for penetrating abdominal trauma: a multicenter experience. *J Trauma* 1997;42(5):825-829.

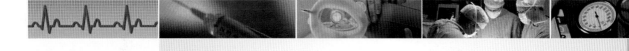

▶▶ Interactive Skill Procedure

Note: **Standard precautions are required when caring for trauma patients.**

The preferred skill procedure for peritoneal lavage is the open technique, which avoids injury to underlying structures. If an individual does not routinely perform an open DPL, use of the Seldinger technique is an acceptable alternative for doctors trained in the technique.

THE FOLLOWING PROCEDURES ARE INCLUDED IN THIS SKILL STATION:

▶▶ **Skill VIII-A:** Diagnostic Peritoneal Lavage: Open Technique

▶▶ **Skill VIII-B:** Diagnostic Peritoneal Lavage: Closed Technique

Performance at this skill station will allow the participant to practice and demonstrate the technique of diagnostic peritoneal lavage (DPL) on a live, anesthetized animal; a fresh, human cadaver; or an anatomic human body manikin. Specifically, the doctor will be able to:

OBJECTIVES

1 Identify the indications and contraindications of DPL.

2 Perform the Seldinger procedure and the open procedure for DPL.

3 Describe the complications of DPL.

▶ Skill VIII-A: Diagnostic Peritoneal Lavage: Open Technique

STEP 1. Decompress the urinary bladder by inserting a urinary catheter.

STEP 2. Decompress the stomach by inserting a gastric tube.

STEP 3. Surgically prepare the abdomen (costal margin to the pubic area and flank to flank, anteriorly).

STEP 4. Inject local anesthetic at the midline, just below the umbilicus. Use lidocaine with epinephrine to avoid blood contamination from skin and subcutaneous tissue.

STEP 5. Vertically incise the skin and subcutaneous tissues to the fascia.

STEP 6. Grasp the fascial edges with clamps, and elevate and incise the fascia down to the peritoneum. Make a small nick in the peritoneum, entering the peritoneal cavity.

STEP 7. Insert a peritoneal dialysis catheter into the peritoneal cavity.

STEP 8. Advance the catheter into the pelvis.

STEP 9. Connect the dialysis catheter to a syringe, and aspirate.

STEP 10. If gross blood is not obtained, instill 1 L of warmed isotonic crystalloid solution/normal saline (10 mL/kg in a child) into the peritoneum through the intravenous tubing attached to the dialysis catheter.

STEP 11. Gently agitate the abdomen to distribute the fluid throughout the peritoneal cavity and increase mixing with the blood.

STEP 12. If the patient's condition is stable, let the fluid remain a few minutes before placing the crystalloid container on the floor and allowing the peritoneal fluid to drain from the abdomen. Make sure the container is vented to promote flow of the fluid from the abdomen; adequate fluid return is >30% of the infused volume.

STEP 13. After the fluid returns, send a sample to the laboratory for Gram staining and erythrocyte and leukocyte counts (unspun). Positive test results and the need for surgical intervention are indicated by 100,000 red cells per cubic millimeter or more, more than 500 white cells per cubic millimeter, or a positive Gram stain for food fibers or bacteria. A negative lavage does not exclude retroperitoneal injuries, such as pancreatic and duodenal injuries or diaphragmatic tears.

▶▶ COMPLICATIONS OF PERITONEAL LAVAGE

- Hemorrhage, secondary to injection of local anesthetic or incision of the skin or subcutaneous tissues, which produces false positive results
- Peritonitis due to intestinal perforation from the catheter
- Laceration of urinary bladder (if bladder not evacuated prior to procedure)
- Injury to other abdominal and retroperitoneal structures requiring operative care
- Wound infection at the lavage site (late complication)

▶ Skill VIII-B: Diagnostic Peritoneal Lavage: Closed Technique

STEP 1. Decompress the urinary bladder by inserting a urinary catheter.

STEP 2. Decompress the stomach by inserting a gastric tube.

STEP 3. Surgically prepare the abdomen (costal margin to the pubic area and flank to flank, anteriorly).

STEP 4. Inject local anesthetic at the midline, just below the umbilicus. Use lidocaine with epinephrine to avoid blood contamination from skin and subcutaneous tissue.

STEP 5. Elevate the skin on either side of the proposed needle insertion site with the fingers or forceps.

STEP 6. Insert an 18-gauge beveled needle attached to a syringe through the skin and subcutaneous tissue. Resistance is encountered when traversing the fascia and again when penetrating the peritoneum.

STEP 7. Pass the flexible end of the guidewire through the 18-gauge needle until resistance is met or 3 cm is still showing outside the needle. Remove the needle from the abdominal cavity so that only the guidewire remains.

STEP 8. Make a small skin incision at the entrance site of the catheter, and insert the peritoneal lavage catheter over the guidewire and into the peritoneal cavity. Remove the guidewire from the abdominal cavity so that only the lavage catheter remains.

STEP 9. Connect the dialysis catheter to a syringe, and aspirate.

STEP 10. If gross blood is not obtained, instill 1 L of warmed isotonic crystalloid solution (10 mL/kg in a child) into the peritoneum through the intravenous tubing attached to the dialysis catheter.

STEP 11. Gently agitate the abdomen to distribute the fluid throughout the peritoneal cavity and increase mixing with the blood.

STEP 12. If the patient's condition is stable, let the fluid remain a few minutes before placing the crystalloid container on the floor and allowing the peritoneal fluid to drain from the abdomen. Make sure the container is vented to promote flow of the fluid from the abdomen; adequate fluid return is >30% of the infused volume.

STEP 13. After the fluid has returned, send a sample to the laboratory for Gram staining and erythrocyte and leukocyte counts (unspun). A positive test and the need for surgical intervention are indicated by 100,000 red cells per cubic millimeter or more, more than 500 white cells per cubic millimeter, or a positive Gram stain for food fibers or bacteria. A negative lavage does not exclude retroperitoneal injuries, such as pancreatic and duodenal injuries or diaphragmatic tears.

▶▶ COMPLICATIONS OF PERITONEAL LAVAGE

- Hemorrhage, secondary to injection of local anesthetic or incision of the skin or subcutaneous tissues, which produces false positive results
- Peritonitis due to intestinal perforation from the catheter
- Laceration of urinary bladder (if bladder not evacuated prior to procedure)
- Injury to other abdominal and retroperitoneal structures requiring operative care
- Wound infection at the lavage site (late complication)

CHAPTER **6** **Head Trauma**

Upon completion of this topic, the student will demonstrate the ability to apply the techniques of assessment and explain the emergency management of head trauma. Specifically, the doctor will be able to:

OBJECTIVES

1 Describe basic intracranial physiology.

2 Evaluate patients with head and brain injuries.

3 Perform a focused neurologic examination.

4 Explain the importance of adequate resuscitation in limiting secondary brain injury.

5 Determine the need for patient transfer, admission, consultation, or discharge.

Introduction

Head injuries are among the most common types of trauma seen in North American emergency departments (EDs), with an estimated 1 million cases seen annually. Many patients with severe brain injuries die before reaching a hospital, and almost 90% of prehospital trauma-related deaths involve brain injury. About 70% of patients with brain injuries who receive medical attention can be categorized as having minor injuries, 15% as moderate, and 15% as severe. In 2003 there were an estimated 1,565,000 traumatic brain injuries (TBIs) in the United States, including 1,224,000 ED visits, 290,000 hospitalizations, and 51,000 deaths. Survivors of TBI are often left with neuropsychologic impairments that result in disabilities affecting work and social activity. Every year, an estimated 80,000 to 90,000 people in the United States experience the onset of long-term disability from brain injury. In an average European country (Denmark), 363 per million inhabitants suffer moderate to severe head injuries yearly, with more than one-third of these requiring brain injury rehabilitation. Therefore, even a small reduction in the mortality and morbidity resulting from brain injury should have a major impact on public health.

The primary focus of treatment for patients in whom a severe brain injury is suspected should be to prevent secondary brain injury. Providing adequate oxygenation and maintaining a blood pressure that is sufficient to perfuse the brain are the most important ways to limit secondary brain damage and thereby improve the patient's outcome. Subsequent to managing the ABCDEs, identification of a mass lesion requiring surgical evacuation is critical, and this is best achieved by immediately obtaining a computed tomographic (CT) scan of the head. However, obtaining a CT scan should not delay patient transfer to a trauma center capable of immediate and definitive neurosurgical intervention.

The triage of a patient with brain injury depends on the severity of the injury and the facilities available within a particular community. For facilities without neurosurgical coverage, prearranged transfer agreements with higher-level facilities should be in place. Consultation with a neurosurgeon early in the course of treatment is strongly recommended, especially if the patient is comatose or brain injury is otherwise suspected.

In consulting a neurosurgeon about a patient with a brain injury, the following information is relayed:

- Age of patient and mechanism and time of injury

- Respiratory and cardiovascular status (particularly blood pressure and oxygen saturation)

- The neurologic examination, consisting of the Glasgow Coma Scale (GCS) score (with particular emphasis on the motor response) and pupil size and reaction to light

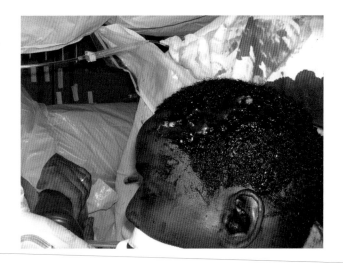

- Presence and type of associated injuries

- Results of diagnostic studies, particularly CT scan (if available)

- Treatment of hypotension or hypoxia

Do not delay patient transfer to obtain a CT scan or other diagnostic tests.

Anatomy

? *What are the unique features of brain anatomy and physiology, and how do they affect patterns of brain injury?*

A review of cranial anatomy includes the scalp, skull, meninges, brain, ventricular system, cerebrospinal fluid, and tentorium (Figure 6-1).

SCALP

The scalp is made up of five layers of tissue (mnemonic: SCALP) that cover the skull: (1) skin, (2) connective tissue, (3) aponeurosis or galea aponeurotica, (4) loose areolar tissue, and (5) pericranium. Loose areolar tissue separates the galea from the pericranium and is the site of subgaleal hematomas. Because of the scalp's generous blood supply, scalp lacerations may result in major blood loss, especially in infants and children.

SKULL

The skull is composed of the cranial vault (calvaria) and the base. The calvaria is especially thin in the temporal regions, but is cushioned here by the temporalis muscle. The base of the skull is irregular, which may contribute to injury as the brain moves within the skull during acceleration and decel-

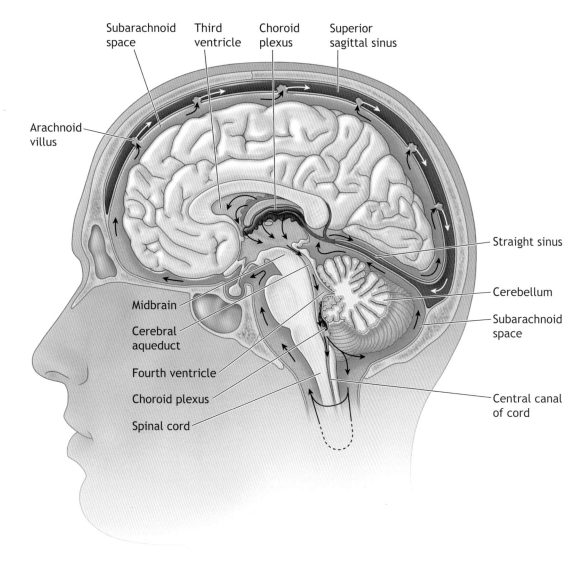

Subarachnoid space | Third ventricle | Choroid plexus | Superior sagittal sinus

Arachnoid villus

Straight sinus

Cerebellum

Subarachnoid space

Midbrain

Cerebral aqueduct

Fourth ventricle

Choroid plexus

Spinal cord

Central canal of cord

■ **Figure 6-1 Overview of Cranial Anatomy.**

eration. The floor of the cranial cavity is divided into three distinct regions: the anterior, middle, and posterior cranial fossae. Simply put, the anterior fossa houses the frontal lobes, the middle fossa the temporal lobes, and the posterior fossa the lower brainstem and the cerebellum.

MENINGES

The meninges cover the brain, and consist of three layers: the dura mater, arachnoid, and pia mater (Figure 6-2). The dura mater is a tough, fibrous membrane that adheres firmly to the internal surface of the skull. At specific sites the dura splits into two leaves that enclose the large venous sinuses that provide the major venous drainage from the brain. The midline superior sagittal sinus drains into the bilateral transverse and sigmoid sinuses, which are usually larger on the right side. Laceration of these venous sinuses may result in massive hemorrhage.

Meningeal arteries lie between the dura and the internal surface of the skull (the epidural space). Overlying skull fractures may lacerate these arteries and cause an epidural hematoma. The most commonly injured meningeal vessel is the middle meningeal artery, which is located over the temporal fossa. An expanding hematoma from arterial injury in this location may lead to rapid deterioration and death. Epidural hematomas may also result from injury to dural sinuses and from skull fractures, which tend to expand more slowly and to put less pressure on the underlying brain. However, most epidural hematomas represent a life-threatening emergency, and must be evaluated by a neurosurgeon as soon as possible.

Beneath the dura is a second meningeal layer, the thin transparent arachnoid membrane. Because the dura is not attached to the underlying arachnoid, a potential space between these layers exists (the subdural space), into which hemorrhage may occur. In brain injury, bridging veins that

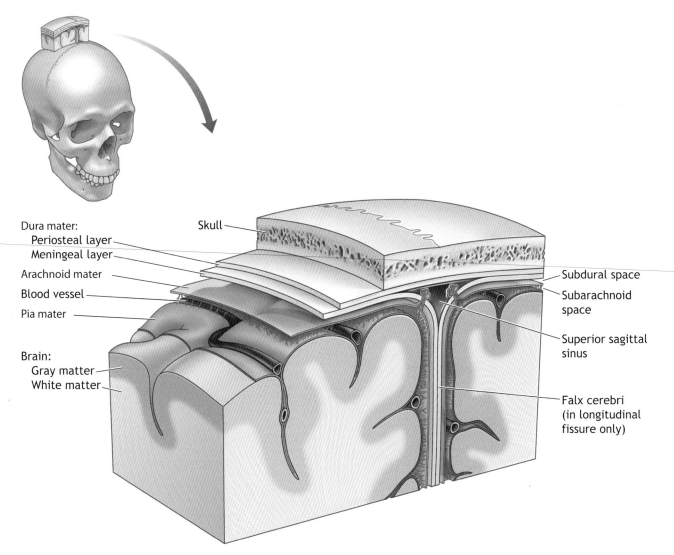

Dura mater:
  Periosteal layer
  Meningeal layer
Arachnoid mater
Blood vessel
Pia mater

Brain:
  Gray matter
  White matter

Skull

Subdural space

Subarachnoid space

Superior sagittal sinus

Falx cerebri (in longitudinal fissure only)

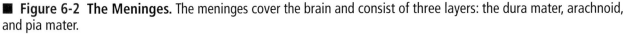

■ **Figure 6-2 The Meninges.** The meninges cover the brain and consist of three layers: the dura mater, arachnoid, and pia mater.

travel from the surface of the brain to the venous sinuses within the dura may tear, leading to the formation of a subdural hematoma.

The third layer, the pia mater, is firmly attached to the surface of the brain. Cerebrospinal fluid (CSF) fills the space between the watertight arachnoid and the pia mater (the subarachnoid space), cushioning the brain and spinal cord. Hemorrhage into this fluid-filled space (subarachnoid hemorrhage) is frequently seen in brain contusion or injury to major blood vessels at the base of the brain.

BRAIN

The brain consists of the cerebrum, cerebellum, and brainstem (see Figure 6-1). The cerebrum is composed of right and left hemispheres that are separated by the falx cerebri—a downward dural reflection from the inferior aspect of the midline superior sagittal sinus. The left hemisphere contains the language centers in virtually all right-handed people and

in more than 85% of left-handed people. The hemisphere that contains the language centers is referred to as the dominant hemisphere. The frontal lobe controls executive function, emotions, motor function, and, on the dominant side, expression of speech (motor speech areas). The parietal lobe directs sensory function and spatial orientation. The temporal lobe regulates certain memory functions. In virtually all right-handed and the majority of left-handed people, the left temporal lobe contains areas responsible for speech reception and integration. The occipital lobe is responsible for vision.

The brainstem is composed of the midbrain, pons, and medulla. The midbrain and upper pons contain the reticular activating system, which is responsible for the state of alertness. Vital cardiorespiratory centers reside in the medulla, which continues on to form the spinal cord. Even small lesions in the brainstem may be associated with severe neurologic deficits.

The cerebellum, responsible mainly for coordination and balance, projects posteriorly in the posterior fossa and forms connections with the spinal cord, brainstem, and ultimately, the cerebral hemispheres.

VENTRICULAR SYSTEM

The ventricles are a system of CSF-filled spaces and aqueducts within the brain. Located in the roof of the left and right lateral ventricles and midline third ventricle is a lacy structure called the choroid plexus. The choroid produces CSF at a rate of approximately 20 mL/hr. The CSF circulates from the lateral ventricles of the brain through the foramina of Monro, the third ventricle, and the aqueduct of Sylvius into the fourth ventricle in the posterior fossa. It then exits from the ventricular system into the subarachnoid space overlying the brain and spinal cord and is reabsorbed into the venous circulation through arachnoid granulations that project into the superior sagittal sinus. The presence of blood in the CSF may impair CSF reabsorption, resulting in increased intracranial pressure and enlarging ventricles (posttraumatic communicating hydrocephalus). Edema and mass lesions (eg, hematomas) may cause effacement or shifting of the usually symmetric ventricles that can be easily identified on CT scans of the brain.

TENTORIUM

The tentorium cerebelli divides the head into the supratentorial compartment (comprising the anterior and middle fossae of the skull) and the infratentorial compartment (containing the posterior fossa). The midbrain connects the cerebral hemispheres to the rest of the brainstem (pons and medulla oblongata) as it passes through a large aperture in the tentorium known as the tentorial incisura. The oculomotor (cranial nerve III) nerve runs along the edge of the tentorium and may become compressed against it during temporal lobe herniation, which most commonly results from a supratentorial mass or edema. Parasympathetic fibers that constrict the pupil lie on the surface of the third cranial nerve. Compression of these superficial fibers during herniation causes pupillary dilation due to unopposed sympathetic activity, often referred to as a "blown" pupil.

The part of the brain that usually herniates through the tentorial notch is the medial part of the temporal lobe, known as the uncus. Uncal herniation also causes compression of the corticospinal (pyramidal) tract in the midbrain. The motor tract crosses to the opposite side at the foramen magnum, so compression at the level of the midbrain results in weakness of the opposite side of the body (contralateral hemiparesis). Ipsilateral pupillary dilation associated with contralateral hemiparesis is the classic syndrome of uncal herniation. Infrequently, the mass lesion may push the opposite side of the midbrain against the tentorial edge, resulting in hemiparesis and a dilated pupil on the same side as the hematoma (Kernohan's notch syndrome).

Physiology

Physiologic concepts that relate to head trauma include intracranial pressure, the Monro-Kellie doctrine, and cerebral blood flow.

INTRACRANIAL PRESSURE

Several pathologic processes that affect the brain may cause elevation of intracranial pressure (ICP). Elevated ICP may reduce cerebral perfusion and cause or exacerbate ischemia. The normal ICP in the resting state is approximately 10 mm Hg. Pressures greater than 20 mm Hg, particularly if sustained and refractory to treatment, are associated with poor outcomes.

MONRO-KELLIE DOCTRINE

The Monro-Kellie Doctrine is a simple, yet vitally important, concept related to the understanding of ICP dynamics. It states that the total volume of the intracranial contents must remain constant, because the cranium is a rigid, nonexpansile container. Venous blood and cerebrospinal fluid may be compressed out of the container, providing a degree of pressure buffering (Figure 6-3 and Figure 6-4). Thus, very early after injury, a mass such as a blood clot may enlarge while the ICP remains normal. However, once the limit of displacement of CSF and intravascular blood has been reached, ICP rapidly increases.

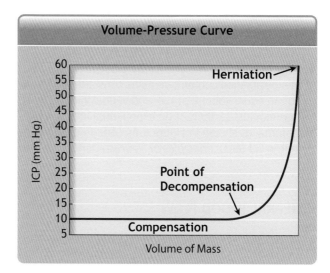

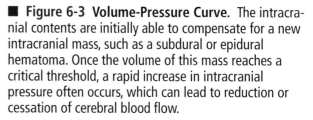

■ **Figure 6-3 Volume-Pressure Curve.** The intracranial contents are initially able to compensate for a new intracranial mass, such as a subdural or epidural hematoma. Once the volume of this mass reaches a critical threshold, a rapid increase in intracranial pressure often occurs, which can lead to reduction or cessation of cerebral blood flow.

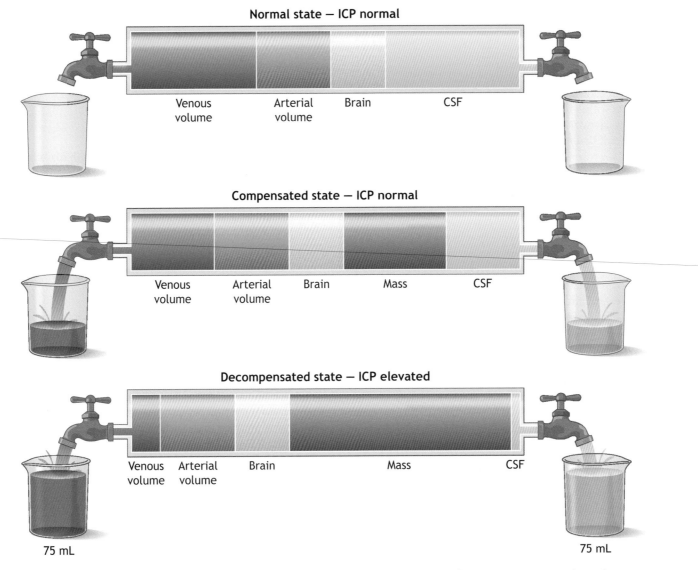

Normal state — ICP normal

Venous volume · Arterial volume · Brain · CSF

Compensated state — ICP normal

Venous volume · Arterial volume · Brain · Mass · CSF

Decompensated state — ICP elevated

Venous volume · Arterial volume · Brain · Mass · CSF

75 mL   75 mL

■ **Figure 6-4 The Monro-Kellie Doctrine** regarding intracranial compensation for expanding mass. The volume of the intracranial contents remains constant. If the addition of a mass such as a hematoma results in the squeezing out of an equal volume of CSF and venous blood, the ICP remains normal. However, when this compensatory mechanism is exhausted, there is an exponential increase in ICP for even a small additional increase in the volume of the hematoma, as shown in Figure 6-4. (Adapted with permission from Narayan RK: Head Injury, in Grossman RG, Hamilton WJ (eds): *Principles of Neurosurgery.* New York, Raven Press, 1991.)

CEREBRAL BLOOD FLOW

In healthy adults, cerebral blood flow (CBF) is 50 to 55 mL/100 g of brain tissue per minute. In children, CBF may be much higher, depending on age. At 1 year of age, CBF approximates adult levels, but at 5 years of age, normal CBF is approximately 90 mL/100 g/min and then gradually declines to adult levels by the mid to late teens.

Brain injury severe enough to cause coma may cause a marked reduction in CBF during the first few hours after injury. It usually increases over the next 2 to 3 days, but for patients who remain comatose, CBF remains below normal for days or weeks after injury. There is increasing evidence that such low levels of CBF are inadequate to meet the metabolic demands of the brain early after injury and that regional, even global, cerebral ischemia is common.

The precapillary cerebral vasculature normally has the ability to reflexively constrict or dilate in response to changes in cerebral perfusion pressure (CPP), which for clinical purposes is defined as mean arterial blood pressure minus intracranial pressure. A CPP of 50 to 150 mm Hg is required to maintain a constant CBF (pressure autoregulation). These vessels also normally constrict or dilate in response to changes in the PaO_2 or $PaCO_2$ of the blood (chemical autoregulation). Severe traumatic brain injury may disrupt both of these autoregulatory mechanisms.

Consequently, the traumatized brain is vulnerable to ischemia and infarction due to the severe reduction in blood flow caused by the traumatic insult itself. This preexisting ischemia may easily be exacerbated by the secondary insults of hypotension, hypoxia, and hypocapnia, such as that caused iatrogenically by overly aggressive hyperventilation. **Therefore, every effort should be made to enhance cerebral perfusion and blood flow by reducing the elevated ICP, maintaining normal intravascular volume, maintaining a normal mean arterial blood pressure (MAP), and restoring normal oxygenation and normocapnia. Hematomas and other lesions that increase intracranial volume should be evacuated early.** Maintaining the cerebral perfusion pressure above 60 mm Hg helps to improve CBF (although significantly higher pressures have been implicated in worsening pulmonary outcomes). Once compensatory mechanisms are exhausted and there is an exponential increase in ICP, brain perfusion is compromised, especially in patients with hypotension. Additional insults contribute to the potentially devastating "secondary injury" that may occur in otherwise salvageable brain tissue during the first few days after severe TBI. This pathophysiologic state is characterized by progressive inflammation, vascular permeability, and brain tissue edema, culminating in intractably elevated ICP and death.

Classifications of Head Injuries

Head injuries are classified in several ways. For practical purposes, the following three descriptions are useful: (1) mechanism, (2) severity, and (3) morphology (Table 6-1).

MECHANISM OF INJURY

Brain injury may be broadly classified as blunt or penetrating. For practical purposes, the term *blunt brain injury* usually is associated with automobile collisions, falls, and assaults with blunt weapons. Penetrating brain injury usually results from gunshot and stab wounds.

TABLE 6-1 ■ Classifications of Brain Injury	
Mechanism	
• Blunt	High velocity (automobile collision)
	Low velocity (fall, assault)
• Penetrating	Gunshot wounds
	Other penetrating injuries
Severity	
• Minor	GCS score 13–15
• Moderate	GCS score 9–12
• Severe	GCS score 3–8
Morphology	
• Skull fractures	
• Vault	Linear vs. stellate
	Depressed/nondepressed
	Open/closed
• Basilar	With/without CSF leak
	With/without seventh-nerve palsy
• Intracranial lesions	
• Focal	Epidural
	Subdural
	Intracerebral
• Diffuse	Concussion
	Multiple contusions
	Hypoxic/ischemic injury

Adapted with permission from Valadka AB, Narayan RK. Emergency room management of the head-injured patient. In: Narayan RK, Wilberger JE, Povlishock JT, eds. *Neurotrauma.* New York, NY: McGraw-Hill; 1996:120.

SEVERITY OF INJURY

The GCS score is used as an objective clinical measure of the severity of brain injury. Patients who open their eyes spontaneously, obey commands, and are oriented score a total of 15 points on the GCS, whereas flaccid patients who do not open their eyes or vocalize sounds score the minimum (3 points) (Table 6-2). **A GCS score of 8 or less has become the generally accepted definition of coma or severe brain injury.** Patients with a brain injury who have a GCS score of 9 to 12 are categorized as "moderate," and those with a GCS score of 13 to 15 are designated as "minor." **In assessing the GCS score, when there is right/left asymmetry, it is important to use the best motor response in calculating the score because this is the most reliable predictor of outcome.** However, one must record the actual response on both sides.

MORPHOLOGY

Head trauma may include fractures, contusions, hematomas, and diffuse injuries.

Skull Fractures

Skull fractures may be seen in the cranial vault or skull base. They may be linear or stellate, and open or closed. Basal skull fractures usually require CT scanning with bone-window settings for identification. The presence of clinical signs of a basal skull fracture should increase the index of suspicion

and help in its identification. These signs include periorbital ecchymosis (raccoon eyes), retroauricular ecchymosis (Battle sign), CSF leakage from the nose (rhinorrhea) or ear (otorrhea), and seventh- and eighth-nerve dysfunction (facial paralysis and hearing loss), which may occur immediately or a few days after the initial injury. In general, the prognosis for the recovery of seventh-nerve function is better in the delayed-onset variety, but the prognosis for recovery of eighth-nerve function is poor. Basal skull fractures that traverse the carotid canals may damage the carotid arteries (dissection, pseudoaneurysm, or thrombosis), and consideration should be given to cerebral arteriography.

Open or compound skull fractures may provide a direct communication between the scalp laceration and the cerebral surface, because the dura may be torn. **The significance of a skull fracture should not be underestimated, since it takes considerable force to fracture the skull.** A linear vault fracture in conscious patients increases the likelihood of an intracranial hematoma by about 400 times.

Intracranial Lesions

Intracranial lesions may be classified as diffuse or focal, although these two forms frequently coexist. Focal lesions include epidural hematomas, subdural hematomas, contusions, and intracerebral hematomas (see Table 6-1 and Figure 6-5).

Diffuse Brain Injuries   Diffuse brain injuries range from mild concussions, in which the CT scan of the head is usually normal, to severe hypoxic ischemic injuries. With a concussion, the patient has a transient, nonfocal neurologic disturbance that often includes loss of consciousness. Severe diffuse injuries often result from a hypoxic, ischemic insult to the brain due to prolonged shock or apnea occurring immediately after the trauma. In such cases, the CT scan may initially appear normal, or the brain may appear diffusely swollen, with loss of the normal gray-white distinction. Another diffuse pattern, often seen in high-velocity impact or deceleration injuries, may produce multiple punctate hemorrhages throughout the cerebral hemispheres, which are often seen in the border between the gray matter and white matter. These "shearing injuries," referred to as diffuse axonal injury (DAI), previously defined a clinical syndrome of severe brain injury with uniformly poor outcome. However, it may be more appropriate to restrict the use of this term to cases in which there is microscopic evidence of cerebral axonal injury, which may be seen in a wide spectrum of clinical presentations.

Epidural Hematomas   Epidural hematomas are relatively uncommon, occurring in about 0.5% of patients with brain injuries and in 9% of those who are comatose. These hematomas typically become biconvex or lenticular in shape as they push the adherent dura away from the inner table of the skull. They are most often located in the temporal or tem-

TABLE 6-2 ■ Glasgow Coma Scale (GCS)

ASSESSMENT AREA	SCORE
Eye opening (E)	
• Spontaneous	4
• To speech	3
• To pain	2
• None	1
Best motor response (M)	
• Obeys commands	6
• Localizes pain	5
• Normal flexion (withdrawal)	4
• Abnormal flexion (decorticate)	3
• Extension (decerebrate)	2
• None (flaccid)	1
Verbal response (V)	
• Oriented	5
• Confused conversation	4
• Inappropriate words	3
• Incomprehensible sounds	2
• None	1

GCS score = (E + M + V); best possible score = 15; worst possible score = 3.

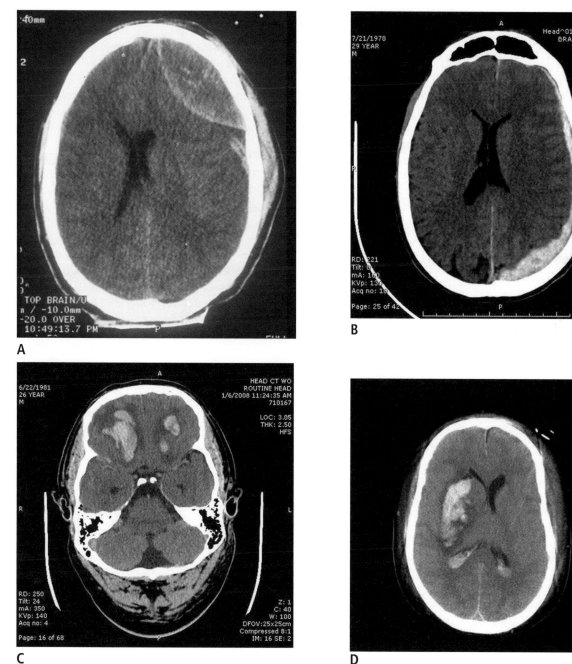

■ **Figure 6-5 CT Scans of Intracranial Hematomas. (A)** Epidural hematoma. **(B)** Subdural hematoma. **(C)** Bilateral contusions with hemorrhage. **(D)** Right intraparenchymal hemorrhage with right to left midline shift. Associated biventricular hemorrhages.

poroparietal region and often result from a tear of the middle meningeal artery as the result of a fracture. These clots are classically arterial in origin; however, they also may result from disruption of a major venous sinus or bleeding from a skull fracture.

Subdural Hematomas Subdural hematomas are more common than epidural hematomas, occurring in approximately 30% of severe brain injuries. They often develop from the shearing of small surface or bridging blood vessels of the

cerebral cortex. In contrast to the lenticular shape of an epidural hematoma on CT scan, subdural hematomas more often appear to conform to the contours of the brain. Subdural hematomas may grow to cover the entire surface of the hemisphere. Furthermore, the brain damage underlying an acute subdural hematoma is typically much more severe than that with epidural hematomas.

Contusions and Intracerebral Hematomas Cerebral contusions are fairly common (present in about 20% to 30%

of severe brain injuries). The majority of contusions occur in the frontal and temporal lobes, although they may occur in any part of the brain. Contusions may, in a period of hours or days, evolve to form an intracerebral hematoma or a coalescent contusion with enough mass effect to require immediate surgical evacuation. This occurs in as many as 20% of patients presenting with contusions on initial CT scan of the head. **For this reason, patients with contusions should undergo repeat CT scanning to evaluate for changes in the pattern of contusion 12 to 24 hours after the initial scan.**

Management of Minor Brain Injury (GCS Score 13–15)

? What is the optimal treatment for patients with brain injuries?

An estimated 1 million patients with head injuries are seen in North American EDs annually. Approximately 80% of these patients are categorized as having a minor brain injury. Minor traumatic brain injury (MTBI) is defined by a history of disorientation, amnesia, or transient loss of consciousness in a patient who is conscious and talking. This correlates with a GCS score of 13 to 15. The definition of MTBI has often been distinguished from the term *concussion*, which has been broadly defined as "a complex pathophysiologic process affecting the brain, induced by traumatic biomechanical forces." The history of a brief loss of consciousness can be difficult to confirm, and the picture often is confounded by alcohol or other intoxicants. The management of patients with minor brain injury is described in Figure 6-6.

Most patients with minor brain injury make uneventful recoveries. About 3% have unexpected deterioration, possibly resulting in severe neurologic dysfunction unless the decline in mental status is detected early. Others struggle with persistent morbidity, including chronic headaches or memory and sleep disturbances.

The secondary survey is particularly important in evaluating patients with MTBI. Note the mechanism of injury,

PITFALL

Patients with minor traumatic brain injuries may appear neurologically normal but continue to be symptomatic for some time. Be sure that these patients avoid any unnecessary risk of a "second impact" during the symptomatic period that can result in devastating brain edema. Emphasize the need for competent follow-up and clearance before resuming normal activities, especially contact sports.

with particular attention to any loss of consciousness, including the length of time the patient was unresponsive, any seizure activity, and the subsequent level of alertness. Determine the duration of amnesia both before (retrograde) and after (antegrade) the accident. Grade the severity of headache and note the length of time the patient requires to return to a GCS score of 15 using serial examinations.

CT scanning is the preferred method of imaging. A CT scan should be obtained in all patients with brain injury who fail to reach a GCS score of 15 within 2 hours of injury; who have a clinically suspected open skull fracture, any sign of basal skull fracture, or more than two episodes of vomiting; or who are older than 65 years (Table 6-3). CT should also be considered if the patient has had a loss of consciousness for longer than 5 minutes, retrograde amnesia for longer than 30 minutes, a dangerous mechanism of injury, severe headaches, or a focal neurologic deficit attributable to the brain. Caution should be applied in assessing patients with TBI who are anticoagulated. The international normalized ratio (INR) should be obtained and a CT should be performed expeditiously in these patients when indicated.

Applying these parameters to patients with a GCS score of 13, approximately 25% will have a CT finding indicative of trauma, and 1.3% will require neurosurgical intervention. Using these rules in patients with a GCS score of 15, 10% will have the CT findings and 0.5% will require neurosurgery. Based on current best evidence, no patients with clinically important brain injury or patients requiring neurosurgical intervention will be missed.

If CT scanning is not available, skull x-ray films may be obtained for blunt or penetrating head injury. If a skull x-ray film is obtained, look for the following features: (1) linear or depressed skull fractures, (2) midline position of the pineal gland (if calcified), (3) air–fluid levels in the sinuses, (4) pneumocephalus, (5) facial fractures, and (6) foreign bodies. **Obtaining CT scans or skull films should not delay transfer of the patient.**

If abnormalities are observed on the CT scan, or if the patient remains symptomatic or continues to have neurologic abnormalities, he or she should be admitted to the hospital and a neurosurgeon consulted.

If patients are asymptomatic, are fully awake and alert, and have no neurologic abnormalities, they may be observed for several hours, reexamined, and, if still normal, safely discharged. Ideally, the patient is discharged to the care of a companion who can observe the patient continually over the next 24 hours. An instruction sheet directs both the patient and the companion to continue close observation and to return to the ED if headaches develop, there is a decline in mental status, or focal neurologic deficits develop. In all cases, written discharge instructions should be supplied to and carefully reviewed with the patient and/or companion (Figure 6-7). If the patient is not alert or oriented enough to clearly understand the written and verbal instructions, the decision for discharge should be reconsidered.

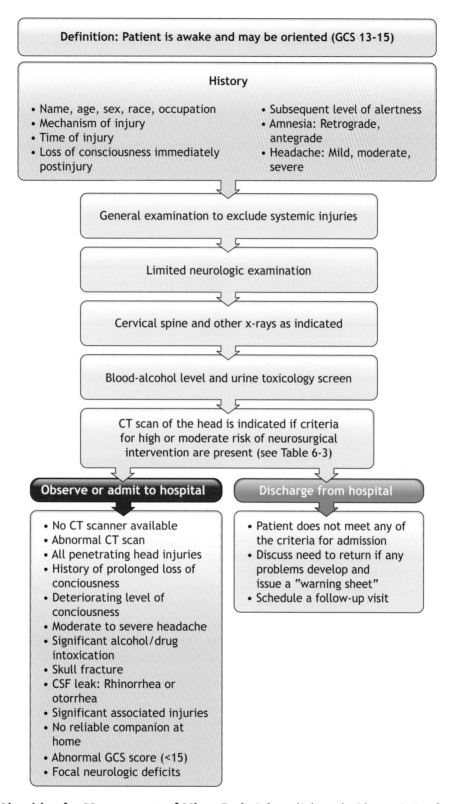

Definition: Patient is awake and may be oriented (GCS 13-15)

History

- Name, age, sex, race, occupation
- Mechanism of injury
- Time of injury
- Loss of consciousness immediately postinjury

- Subsequent level of alertness
- Amnesia: Retrograde, antegrade
- Headache: Mild, moderate, severe

General examination to exclude systemic injuries

Limited neurologic examination

Cervical spine and other x-rays as indicated

Blood-alcohol level and urine toxicology screen

CT scan of the head is indicated if criteria for high or moderate risk of neurosurgical intervention are present (see Table 6-3)

Observe or admit to hospital

- No CT scanner available
- Abnormal CT scan
- All penetrating head injuries
- History of prolonged loss of conciousness
- Deteriorating level of conciousness
- Moderate to severe headache
- Significant alcohol/drug intoxication
- Skull fracture
- CSF leak: Rhinorrhea or otorrhea
- Significant associated injuries
- No reliable companion at home
- Abnormal GCS score (<15)
- Focal neurologic deficits

Discharge from hospital

- Patient does not meet any of the criteria for admission
- Discuss need to return if any problems develop and issue a "warning sheet"
- Schedule a follow-up visit

■ **Figure 6-6 Algorithm for Management of Minor Brain Injury.** (Adapted with permission from Valadka AB, Narayan RK: Emergency room management of the head-injured patient, in Narayan RK, Wilberger JE, Povlishock JT (eds): *Neurotrauma.* New York, McGraw-Hill, 1996.)

TABLE 6-3 ■ Indications for CT Scanning in MTBI

Head CT is required for patients with minor head injuries (ie, witnessed loss of consciousness, definite amnesia, or witnessed disorientation in a patient with a GCS score of 13 to 15) *and* any one of the following:

High risk for neurosurgical intervention:	Moderate risk for brain injury on CT:
• GCS score less than 15 at 2 hours after injury • Suspected open or depressed skull fracture • Any sign of basal skull fracture (eg, hemotympanum, raccoon eyes, CSF otorrhea or rhinorrhea, Battle sign) • Vomiting (more than two episodes) • Age greater than 65 years	• Amnesia before impact (more than 30 minutes) • Dangerous mechanism (eg, pedestrian struck by motor vehicle, occupant ejected from motor vehicle, fall from height more than 3 feet or five stairs)

Adapted from Stiell IG, Wells GA, Vandemheen K, et al. The Canadian CT Head Rule for patients with minor head injury. *Lancet* 2001;357:1294.

Management of Moderate Brain Injury (GCS Score 9–12)

Approximately 10% of patients with brain injury who are seen in the ED have a moderate injury. They still are able to follow simple commands, but usually are confused or somnolent and can have focal neurologic deficits such as hemiparesis. Approximately 10% to 20% of these patients deteriorate and lapse into coma. For this reason, serial neurologic examinations are critical to treat these patients.

The management of patients with moderate brain injury is described in Figure 6-8.

On admission to the ED, a brief history is obtained and cardiopulmonary stability is ensured before neurologic assessment. A CT scan of the head is obtained, and a neurosurgeon is contacted. All of these patients require admission for observation in an intensive care unit (ICU) or a similar unit capable of close nursing observation and frequent neurologic reassessment for at least the first 12 to 24 hours. A follow-up CT scan in 12 to 24 hours is recommended if the initial CT scan is abnormal, sooner if there is deterioration of the patient's neurologic status.

PITFALL

Patients with moderate brain injury can have rapid deterioration with hypoventilation or a subtle loss of their ability to protect their airway from declining mental status. Narcotic analgesics must be used with caution. Avoid hypercapnia with close monitoring of respiratory status and the ability of patients to manage their airway. Urgent intubation may become a necessity under these circumstances.

Management of Severe Brain Injury (GCS Score 3–8)

Patients who have sustained a severe brain injury are unable to follow simple commands, even after cardiopulmonary stabilization. Although this definition includes a wide spectrum of brain injury, it identifies the patients who are at greatest risk of suffering significant morbidity and mortality. A "wait and see" approach in such patients can be disastrous, and prompt diagnosis and treatment are extremely important. **Do not delay patient transfer to obtain a CT scan.**

The initial management of severe brain injury is outlined in Figure 6-9.

PRIMARY SURVEY AND RESUSCITATION

Brain injury often is adversely affected by secondary insults. The mortality rate for patients with severe brain injury who have hypotension on admission is more than double that of patients who do not have hypotension. The presence of hypoxia in addition to hypotension is associated with mortality of approximately 75%. **Therefore, it is imperative that cardiopulmonary stabilization be achieved rapidly in patients with severe brain injury.** See Box 6-1 for the priorities of the initial evaluation and triage of patients with severe brain injuries. ■ See Skill Station IX: Head and Neck Trauma: Assessment and Management, Skill IX-A: Primary Survey.

Airway and Breathing

Transient respiratory arrest and hypoxia are common and may cause secondary brain injury. **Early endotracheal intubation should be performed in comatose patients.**

The patient should be ventilated with 100% oxygen until blood gas measurements are obtained, and then appropriate adjustments to the fraction of inspired oxygen (FiO_2) are made. Pulse oximetry is a useful adjunct, and oxygen saturations of >98% are desirable. Hyperventilation

County General Hospital

Mild Traumatic Brain Injury Warning Discharge Instructions

Patient Name: _____

Date: _____

We have found no evidence to indicate that your head injury was serious. However, new symptoms and unexpected complications can develop hours or even days after the injury. The first 24 hours are the most crucial and you should remain with a reliable companion at least during this period. If any of the following signs develop, call your doctor or come back to the hospital.

1 *Drowsiness or increasing difficulty in awakening patient (awaken every 2 hours during period of sleep)*
2 *Nausea or vomiting*
3 *Convulsions or fits*
4 *Bleeding or watery drainage from the nose or ear*
5 *Severe headaches*
6 *Weakness or loss of feeling in the arm or leg*
7 *Confusion or strange behavior*
8 *One pupil (black part of eye) much larger than the other; peculiar movements of the eyes, double vision, or other visual disturbances*
9 *A very slow or very rapid pulse, or an unusual breathing pattern.*

If there is swelling at the site of the injury, apply an ice pack, making sure that there is a cloth or towel between the ice pack and the skin. If swelling increases markedly in spite of the ice pack application, call us or come back to the hospital.

You may eat or drink as usual if you so desire. However, you should NOT drink alcoholic beverages for at least 3 days after your injury.

Do not take any sedatives or any pain relievers stronger than acetaminophen, at least for the first 24 hours. Do not use aspirin-containing medicines.

If you have any further questions, or in case of emergency, we can be reached at: <telephone number>

Physician's Signature _____

■ **Figure 6-7 Example of Head Injury Warning Discharge Instructions.**

should be used cautiously in patients with severe brain injury and only when acute neurologic deterioration has occurred.

Circulation

Hypotension usually is not due to the brain injury itself, except in the terminal stages when medullary failure supervenes. Intracranial hemorrhage cannot cause hemorrhagic shock. Euvolemia should be established as soon as possible if the patient has hypotension.

Hypotension is a marker of severe blood loss, which is not always obvious. Associated spinal cord injury (neurogenic shock), cardiac contusion or tamponade, and tension pneumothorax are also possible causes.

While efforts are in progress to determine the cause of hypotension, volume replacement should be initiated. **FAST or DPL is used routinely in comatose patients with hypotension, because a clinical examination for abdominal tenderness is not possible in such patients.** See Chapter 3: Shock. It must be emphasized that the neurologic examination of patients with hypotension is unreliable. Even if severe

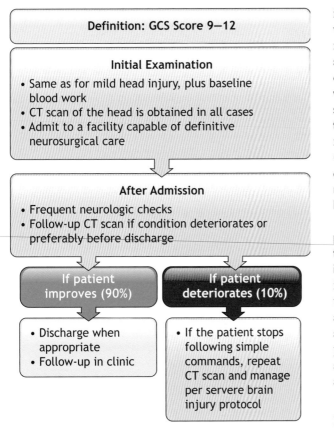

Definition: GCS Score 9–12

Initial Examination
- Same as for mild head injury, plus baseline blood work
- CT scan of the head is obtained in all cases
- Admit to a facility capable of definitive neurosurgical care

After Admission
- Frequent neurologic checks
- Follow-up CT scan if condition deteriorates or preferably before discharge

If patient improves (90%)
- Discharge when appropriate
- Follow-up in clinic

If patient deteriorates (10%)
- If the patient stops following simple commands, repeat CT scan and manage per severe brain injury protocol

■ **Figure 6-8 Algorithm for Management of Moderate Brain Injury.** (Adapted with permission from Valadka AB, Narayan RK: Emergency room management of the head-injured patient, in Narayan RK, Wilberger JE, Povlishock JT (eds): Neurotrauma. New York, McGraw-Hill, 1996.)

brain injury exists, hypotension is a well-known cause of secondary brain injury. Patients with hypotension who are unresponsive to any form of stimulation may revert to near-normal neurologically soon after normal blood pressure is restored, and the primary source of the hypotension must be urgently sought and treated.

Neurologic Examination
? *What is a focused neurological examination?*

As soon as the patient's cardiopulmonary status is corrected, a rapid and directed neurologic examination is performed. It consists primarily of determining the GCS score and the pupillary light response. It is important to recognize confounding issues in the evaluation of traumatic brain injury, including the presence of drugs, alcohol, and intoxicants and other injuries. Do not overlook a severe brain injury because the patient is also

intoxicated. The postictal state after a traumatic seizure will typically worsen the patient's responsiveness for minutes or hours. In a comatose patient, motor responses may be elicited by pinching the trapezius muscle or with nail-bed pressure. **If a patient demonstrates variable responses to stimulation, the best motor response elicited is a more accurate prognostic indicator than the worst response.** Testing for doll's eye movements (oculocephalic), the caloric test with ice water (oculovestibular), and testing of corneal responses are deferred to a neurosurgeon. **Doll's eye testing should never be attempted until an unstable cervical spine injury has been ruled out.**

It is important to obtain the GCS score and to perform a pupillary examination prior to sedating or paralyzing the patient, because knowledge of the patient's clinical condition is important for determining subsequent treatment. Long-acting paralytic and sedating agents should not be used during the primary survey. Sedation should be avoided except when a patient's agitated state may place him or her at risk. The shortest-acting agents available are recommended when pharmacologic paralysis or brief sedation is necessary for safe endotracheal intubation or obtaining good quality diagnostic studies.

SECONDARY SURVEY

Serial examinations (GCS score, lateralization, and pupillary reaction) should be performed to detect neurologic deterioration as early as possible. A well-known early sign of temporal lobe (uncal) herniation is dilation of the pupil and loss of the pupillary response to light. Direct trauma to the eye also is a potential cause of abnormal pupillary response and may make pupil evaluation difficult. However, in the setting of brain trauma, brain injury should be considered first. ▪ See Skill Station IX: Head and Neck Trauma: Assessment and Management, Skill IX-B: Secondary Survey and Management.

DIAGNOSTIC PROCEDURES

An emergency head CT scan must be obtained as soon as possible after hemodynamic normalization. CT scanning

PITFALL

In the past, severe traumatic brain injury was often considered "unrecoverable," and a sense of nihilism had frequently prevailed. Vigorous management and improved understanding of the pathophysiology of severe head injury, especially the role of hypotension, hypoxia, and cerebral perfusion, has made a significant impact on patient outcomes. Do not give up too soon.

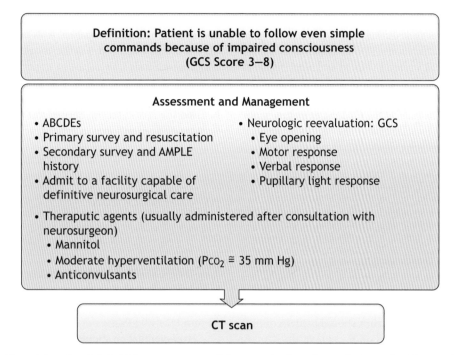

Definition: Patient is unable to follow even simple commands because of impaired consciousness (GCS Score 3–8)

Assessment and Management

- ABCDEs
- Primary survey and resuscitation
- Secondary survey and AMPLE history
- Admit to a facility capable of definitive neurosurgical care

- Neurologic reevaluation: GCS
  - Eye opening
  - Motor response
  - Verbal response
  - Pupillary light response

- Theraputic agents (usually administered after consultation with neurosurgeon)
  - Mannitol
  - Moderate hyperventilation ($Pco_2 \cong 35$ mm Hg)
  - Anticonvulsants

CT scan

■ **Figure 6-9 Algorithm for Initial Management of Severe Brain Injury.** (Adapted with permission from Valadka AB, Narayan RK: Emergency room management of the head-injured patient, in Narayan RK, Wilberger JE, Povlishock JT (eds): *Neurotrauma.* New York, McGraw-Hill, 1996.)

Box 6-1
Priorities for the Initial Evaluation and Triage of Patients with Severe Brain Injuries

1 All comatose patients with brain injuries should undergo resuscitation (ABCDEs) on arrival in the ED.

2 As soon as the blood pressure (BP) is normalized, a neurologic exam is performed (GCS score and pupillary reaction). If the BP cannot be normalized, the neurologic examination is still performed, and the hypotension recorded.

3 If the patient's systolic BP cannot be brought up to >100 mm Hg despite aggressive fluid resuscitation, the priority is to establish the cause of the hypotension, with the neurosurgical evaluation taking second priority. In such cases, the patient undergoes a DPL or ultrasound in the ED and may need to go directly to the operating room (OR) for a laparotomy. CT scans of the head are obtained after the laparotomy. If there is clinical evidence of an in-

tracranial mass, diagnostic burr holes or craniotomy may be undertaken in the OR while the laparotomy is being performed.

4 If the patient's systolic BP is >100 mm Hg after resuscitation and the patient has clinical evidence of a possible intracranial mass (unequal pupils, asymmetric results on motor exam), the first priority is to obtain a CT head scan. A DPL or FAST exam may be performed in the ED, CT area, or OR, but the patient's neurologic evaluation or treatment should not be delayed.

5 In borderline cases—i.e., when the systolic BP can be temporarily corrected but tends to slowly decrease—every effort should be made to get a head CT prior to taking the patient to the OR for a laparotomy or thoracotomy. Such cases call for sound clinical judgment and cooperation between the trauma surgeon and neurosurgeon.

also should be repeated whenever there is a change in the patient's clinical status and routinely at 12 to 24 hours after injury for patients with a contusion or hematoma on the initial scan. ◾ See Skill Station IX: Head and Neck Trauma: Assessment and Management, Skill IX-C: Evaluation of CT Scans of the Head.

Findings of significance on the CT images include scalp swelling or subgaleal hematomas at the region of impact. Skull fractures may be seen better with bone windows, but are often apparent even on the soft-tissue windows. The crucial findings on the CT scan are intracranial hematoma, contusions, and shift of the midline (mass effect) (see Figure 6-5: CT Scans of Intracranial Hematomas). The septum pellucidum, which lies between the two lateral ventricles, should be located in the midline. The midline can be determined by drawing a line from the crista galli anteriorly to the insertion of the falx at the internal occipital protuberance posteriorly. The degree of displacement of the septum pellucidum away from the side of the hematoma should be noted, and the actual degree of shift should be determined by using the scale that is printed on the side of the scan. **A shift of 5 mm or greater is often indicative of the need for surgery to evacuate the blood clot or contusion causing the shift.** There is some evidence that the addition of CT angiography (CT-A) or cerebral arteriography may uncover unsuspected vascular injury to the skull base that could place the patient at risk for stroke. These studies should be considered when a high-energy mechanism of injury is present. ◾ See Chapter 7: Spine and Spinal Cord Trauma for specific criteria.

In patients whose blood pressure can be normalized, every effort should be made to obtain a head CT scan prior to taking the patient to the operating room. Such cases require sound clinical judgment and cooperation between the trauma surgeon and the neurosurgeon (see Figure 6-9).

Table 6-4 provides an overview of the management of traumatic brain injury.

Medical Therapies for Brain Injury

The primary aim of intensive care protocols is to prevent secondary damage to an already injured brain. **The basic principle is that if injured neural tissue is provided an optimal milieu in which to recover, it may go on to regain normal function.** However, if the neural tissue is provided with a suboptimal or hostile milieu, it may die. Medical therapies for brain injury are primarily aimed at maintaining cerebral perfusion.

INTRAVENOUS FLUIDS

Intravenous fluids should be administered as required to resuscitate the patient and maintain normovolemia.

Hypovolemia in these patients is harmful. Care should also be taken not to overload the patient with fluids. Hypotonic fluids should not be used. Furthermore, the use of glucose-containing fluids may result in hyperglycemia, which has been shown to be harmful to the injured brain. Therefore, it is recommended Ringer's lactate solution *or* normal saline be used for resuscitation. Serum sodium levels need to be very carefully monitored in patients with head injuries. Hyponatremia is associated with brain edema and should be prevented.

HYPERVENTILATION

In most patients, normocarbia is preferred. Hyperventilation acts by reducing $PaCO_2$ and causing cerebral vasoconstriction. Aggressive and prolonged hyperventilation may actually produce cerebral ischemia by causing severe cerebral vasoconstriction and thus impaired cerebral perfusion. This is particularly true if the $PaCO_2$ is allowed to fall below 30 mm Hg (4.0 kPa).

Hyperventilation should be used only in moderation and for as limited a period as possible. In general, it is preferable to keep the $PaCO_2$ at 35 mm Hg or above. Brief periods of hyperventilation ($PaCO_2$ 25 to 30 mm Hg) are acceptable if necessary for acute neurologic deterioration while other treatments are initiated.

MANNITOL

Mannitol is used to reduce elevated ICP. The preparation most commonly used is a 20% solution. The most widely accepted regimen is 0.25 to 1 g/kg administered intravenously as a bolus. Large doses of mannitol should not be

PITFALLS

- It is important to monitor the ICP if active ICP management is being undertaken. For example, mannitol may have a significant rebound effect on ICP, and additional therapies may be indicated if ongoing management is required. Hypertonic saline is being studied as a possibly safer and/or more effective alternative.

- It is important to remember that seizures are *not* controlled with muscle relaxants. Prolonged seizures in a patient whose muscles are relaxed pharmacologically can still be devastating to brain function, and may go undiagnosed and untreated if tonic-clonic muscle contractions are masked by a neuromuscular blocker such as vecuronium or succinylcholine. In a patient with a witnessed seizure, make sure appropriate antiseizure therapy is being initiated and that the seizure is under control before initiating neuromuscular blockade if at all possible.

TABLE 6-4 ■ Management Overview of Traumatic Brain Injury

ALL PATIENTS: PERFORM ABCDEs WITH SPECIAL ATTENTION TO HYPOXIA AND HYPOTENSION

GCS CLASSIFICATION	13 TO 15 MILD TRAUMATIC BRAIN INJURY		9 TO 12 MODERATE TRAUMATIC BRAIN INJURY	3 TO 8 SEVERE TRAUMATIC BRAIN INJURY
	May discharge if admission criteria not met	Admit for indications below:	Neurosurgery eval required	Urgent neurosurgery consult required
Initial Management	*AMPLE History and neurologic exam:		*Primary survey and resuscitation	*Primary survey and resuscitation
	Determine mechanism, times of injury, initial GCS, confusion, amnestic interval, seizure, headache severity, etc.	No CT available, CT abnormal, skull fracture, CSF leak	*Arrange for transfer to definitive neurosurgical evaluation and management	*Intubation & ventilation for airway protection *Treat hypotension, hypovolemia and hypoxia
	*Secondary survey including focused neurologic exam	Focal neurologic deficit GCS does not return to 15 within 2 hours	*Focused neuro exam *Secondary survey and AMPLE history	*Focused neuro exam *Secondary survey and AMPLE history
Diagnostic	*CT scanning as determined by head CT rules (Table 3)	CT not available, CT abnormal, skull fracture	*CT scan in all cases *Evaluate carefully for other injuries	CT scan in all cases *Evaluate carefully for other injuries
	*Blood/Urine EtOH & tox screens	Significant intoxication (admit or observe)	*Full preop labs & x-rays	*Full preop labs & x-rays
Secondary MGMT	*Serial examinations until GCS is 15 and patient has no perseveration or memory deficit	*Perform serial examinations *Perform follow-up CT scan if 1st is abnormal or GCS remains less than 15	*Serial exams *Consider follow-up CT in 12–18 h	*Frequent serial neuro examinations w/GCS *Pco$_2$ 35+/-3 *Mannitol, Pco$_2$ 28-32 for deterioration *Avoid Pco$_2$ <28
	*rule out indication for CT (Table 3)	*repeat CT if neuro exam deteriorates		*Address intracranial lesions appropriately
Disposition	*Home if patient does not meet criteria for admission	Obtain neurosurgical eval if CT or neurologic exam is abnormal or patient deteriorates	*Repeat CT immediately for deterioration and manage as in severe brain injury (10%)	*Transfer as soon as possible to definitive neurosurgical care
	*Discharge with head injury warning sheet and followup arranged	*Arrange for medical followup and neuropsych evaluation as required (may be done as outpatient)	*Discharge with medical and neuropsychological followup arranged when stable GCS 15 (90%)	

*Asterisk denotes action required.

given to patients with hypotension, because mannitol is a potent osmotic diuretic. Acute neurologic deterioration, such as the development of a dilated pupil, hemiparesis, or loss of consciousness while the patient is being observed, is a strong indication for administering mannitol. In this setting, a bolus of mannitol (1 g/kg) should be given rapidly (over 5 minutes) and the patient transported immediately to

the CT scanner or directly to the operating room if the causative lesion already has been identified.

STEROIDS

Studies have not demonstrated any beneficial effect of steroids in controlling increased ICP or improving outcome from severe brain injury. Some studies have demonstrated an increase in mortality and complications associated with the use of steroids in this setting. Therefore, steroids are not recommended in the management of acute brain injury.

BARBITURATES

Barbiturates are effective in reducing ICP refractory to other measures. They should not be used in the presence of hypotension or hypovolemia. Furthermore, hypotension often results from their use. Therefore, barbiturates are not indicated in the acute resuscitative phase.

ANTICONVULSANTS

Posttraumatic epilepsy occurs in about 5% of patients admitted to the hospital with closed head injuries and in 15% of those with severe head injuries. Three main factors are linked to a high incidence of late epilepsy: (1) seizures occurring within the first week, (2) an intracranial hematoma, and (3) a depressed skull fracture. A double-blind study found that prophylactic phenytoin reduced the incidence of seizures in the first week of injury, but not thereafter. Currently, phenytoin or fosphenytoin is the agent usually used in the acute phase. For adults, the usual loading dose is 1 g of phenytoin given intravenously at a rate no faster than 50 mg/min. The usual maintenance dose is 100 mg/8 hours, with the dose titrated to achieve therapeutic serum levels. For patients with prolonged seizures, diazepam or lorazepam are used in addition to phenytoin until the seizure stops. Control of continuous seizures may require general anesthesia. It is imperative that the seizure be controlled as soon as possible because prolonged seizures (30 to 60 minutes) may cause secondary brain injury.

Surgical Management

Surgical management may be necessary for scalp wounds, depressed skull fractures, intracranial mass lesions, and penetrating brain injuries.

SCALP WOUNDS

It is important to clean the wound thoroughly before suturing. The most common cause of infected scalp wounds is inadequate cleansing and debridement. Blood loss from scalp wounds may be extensive, especially in children. Scalp hemorrhage usually can be controlled by applying direct pressure and cauterizing or ligating large vessels. Appropriate sutures, clips, or staples may then be applied. Carefully inspect the wound under direct vision for signs of a skull fracture or foreign material. CSF leakage indicates that there is an associated dural tear. A neurosurgeon should be consulted in all cases of open or depressed skull fractures. Not infrequently, a subgaleal collection of blood can feel like a skull fracture. In such cases, the presence of a fracture can be confirmed or excluded by plain x-ray examination of the region and/or a CT scan.

DEPRESSED SKULL FRACTURES

Generally, a depressed skull fracture needs operative elevation if the degree of depression is greater than the thickness of the adjacent skull, or if it is open and grossly contaminated. Less significant depressed fractures can often be managed with closure of the overlying scalp laceration, if present. A CT scan is valuable in identifying the degree of depression, but more importantly in excluding the presence of an intracranial hematoma or contusion.

INTRACRANIAL MASS LESIONS

Intracranial mass lesions typically are evacuated or treated by a neurosurgeon. If a neurosurgeon is not available in the facility initially receiving the patient with an intracranial mass lesion, early transfer to a hospital with a neurosurgeon is essential. In very exceptional circumstances, a rapidly expanding intracranial hematoma may be imminently life-threatening and may not allow time for transfer if neurosurgical care is some distance away. Although this circumstance is rare in urban settings, it may occur in rural areas. Under such conditions, emergency craniotomy may be considered if a surgeon properly trained in the procedure is available. This procedure is especially important in a patient whose neurologic status is rapidly deteriorating and does not respond to nonsurgical measures. Emergency craniotomy by a non-neurosurgeon should be considered only in extreme circumstances, and the procedure should be done only with the advice of a neurosurgeon.

The indications for a craniotomy performed by a non-neurosurgeon are few, and widespread use as a desperation maneuver is neither recommended nor supported by the Committee on Trauma. This procedure is justified only when definitive neurosurgical care is unavailable. The Committee on Trauma strongly recommends that those who anticipate the need for this procedure receive proper training from a neurosurgeon.

PENETRATING BRAIN INJURIES

CT scanning of the head is strongly recommended to evaluate patients with penetrating brain injury. Plain radiographs of the head can be helpful in assessing bullet trajectory and the presence of large foreign bodies and intracranial air. However, when CT is available, plain radiographs are not essential. CT-A and/or conventional angiography is recommended when vascular injury is sus-

PITFALL

Burr hole craniostomy—placing a 10-to-15-mm drill hole in the skull—has been advocated as a method of emergently addressing hematomas in patients with rapid deterioration when neurosurgeons are not readily available. Unfortunately, even in very experienced hands, these drill holes are easily placed incorrectly, and they seldom result in draining enough of the hematoma to make a clinical difference. In patients who need an evacuation, bone flap craniotomy (and not a simple burr hole) is the definitive lifesaving procedure to decompress the brain, and every attempt should be made to have a practitioner trained and experienced in doing the procedure perform it in a timely fashion.

pected, such as when a trajectory passes through or near the skull base or a major dural venous sinus. Substantial subarachnoid hemorrhage or delayed hematoma should also prompt consideration of vascular imaging. Patients with a penetrating injury involving the orbitofacial or pterional regions should undergo angiography to identify a traumatic intracranial aneurysm or arteriovenous (AV) fistula. When an aneurysm or AV fistula is identified, surgical or endovascular management is recommended. MRI can play a role in evaluating injuries from penetrating wooden or other nonmagnetic objects, but it is generally not necessary in the evaluation of missile-induced injury. The presence on CT of large contusions, hematomas, or intraventricular hemorrhage is associated with increased mortality, especially when both hemispheres are involved.

Prophylactic broad-spectrum antibiotics are appropriate for patients with penetrating brain injury. Antiseizure medication in the first week after the injury is recommended to prevent early posttraumatic seizures. Prophylactic treatment with anticonvulsants beyond the first week after injury has not been shown to prevent new seizures, and is not recommended. Early ICP monitoring is recommended when the clinician is unable to assess the neurologic examination accurately; the need to evacuate a mass lesion is unclear; or imaging studies suggest elevated ICP.

It is appropriate to treat small bullet entrance wounds to the head with local wound care and closure in patients whose scalp is not devitalized and who have no major intracranial pathology.

Objects that penetrate the intracranial compartment or infratemporal fossa must be left in place until possible vascular injury has been evaluated and definitive neurosurgical management established. Disturbing or removing penetrating objects prematurely can lead to fatal vascular injury or intracranial hemorrhage. More extensive wounds with nonviable scalp, bone, or dura are carefully debrided before primary closure or grafting to secure a watertight wound. In patients with significant fragmentation of the skull, de-

bridement of the cranial wound with opening or removing a portion of the skull is necessary. Significant mass effect is addressed by evacuation of intracranial hematomas and debridement of necrotic brain tissue and safely accessible bone fragments. In the absence of significant mass effect, surgical debridement of the missile track in the brain, routine surgical removal of fragments distant from the entry site, and reoperation solely to remove retained bone or missile fragments do not measurably improve outcome and are not recommended. Repair of open-air sinus injuries and CSF leaks that do not close spontaneously (or with temporary CSF diversion) is recommended, using careful watertight closure of the dura. During the primary surgery, every effort should be made to close the dura and prevent CSF leaks.

Prognosis

All patients should be treated aggressively pending consultation with a neurosurgeon. This is particularly true of children, who occasionally have a remarkable ability to recover from seemingly devastating injuries.

Brain Death

? How do I diagnose brain death?

The diagnosis of "brain death" implies that there is no possibility for recovery of brain function. Most experts agree that the following criteria should be satisfied for the diagnosis of brain death:

- Glasgow Coma Scale score = 3

- Nonreactive pupils

- Absent brainstem reflexes (eg, oculocephalic, corneal, and Doll's eyes and no gag reflex)

- No spontaneous ventilatory effort on formal apnea testing

Ancillary studies that may be used to confirm the diagnosis of brain death include:

- Electroencephalography: No activity at high gain

- CBF studies: No CBF (eg, isotope studies, Doppler studies, xenon CBF studies)

- ICP: Exceeds MAP for 1 hour or longer

- Cerebral angiography

Certain reversible conditions, such as hypothermia or barbiturate coma, may mimic the appearance of brain death; therefore, this diagnosis should be considered only after all physiologic parameters are normalized and CNS function is not potentially affected by medications. The remarkable ability of children to recover from seemingly devastating brain injuries should be carefully considered prior to diagnosing brain death in children. If any doubt exists, especially in children, multiple serial exams spaced several hours apart are useful in confirming the initial clinical impression. Local organ-procurement agencies should be notified about all patients with the diagnosis or impending diagnosis of brain death prior to discontinuing artificial life support measures.

CHAPTER SUMMARY

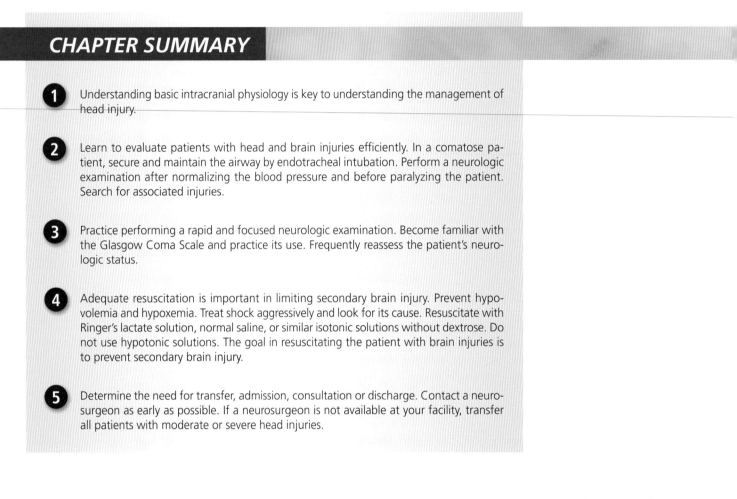

1 Understanding basic intracranial physiology is key to understanding the management of head injury.

2 Learn to evaluate patients with head and brain injuries efficiently. In a comatose patient, secure and maintain the airway by endotracheal intubation. Perform a neurologic examination after normalizing the blood pressure and before paralyzing the patient. Search for associated injuries.

3 Practice performing a rapid and focused neurologic examination. Become familiar with the Glasgow Coma Scale and practice its use. Frequently reassess the patient's neurologic status.

4 Adequate resuscitation is important in limiting secondary brain injury. Prevent hypovolemia and hypoxemia. Treat shock aggressively and look for its cause. Resuscitate with Ringer's lactate solution, normal saline, or similar isotonic solutions without dextrose. Do not use hypotonic solutions. The goal in resuscitating the patient with brain injuries is to prevent secondary brain injury.

5 Determine the need for transfer, admission, consultation or discharge. Contact a neurosurgeon as early as possible. If a neurosurgeon is not available at your facility, transfer all patients with moderate or severe head injuries.

Bibliography

1. Amirjamshidi A, Abbassioun K, Rahmat H. Minimal debridement or simple wound closure as the only surgical treatment in war victims with low-velocity penetrating head injuries. Indications and management protocol based upon more than 8 years follow-up of 99 cases from Iran-Iraq conflict. *Surg Neurol* 2003;60(2):105-110; discussion 110-111.

2. Andrews BT, Chiles BW, Olsen WL, et al. The effect of intracerebral hematoma location on the risk of brainstem compression and on clinical outcome. *J Neurosurg* 1988;69:518-522.

3. Aubry M, Cantu R, Dvorak J, et al. Summary and agreement statement of the first International Conference on Concussion in Sport, Vienna 2001. *Phys Sportsmed* 2002;30:57-62 (co-published in *Br J Sports Med* 2002;36:3-7 and *Clin J Sport Med* 2002;12:6-12).

4. Boyle A, Santarius L, Maimaris C. Evaluation of the impact of the Canadian CT head rule on British practice. *Emerg Med J* 2004; 21(4):426-428.

5. Brain Trauma Foundation. *Early Indicators of Prognosis in Severe Traumatic Brain Injury.* http://www2.braintrauma.org/guidelines/downloads/btf_prognosis_guidelines.pdf?BrainTrauma_Session=1157580cb4d126eb381748a50424bb99. Accessed September 8, 2007.

6. Brain Trauma Foundation. *Guidelines for the Management of Severe Traumatic Brain Injury.* http://www2.braintrauma.org/guidelines/downloads/JON_24_Supp1.pdf?BrainTrauma_Session=1157580cb4d126eb381748a50424bb99. Accessed September 8, 2007.

7. Chestnut RM, Marshall LF, Klauber MR, et al. The role of secondary brain injury in determining outcome from severe head injury. *J Trauma* 1993;34:216-222.

8. Chibbaro S, Tacconi L. Orbito-cranial injuries caused by penetrating non-missile foreign bodies. Experience with eighteen patients. *Acta Neurochir (Wien)* 2006; 148(9), 937-941; discussion 941-942.

9. Clement CM, Stiell IG, Schull MJ, et al. Clinical features of head injury patients presenting with a Glasgow Coma Scale score of 15 and who require neurosurgical intervention. *Ann Emerg Med* 2006; 48(3):245-251.

10. Eisenberg HM, Frankowski RF, Contant CR, et al. High-dose barbiturates control elevated intracranial pressure in patients with severe head injury. *J Neurosurg* 1988;69:15-23.

11. Giri BK, Krishnappa IK, Bryan RMJ, et al. Regional cerebral blood flow after cortical impact injury complicated by a secondary insult in rats. *Stroke* 2000;31:961-967.

12. Gonul E, Erdogan E, Tasar M, et al. Penetrating orbitocranial gunshot injuries. *Surg Neurol* 2005;63(1):24-30; discussion 31.

13. Gopinath SP, Robertson CS, Contant CF, et al. Jugular venous desaturation and outcome after head injury. *J Neurol Neurosurg Psychiatry* 1994;57:717-723.

14. Marion DW, Carlier PM. Problems with initial Glasgow Coma Scale assessment caused by prehospital treatment of patients with head injuries: results of a national survey. *J Trauma* 1994;36(1):89-95.

15. Marion DW, Spiegel TP. Changes in the management of severe traumatic brain injury: 1991-1997. *Crit Care Med* 2000;28:16-18.

16. McCrory, P, Johnston, K, Meeuwisse, W, et al. Summary and agreement statement of the 2nd International Conference on Concussion in Sport, Prague 2004. *Br J Sports Med* 2005;39:196-204.

17. Muizelaar JP, Marmarou A, Ward JD, et al. Adverse effects of prolonged hyperventilation in patients with severe head injury: a randomized clinical trial. *J Neurosurg* 1991;75:731-739.

18. Neuroimaging in the management of penetrating brain injury. *J Trauma* 2001;51(2 Suppl):S7-S11.

19. Part 1: Guidelines for the management of penetrating brain injury. Introduction and methodology. *J Trauma* 2001;51(2 Suppl):S3-S6.

20. Part 2: Prognosis in penetrating brain injury. *J Trauma* 2001;51(2 Suppl):S44-S86.

21. Robertson CS, Valadka AB, Hannay HJ, et al. Prevention of secondary ischemic insults after severe head injury. *Crit Care Med* 1999;27:2086-2095.

22. Rosner MJ, Rosner SD, Johnson AH. Cerebral perfusion pressure management protocols and clinical results. *J Neurosurg* 1995;83:949-962.

23. Smits M, Dippel DW, de Haan GG, et al. External validation of the Canadian CT Head Rule and the New Orleans Criteria for CT scanning in patients with minor head injury. *JAMA* 2005;294(12):1519-1525.

24. Stiell IG, Clement CM, Rowe BH, et al. Comparison of the Canadian CT Head Rule and the New Orleans Criteria in patients with minor head injury. *JAMA* 2005;294(12):1511-1518.

25. Stiell IG, Lesiuk H, Wells GA, et al. Canadian CT head rule study for patients with minor head injury: methodology for phase II (validation and economic analysis). *Ann Emerg Med* 2001;38(3):317-322.

26. Stiell IG, Lesiuk H, Wells GA, et al. The Canadian CT Head Rule Study for patients with minor head injury: rationale, objectives, and methodology for phase I (derivation). *Ann Emerg Med 2001; 38(2):160-169.*

27. *Stiell IG, Wells GA, Vandemheen K, et al. The Canadian CT Head Rule for patients with minor head injury. Lancet 2001; 357(9266):1391-1396.*

28. Sultan HY, Boyle A, Pereira M, Antoun N, Maimaris C. Application of the Canadian CT head rules in managing minor head injuries in a UK emergency department: implications for the implementation of the NICE guidelines. *Emerg Med J* 2004; 21(4):420-425.

29. Surgical management of penetrating brain injury. *J Trauma* 2001; 51(2 Suppl), S16-25.

30. Temkin NR, Dikman SS, Wilensky AJ, et al. A randomized, double-blind study of phenytoin for the prevention of post-traumatic seizures. *N Engl J Med* 1990;323:497-502.

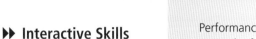

▶▶ Interactive Skills Procedure

***Note:* Standard precautions are required when caring for trauma patients.**

A series of scenarios accompanies some of the skills procedures for this station. The scenarios are provided at the conclusion of the procedures for your review and preparation for this station.

THE FOLLOWING PROCEDURES ARE INCLUDED IN THIS SKILLS STATION:

▶▶ **Skill IX-A:** Primary Survey

▶▶ **Skill IX-B:** Secondary Survey and Management

▶▶ **Skill IX-C:** Evaluation of CT Scans of the Head

▶▶ **Skill IX-D:** Helmet Removal

Performance at this station will allow the participant to practice and demonstrate the following activities in a simulated clinical situation:

OBJECTIVES

1 Demonstrate assessment and diagnostic skills in determining the type and extent of injuries with a head trauma manikin.

2 Describe the significance of clinical signs and symptoms of brain trauma found through assessment.

3 Establish priorities for the initial treatment of patients with brain trauma.

4 Identify diagnostic aids that can be used to determine the area of injury within the brain and the extent of the injury.

5 Demonstrate proper helmet removal while protecting the patient's cervical spine.

6 Perform a complete secondary assessment and determine the patient's Glasgow Coma Scale (GCS) score through the use of scenarios and interactive dialogue with the instructor.

7 Differentiate between normal and abnormal computed tomographic (CT) scans of the head, and identify injury patterns.

▶ Skill IX-A: Primary Survey

STEP 1. ABCDEs

STEP 2. Immobilize and stabilize the cervical spine.

STEP 3. Perform a brief neurologic examination, looking for:
- A. Pupillary response
- B. GCS score determination

▶ Skill IX-B: Secondary Survey and Management

STEP 1. Inspect the entire head, including the face, looking for:
- A. Lacerations
- B. Nose and ears for presence of cerebrospinal fluid (CSF) leakage

STEP 2. Palpate the entire head, including the face, looking for:
- A. Fractures
- B. Lacerations and underlying fractures

STEP 3. Inspect all scalp lacerations, looking for:
- A. Brain tissue
- B. Depressed skull fractures
- C. Debris
- D. CSF leaks

STEP 4. Determine the GCS score and pupillary response, including:
- A. Eye-opening response
- B. Best limb motor response
- C. Verbal response
- D. Pupillary response

STEP 5. Examine the cervical spine.
- A. Palpate for tenderness/pain and apply a semirigid cervical collar, if needed.
- B. Perform a cross-table lateral cervical spine x-ray examination as needed

STEP 6. Determine the extent of injury.

STEP 7. Reassess the patient continuously, observing for signs of deterioration.
- A. Frequency
- B. Parameters to be assessed
- C. Serial GCS scores and extremity motor assessment
- D. Remember, reassess ABCDEs

▶ Skill IX-C: Evaluation of CT Scans of the Head

Diagnosis of abnormalities seen on CT scans of the head can be very subtle and difficult. Because of the inherent complexity in interpreting these scans, early review by a neurosurgeon or radiologist is important. The steps outlined here for evaluating a CT scan of the head provide one approach to assessing for significant, life-threatening pathology. Remember, obtaining a CT scan of the head should not delay resuscitation or transfer of the patient to a trauma center.

STEP 1. Follow the process for initial review of CT scans of the head.
- A. Confirm that the images being reviewed are of the correct patient.
- B. Ensure that the CT scan of the head was done without an intravenous contrast agent.
- C. Use the patient's clinical findings to focus the review of the CT scan, and use the image findings to enhance further physical evaluation.

STEP 2. Assess the scalp component for contusion or swelling that can indicate the site of external trauma.

STEP 3. Assess for skull fractures. Keep in mind that:
- A. Suture lines (joining of the bones of the cranial vault) may be mistaken for fractures.
- B. Depressed skull fractures (thickness of skull) require neurosurgical consultation.
- C. Open fractures require neurosurgical consultation. Missile wound tracts may appear as linear areas of low attenuation.

STEP 4. Assess the gyri and sulci for symmetry. If asymmetry exists, consider these diagnoses:
- A. Acute subdural hematoma:
  - Typically are areas of increased density covering and compressing the gyri and sulci over the entire hemisphere
  - Appear within the skull

- Can cause a shift of the underlying ventricles across the midline
- Occur more commonly than epidural hematomas
- Can have associated cerebral contusions and intracerebral hematomas

B. Acute epidural hematoma:
- Typically are lenticular or biconvex areas of increased density
- Appear within the skull and compress the underlying gyri and sulci
- Can cause a shift of the underlying ventricles across the midline
- Most often are located in the temporal or temporoparietal region

STEP 5. Assess the cerebral and cerebellar hemispheres.
- **A.** Compare both cerebral and cerebellar hemispheres for similar density and symmetry.
- **B.** Intracerebral hematomas appear as large areas of high density.
- **C.** Cerebral contusions appear as punctate areas of high density.
- **D.** Diffuse axonal injury can appear normal or have scattered, small areas of cerebral contusion and areas of low density.

STEP 6. Assess the ventricles.
- **A.** Check size and symmetry
- **B.** Significant mass lesions compress and distort the ventricles, especially the lateral ventricles.

- **C.** Significant intracranial hypertension is often associated with decreased ventricular size.
- **D.** Intraventricular hemorrhage appears as regions of increased density (bright spots) in the ventricles.

STEP 7. Determine the shifts. Midline shifts may be caused by a hematoma or swelling that causes the septum pellucidum, between the two lateral ventricles, to shift away from the midline. The midline is a line extending from the crista galli anteriorly to the tentlike projection posteriorly (inion). After measuring the distance from the midline to the septum pellucidum, the actual shift is determined by correcting against the scale on the CT print. A shift of 5 mm or more is considered indicative of a mass lesion and the need for surgical decompression.

STEP 8. Assess the maxillofacial structures.
- **A.** Assess the facial bones for fracture-related crepitus.
- **B.** Assess the sinuses and mastoid air cells for air-fluid levels.
- **C.** Facial bone fractures, sinus fractures, and sinus or mastoid air-fluid levels may indicate basilar skull or cribriform plate fractures.

STEP 9. Look for the four Cs of increased density:
- **A.** Contrast
- **B.** Clot
- **C.** Cellularity (tumor)
- **D.** Calcification (pineal gland, choroid plexus)

▶ Skill IX-D: Helmet Removal

Patients wearing a helmet who require airway management should have the head and neck held in a neutral position while the helmet is removed using the two-person procedure. *Note:* A poster titled "Techniques of Helmet Removal from Injured Patients" is available from the American College of Surgeons (www.facs.org/trauma/publications/helmet.pdfP). This poster provides a pictorial and narrative description of helmet removal. There are some varieties of helmet that have special removal mechanisms that should be used in accordance with the specific helmet.

STEP 1. One person stabilizes the patient's head and neck by placing one hand on either side of the helmet with the fingers on the patient's mandible. This position prevents slippage if the strap is loose.

STEP 2. The second person cuts or loosens the helmet strap at the D-rings.

STEP 3. The second person then places one hand on the mandible at the angle, with the thumb on one

side and the fingers on the other. The other hand applies pressure from under the head at the occipital region. This maneuver transfers the responsibility for in-line immobilization to the second person.

STEP 4. The first person then expands the helmet laterally to clear the ears and carefully removes the helmet. If the helmet has a face cover, this device must be removed first. If the helmet provides full facial coverage, the patient's nose will impede helmet removal. To clear the nose, the helmet must be tilted backward and raised over the patient's nose.

STEP 5. During this process, the second person must maintain in-line immobilization from below to prevent head tilt.

STEP 6. After the helmet is removed, in-line manual immobilization is reestablished from above, and the patient's head and neck are secured during airway management.

STEP 7. If attempts to remove the helmet result in pain and paresthesia, the helmet should be removed with a cast cutter. The helmet also should be removed with a cast cutter if there is evidence of a cervical spine injury on x-ray film. The head and neck must be stabilized during this procedure, which is accomplished by dividing the helmet in the coronal plane through the ears. The outer rigid layer is removed easily, and the inside Styrofoam® layer is then incised and removed anteriorly. Maintaining neutral alignment of the head and neck, the posterior portions are removed.

▶ SCENARIOS

SCENARIO IX-1

A 17-year-old high-school football player, involved in a crushing tackle with a brief loss of consciousness, reports neck pain and paresthesia in his left arm. He is immobilized on a long spine board with his helmet in place and transported to the emergency department (ED). He is not in respiratory distress, talks coherently, and is awake and alert.

SCENARIO IX-2

A 25-year-old man is transported to the ED after a car crash while driving home from a tavern. His airway is clear, he is breathing spontaneously without difficulty, and he has no hemodynamic abnormalities. He has a scalp contusion over the left side of his head. There is a strong odor of alcohol on his breath, but he is able to answer questions appropriately. His eyes are open, but he appears confused and pushes away the examiner's hands when examined for response to pain. He is thought to have suffered a concussion and to have alcohol intoxication. He is kept in the ED for observation.

One hour later, the patient is more somnolent, briefly opens his eyes to painful stimuli, and demonstrates an abnormal flexion response to painful stimuli on the right and withdrawal on the left. His left pupil is now 2 mm larger than his right. Both pupils react sluggishly to light. His verbal response consists of incomprehensible sounds.

SCENARIO IX-3

A 21-year-old man was thrown from and then kicked in the face by a horse. He was initially unconscious for at least 5 minutes. He now opens his eyes to speech, moves only to painful stimuli by withdrawing his extremities, and utters inappropriate words. His blood pressure is 180/80 mm Hg, and heart rate 64 beats/min.

SCENARIO IX-4

A 40-year-old motorcyclist is brought to the ED with obvious, isolated head trauma. The prehospital personnel report that he has unequal pupils and responds only to painful stimuli by abnormally flexing his arms, opening his eyes, and speaking incomprehensibly. When not stimulated, his respirations are very sonorous.

CHAPTER 7

Spine and Spinal Cord Trauma

Upon completion of this topic, the student will be able to demonstrate the techniques of assessment and explain the emergency management of spine and spinal cord trauma. Specifically, the doctor will be able to:

OBJECTIVES

1 Describe the basic spinal anatomy and physiology.

2 Evaluate a patient with suspected spinal injury.

3 Identify the common types of spinal injuries and their x-ray features.

4 Appropriately treat patients with spinal injuries during the first hour after injury.

5 Determine the appropriate disposition of patients with spine trauma.

Introduction

Vertebral column injury, with or without neurologic deficits, must always be considered in patients with multiple injuries. Approximately 5% of patients with brain injury have an associated spinal injury, whereas 25% of patients with spinal injury have at least a mild brain injury. Approximately 55% of spinal injuries occur in the cervical region, 15% in the thoracic region, 15% at the thoracolumbar junction, and 15% in the lumbosacral area. **Approximately 10% of patients with a cervical spine fracture have a second, noncontiguous vertebral column fracture.**

Doctors and other medical personnel who care for patients with spine injuries must be constantly aware that excessive manipulation and inadequate immobilization of such patients may cause additional neurologic damage and worsen the patient's outcome. At least 5% of patients experience the onset of neurologic symptoms or the worsening of preexisting symptoms after reaching the emergency department. This is usually due to ischemia or progression of spinal cord edema, but it may also be the result of failure to provide adequate immobilization. **As long as the patient's spine is protected, evaluation of the spine and exclusion of spinal injury may be safely deferred, especially in the presence of systemic instability, such as hypotension and respiratory inadequacy.**

Excluding the presence of a spinal injury is simple in a patient who is awake and alert. In a neurologically intact patient, the absence of pain or tenderness along the spine virtually excludes the presence of a significant spinal injury. However, in a patient who is comatose or has a depressed level of consciousness, the process is not as simple. In this case, it is incumbent on the doctor to obtain the appropriate x-ray films to exclude a spinal injury. If the x-rays are inconclusive, the patient's spine should remain protected until further testing can be performed.

Although the dangers of inadequate immobilization have been fairly well documented, there also is some danger in prolonged immobilization of patients on a hard surface such as a backboard. In addition to causing severe discomfort in an awake patient, prolonged immobilization may lead to the formation of serious decubitus ulcers in patients with spinal cord injuries. Therefore, the long backboard should be used only as a patient transportation device, and every effort made to have the patient evaluated by the appropriate specialists and removed from the spine board as quickly as possible. If this is not feasible within 2 hours, the patient should be removed from the spine board and then logrolled every 2 hours, while maintaining the integrity of the spine, to reduce the risk of the formation of decubitus ulcers.

Anatomy and Physiology

The following review of the anatomy and physiology of the spine and spinal cord includes the spinal column, spinal cord anatomy, sensory and motor examination, myotomes, neurogenic and spinal shock, and the effects on other organ systems.

SPINAL COLUMN

The spinal column consists of 7 cervical, 12 thoracic, and 5 lumbar vertebrae, as well as the sacrum and the coccyx (Figure 7-1). The typical vertebra consists of the anteriorly placed vertebral body, which forms the main weight-bearing column. The vertebral bodies are separated by intervertebral disks, and are held together anteriorly and posteriorly by the anterior and posterior longitudinal ligaments, respectively. Posterolaterally, two pedicles form the pillars on which the roof of the vertebral canal (ie, the lamina) rests. The facet joints, interspinous ligaments, and paraspinal muscles all contribute to the stability of the spine.

The cervical spine is the most vulnerable to injury, because of its mobility and exposure. The cervical canal is wide in the upper cervical region—that is, from the foramen magnum to the lower part of C2. The majority of patients with injuries at this level who survive are neurologically intact on arrival at the hospital. However, approximately one-third of patients with upper cervical spine injuries die at the injury scene from apnea caused by loss of central innervation of the phrenic nerves caused by spinal cord injury at C1. Below the level of C3 the diameter of the spinal canal is much smaller relative to the diameter of the spinal cord, and vertebral column injuries are much more likely to cause spinal cord injuries.

The mobility of the thoracic spine is much more restricted than that of the cervical spine, and it has additional support from the rib cage. Hence, the incidence of thoracic fractures is much lower, with most thoracic spine fractures being wedge compression fractures that are not associated with spinal cord injury. However, when a fracture-dislocation in the thoracic spine does occur, it almost always results in a complete spinal cord injury because of the relatively narrow thoracic canal. The thoracolumbar junction is a fulcrum between the inflexible thoracic region and the stronger lumbar levels. This makes it more vulnerable to injury, and 15% of all spinal injuries occur in this region.

SPINAL CORD ANATOMY

The spinal cord originates at the caudal end of the medulla oblongata at the foramen magnum. In adults, it usually ends around the L1 bony level as the conus medullaris. Below this level is the cauda equina, which is somewhat more resilient to injury. Of the many tracts in the spinal cord, only three can be readily assessed clinically: (1) the corticospinal tract, (2) the spinothalamic tract, and (3) the posterior columns (Figure 7-2). Each is a paired tract that may be injured on one or both sides of the cord.

The corticospinal tract, which lies in the posterolateral segment of the cord, controls motor power on the same side

A

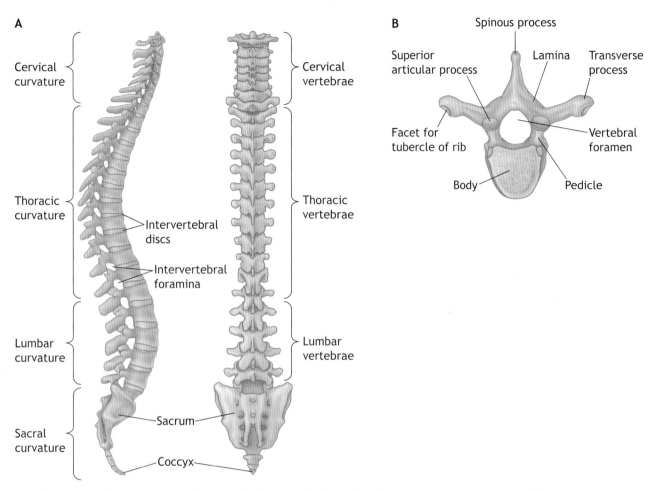

Cervical curvature

Thoracic curvature

Intervertebral discs

Intervertebral foramina

Lumbar curvature

Sacral curvature

Sacrum

Coccyx

Cervical vertebrae

Thoracic vertebrae

Lumbar vertebrae

B

Spinous process

Superior articular process

Lamina

Transverse process

Facet for tubercle of rib

Vertebral foramen

Body

Pedicle

■ **Figure 7-1 The Spine. (A)** The spinal column, right lateral and posterior views. **(B)** A typical thoracic vertebra, superior view.

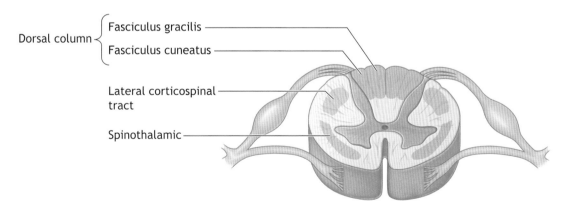

Dorsal column

Fasciculus gracilis

Fasciculus cuneatus

Lateral corticospinal tract

Spinothalamic

■ **Figure 7-2** Of the many tracts in the spinal cord, only three can be readily assessed clinically: (1) the corticospinal tract, (2) the spinothalamic tract, and (3) the posterior columns. Each is a paired tract that can be injured on one or both sides of the cord.

of the body and is tested by voluntary muscle contractions or involuntary response to painful stimuli. The spinothalamic tract, in the anterolateral aspect of the cord, transmits pain and temperature sensation from the opposite side of the body. In general, it is tested by pinprick and light touch. The posterior columns carry position sense (proprioception), vibration sense, and some light-touch sensation from the same side of the body. These columns are tested by position sense in the toes and fingers or vibration sense using a tuning fork.

The state of no demonstrable sensory or motor function below a certain level is referred to as a complete spinal cord injury. During the first weeks after injury, this diagnosis cannot be made with certainty, because of the possibility of spinal shock. ▪See Chapter 3: Shock. An incomplete injury is one in which any motor or sensory function remains; the prognosis for recovery is significantly better than that for complete spinal cord injury. Sparing of sensation in the perianal region (sacral sparing) may be the only sign of residual function. Sacral sparing can be demonstrated by preservation of some sensory perception in the perianal region and/or voluntary contraction of the rectal sphincter.

SENSORY EXAMINATION

❓ *How do I assess the patient's neurologic status?*

A dermatome is the area of skin innervated by the sensory axons within a particular segmental nerve root. Knowledge of some of the major dermatome levels is invaluable in determining the level of injury and assessing neurologic improvement or deterioration. The sensory level is the lowest dermatome with normal sensory function and can often differ on the two sides of the body. For practical purposes, the upper cervical dermatomes (C1 to C4) are somewhat variable in their cutaneous distribution and are not commonly used for localization. However, it should be remembered that the supraclavicular nerves (C2 through C4) provide sensory innervation to the region overlying the pectoralis muscle (cervical cape). The presence of sensation in this region may confuse the examiner when he or she is trying to determine the sensory level in patients with lower cervical injuries. The key sensory points are (Figure 7-3):

- C5—Area over the deltoid
- C6—Thumb
- C7—Middle finger
- C8—Little finger
- T4—Nipple
- T8—Xiphisternum
- T10—Umbilicus

PITFALLS

- Sensory examination may be confounded by pain.
- Patients sometimes observe the examination itself, which may alter the findings.
- Altered level of consciousness limits the ability to perform a definitive neurologic examination.

- T12—Symphysis pubis
- L4—Medial aspect of the calf
- L5—Web space between the first and second toes
- S1—Lateral border of the foot
- S3—Ischial tuberosity area
- S4 and S5—Perianal region

MYOTOMES

Each segmental nerve (root) innervates more than one muscle, and most muscles are innervated by more than one root (usually two). Nevertheless, for the sake of simplicity, certain muscles or muscle groups are identified as representing a single spinal nerve segment. The important key muscle(s) are (Figure 7-4):

- C5—Deltoid
- C6—Wrist extensors (biceps, extensor carpi radialis longus and brevis)
- C7—Elbow extensors (triceps)
- C8—Finger flexors to the middle finger (flexor digitorum profundus)
- T1—Small finger abductors (abductor digiti minimi)
- L2—Hip flexors (iliopsoas)
- L3, L4—Knee extensors (quadriceps, patellar reflexes)
- L4, L5 to S1—Knee flexion (hamstrings)
- L5—Ankle and big toe dorsiflexors (tibialis anterior and extensor hallucis longus)
- S1—Ankle plantar flexors (gastrocnemius, soleus)

The key muscles should be tested for power on both sides. Each muscle is graded on a six-point scale from normal strength to paralysis (Table 7-1). Documentation of the power in key muscle groups helps to assess neurologic improvement or deterioration on subsequent examinations. In addition, the external anal sphincter should be tested for voluntary contraction by digital examination.

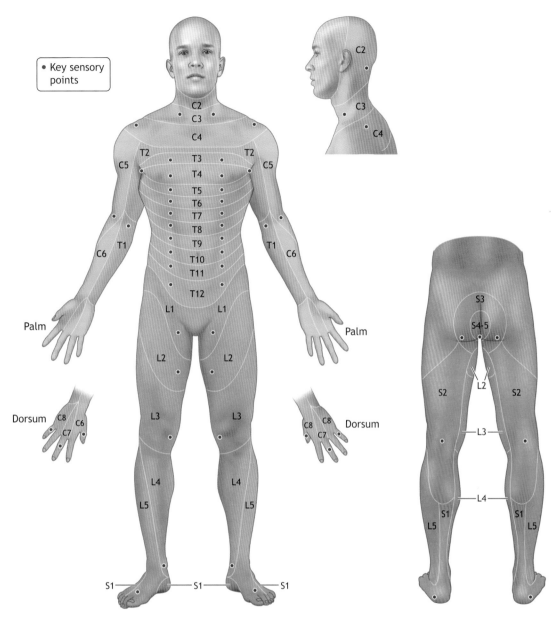

• Key sensory points

■ **Figure 7-3 Key Sensory Points by Spinal Dermatomes.** (Adapted from American Spinal Injury Association: International *Standards for Neurological Classification of Spinal Cord Injury,* revised 2002. Chicago, IL: American Spinal Injury Association; 2002.

NEUROGENIC SHOCK VERSUS SPINAL SHOCK

? *How do I identify and treat neurogenic and spinal shock?*

Neurogenic shock results from impairment of the descending sympathetic pathways in the cervical or upper thoracic spinal cord. This condition results in the loss of vasomotor tone and in sympathetic innervation to the heart. The former causes vasodilation of visceral and lower-extremity blood vessels, pooling of blood, and, consequently, hypotension. Loss of cardiac sympathetic tone may cause the development of bradycardia or at least a failure of tachycardia in response to hypovolemia. In this condition, the blood pressure may not be restored by fluid infusion alone, and massive fluid resuscitation may result in fluid overload and pulmonary edema. The blood pressure may often be restored by the judicious use of vasopressors after moderate volume replacement. Atropine may be used to counteract hemodynamically significant bradycardia.

"Spinal shock" refers to the flaccidity (loss of muscle tone) and loss of reflexes seen after spinal cord injury. The "shock" to the injured cord may make it appear completely nonfunctional, although all areas are not necessarily destroyed. The duration of this state is variable.

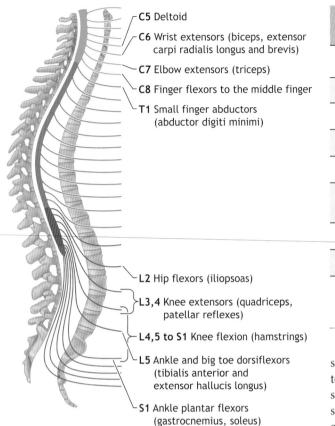

C5 Deltoid
C6 Wrist extensors (biceps, extensor carpi radialis longus and brevis)
C7 Elbow extensors (triceps)
C8 Finger flexors to the middle finger
T1 Small finger abductors (abductor digiti minimi)

L2 Hip flexors (iliopsoas)
L3,4 Knee extensors (quadriceps, patellar reflexes)
L4,5 to S1 Knee flexion (hamstrings)
L5 Ankle and big toe dorsiflexors (tibialis anterior and extensor hallucis longus)
S1 Ankle plantar flexors (gastrocnemius, soleus)

■ **Figure 7-4 Key Myotomes.**

TABLE 7-1	■ Muscle Strength Grading
SCORE	**RESULTS OF EXAMINATION**
0	Total paralysis
1	Palpable or visible contraction
2	Full range of motion with gravity eliminated
3	Full range of motion against gravity
4	Full range of motion, but less than normal strength
5	Normal strength
NT	Not testable

Adapted with permission from Kirshblum SC, Memmo P, Kim N, Campagnolo D, Millis S. Comparison of the revised 2000 American Spinal Injury Association classification standards with the 1996 guidelines. *Am J Phys Med Rehabil* 2002;81:502-505.

EFFECTS ON OTHER ORGAN SYSTEMS

Hypoventilation due to paralysis of the intercostal muscles may result from an injury involving the lower cervical or upper thoracic spinal cord. If the upper or middle cervical cord is injured, the diaphragm also is paralyzed because of involvement of the C3 to C5 segments, which innervate the diaphragm via the phrenic nerve. **The inability to perceive pain may mask a potentially serious injury elsewhere in the body, such as the usual signs of an acute abdomen.**

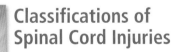

Classifications of Spinal Cord Injuries

❓ *When do I suspect spine injury?*

Spinal cord injuries can be classified according to (1) level, (2) severity of neurologic deficit, (3) spinal cord syndrome, and (4) morphology.

LEVEL

The neurologic level is the most caudal segment of the spinal cord that has normal sensory and motor function on both sides of the body. When the term *sensory level* is used, it refers to the most caudal segment of the spinal cord with normal sensory function. The *motor level* is defined similarly with respect to motor function as the lowest key muscle that has a grade of at least 3/5 (see Table 7-1). In complete injuries, when some impaired sensory and/or motor function is found just below the lowest normal segment, this is referred to as the zone of partial preservation. As described previously, the determination of the level of injury on both sides is important.

A broad distinction may be made between lesions above and below T1. Injuries of the first eight cervical segments of the spinal cord result in quadriplegia, and lesions below the T1 level result in paraplegia. The *bony level of injury* is the vertebra at which the bones are damaged, causing injury to the spinal cord. The *neurologic level of injury* is determined primarily by clinical examination. Frequently, there is a discrepancy between the bony and the neurologic levels because the spinal nerves enter the spinal canal through the foramina and ascend or descend inside the spinal canal before actually entering the spinal cord. The further caudal the injury is, the more pronounced this discrepancy becomes. Apart from the initial management to stabilize the bony injury, all subsequent descriptions of the level of injury are based on the neurologic level.

SEVERITY OF NEUROLOGIC DEFICIT

Spinal cord injury may be categorized as:

- Incomplete paraplegia (incomplete thoracic)
- Complete paraplegia (complete thoracic)
- Incomplete quadriplegia (incomplete cervical)
- Complete quadriplegia (complete cervical injury)

It is important to assess for any sign of preservation of function of the long tracts of the spinal cord. Any motor or sensory function below the level of the injury constitutes an incomplete injury. Signs of an incomplete injury include any sensation (including position sense) or voluntary movement in the lower extremities, sacral sparing (ie, perianal sensation), voluntary anal sphincter contraction, and voluntary toe flexion. Sacral reflexes, such as the bulbocavernosus reflex or anal wink, do not qualify as sacral sparing.

SPINAL CORD SYNDROMES

Certain characteristic patterns of neurologic injury are frequently seen in patients with spinal cord injuries. These patterns should be recognized so they do not confuse the examiner.

Central cord syndrome is characterized by a disproportionately greater loss of motor power in the upper extremities than in the lower extremities, with varying degrees of sensory loss. Usually this syndrome is seen after a hyperextension injury in a patient with preexisting cervical canal stenosis (often due to degenerative osteoarthritic changes). The history is commonly that of a forward fall that resulted in a facial impact. It may occur with or without cervical spine fracture or dislocation. Recovery usually follows a characteristic pattern, with the lower extremities recovering strength first, bladder function next, and the proximal upper extremities and hands last. The prognosis for recovery in central cord injuries is somewhat better than with other incomplete injuries. Central cord syndrome is thought to be due to vascular compromise of the cord in the distribution of the anterior spinal artery. This artery supplies the central portions of the cord. Because the motor fibers to the cervical segments are topographically arranged toward the center of the cord, the arms and hands are the most severely affected.

Anterior cord syndrome is characterized by paraplegia and a dissociated sensory loss with a loss of pain and temperature sensation. Posterior column function (position, vibration, and deep pressure sense) is preserved. Usually, anterior cord syndrome is due to infarction of the cord in the territory supplied by the anterior spinal artery. This syndrome has the poorest prognosis of the incomplete injuries.

Brown-Séquard syndrome results from hemisection of the cord, usually as a result of a penetrating trauma; it is rarely seen. Nevertheless, variations on the classic picture are not uncommon. In its pure form, the syndrome consists of ipsilateral motor loss (corticospinal tract) and loss of position sense (posterior column), associated with contralateral loss of pain and temperature sensation beginning one to two levels below the level of injury (spinothalamic tract). Even if the syndrome is caused by a direct penetrating injury to the cord, some recovery is usually seen.

MORPHOLOGY

Spinal injuries can be described as fractures, fracture-dislocations, spinal cord injury without radiographic abnormalities (SCIWORA), and penetrating injuries. Each of these categories may be further described as stable or unstable. However, determining the stability of a particular type of injury is not always simple and, indeed, even experts may disagree. **Hence, especially in the initial treatment, all patients with radiographic evidence of injury and all those with neurologic deficits should be considered to have an unstable spinal injury.** These patients should be immobilized until after consultation with an appropriately qualified doctor, usually a neurosurgeon or orthopedic surgeon.

Specific Types of Spinal Injuries

Cervical spine injuries can result from one or a combination of the following mechanisms of injury:

- Axial loading
- Flexion
- Extension
- Rotation
- Lateral bending
- Distraction

The injuries identified in this chapter all involve the spinal column. They are listed in anatomic sequence (not in order of frequency), progressing from the cranial to the caudal end of the spine.

ATLANTO-OCCIPITAL DISLOCATION

Craniocervical disruption injuries are uncommon and result from severe traumatic flexion and distraction. Most of these patients die of brainstem destruction and apnea or have profound neurologic impairments (are ventilator-dependent and quadriplegic). An occasional patient may survive if prompt resuscitation is available at the injury scene. This injury may be identified in up to 19% of patients with fatal cervical spine injuries and is a common cause of death in cases of shaken baby syndrome in which the infant dies immediately after shaking. Cervical traction is not used in patients with craniocervical dislocation. Spinal immobilization is recommended initially. ◾ Aids to the identification of atlanto-occipital dislocation on spine films, including Power's ratio, are included in Skill Station X: X-Ray Identification of Spine Injuries.

ATLAS FRACTURE (C1)

The atlas is a thin, bony ring with broad articular surfaces. Fractures of the atlas represent approximately 5% of acute cervical spine fractures. Approximately 40% of atlas fractures are associated with fractures of the axis (C2). The most common C1 fracture is a burst fracture (Jefferson fracture). The usual mechanism of injury is axial loading, which occurs when a large load falls vertically on the head or a patient lands on the top of his or her head in a relatively neutral position. The Jefferson fracture involves disruption of both the anterior and posterior rings of C1 with lateral displacement of the lateral masses. The fracture is best seen on an open-mouth view of the C1 to C2 region and axial CT scans (Figure 7-5). In patients who survive, these fractures usually are not associated with spinal cord injuries. However, they are unstable and should be initially treated with a cervical collar. Unilateral ring or lateral mass fractures are not uncommon and tend to be stable injuries. However, they are treated as unstable until the patient is examined by an appropriately qualified doctor, usually a neurosurgeon or orthopedic surgeon.

C1 ROTARY SUBLUXATION

C1 rotary subluxation injury is most often seen in children. It may occur spontaneously, after major or minor trauma, with an upper respiratory infection, or with rheumatoid arthritis. The patient presents with a persistent rotation of the head (torticollis). This injury is also best diagnosed with an open-mouth odontoid view, although the x-ray findings may be confusing. In this injury, the odontoid is not equidistant from the two lateral masses of C1. The patient should not be forced to overcome the rotation, but should be immobilized in the rotated position and referred for further specialized treatment.

AXIS (C2) FRACTURES

The axis is the largest cervical vertebra and is the most unusual in shape. Therefore, it is susceptible to various fractures depending on the force and direction of the impact. Acute fractures of C2 represent approximately 18% of all cervical spine injuries.

Odontoid Fractures

Approximately 60% of C2 fractures involve the odontoid process, a peg-shaped bony protuberance that projects upward and is normally positioned in contact with the anterior arch of C1. The odontoid process is held in place primarily by the transverse ligament. Odontoid fractures are initially identified by a lateral cervical spine film or on open-mouth odontoid views. However, a CT scan usually is required for further delineation. Type I odontoid fractures typically involve the tip of the odontoid and are relatively uncommon. Type II odontoid fractures occur through the base of the dens and are the most common odontoid fracture (Figure 7-6). In children younger than 6 years of age, the epiphysis may be prominent and may look like a fracture at this level. Type III odontoid fractures occur at the base of the dens and extend obliquely into the body of the axis.

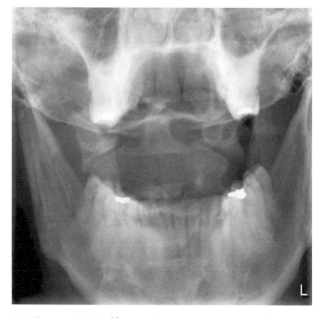

■ **Figure 7-5 Jefferson Fracture.** Open-mouth view radiograph showing a Jefferson fracture.

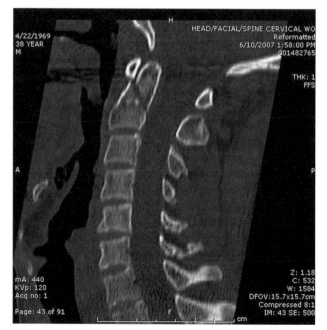

■ **Figure 7-6 Odontoid Fracture.** CT view of a Type II odontoid fracture.

Posterior Element Fractures of C2

A hangman's fracture involves the posterior elements of C2—that is, the pars interarticularis (Figure 7-7). This type of fracture represents approximately 20% of all axis fractures and usually is caused by an extension-type injury. Patients with this fracture should be maintained in external immobilization until specialized care is available.

Variations of a hangman's fracture include bilateral fractures through the lateral masses or pedicles. Approximately 20% of all axis fractures are nonodontoid and non-hangman's. These include fractures through the body, pedicle, lateral mass, laminae, and spinous process.

FRACTURES AND DISLOCATIONS (C3 THROUGH C7)

A fracture of C3 is very uncommon, possibly because it is positioned between the more vulnerable axis and the more mobile "relative fulcrum" of the cervical spine—that is, C5 and C6—where the greatest flexion and extension of the cervical spine occur. In adults, the most common level of cervical vertebral fracture is C5, and the most common level of subluxation is C5 on C6. The most common injury patterns identified at these levels are vertebral body fractures with or without subluxation, subluxation of the articular processes (including unilateral or bilateral locked facets), and fractures of the laminae, spinous processes, pedicles, or lateral masses. Rarely, ligamentous disruption occurs without fractures or facet dislocations.

The incidence of neurologic injury increases dramatically with facet dislocations. In the presence of unilateral facet dislocation, 80% of patients have a neurologic injury—approximately 30% have root injuries only, 40% incomplete spinal cord injuries, and 30% complete spinal cord injuries. In the presence of bilateral locked facets, the morbidity is much worse, with 16% incomplete and 84% complete spinal cord injuries.

THORACIC SPINE FRACTURES (T1 THROUGH T10)

Thoracic spinal fractures may be classified into four broad categories:

- Anterior wedge compression injuries
- Burst injuries
- Chance fractures (Figure 7-8)
- Fracture-dislocations

Axial loading with flexion produces an anterior wedge compression injury. The amount of wedging usually is quite small, and the anterior portion of the vertebral body rarely is more than 25% shorter than the posterior body. Because of the rigidity of the rib cage, most of these fractures are stable. The second type of thoracic fracture is the burst injury, which is caused by vertical-axial compression. Chance fractures are transverse fractures through the vertebral body. They are caused by flexion about an axis anterior to the vertebral column and are most frequently seen following motor vehicle crashes in which the patient was restrained by only a lap belt. Chance fractures may be associated with retroperitoneal and abdominal visceral injuries. Fracture-dislocations are relatively uncommon in the thoracic and lumbar spine because of the orientation of the facet joints. These injuries almost always are due to extreme flexion or severe blunt trauma to the spine, which causes disruption of the posterior elements (pedicles, facets, and lamina) of the vertebra. The thoracic spinal canal is narrow in relation to the spinal cord, so fracture subluxations in the thoracic spine commonly result in complete neurologic deficits.

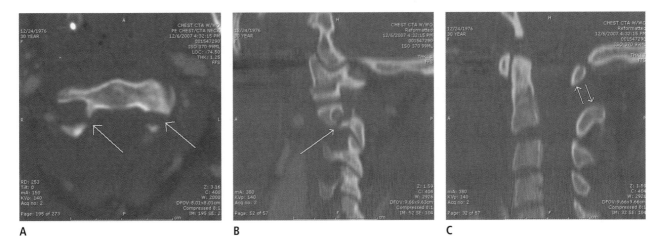

A   **B**   **C**

■ **Figure 7-7 Hangman's Fracture** (arrows) demonstrated in axial **(A)**, sagittal paramedian **(B)**, and sagittal midline **(C)** CT reconstructions. Note the anterior angulation and excessive distance between the spinous processes of C1 and C2 (double arrows).

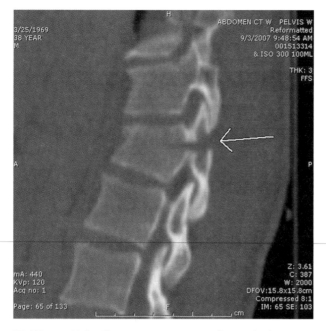

Figure 7-8 Chance Fracture. Radiograph showing the Chance fracture.

Simple compression fractures are usually stable and often treated with a rigid brace. Burst fractures, Chance fractures, and fracture-dislocations are extremely unstable and almost always require internal fixation.

THORACOLUMBAR JUNCTION FRACTURES (T11 THROUGH L1)

Fractures at the level of the thoracolumbar junction are due to the relative immobility of the thoracic spine as compared with the lumbar spine. They most often result from a combination of acute hyperflexion and rotation, and, consequently, they are usually unstable. People who fall from a height and restrained drivers who sustain severe flexion energy transfer are at particular risk for this type of injury.

The spinal cord terminates as the conus medullaris at approximately the level of L1, and injury to this part of the cord commonly results in bladder and bowel dysfunction, as well as in decreased sensation and strength in the lower extremities. **Patients with thoracolumbar fractures are particularly vulnerable to rotational movement.** Therefore, logrolling should be performed with extreme care.

LUMBAR FRACTURES

The radiographic signs associated with a lumbar fracture are similar to those of thoracic and thoracolumbar fractures. However, because only the cauda equina is involved, the probability of a complete neurologic deficit is much less with these injuries.

PENETRATING INJURIES

The most common types of penetrating injuries are those caused by gunshot wounds or stabbings. It is important to determine the path of the bullet or knife. This can be done

PITFALLS

- An inadequate secondary assessment may result in the failure to recognize a spinal cord injury, particularly an incomplete spinal cord injury.
- Patients with a diminished level of consciousness and those who arrive in shock are often difficult to assess for the presence of spinal cord injury. These patients require careful repeat assessment once initial life-threatening injuries have been managed.

by combining information from the history, clinical examination (entry and exit sites), plain x-ray films, and CT scans. If the path of injury passes directly through the vertebral canal, a complete neurologic deficit usually results. Complete deficits also may result from energy transfer associated with a high-velocity missile (eg, bullet) passing close to the spinal cord rather than through it. Penetrating injuries of the spine usually are stable injuries unless the missile destroys a large portion of the vertebra.

BLUNT CAROTID AND VERTEBRAL VASCULAR INJURIES

Blunt trauma to the head and neck has been recognized as a risk factor for carotid and vertebral arterial injuries. Early recognition and treatment of these injuries may reduce the risk of stroke. Indications for screening are evolving, but suggested criteria for screening include:

- C1–C3 fracture
- Cervical spine fracture with subluxation
- Fractures involving the foramen transversarium

Approximately one-third of these patients will be shown to have blunt carotid and vertebral vascular injury (BCVI) on CT angiography of the neck (Figure 7-9). The treatment of these injuries is evolving, and the impact of treatment is not well defined.

X-Ray Evaluation

? How do I confirm the presence or absence of a significant spine injury?

Both careful clinical examination and thorough radiographic assessment are critical in identifying significant spine injury. ◢▪ See Skill Station X: X-Ray Identification of Spine Injuries.

CERVICAL SPINE

Cervical spine radiography is indicated for all trauma patients who have midline neck pain, tenderness on palpation,

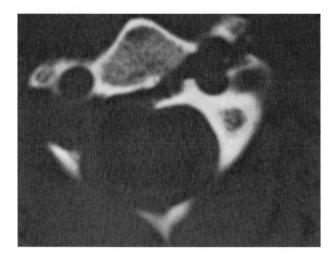

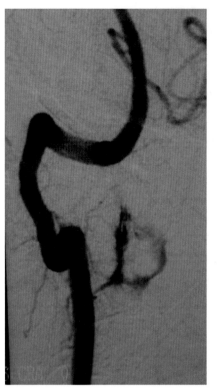

■ **Figure 7-9 Blunt Vertebral Artery Injury.** CT and angiogram of blunt vertebral artery injury.

neurologic deficits referable to the cervical spine, or an altered level of consciousness or in whom intoxication is suspected. Lateral, anteroposterior (AP) and open-mouth odontoid views should be obtained.

On the lateral view, the base of the skull, all seven cervical vertebrae, and the first thoracic vertebra must be visualized. The patient's shoulders may need to be pulled down when obtaining the lateral cervical spine x-ray film, to avoid missing fractures or fracture-dislocations in the lower cervical spine. If all seven cervical vertebrae are not visualized on the lateral x-ray film, a swimmer's view of the lower cervical and upper thoracic area should be obtained.

The open-mouth odontoid view should include the entire odontoid process and the right and left C1, C2 articulations. The AP view of the c-spine assists in the identification of a unilateral facet dislocation in cases in which little or no dislocation is identified on the lateral film. Axial CT scans at 3-mm intervals also should be obtained through suspicious areas identified on the plain films or through the lower cervical spine if it is not adequately visualized on the plain films. Axial CT images through C1 and C2 may also be more sensitive than plain films for detection of fractures of these vertebrae. If these films are of good quality and are properly interpreted, unstable cervical spine injuries can be detected with a sensitivity of greater than 97%. **The complete series of cervical spine radiographs must be reviewed by a doctor experienced in the proper interpretation of these films before the spine is considered normal and the cervical collar is removed. CT scans may be used in lieu of plain images to evaluate the cervical spine.**

If the screening radiographs described above are normal, flexion-extension x-ray films of the cervical spine may be obtained in injured patients without an altered level of consciousness, or in those who report neck pain, to detect occult instability or determine the stability of a known fracture, such as a laminar or compression fracture. It is possible for patients to have a purely ligamentous spine injury that results in instability without associated fracture, although some studies suggest that if plain three-view cervical spine radiographs with CT supplementation are truly normal (ie, no anterior soft-tissue swelling, no abnormal angulation), then significant instability is unlikely.

In some patients with significant soft-tissue injury, paraspinal muscle spasm may severely limit the degree of flexion and extension that the patient allows. In such cases, the patient is treated with a semirigid cervical collar for 2 to 3 weeks before another attempt is made to obtain flexion-extension views. Under no circumstances should the patient's neck be forced into a position that elicits pain. All movements must be voluntary. These films should be obtained under the direct supervision and control of a doctor experienced in the interpretation of such films.

Approximately 10% of patients with a cervical spine fracture have a second, noncontiguous vertebral column fracture. This warrants a complete radiographic screening of the entire spine in patients with a cervical spine fracture. Such screening also is advisable in all comatose trauma patients.

In the presence of neurologic deficits, magnetic resonance imaging (MRI) is recommended to detect any soft tissue compressive lesion, such as a spinal epidural hematoma or traumatized herniated disk, which cannot be detected with plain films. MRI may also detect spinal cord contusions or disruption, and paraspinal ligamentous and soft tissue injury. However, MRI is frequently not feasible in patients with hemodynamic instability. When MRI is not available or appropriate, CT myelography may be used to exclude the presence of acute spinal cord compression caused by a traumatic herniated disk or epidural hematoma. These specialized studies usually are performed at the discretion of a spine surgery consultant. Box 7-1 presents guidelines for screening trauma patients with suspected spine injury, and may serve as a model for the development of hospital policies.

THORACIC AND LUMBAR SPINE

The indications for screening radiography of the thoracic and lumbar spine are the same as those for the cervical spine. AP and lateral plain radiographs with axial CT scans at 3-mm intervals through suspicious areas can detect more than 99% of unstable injuries. On the AP views, the vertical alignment of the pedicles and the distance between pedicles of each thoracic and lumbar vertebra should be observed. Unstable fractures commonly cause widening of the interpedicular distance. The lateral films detect subluxations, compression fractures, and Chance fractures. CT scanning is particularly useful for detecting fractures of the posterior elements (pedicles, lamina, and spinous processes) and determining the degree of canal compromise caused by burst fractures. Sagittal reconstructions of axial CT images or plain tomography may be needed to adequately characterize Chance fractures. **As with the cervical spine, a complete series of good quality radiographs must be properly interpreted as normal by an experienced doctor before spine precautions are discontinued.**

General Management

? *How do I treat patients with spinal cord injury and limit secondary injury?*

General management spine and spinal cord trauma includes immobilization, intravenous fluids, medications, and transfer, if appropriate. ◼ See Skill Station XI: Spinal Cord Injury: Assessment and Management.

IMMOBILIZATION

? *How do I protect the spine during evaluation and transport?*

Prehospital care personnel usually immobilize patients before their transport to the emergency department. Any patient with a suspected spine injury should be immobilized above and below the suspected injury site until a fracture is excluded by x-ray examination. Remember, spinal protection should be maintained until a cervical spine injury is excluded. Proper immobilization is achieved with the patient in the neutral position—that is, supine without rotating or

bending the spinal column. No effort should be made to reduce an obvious deformity. Children may have torticollis, and the elderly may have severe degenerative spine disease that causes them to have a nontraumatic kyphotic or angulation deformity of the spine. Such patients should be immobilized on a backboard in a position of comfort. Supplemental padding is often necessary. **Attempts to align the spine for the purpose of immobilization on the backboard are not recommended if they cause pain.**

Immobilization of the neck with a semirigid collar does not ensure complete stabilization of the cervical spine. Immobilization using a spine board with appropriate bolstering devices is more effective in limiting certain neck motions. The use of long spine boards is recommended. **Cervical spine injury requires continuous immobilization of the entire patient with a semirigid cervical collar, head immobilization, backboard, tape, and straps before and during transfer to a definitive-care facility (Figure 7-10).** Extension or flexion of the neck should be avoided because these movements are the most dangerous to the spinal cord. The airway is of critical importance in patients with spinal cord injury, and early intubation should be accomplished if there is evidence of respiratory compromise. During intubation, the neck must be maintained in a neutral position.

Of special concern is the maintenance of adequate immobilization of restless, agitated, or violent patients. This condition can be due to pain, confusion associated with hypoxia or hypotension, alcohol or drug use, or simply a personality disorder. The doctor should search for and correct the cause, if possible. If necessary, a sedative or paralytic agent may be administered, keeping in mind the need for adequate airway protection, control, and ventilation. The use of sedatives or paralytic agents in this setting requires considerable clinical judgment, skill, and experience. The use of short-acting, reversible agents is advised.

Once the patient arrives at the emergency department, every effort should be made to remove the rigid spine board as early as possible to reduce the risk of decubitus ulcer formation. Removal of the board is often done as part of the secondary survey when the patient is logrolled for inspection and palpation of the back. It should not be delayed solely for the purpose of obtaining definitive spine radiographs, particularly if radiographic evaluation may not be completed for several hours.

The safe movement, or logrolling, of a patient with an unstable or potentially unstable spine, requires planning and the assistance of four or more individuals, depending on the size of the patient (Figure 7-11). Neutral anatomic alignment of the entire vertebral column must be maintained while rolling or lifting the patient. One person is assigned to maintain in-line immobilization of the head and neck. Individuals positioned on the same side of the patient's torso manually prevent segmental rotation, flexion, extension, lateral bending, or sagging of the chest or abdomen during transfer of the patient. A fourth person is responsible for moving the legs and removing the spine board and examining the patient's back.

BOX 7-1
Guidelines for Screening Patients with Suspected Spine Injury

Suspected Cervical Spine Injury

1 The presence of paraplegia or quadriplegia is presumptive evidence of spinal instability.

2 *Patients who are awake, alert, sober, and neurologically normal, and have no neck pain or midline tenderness:* These patients are extremely unlikely to have an acute c-spine fracture or instability. With the patient in a supine position, remove the c-collar and palpate the spine. If there is no significant tenderness, ask the patient to voluntarily move his or her neck from side to side. **Never force the patient's neck.** When performed voluntarily by the patient, these maneuvers are generally safe. If there is no pain, have the patient voluntarily flex and extend his or her neck.

Again, if there is no pain, c-spine films are not necessary.

3 *Patients who are awake and alert, neurologically normal, cooperative, and able to concentrate on their spine but do have neck pain or midline tenderness:* The burden of proof is on the doctor to exclude a spinal injury. All such patients should undergo lateral, AP, and open-mouth odontoid x-ray examinations of the c-spine with axial CT images of suspicious areas or of the lower cervical spine if not adequately visualized on the plain films. Assess the c-spine films for: (a) bony deformity, (b) fracture of the vertebral body or processes, (c) loss of alignment of the posterior aspect of the vertebral bodies (anterior extent of the vertebral canal), (d) increased distance between the spinous processes at one level, (e) narrowing of the vertebral canal, and (f) increased prevertebral soft tissue space. If these films are normal, remove the c-collar. Under the care of a knowledgeable doctor, obtain flexion and extension, lateral cervical spine films with the patient voluntarily flexing and extending his/her neck. If the films show no subluxation, the patient's c-spine can be cleared and the c-collar removed. However, if any of these films are suspicious or unclear, replace the collar and obtain consultation from a spine specialist.

4 *Patients who have an altered level of consciousness or are too young to describe their symptoms:* Lateral, AP, and open-mouth odontoid films with CT supplementation through suspicious areas (eg, C1 and C2, and through the lower cervical spine if areas are not adequately visualized on the plain films) should be obtained for all such patients. In children, CT supplementation is optional. If the entire c-spine can be visualized and is found to be normal, the collar can be removed after appropriate evaluation by a doctor/consultant skilled in the evaluation/management of patients with spine injuries. Clearance of the c-spine is particularly important if pulmonary or other care of the patient is compromised by an inability to mobilize the patient.

5 When in doubt, leave the collar on.

6 *Consult:* Doctors who are skilled in the evaluation and management of patients with spine injuries should be consulted in all cases in which a spine injury is detected or suspected.

7 *Backboards:* Patients who have neurologic deficits (quadriplegia or paraplegia) should be evaluated quickly and taken off the backboard as soon as possible. **A paralyzed patient who is allowed to lie on a hard board for more than 2 hours is at high risk for serious decubitus ulcers.**

8 *Emergency situations:* Trauma patients who require emergency surgery before a complete workup of the spine can be accomplished should be transported carefully, assuming that an unstable spine injury is present. The c-collar should be left on and the patient logrolled when moved to and from the operating table. The patient should not be left on a rigid backboard during surgery. The surgical team should take particular care to protect the neck as much as possible during the operation. The

Continued

BOX 7-1
Continued

anesthesiologist should be informed of the status of the workup.

Suspected Thoracolumbar Spine Injury

1 **The presence of paraplegia or a level of sensory loss on the chest or abdomen is presumptive evidence of spinal instability.**

2 *Patients who are awake, alert, sober, neurologically normal, and have no midline thoracic or lumbar back pain or tenderness:* The entire extent of the spine should be palpated and inspected. If there is no tenderness on palpation or ecchymosis over the spinous processes, an unstable spine fracture is unlikely, and thoracolumbar radiographs may not be necessary.

3 *Patients who have spine pain or tenderness on palpation, neurologic deficits, or an altered level of consciousness or in whom intoxication is suspected:* AP and lateral radiographs of the entire thoracic and lumbar spine should be obtained. Axial CT images at 3-mm intervals should be obtained through suspicious areas identified on the plain films. **All images must be of good quality and interpreted as normal by an experienced doctor before discontinuing spine precautions.**

4 *Consult* a doctor skilled in the evaluation and management of spine injuries if a spine injury is detected or suspected.

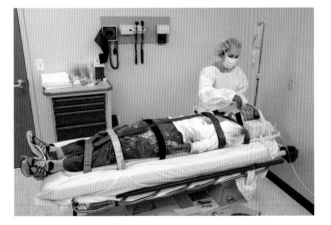

■ **Figure 7-10** Cervical spine injury requires continuous immobilization of the entire patient with a semi-rigid cervical collar, head immobilization, backboard, tape, and straps before and during transfer to a definitive-care facility.

INTRAVENOUS FLUIDS

In patients in whom spine injury is suspected, intravenous fluids are administered as they would usually be for resuscitation of the trauma patient. If active hemorrhage is not detected or suspected, persistent hypotension despite the administration of 2 L or more of fluid should raise the suspicion of neurogenic shock. Patients with hypovolemic shock usually have tachycardia, whereas those with neurogenic shock classically have bradycardia. If the blood pressure does not improve after a fluid challenge, the judicious use of vasopressors may be indicated. Phenylephrine hydrochloride, dopamine, or norepinephrine is recommended. Overzealous fluid administration may cause pulmonary edema in patients with neurogenic shock. When the fluid status is uncertain, the use of invasive monitoring may be helpful. A urinary catheter is inserted to monitor urinary output and prevent bladder distention.

MEDICATIONS

At present, there is insufficient evidence to support the routine use of steroids in spinal cord injury.

PITFALL

Patients being transported to a trauma center may have unrecognized spinal injuries. These patients should be maintained in complete spinal immobilization.

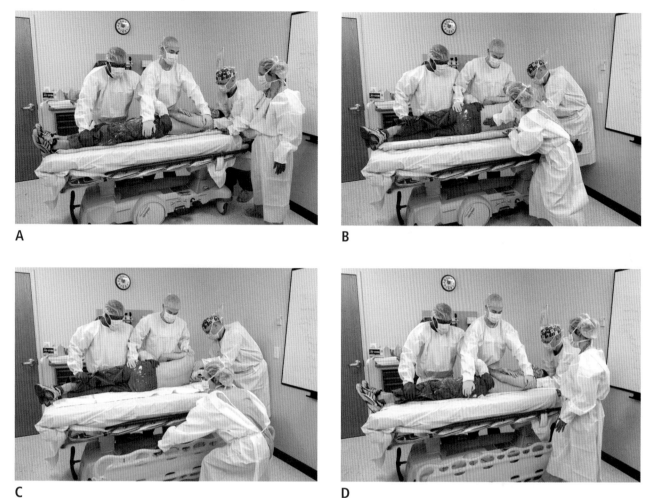

■ Figure 7-11 Four-Person Logroll. Logrolling a patient to remove a spine board and/or examine the back should be accomplished using four people. One person stands at the patient's head to control the head and c-spine, and two are along the patient's sides to control the body and extremities **(A)**. As the patient is rolled, these three people maintain alignment of the spine, while the fourth person removes the board and examines the back **(B** and **C)**. Once the board is removed, the patient is returned to the supine position, while maintaining alignment of the spine **(D)**.

TRANSFER

Patients with spine fractures or neurologic deficit should be transferred to a definitive-care facility. The safest procedure is to transfer the patient after telephone consultation with a spine specialist. Avoid unnecessary delay. Stabilize the patient's condition, and apply the necessary splints, backboard, and/or semirigid cervical collar. **Remember, cervical spine injuries above C6 can result in partial or total loss of respiratory function.** If there is any concern about the adequacy of ventilation, the patient should be intubated prior to transfer.

CHAPTER SUMMARY

1 The spinal column consists of cervical, thoracic and lumbar vertebrae. The spinal cord contains three important tracts: the corticospinal tract, the spinothalamic tract and the posterior columns.

2 Obtain lateral, AP, and open-mouth odontoid c-spine x-ray films, when indicated, as soon as life-threatening injuries are controlled. Document the patient's history and physical examination so as to establish a baseline for any changes in the patient's neurologic status.

3 Spinal cord injuries may be complete or incomplete and may involve any level of the spinal cord.

4 Attend to life-threatening injuries first, minimizing movement of the spinal column. Establish and maintain proper immobilization of the patient until vertebral fractures or spinal cord injuries have been excluded. Obtain early consultation with a neurosurgeon and/or orthopedic surgeon whenever a spinal injury is suspected or detected.

5 Transfer patients with vertebral fractures or spinal cord injuries to a definitive-care facility.

Bibliography

1. Bach CM, Steingruber IE, Peer S, Peer-Kuhberger R, Jaschke W, Ogon M. Radiographic evaluation of cervical spine trauma. Plain radiography and conventional tomography versus computed tomography. *Arch Orthop Trauma Surg* 2001; 121(7):385-387.

2. Bachulis BL, Long WI, Hynes GD, et al. Clinical indications for cervical spine radiographs in the traumatized patient. *Am J Surg* 1987;153:473-477.

3. Berne JD, Reuland KS, Villarreal DH, McGovern TM, Rowe SA, Norwood SH. Sixteen-slice multi-detector computed tomographic angiography improves the accuracy of screening for blunt cerebrovascular injury. *J Trauma* 2006;60(6):1204-1209; discussion 1209-1210.

4. Biffl WL, Egglin T, Benedetto B, Gibbs F, Cioffi WG. Sixteen-slice computed tomographic angiography is a reliable noninvasive screening test for clinically significant blunt cerebrovascular injuries. *J Trauma* 2006;60(4):745-751; discussion 751-752.

5. Bracken MB, Shepard MJ, Collins WF, et al. A randomized, controlled trial of methylprednisolone or naloxone in the treatment of spinal cord injury: results of the second National Spinal Cord Injury Study. *N Engl J Med* 1990;322:1405-1411.

6. Bracken MB, Shepard MJ, Holford TR, et al. Methylprednisolone or tirlazad mesylate administration after acute spinal cord injury: 1-year follow up: results of the third national Acute Spinal Cord Injury Randomized Controlled Trial. *J Neurosurg* 1998;89:699-706.

7. Brown CV, Antevil JL, Sise MJ, Sack DI. Spiral computed tomography for the diagnosis of cervical, thoracic, and lumbar spine fractures: its time has come. *J Trauma* 2005; 58(5):890-895; discussion 895-896.

8. Coleman WP, Benzel D, Cahill DW, et al. A critical appraisal of the reporting of the National Acute Spinal Cord Injury Studies (II and III) of methylprednisolone in acute spinal cord injury. *J Spinal Disord* 2000; 13(3):185-199.

9. Cooper C, Dunham CM, Rodriguez A. Falls and major injuries are risk factors for thoracolumbar fractures: cognitive impairment and multiple injuries impede the detection of back pain and tenderness. *J Trauma* 1995;38:692-696.

10. Cothren CC, Moore EE, Biffl WL, et al. Anticoagulation is the gold standard therapy for blunt carotid injuries to reduce stroke rate. *Arch Surg* 2004;139(5):540-545; discussion 545-546.

11. Cothren CC, Moore EE, Biffl WL, et al. Cervical spine fracture patterns predictive of blunt vertebral artery injury. *J Trauma* 2003;55(5):811-813.

12. Cothren CC, Moore EE, Ray CE, Johnson JL, Moore JB, Burch JM. Cervical spine fracture patterns mandating screening to rule out blunt cerebrovascular injury. *Surgery* 2007;141(1):76-82.

13. Daffner RH, Sciulli RL, Rodriguez A, Protetch J. Imaging for evaluation of suspected cervical spine trauma: a 2-year analysis. *Injury* 2006;37(7):652-658.

14. Dziurzynski K, Anderson PA, Bean DB, et al. A blinded assessment of radiographic criteria for atlanto-occipital dislocation. *Spine* 2005;30(12):1427-1432.

15. Eastman AL, Chason DP, Perez CL, McAnulty AL, Minei JP. Computed tomographic angiography for the diagnosis of blunt cervical vascular injury: is it ready for primetime? *J Trauma* 2006;60(5),:925-929; discussion 929.

16. Gale SC, Gracias VH, Reilly PM, Schwab CW. The inefficiency of plain radiography to evaluate the cervical spine after blunt trauma. *J Trauma* 2005;59(5):1121-1125.

17. Ghanta MK, Smith LM, Polin RS, Marr AB, Spires WV. An analysis of Eastern Association for the Surgery of Trauma practice guidelines for cervical spine evaluation in a series of patients with multiple imaging techniques. *Am Surg* 2002;68(6):563-567; discussion 567-568.

18. Grogan EL, Morris JA, Dittus RS, et al. Cervical spine evaluation in urban trauma centers: lowering institutional costs and complications through helical CT scan. *J Am Coll Surg* 2005;200(2):160-165.

19. Hadley MN, Fitzpatrick B, Browner C, et al. Facet fracture-dislocation injuries of the cervical spine. *J Neurosurgery* 1992;30:661-666.

20. Hall ED, Springer JE. Neuroprotection and acute spinal cord injury: a reappraisal. *NeuroRx* 2004;1(1):80-100.

21. Harris JH, Carson GC, Wagner LK, Kerr N. Radiologic diagnosis of traumatic occipitovertebral dissociation: 2. Comparison of three methods of detecting occipitovertebral relationships on lateral radiographs of supine subjects. *AJR Am J Roentgenol* 1994;162(4):887-892.

22. Holmes JF, Akkinepalli R. Computed tomography versus plain radiography to screen for cervical spine injury: a meta-analysis. *J Trauma* 2005;58(5):902-905.

23. Hugenholtz H, Cass DE, Dvorak MF, et al. High-dose methylprednisolone for acute closed spinal cord injury—only a treatment option. *Can J Neurol Sci* 2002;29(3): 227-235.

24. Hurlbert RJ. Methylprednisolone for acute spinal cord injury: an inappropriate standard of care. *J Neurosurg* 2000;93(1 Suppl):1-7.

25. Hurlbert RJ. Strategies of medical intervention in the management of acute spinal cord injury. *Spine* 2006;31(11 Suppl):S16-S21; discussion S36.

26. Hurlbert RJ. The role of steroids in acute spinal cord injury: an evidence-based analysis. *Spine* 2001;26(24 Suppl):S39-S46.

27. *International Standards for Neurological and Functional Classification of Spinal Cord Injury.* Atlanta, GA: American Spinal Injury Association and International Medical Society of Paraplegia (ASIA/IMSOP);1996.

28. Kronvall E, Sayer FT, Nilsson OG. [Methylprednisolone in the treatment of acute spinal cord injury has become more and more questioned]. *Lakartidningen* 2005;102(24-25):1887-1888, 1890.

29. Macdonald RL, Schwartz ML, Mirich D, et al. Diagnosis of cervical spine injury in motor vehicle crash victims: how many x-rays are enough? *J Trauma* 1990;30:392-397.

30. Marion DW, Pryzybylski G. Injury to the vertebrae and spinal cord. In: Mattox KL, Feliciano DV, Moore EE, eds. *Trauma.* New York, NY: McGraw-Hill; 2000:451-471.

31. McGuire RA, Neville S, Green BA, et al. Spine instability and the log-rolling maneuver. *J Trauma* 1987;27:525-531.

32. Michael DB, Guyot DR, Darmody WR. Coincidence of head and cervical spine injury. *J Neurotrauma* 1989;6:177-189.

33. Mower WR, Hoffman JR, Pollack CV, Zucker MI, Browne BJ, Wolfson AB. Use of plain radiography to screen for cervical spine injuries. *Ann Emerg Med* 2001;38(1):1-7.

34. Nesathurai S. Steroids and spinal cord injury: revisiting the NASCIS 2 and NASCIS 3 trials. *J Trauma* 1998;45(6):1088-1093.

35. Pasquale M, Marion DW, Domeier R, et al. Practice management guidelines for trauma: identifying cervical spine instability after trauma. *J Trauma* 1998;44:945-946.

36. Sanchez B, Waxman K, Jones T, Conner S, Chung R, Becerra S. Cervical spine clearance in blunt trauma: evaluation of a computed tomography-based protocol. *J Trauma* 2005;59(1):179-183.

37. Sayer FT, Kronvall E, Nilsson OG. Methylprednisolone treatment in acute spinal cord injury: the myth challenged through a structured analysis of published literature. *Spine J* 2006;6(3):335-343.

38. Schenarts PJ, Diaz J, Kaiser C, Carrillo Y, Eddy V, Morris JA. Prospective comparison of admission computed tomographic scan and plain films of the upper cervical spine in trauma patients with altered mental status. *J Trauma* 2001;51(4):663-668; discussion 668-669.

39. Short D. Is the role of steroids in acute spinal cord injury now resolved? *Curr Opin Neurol* 2001;14(6):759-763.

40. Short DJ, El MWS, Jones PW. High dose methylprednisolone in the management of acute spinal cord injury - a systematic review from a clinical perspective. *Spinal Cord* 2000;38(5):273-286.

41. Tator CH, Fehlings MG. Review of the secondary injury theory of acute spinal cord trauma with special emphasis on vascular mechanisms. *J Neurosurg* 1991;75:15-26.

42. Widder S, Doig C, Burrowes P, Larsen G, Hurlbert RJ, Kortbeek JB. Prospective evaluation of computed tomographic scanning for the spinal clearance of obtunded trauma patients: preliminary results. *J Trauma* 2004;56(6):1179-1184.

X-Ray Identification of Spine Injuries

▶▶ Interactive Skill Procedure

THE FOLLOWING PROCEDURES ARE INCLUDED IN THIS SKILL STATION:

▶▶ **Skill X-A:** Cervical Spine X-Ray Assessment

▶▶ **Skill X-B:** Atlanto-Occipital Joint Assessment

▶▶ **Skill X-C:** Thoracic and Lumbar X-Ray Assessment

▶▶ **Skill X-D:** Review Spine X-Rays

Performance at this skill station will allow the participant to:

OBJECTIVES

1 Identify various spine injuries by using specific anatomic guidelines for examining a series of spine x-rays.

2 Given a series of spine x-rays and scenarios,

Define limitations of examination.
Diagnose fractures.
Delineate associated injuries.
Define other areas of possible injury.

▶ Skill X-A: Cervical Spine X-Ray Assessment
(See Figures X-1, X-2, and X-3)

STEP 1. Assess adequacy and alignment (Figure X-1).
   A. Identify the presence of all 7 cervical vertebrae and the superior aspect of T1.
   B. Identify the:
   - Anterior vertebral line (Fig. X-1, line A)
   - Anterior spinal line (Fig. X-1, line B)
   - Posterior spinal line (Fig. X-1, line C)
   - Spinous processes (Fig. X-1, line D)

STEP 2. Assess the bone (Figure X-2).
   A. Examine all vertebrae for preservation of height and integrity of the bony cortex.
   B. Examine facets.
   C. Examine spinous processes.

STEP 3. Assess the cartilage, including examining the cartilaginous disk spaces for narrowing or widening (see Figure X-2).

STEP 4. Assess the dens (Figure X-3).
   A. Examine the outline of the dens.
   B. Examine the predental space (3 mm).
   C. Examine the clivus; it should point to the dens.

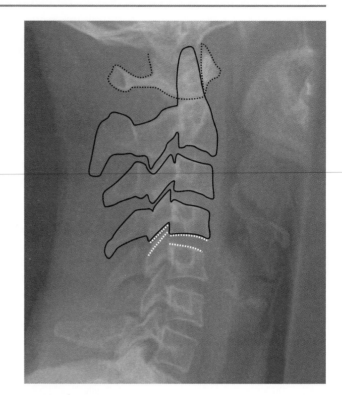

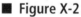

■ Figure X-2

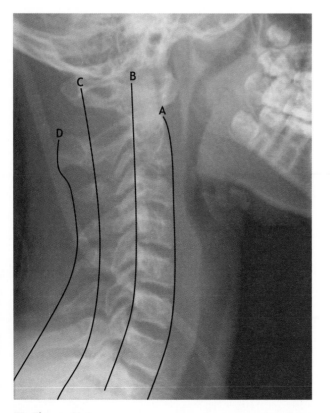

■ Figure X-1

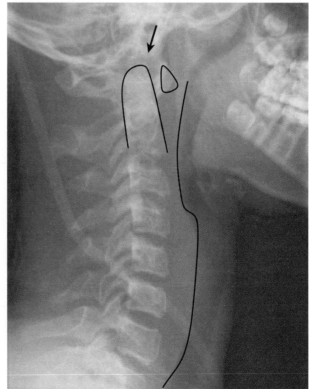

■ Figure X-3

STEP 5. Assess the extraaxial soft tissues.
    A. Examine the extraaxial space and soft tissues
- 7 mm at C3
- 3 cm at C7

B. Examine the distances between the spinous processes.

▶ Skill X-B: Atlanto-Occipital Joint Assessment
(See Figures X-4 and X-5)

Detection of an atlanto-occipital dislocation can be challenging. Two useful findings include a Power's ratio >1 (BC/OA, where BC is the distance from the basion [B] to the posterior arch [C] of C1 and OA is the distance from the anterior arch of C1 [A] to the opisthion [O-the posterior margin of the foramen magnum]). Wackenheim's line runs along the posterior clivus and passes tangentially to the posterior tip of the dens. If an atlanto-occipital injury is suspected, spinal immobilization should be preserved, and expert radiologic interpretation should be obtained.

NORMAL

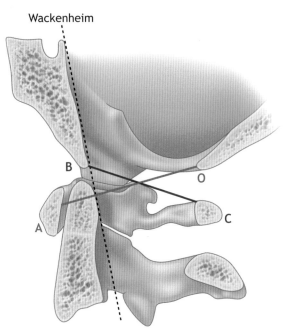

BC/AO (Power's ratio) ≤ 1

C0-C1 INSTABILITY

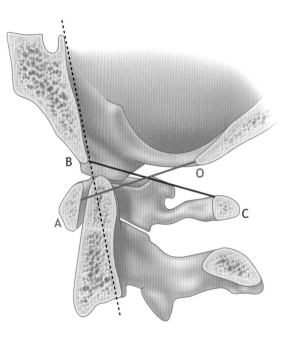

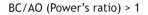

BC/AO (Power's ratio) > 1

■ **Figure X-4**

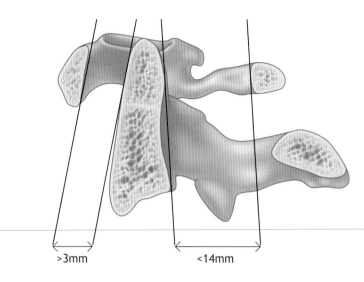

>3mm   <14mm

■ **Figure X-5**

▶ Skill X-C: Thoracic and Lumbar X-Ray Assessment

▶▶ ANTEROPOSTERIOR VIEW

STEP 1. Assess for:
  A. Alignment
  B. Symmetry of pedicles
  C. Contour of bodies
  D. Height of disk spaces
  E. Central position of spinous processes

▶▶ LATERAL VIEW

STEP 2. Assess for:
  A. Alignment of bodies/angulation of spine
  B. Contour of bodies
  C. Presence of disk spaces
  D. Encroachment of body on canal

▶ Skill X-D: Review Spine X-Rays

Instructor will display a series of films to be interpreted and discussed with students.

▶ SPINE X-RAY SCENARIOS

PATIENT X-1

28-year-old male fell while mountain biking. No neurologic deficit.

PATIENT X-2

54-year-old male hit a tree while driving his car. Symptoms are only slight discomfort of his neck and some numbness in his digit V, left side.

PATIENT X-3

8-year-old child fell down the stairs and is crying. No neurologic deficit.

PATIENT X-4

62-year-old male hit an abutment while driving his car. There is no neurologic deficit, but patient is unable to actively move his neck because of pain.

PATIENT X-5

19-year-old female with head and neck trauma as the result of an assault.

PATIENT X-6

22-year-old male struck a tree while riding his motorcycle. No neurologic deficit.

PATIENT X-7

Box fell on head. Painful neck, no neurologic deficit.

PATIENT X-8

45-year-old woman attempted to hang herself. GCS score of 7.

PATIENT X-9

30-year-old male in motor vehicle crash versus tree. Patient was restrained, but there was no airbag. GCS score of 15; neurologic exam intact; patient reports neck pain.

PATIENT X-10

36-year-old male fell from a height greater than 3 meters and has back pain.

PATIENT X-11

30-year-old male involved in motorcycle crash. On examination, he appears to have a sensory and motor deficit involving both legs. Deep-tendon reflexes are absent.

PATIENT X-12

25-year-old female involved in motor vehicle crash. Patient was wearing a lap belt without shoulder harness. No neurologic deficit.

Spinal Cord Injury:
Assessment and Management

▶▶ Interactive Skill Procedure

Note: Standard precautions are required when caring for trauma patients. This Skill Station includes scenarios and related x-rays for use in making evaluation and management decisions based on the findings.

THE FOLLOWING PROCEDURES ARE INCLUDED IN THIS SKILL STATION:

▶▶ **Skill XI-A:** Primary Survey and Resuscitation—Assessing Spine Injuries

▶▶ **Skill XI-B:** Secondary Survey—Neurologic Assessment

▶▶ **Skill XI-C:** Examination for Level of Spinal Cord Injury

▶▶ **Skill XI-D:** Treatment Principles for Patients with Spinal Cord Injuries

▶▶ **Skill XI-E:** Principles of Spine Immobilization and Logrolling

Performance at this skill station will allow the participant to:

OBJECTIVES

1 Demonstrate the examination of a patient in whom spine and/or spinal cord injuries are suspected.

2 Explain the principles for immobilizing and logrolling patients with neck and/or spinal injuries, including the indications for removing protective devices.

3 Perform a neurologic examination and determine the level of spinal cord injury.

4 Determine the need for neurosurgical consultation.

5 Determine the need for interhospital or intrahospital transfer, and describe how the patient should be properly immobilized for transfer.

▶ Skill XI-A: Primary Survey and Resuscitation—Assessing Spine Injuries

Note: The patient should be maintained in a supine, neutral position using proper immobilization techniques.

STEP 1. Airway :
  A. Assess the airway while protecting the cervical spine.
  B. Establish a definitive airway as needed.

STEP 2. Breathing: Assess and provide adequate oxygenation and ventilatory support as needed.

STEP 3. Circulation:
  A. If the patient has hypotension, differentiate hypovolemic shock (decreased blood pressure, increased heart rate, and cool extremities) from neurogenic shock (decreased blood pressure, decreased heart rate, and warm extremities).

  B. Replace fluids for hypovolemia.
  C. If spinal cord injury is present, fluid resuscitation should be guided by monitoring central venous pressure (CVP). (*Note:* Some patients may need inotropic support.)
  D. When performing a rectal examination before inserting the urinary catheter, assess for rectal sphincter tone and sensation.

STEP 4. Disability—Brief Neurologic Examination:
  A. Determine level of consciousness and assess pupils.
  B. Determine Glasgow Coma Scale (GCS) score.
  C. Recognize paralysis/paresis.

▶ Skill XI-B: Secondary Survey—Neurologic Assessment

STEP 1. Obtain AMPLE History
  A. History and mechanism of injury
  B. Medical history
  C. Identify and record drugs given prior to patient's arrival and during assessment and management phases

STEP 2. Reassess level of consciousness and pupils.

STEP 3. Reassess GCS score.

STEP 4. Assess the spine (See Skill XI-C: Examination for Level of Spinal Cord Injury)
  A. Palpate the entire spine posteriorly by carefully logrolling the patient and assessing for:
    • Deformity and/or swelling
    • Grating crepitus
    • Increased pain with palpation

    • Contusions and lacerations/penetrating wounds
  B. Assess for pain, paralysis, and paresthesia:
    • Presence/absence
    • Location
    • Neurologic level
  C. Test sensation to pinprick in all dermatomes and record the most caudal dermatome that feels the pinprick.
  D. Assess motor function.
  E. Measure deep tendon reflexes (least informative in the emergency setting).
  F. Document and repeat—record the results of the neurologic examination and repeat motor and sensory examinations regularly until consultation is obtained.

STEP 5. Reevaluate—Assess for associated/occult injuries.

▶ Skill XI-C: Examination for Level of Spinal Cord Injury

A patient with a spinal cord injury may have varying levels of neurologic deficit. The level of motor function and sensation must be reassessed frequently and carefully documented, because changes in the level of function can occur.

STEP 1. Best Motor Examination
  A. Determining the level of quadriplegia, nerve root level:

    • Raises elbow to level of shoulder—deltoid, C5
    • Flexes forearm—biceps, C6
    • Extends forearm—triceps, C7
    • Flexes wrist and fingers, C8
    • Spreads fingers, T1
  B. Determining the level of paraplegia, nerve root level:

- Flexes hip—iliopsoas, L2
- Extends knee—quadriceps, L3-L4
- Flexes knee—hamstrings, L4-L5 to S1
- Dorsiflexes big toe—extensor hallucis longus, L5
- Plantar flexes ankle—gastrocnemius, S1

STEP 2. Sensory Examination: Determining the level of sensation is done primarily by assessing the dermatomes. ▪ See Figure 7-3 in Chapter 7:

Spine and Spinal Cord Trauma. Remember, the cervical sensory dermatomes of C2 through C4 form a cervical cape or mantle that can extend down as far as the nipples. Because of this unusual pattern, the examiner should not depend on the presence or absence of sensation in the neck and clavicular area, and the level of sensation must be correlated with the motor response level.

▶ Skill XI-D: Treatment Principles for Patients with Spinal Cord Injuries

STEP 1. Patients with suspected spine injury must be protected from further injury. Such protection includes applying a semirigid cervical collar and long back board, performing a modified logroll to ensure neutral alignment of the entire spine, and removing the patient from the long spine board as soon as possible. Paralyzed patients who are immobilized on a long spine board are at particular risk for pressure points and decubitus ulcers. Therefore, paralyzed patients should be removed from the long spine board as soon as possible after a spine injury is diagnosed, ie, within 2 hours.

STEP 2. Fluid Resuscitation and Monitoring:
  A. CVP monitoring: Intravenous fluids usually are limited to maintenance levels unless

specifically needed for the management of shock. A central venous catheter should be inserted to carefully monitor fluid administration.
  B. Urinary catheter: A urinary catheter should be inserted during the primary survey and resuscitation phases to monitor urinary output and prevent bladder distention.
  C. Gastric catheter: A gastric catheter should be inserted in all patients with paraplegia and quadriplegia to prevent gastric distention and aspiration.

▶ Skill XI-E: Principles of Spine Immobilization and Logrolling

▶▶ ADULT PATIENT

Four people are needed to perform the modified logrolling procedure and to immobilize the patient—for example, on a long spine board: one person to maintain manual, in-line immobilization of the patient's head and neck; one for the torso (including the pelvis and hips); one for the pelvis and legs; and one to direct the procedure and move the spine board. This procedure maintains the patient's entire body in neutral alignment, thereby minimizing any untoward movement of the spine. This procedure assumes that any extremity suspected of being fractured has already been immobilized.

STEP 1. Place the long spine board with straps next to the patient's side. Position the straps for fastening later across the patient's thorax, just above the iliac crests, across the thighs, and just above the ankles. Straps or tape can be used to secure the patient's head and neck to the long board.

STEP 2. Apply gentle, in-line manual immobilization to the patient's head and apply a semirigid cervical collar.

STEP 3. Gently straighten and place the patient's arms (palm in) next to the torso.

STEP 4. Carefully straighten the patient's legs and place them in neutral alignment with the patient's spine. Tie the ankles together with a roller-type dressing or cravat.

STEP 5. While maintaining alignment of the patient's head and neck, another person reaches across and grasps the patient at the shoulder and wrist. A third person reaches across and grasps the patient's hip just distal to the wrist with one hand and with the other hand firmly grasps the roller bandage or cravat that is securing the ankles together.

STEP 6. At the direction of the person who is maintaining immobilization of the patient's head and neck, cautiously logroll the patient as a unit toward the two assistants at the patient's side, but only to the least degree necessary to position the board under the patient. Maintain neutral alignment of the entire body during this procedure.

STEP 7. Place the spine board beneath the patient and carefully logroll the patient in one smooth movement onto the spine board. The spine board is used only for transferring the patient and should not be left under the patient for any length of time.

STEP 8. Consider padding under the patient's head to avoid hyperextension of the neck and for patient comfort.

STEP 9. Place padding, rolled blankets, or similar bolstering devices on both sides of the patient's head and neck, and firmly secure the patient's head to the board. Tape the cervical collar, further securing the patient's head and neck to the long board.

▶▶ PEDIATRIC PATIENT

A pediatric-sized long spine board is preferable when immobilizing a small child. If only an adult-sized board is available, place blanket rolls along the entire sides of the child to prevent lateral movement. A child's head is proportionately larger than an adult's. Therefore, padding should be placed under the shoulders to elevate the torso so that the large occiput of the child's head does not produce flexion of the cervical spine; this maintains neutral alignment of the child's spine. Such padding extends from the child's lumbar spine to the top of the shoulders and laterally to the edges of the board.

▶▶ COMPLICATIONS

If left immobilized for any length of time (approximately 2 hours or longer) on the long spine board, pressure sores may develop at the occiput, scapulae, sacrum, and heels. Therefore, padding should be applied under these areas as soon as possible, and the patient should be removed from the long spine board as soon as his or her condition permits.

▶▶ REMOVAL FROM A LONG SPINE BOARD

Movement of a patient with an unstable vertebral spine injury can cause or worsen a spinal cord injury. To reduce the risk of spinal cord damage, mechanical protection is necessary for all patients at risk. Such protection should be maintained until an unstable spine injury has been excluded.

STEP 1. As previously described, properly secure the patient to a long spine board, which is the basic technique for splinting the spine. In general, this is done in the prehospital setting, and the patient arrives at the hospital already immobilized. The long spine board provides an effective splint and permits safe transfers of the patient with a minimal number of assistants. However, unpadded spine boards can soon become uncomfortable for conscious patients and pose a significant risk for pressure sores on posterior bony prominences (occiput, scapulae, sacrum, and heels). Therefore, the patient should be transferred from the spine board to a firm, well-padded gurney or equivalent surface as soon as it can be done safely. Before removing the patient from the spine board, c-spine, chest, and pelvis x-ray films should be obtained as indicated, because the patient can be easily lifted and the x-ray plates placed beneath the spine board. While the patient is immobilized on the spine board, it is very important to maintain immobilization of the head and the body continuously. The straps used to immobilize the patient on the board should not be removed from the body while the head remains taped to the upper portion of the spine board.

STEP 2. Remove the patient from the spine board as early as possible. Preplanning is required. A good time to remove the board from under the patient is when the patient is logrolled to evaluate the back.

STEP 3. Safe movement of a patient with an unstable or potentially unstable spine requires continuous maintenance of anatomic alignment of the vertebral column. Rotation, flexion, extension, lateral bending, and shearing-type movements in any direction must be avoided. Manual, in-line immobilization best controls the head and neck. No part of the patient's body should be allowed to sag as the patient is lifted off the supporting surface. The transfer options listed below may be used, depending on available personnel and equipment resources.

STEP 4. Modified Logroll Technique: The modified logroll technique, previously outlined, is reversed to remove the patient from the long spine board. Four assistants are required: one to maintain manual, in-line immobilization of the patient's head and neck; one for the torso (including the pelvis and hips); one for the pelvis and legs; and one to direct the procedure and remove the spine board.

STEP 5. Scoop Stretcher: The scoop stretcher is an alternative to using the modified logrolling techniques for patient transfer. The proper use of this device can provide rapid, safe transfer of the patient from the long spine board onto a firm, padded patient gurney. For example, this device can be used to transfer the patient from one transport device to another or to a designated place, eg, x-ray table.

The patient must remain securely immobilized until a spine injury is excluded. After the patient is transferred from the backboard to the gurney (stretcher) and the scoop stretcher is removed, the patient must again be immobilized securely on the gurney (stretcher). The scoop stretcher is *not* a device on which the patient is immobilized. In addition, the scoop stretcher is not used to transport the patient, nor should the patient be transferred to the gurney by picking up only the foot and head ends of the scoop stretcher. Without firm support under the stretcher, it can sag in the middle and result in loss of neutral alignment of the spine.

▶▶ IMMOBILIZATION OF THE PATIENT WITH POSSIBLE SPINE INJURY

Patients frequently arrive in the ED with spinal protective devices in place. These devices should cause the examiner to suspect that a c-spine and/or thoracolumbar spine injury may exist, based on mechanism of injury. In patients with multiple injuries with a diminished level of consciousness, protective devices should be left in place until a spine injury is excluded by clinical and x-ray examinations. ▪ See Chapter 7: Spine and Spinal Cord Trauma. If a patient is immobilized on a spine board and is paraplegic, spinal instability should be presumed and all appropriate x-ray films obtained to determine the site of spinal injury. However, if the patient is awake, alert, sober, neurologically normal; is not experiencing neck or back pain; and does not have tenderness to spine palpation, spine x-ray examination and immobilization devices are not needed.

Patients who sustain multiple injuries and are comatose should be kept immobilized on a padded gurney (stretcher) and logrolled to obtain the necessary x-ray films to exclude a fracture. Then, using one of the aforementioned procedures, they can be transferred carefully to a bed for better ventilatory support.

▶ SCENARIOS

SCENARIO XI-1

A 15-year-old boy is riding his bicycle through a parking lot. He is distracted and hits a car at low speed when it backs out of a parking space. He is thrown from his bicycle across the trunk of the car and sustains a mild abrasion and an angled deformity of the left wrist. He is brought to the ED immobilized on a long spine board and with a semirigid cervical collar in place. He is alert and cooperative and has no hemodynamic abnormalities.

SCENARIO XI-2

A 75-year-old male is walking to the store when he trips and falls forward, striking his chin on a parked car. He is transported to the ED immobilized on a long spine board with a semirigid cervical collar applied. He has an abrasion on his chin and is alert and appropriately responsive. Physical examination reveals paralysis of his hands, with very little finger motion. He has some upper-extremity movement (grade 2/5), but is clearly weak bilaterally. Examination of the lower extremities reveals weakness, but he is able to flex and extend both his legs at the hip and knee. He has various areas of hypesthesia over his body.

SCENARIO XI-3

A 25-year-old male passenger sustains multiple injuries in a car collision. The driver died at the scene of the injury. The patient is transported to the ED immobilized on a long spine board with a semirigid cervical collar applied. Oxygen is being administered, and administration of warmed crystalloid fluids with two large-caliber intravenous lines is initiated. His blood pressure is 85/40 mm Hg, his heart rate 130 beats/min, and his respiratory rate 40 breaths/min. His respirations are shallow, and there is a contusion over the chest wall. His eyes are open, and his verbal response is appropriate. He is able to shrug his shoulders, but is unable to raise his elbow to the shoulder level or move his legs.

SCENARIO XI-4

This scenario is essentially the same as Scenario XI-3, but the instructor will make changes in the patient's neurologic status as the student examines the patient.

A 25-year-old passenger sustains multiple injuries in a car collision. The driver died at the scene of the injury. The passenger is transported to the ED immobilized on a long spine board with a semirigid cervical collar applied. Oxygen is being administered, administration of warmed crystalloid fluids with two large-caliber intravenous lines is initiated.

SCENARIO XI-5

A 6-year-old boy fell off his bicycle and hit the back of his head. In the ED, his head and neck are in a flexed position, and he reports pain in his neck. He is immobilized on an unpadded long spine board without a cervical collar.

CHAPTER 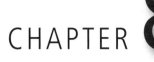 Musculoskeletal
Trauma

CHAPTER OUTLINE

Introduction

Primary Survey and Resuscitation

Adjuncts to Primary Survey
Fracture Immobilization
X-Ray Examination

Secondary Survey
History
Physical Examination

Potentially Life-Threatening Extremity Injuries
Major Pelvic Disruption with Hemorrhage
Major Arterial Hemorrhage
Crush Syndrome (Traumatic Rhabdomyolysis)

Limb-Threatening Injuries
Open Fractures and Joint Injuries
Vascular Injuries, Including Traumatic Amputation
Compartment Syndrome
Neurologic Injury Secondary to Fracture-Dislocation

Other Extremity Injuries
Contusions and Lacerations
Joint Injuries
Fractures

Principles of Immobilization
Femoral Fractures
Knee Injuries
Tibia Fractures
Ankle Fractures
Upper-Extremity and Hand Injuries

Pain Control

Associated Injuries

Occult Skeletal Injuries

Chapter Summary

Bibliography

Upon completion of this topic, the student will be able to initially assess and manage patients with life-threatening and limb-threatening musculoskeletal injuries. Specifically, the doctor will be able to:

OBJECTIVES

1 Explain the significance of musculoskeletal injuries in patients with multiple injuries.

2 Outline priorities in the assessment of musculoskeletal trauma to identify life-threatening and limb-threatening injuries.

3 Explain the proper principles of initial management for musculoskeletal injuries.

Introduction

Injuries to the musculoskeletal system occur in 85% of patients who sustain blunt trauma; they often appear dramatic, but rarely cause an immediate threat to life or limb. However, musculoskeletal injuries must be assessed and managed properly and appropriately so life and limb are not jeopardized. The doctor must recognize the presence of such injuries, be familiar with the anatomy of the injury, protect the patient from further disability, and anticipate and prevent complications.

Major musculoskeletal injuries indicate that significant forces were sustained by the body. For example, a patient with long-bone fractures above and below the diaphragm has an increased likelihood of associated internal torso injuries. Unstable pelvic fractures and open femur fractures may be accompanied by brisk bleeding. Severe crush injuries cause the release of myoglobin, which may precipitate in the renal tubules and result in renal failure. Swelling into an intact musculofascial space may cause an acute compartment syndrome that, if not diagnosed and treated, may lead to lasting impairment and loss of use of the extremities. Fat embolism, an uncommon but highly lethal complication of long-bone fractures, may lead to pulmonary failure and impaired cerebral function.

Musculoskeletal trauma does not warrant a reordering of the priorities of resuscitation (ABCDEs). However, the presence of significant musculoskeletal trauma does pose a challenge to the treating doctor. Musculoskeletal injuries cannot be ignored and treated at a later time. The doctor must treat the whole patient, including musculoskeletal injuries, to ensure an optimal outcome. Despite careful assessment and management of multiple injuries, fractures and soft tissue injuries may not be initially recognized. **Continued reevaluation of the patient is necessary to identify all injuries.**

Primary Survey and Resuscitation

❓ *What impact do musculoskeletal injuries have on the primary survey?*

During the primary survey, it is imperative to recognize and control hemorrhage from musculoskeletal injuries. Deep soft tissue lacerations may involve major vessels and lead to exsanguinating hemorrhage. Hemorrhage control is best effected by direct pressure.

Hemorrhage from long-bone fractures may be significant, and certain femoral fractures may result in up to 4 units of blood loss into the thigh, producing class III shock. Appropriate splinting of the fracture may significantly decrease bleeding by reducing motion and enhancing a tamponade effect of the muscle. If the fracture is open,

> **PITFALL**
>
> Musculoskeletal injuries are a potential source of occult blood loss in patients with hemodynamic abnormalities. Occult sites of hemorrhage are the retroperitoneum from unstable pelvic ring injuries, the thigh from femoral fractures, and any open fracture with major soft tissue involvement in which blood loss may be serious and occurs before the patient reaches the hospital.

application of a sterile pressure dressing usually controls hemorrhage. Aggressive fluid resuscitation is an important supplement to these mechanical measures.

Adjuncts to Primary Survey

Adjuncts to the primary survey of patients with musculoskeletal trauma include fracture immobilization and x-ray examination.

FRACTURE IMMOBILIZATION

The goal of initial fracture immobilization is to realign the injured extremity in as close to anatomic position as possible and to prevent excessive fracture-site motion. This realignment is accomplished by the application of in-line traction to realign the extremity and maintained by an immobilization device. The proper application of a splint helps control blood loss, reduce pain, and prevent further soft tissue injury. If an open fracture is present, the doctor need not be concerned about pulling exposed bone back into the wound because all open fractures require surgical debridement. ■ See Skill Station XII: Musculoskeletal Trauma: As-

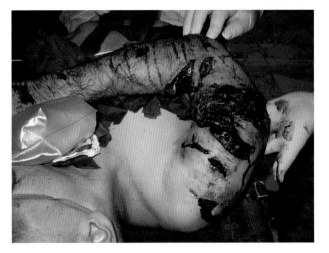

Major musculoskeletal injuries indicate that significant forces were sustained by the body.

sessment and Management, Skill XII-C: Realigning a Deformed Extremity.

Joint dislocations usually require splinting in the position in which they are found. If a closed reduction has successfully relocated the joint, immobilization in an anatomic position may be accomplished in a number of ways: prefabricated splints, pillows, or plaster. These devices will maintain the extremity in its unreduced position.

Splints should be applied as soon as possible, but they must not take precedence over resuscitation. However, splints may be very helpful during this phase to control hemorrhage and pain.

X-RAY EXAMINATION

X-ray examination of most skeletal injuries occurs as the part of the secondary survey. Which x-ray films to obtain and when to obtain them are determined by the patient's initial and obvious clinical findings, the patient's hemodynamic status, and the mechanism of injury. An anteroposterior (AP) view of the pelvis should be obtained early for all patients with multiple injuries for whom a source of bleeding has not been identified.

Secondary Survey

Elements of the secondary survey of patients with musculoskeletal injuries are the history and physical examination.

HISTORY

Key aspects of the patient history are mechanism of injury, environment, preinjury status and predisposing factors, and prehospital observations and care.

Mechanism of Injury

Information obtained from the transport personnel, the patient, relatives, and bystanders at the scene of the injury should be documented and included as a part of the patient's medical record. It is particularly important to determine the mechanism of injury, which may arouse suspicion of injuries that may not be immediately apparent. ▪ See Appendix B: Biomechanics of Injury. The doctor should mentally reconstruct the injury scene, identify other potential injuries that the patient may have sustained, and determine as much of the following information as possible:

1. In a motor vehicle crash, what was the precrash location of the patient in the vehicle—driver or passenger? This fact can indicate the type of fracture—for example, lateral compression fracture of the pelvis resulting from a side impact in a vehicle collision.

2. What was the postcrash location of the patient—inside the vehicle or ejected? Was a seat belt or airbag in use? This information may indicate patterns of injury. If the patient was ejected, determine the distance the patient was thrown and the landing conditions. Ejection generally results in increased injury severity and unpredictable patterns of injury.

3. Was there external damage to the vehicle—for example, deformation to the front of the vehicle from a head-on collision? This information raises the suspicion of a hip dislocation.

4. Was there internal damage to the vehicle—for example, bent steering wheel, deformation to the dashboard, or damage to the windscreen? These findings indicate a greater likelihood of sternal, clavicular, or spinal fractures or hip dislocation.

5. Was the patient wearing a restraint? If so, what type (lap or three-point safety belt)? Was the restraint applied properly? Faulty application of safety restraints may cause spinal fractures and associated intraabdominal visceral injuries. Was an air bag deployed?

6. Did the patient fall? If so, what was the distance of the fall, and how did the patient land? This information helps identify the spectrum of injuries. Landing on the feet may cause foot and ankle injuries with associated spinal fractures.

7. Was the patient crushed by an object? If so, identify the weight of the crushing object, the site of the injury, and duration of weight applied to the site. Depending on whether a subcutaneous bony surface or a muscular area was crushed, different degrees of soft tissue damage may occur, ranging from a simple contusion to a severe degloving extremity injury with compartment syndrome and tissue loss.

8. Did an explosion occur? If so, what was the magnitude of the blast and what was the patient's distance from the blast? An individual close to the explosion may sustain primary blast injury from the force of the blast wave. A secondary blast injury may occur from debris and other objects accelerated by the blast effect (eg, fragments), leading to penetrating wounds, lacerations, and contusions. The patient also may be violently thrown to the ground or against other objects by the blast effect, leading to blunt musculoskeletal and other injuries (tertiary blast effect).

9. Was the patient involved in a vehicle-pedestrian collision? Musculoskeletal injuries may follow predicted patterns (eg, bumper injury to leg) based on the size and age of the patient.

Environment

Ask prehospital care personnel for information about the environment, including:

- Patient exposure to temperature extremes

- Patient exposure to toxic fumes or agents

- Broken glass fragments (which may also injure the examiner)

- Sources of bacterial contamination (eg, dirt, animal feces, fresh or salt water)

This information can help the doctor anticipate potential problems and determine the initial antibiotic treatment.

Preinjury Status and Predisposing Factors

It is important to determine the patient's baseline condition prior to injury, because this information may alter the understanding of the patient's condition, treatment regimen, and outcome. The AMPLE history also should include information about the patient's exercise tolerance and activity level, ingestion of alcohol and/or other drugs, emotional problems or illnesses, and previous musculoskeletal injuries.

Prehospital Observations and Care

Findings at the incident site that may help the doctor identify potential injuries include:

- Position in which the patient was found

- Bleeding or pooling of blood at the scene, including the estimated amount

- Bone or fracture ends that may have been exposed

- Open wounds in proximity to obvious or suspected fractures

- Obvious deformity or dislocation

- Presence or absence of motor and/or sensory function in each extremity

- Delays in extrication procedures or transport

- Changes in limb function, perfusion, or neurologic state, especially after immobilization or during transfer to the hospital

- Reduction of fractures or dislocations during extrication or splinting at the scene

- Dressings and splints applied, with special attention to excessive pressure over bony prominences that may result in peripheral nerve compression injuries, compartment syndromes, or crush syndromes.

The time of the injury also should be noted, especially if there is ongoing bleeding and delay in reaching the hos-

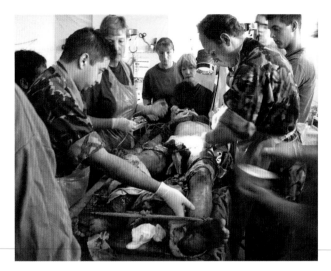

The patient must be completely exposed for adequate assessment.

pital. All prehospital observations and care must be reported and documented.

PHYSICAL EXAMINATION

The patient must be completely undressed for adequate examination. Obvious extremity injuries are often splinted prior to the patient's arrival in the emergency department (ED). There are three goals for the assessment of trauma patients' extremities:

1. Identification of life-threatening injury (primary survey)

2. Identification of limb-threatening injuries (secondary survey)

3. Systematic review to avoid missing any other musculoskeletal injury (continuous reevaluation)

Assessment of musculoskeletal trauma may be achieved by looking at and talking to the patient, as well as by palpation of the patient's extremities and performance of a logical, systematic review of each extremity. The four components that must be assessed are: (1) skin, which protects the patient from excessive fluid loss and infection; (2) neuromuscular function; (3) circulatory status; and (4) skeletal and ligamentous integrity. Using this evaluation process reduces the risk of missing an injury. See Skill Station XII: Musculoskeletal Trauma: Assessment and Management, Skill XII-A: Physical Examination.

Look and Ask

Visually assess the extremities for color and perfusion, wounds, deformity (angulation, shortening), swelling, and discoloration or bruising.

A rapid visual inspection of the entire patient is necessary to identify sites of major external bleeding. A pale or white distal extremity is indicative of a lack of arterial in-flow. Extremities that are swollen in the region of major muscle groups may indicate a crush injury with an impending compartment syndrome. Swelling or ecchymosis in or around a joint and/or over the subcutaneous surface of a bone is a sign of a musculoskeletal injury. Extremity deformity is an obvious sign of major extremity injury (see Table 8-1).

Inspect the patient's entire body for lacerations and abrasions. Open wounds are obvious unless they are located on the dorsum of the body. The patient must be carefully logrolled to assess for an injury or skin laceration. If a bone protrudes or is visualized in the wound, an open fracture exists. Any open wound to a limb with an associated fracture also is considered an open fracture until proven otherwise by a surgeon.

Observe the patient's spontaneous extremity motor function to help identify any neurologic and/or muscular impairment. If the patient is unconscious, absent spontaneous extremity movement may be the only sign of impaired function. With a cooperative patient, active voluntary muscle and peripheral nerve function may be assessed by asking the patient to contract major muscle groups. The ability to move all major joints through a full range of motion usually indicates that the nerve-muscle unit is intact and the joint is stable.

Feel

Palpate the extremities to determine sensation to the skin (neurologic function) and identify areas of tenderness (fracture or deep muscle injury). Loss of sensation to pain and touch demonstrates the presence of a spinal or peripheral nerve injury. Areas of tenderness or pain over muscles may indicate a muscle contusion or fracture. Pain, tenderness, swelling, and deformity over a subcutaneous bony surface usually confirm the diagnosis of a fracture. If pain or tenderness is associated with painful abnormal motion through the bone, fracture is diagnosed. However, attempts to elicit crepitation or demonstrate abnormal motion are not recommended.

At the time of logrolling, palpate the patient's back to identify any lacerations, palpable gaps between the spinous processes, hematomas, or defects in the posterior pelvic region that are indicative of unstable axial skeletal injuries.

Closed soft tissue injuries are more difficult to evaluate. Soft tissue avulsion may shear the skin from the deep fascia, allowing for significant accumulation of blood. Alternatively, the skin may be sheared from its blood supply and undergo necrosis over a few days. This area may have local abrasions or bruised skin that are clues to a more severe degree of muscle damage and potential compartment or crush syndromes. These soft tissue injuries are best evaluated by knowing the mechanism of injury and palpating the specific component involved.

Joint stability may be determined only by clinical examination. Abnormal motion through a joint segment is indicative of a ligamentous rupture. Palpate the joint to identify any swelling and tenderness of the ligaments as well as intraarticular fluid. Following this, cautious stressing of the specific ligaments can be performed. Excessive pain may mask abnormal ligament motion because of guarding of the joint by muscular contraction or spasm; this condition may need to be reassessed later.

Circulatory Evaluation

Palpate the distal pulses in each extremity and assess capillary refill of the digits. If hypotension limits digital examination of the pulse, the use of a Doppler probe may detect blood flow to an extremity. The Doppler signal must have a triphasic quality to ensure no proximal lesion. Loss of sen-

TABLE 8-1 ■ Common Joint Dislocation Deformities

JOINT	DIRECTION	DEFORMITY
Shoulder	Anterior Posterior	Squared off Locked in internal rotation
Elbow	Posterior	Olecranon prominent posteriorly
Hip	Anterior Posterior	Flexed, abducted, externally rotated Flexed, adducted, internally rotated
Knee	Anteroposterior	Loss of normal contour, extended
Ankle	Lateral is most common	Externally rotated, prominent medial malleolus
Subtalar joint	Lateral is most common	Laterally displaced os calcis

PITFALL

Failure to perform a thorough secondary survey can result in missing potential life- and limb-threatening injuries.

sation in a stocking or glove distribution is an early sign of vascular impairment.

In patients with no hemodynamic abnormalities, pulse discrepancies, coolness, pallor, paresthesia, and even motor function abnormalities suggest an arterial injury. Open wounds and fractures in proximity to arteries can be a clue to an arterial injury. A Doppler ankle/brachial index of less than 0.9 is indicative of an abnormal arterial flow secondary to injury or peripheral vascular disease. The ankle/brachial index is determined by taking the systolic blood pressure value as measured by Doppler at the ankle of the injured leg and dividing it by the Doppler-determined systolic blood pressure of the uninjured arm. Auscultation can reveal a bruit with an associated palpable thrill. Expanding hematomas or pulsatile hemorrhage from an open wound also are indicative of arterial injury.

X-Ray Examination

The clinical examination of patients with musculoskeletal injuries often suggests the need for x-ray examination. Any area over a bone that is tender and deformed likely represents a fracture. In patients who have no hemodynamic abnormalities, an x-ray film should be obtained. Joint effusions, abnormal joint tenderness, or joint deformity represent a joint injury or dislocation that also must be x-rayed. The only reason for electing not to obtain an x-ray film prior to treatment of a dislocation or a fracture is the presence of vascular compromise or impending skin breakdown. This is seen commonly with fracture-dislocations of the ankle. If there is going to be a delay in obtaining x-rays, immediate reduction or realignment of the extremity should be performed to reestablish the arterial blood supply and reduce the pressure on the skin. Alignment can be maintained by appropriate immobilization techniques.

Potentially Life-Threatening Extremity Injuries

? *What are my priorities, and what are my management principles?*

Extremity injuries that are considered potentially life-threatening include major pelvic disruption with hemorrhage, major arterial hemorrhage, and crush syndrome.

MAJOR PELVIC DISRUPTION WITH HEMORRHAGE

Injury

Patients with hypotension who have pelvic fractures have a high mortality, and sound decision making is crucial. Pelvic fractures associated with hemorrhage commonly exhibit disruption of the posterior osseous ligamentous (sacroiliac, sacrospinous, sacrotuberous, and the fibromuscular pelvic floor) complex from a sacroiliac fracture and/or dislocation, or from a sacral fracture (Figure 8-1). The force vector opens the pelvic ring, tears the pelvic venous plexus, and occasionally disrupts the internal iliac arterial system (anteroposterior compression injury). This mechanism of pelvic ring injury may be caused by motorcycle crashes and pedestrian-vehicle collisions, direct crushing injury to the pelvis, and falls from heights greater than 12 feet (3.6 meters). Mortality in patients with all types of pelvic fractures is approximately one in six (5%—30%). In patients with closed pelvic fractures and hypotension, mortality rises to approximately one in four (10%—42%). Hemorrhage is the major reversible contributing factor to mortality.

In motor vehicle collisions, a common mechanism of pelvic fracture is force applied to the lateral aspect of the pelvis that tends to rotate the involved hemipelvis internally, closing down the pelvic volume and relieving any tension on the pelvic vascular system (lateral compression injury). This rotational motion drives the pubis into the lower genitourinary system, creating injury to the bladder and/or urethra. Hemorrhage from this injury, or its sequelae, rarely results in death, as it does in the completely unstable pelvic injury. ◾ See Skill Station XII: Musculoskeletal Trauma: Assessment and Management, Skill XII-F: Identification and Management of Pelvic Fractures.

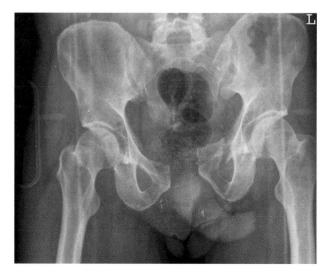

■ **Figure 8-1** Radiograph showing pelvic fracture associated with hemorrhage. Notice the disruption of the posterior osseous-ligamentous complex.

Assessment

Major pelvic hemorrhage occurs rapidly, and the diagnosis must be made quickly so that appropriate resuscitative treatment can be initiated. Unexplained hypotension may be the only initial indication of major pelvic disruption with instability in the posterior ligamentous complex. The most important physical signs are progressive flank, scrotal, or perianal swelling and bruising. This is associated with failure to respond to initial fluid resuscitation. Open fracture wounds about the pelvis (especially if the open area is in the perineum, rectum, or buttocks), a high-riding prostate gland, blood at the urethral meatus, and demonstrable mechanical instability are signs of unstable pelvic ring injury.

Mechanical instability of the pelvic ring is tested by manual manipulation of the pelvis. This procedure should be performed only once during the physical examination, as repeated testing for pelvic instability can result in further hemorrhage. The first indication of mechanical instability is leg-length discrepancy or rotational deformity (usually external) without a fracture of that extremity. The unstable hemipelvis migrates cephalad because of muscular pull and rotates outward secondary to the effect of gravity on the unstable hemipelvis. Because the unstable pelvis is able to rotate externally, the pelvis can be closed by pushing on the iliac crests at the level of the anterior superior iliac spine. Motion can be felt if the iliac crests are grasped and the unstable hemipelvis is pushed inward and then outward (compression distraction maneuver). With posterior disruption, the involved hemipelvis can be pushed cephalad as well as pulled caudally. This translational motion can be felt by palpating the posterior iliac spine and tubercle while pushing and pulling the unstable hemipelvis. The identification of neurologic abnormalities or open wounds in the flank, perineum, and rectum may be evidence of pelvic ring instability. When appropriate, an AP x-ray of the pelvis confirms the clinical examination. ◾ See Skill Station IV: Shock Assessment and Management.

Management

Initial management of a major pelvic disruption associated with hemorrhage requires hemorrhage control and rapid fluid resuscitation. Hemorrhage control is achieved through mechanical stabilization of the pelvic ring and external counterpressure. Patients with these injuries may be initially assessed and treated in hospitals that do not have the resources to definitively manage the degree of associated hemorrhage. Simple techniques can be used to stabilize the pelvis before transferring the patient. Longitudinal traction applied through the skin or the skeleton is a first-line method. Because these injuries externally rotate the hemipelvis, internal rotation of the lower limbs also reduces the pelvic volume. This procedure may be supplemented by applying a support directly to the pelvis.

A sheet, pelvic binder, or other devices may apply sufficient stability for the unstable pelvis. These temporary methods are suitable to gain early pelvic stabilization. Definitive care of patients with hemodynamic abnormalities demands the cooperative efforts of a team that includes a trauma surgeon and an orthopedic surgeon, as well as any other surgeon whose expertise is required because of the patient's injuries. ◾ See Chapter 5: Abdominal and Pelvic Trauma.

Open pelvic fractures with obvious bleeding require pressure dressings to control hemorrhage, which is done by packing the open wounds. Early surgical consultation is essential.

MAJOR ARTERIAL HEMORRHAGE

Injury

Penetrating wounds of an extremity may result in major arterial vascular injury. Blunt trauma resulting in an extremity fracture or joint dislocation in close proximity to an artery also may disrupt the artery. These injuries may lead to significant hemorrhage through the open wound or into the soft tissues. The use of a tourniquet to control bleeding may be of benefit in select patients.

Assessment

Assess injured extremities for external bleeding, loss of a previously palpable pulse, and changes in pulse quality, Doppler tone, and ankle/brachial index. A cold, pale, pulseless extremity indicates an interruption in arterial blood supply. A rapidly expanding hematoma suggests a significant vascular injury. ◾ See Skill Station XII: Musculoskeletal Trauma: Assessment and Management, Skill XII-G: Identification of Arterial Injury.

Management

If a major arterial injury exists or is suspected, immediate consultation with a surgeon is necessary. Management of major arterial hemorrhage includes application of direct pressure to the open wound and aggressive fluid resuscitation.

The judicious use of a pneumatic tourniquet may be helpful and lifesaving (Figure 8-2). It is not advisable to apply vascular clamps into bleeding open wounds while the patient is in the ED, unless a superficial vessel is clearly identified. If a fracture is associated with an open hemorrhaging wound, it should be realigned and splinted while direct pressure is applied to the open wound. A joint dislocation simply requires immobilization; joint reduction may be extremely difficult, and therefore should be managed by emergency surgical intervention. The use of arteriography and other investigations is indicated only in resuscitated patients who have no hemodynamic abnormalities. Urgent consul-

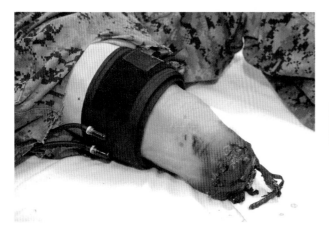

■ **Figure 8-2** Trauma patient with pneumatic tourniquet in place.

tation with a surgeon skilled in vascular and extremity trauma is necessary.

CRUSH SYNDROME (TRAUMATIC RHABDOMYOLYSIS)

Injury

Crush syndrome refers to the clinical effects of injured muscle that, if left untreated, may lead to acute renal failure. This condition is seen in individuals who have sustained a crush injury of a significant muscle mass, most often a thigh or calf. The muscular insult is a combination of direct muscle injury, muscle ischemia, and cell death with release of myoglobin. Muscular trauma is the most common cause of rhabdomyolysis, which ranges from an asymptomatic illness with elevation of the creatine kinase level to a life-threatening condition associated with acute renal failure and disseminated intravascular coagulation (DIC).

Assessment

The myoglobin produces dark amber urine that tests positive for hemoglobin. The myoglobin assay must be specifically requested to confirm the presence of myoglobin. Rhabdomyolysis may lead to hypovolemia, metabolic acidosis, hyperkalemia, hypocalcemia, and DIC.

Management

The initiation of early and aggressive intravenous fluid therapy during the period of resuscitation, along with the administration of sodium bicarbonate and electrolytes, is critical to protecting the kidneys and preventing renal failure. Myoglobin-induced renal failure may be prevented by intravascular fluid expansion and osmotic diuresis to maintain a high tubular volume and urine flow. Alkalization of the urine with sodium bicarbonate reduces intratubular pre-

cipitation of myoglobin and is indicated in most patients. It is recommended to maintain the patient's urinary output at 100 mL/hr until the myoglobinuria is cleared.

Limb-Threatening Injuries

Extremity injuries that are considered potentially limb-threatening include open fractures and joint injuries; vascular injuries, including traumatic amputation; compartment syndrome; and neurologic injury secondary to fracture-dislocation.

OPEN FRACTURES AND JOINT INJURIES

Injury

Open fractures represent a communication between the external environment and the bone (Figure 8-3). Muscle and skin must be injured for this to occur. The degree of soft tissue injury is proportional to the energy applied. This damage, along with bacterial contamination, makes open fractures prone to problems with infection, healing, and function.

Assessment

Diagnosis of an open fracture is based on the history of the incident and physical examination of the extremity that demonstrates an open wound with or without significant muscle damage, contamination, and associated fracture. Management decisions should be based on a complete history of the incident and assessment of the injury.

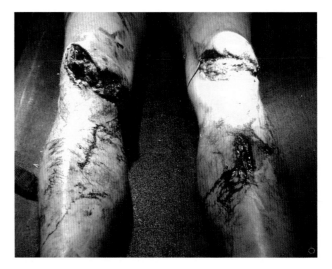

■ **Figure 8-3** Example of an open fracture.

Documentation regarding the open wound begins during the prehospital phase, with the initial description of the injury and any treatment rendered at the scene. If the documentation is adequate, no further inspection of the open wound is warranted. If the documentation or the history is inadequate, the dressing should be removed under as sterile conditions as possible to visually examine the wound. A sterile dressing is then reapplied. At no time should the wound be probed. If a fracture and an open wound exist in the same limb segment, the fracture is considered open until proved otherwise.

If an open wound exists over or near a joint, it should be assumed that this injury connects with or enters the joint, and surgical consultation should be obtained. The insertion of dye, saline, or any other material into the joint to determine whether the joint cavity communicates with the wound is not recommended. The only safe way to determine communication between an open wound and a joint is to surgically explore and debride the wound.

Management

The presence of an open fracture or a joint injury should be promptly determined. Apply appropriate immobilization after an accurate description of the wound is made and associated soft tissue, circulatory, and neurologic involvement is determined. Prompt surgical consultation is necessary. The patient should be adequately resuscitated, with hemodynamic stability achieved if possible. Wounds then may be operatively debrided, fractures stabilized, and distal pulses confirmed. Tetanus prophylaxis should be administered ▪ See Appendix E: Tetanus Immunization. Antibiotics are used only after consultation with a surgeon.

VASCULAR INJURIES, INCLUDING TRAUMATIC AMPUTATION

Injury

A vascular injury should be strongly suspected in the presence of vascular insufficiency associated with a history of blunt, crushing, twisting, or penetrating injury to an extremity.

Assessment

The limb may initially appear viable because extremities often have some collateral circulation that provides enough retrograde flow. Partial vascular injury results in coolness and prolonged capillary refill in the distal part of an extremity, as well as diminished peripheral pulses and an abnormal ankle/brachial index. Alternatively, the distal extremity may have a complete disruption of flow and be cold, pale, and pulseless.

Management

An acutely avascular extremity must be recognized promptly and treated emergently. Although controversial, the use of a tourniquet may occasionally be lifesaving and/or limb-saving in the presence of ongoing hemorrhage uncontrolled by direct pressure. A properly applied tourniquet, while endangering the limb, may save a life. A tourniquet must occlude arterial inflow, as occluding only the venous system can increase hemorrhage. The risks of tourniquet use increase with time. If a tourniquet must remain in place for a prolonged period to save a life, the physician must be cognizant of the fact the choice of life over limb has been made.

Muscle does not tolerate a lack of arterial blood flow for longer than 6 hours before necrosis begins. Nerves also are very sensitive to an anoxic environment. Therefore, early operative revascularization is required to restore arterial flow to the impaired distal extremity. If there is an associated fracture deformity, it can be corrected quickly by gently realigning and splinting the injured extremity.

If an arterial injury is associated with a dislocation of a joint, a doctor who is skilled in joint reduction may attempt *one* gentle reduction maneuver. Otherwise, splinting of the dislocated joint and emergency surgical consultation are necessary. Arteriography must not delay reestablishing arterial blood flow, and is indicated only after consultation with a surgeon. CT angiography may be helpful in institutions in which arteriography is not available.

The potential for vascular compromise also exists whenever an injured extremity is splinted or placed in a cast. Vascular compromise can be identified by the loss of or change in the distal pulse, but excessive pain after cast application also must be investigated. The splint, cast, and any other circumferential dressings must be released promptly and the vascular supply reassessed.

Amputation is a traumatic event for the patient both physically and emotionally. Traumatic amputation, a severe form of open fracture that results in loss of an extremity, may benefit from tourniquet use and requires consultation with and intervention by a surgeon. Certain open fractures with prolonged ischemia, neurologic injury, and muscle damage may require amputation. Amputation of an injured extremity may be lifesaving in patients with hemodynamic abnormalities who are difficult to resuscitate.

Although the potential for replantation should be considered, it must be put into perspective with the patient's other injuries. A patient with multiple injuries who requires intensive resuscitation and emergency surgery is not a candidate for replantation. Replantation usually is performed with an injury of an isolated extremity. A patient with clean, sharp amputations of fingers or of a distal extremity, below the knee or elbow, should be transported to an appropriate surgical team skilled in the decision making for and management of replantation procedures.

The amputated part should be thoroughly washed in isotonic solution (eg, Ringer's lactate) and wrapped in sterile gauze that has been soaked in aqueous penicillin (100,000 units in 50 mL of Ringer's lactate solution). The amputated part is then wrapped in a similarly moistened sterile towel, placed in a plastic bag, and transported with the patient in an insulated cooling chest with crushed ice. Care must be taken not to freeze the amputated part.

COMPARTMENT SYNDROME

Injury

Compartment syndrome develops when the pressure within an osteofascial compartment of muscle causes ischemia and subsequent necrosis. This ischemia may be caused by an increase in compartment size (eg, swelling secondary to revascularization of an ischemic extremity) or by decreasing the compartment size (eg, a constrictive dressing). Compartment syndrome may occur in any site in which muscle is contained within a closed fascial space. (Remember, the skin also may act as a restricting membrane in certain circumstances.) Common areas for compartment syndrome include the lower leg, forearm, foot, hand, gluteal region, and thigh (Figure 8-4).

The end results of unchecked compartment syndrome are catastrophic. They include neurologic deficit, muscle necrosis, ischemic contracture, infection, delayed healing of a fracture, and possible amputation.

Assessment

Any injury to an extremity has the potential to cause a compartment syndrome. However, certain injuries are considered high risk, including:

- Tibial and forearm fractures
- Injuries immobilized in tight dressings or casts
- Severe crush injury to muscle
- Localized, prolonged external pressure to an extremity
- Increased capillary permeability secondary to reperfusion of ischemic muscle
- Burns
- Excessive exercise

The key to the successful treatment of acute compartment syndrome is early diagnosis. A high degree of awareness is important, especially if the patient has an altered mental sensorium and is unable to respond appropriately to pain. ◾ See Skill Station XII: Musculoskeletal Trauma: Assessment and Management, Skill XII-E: Compartment Syndrome: Assessment and Management.

The signs and symptoms of compartment syndrome include:

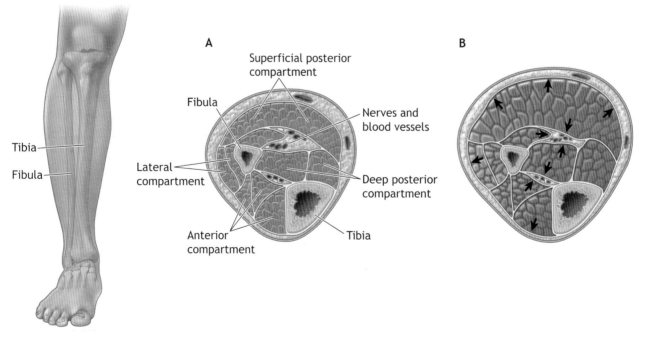

■ **Figure 8-4 Compartment Syndrome.** Develops when the pressure within an osteofascial compartment of muscle causes ischemia and subsequent necrosis. **(A)** Normal calf. **(B)** Calf with compartment syndrome.

- Increasing pain greater than expected and out of proportion to the stimulus

- Palpable tenseness of the compartment

- Asymmetry of the muscle compartments

- Pain on passive stretch of the affected muscle

- Altered sensation

Absence of a palpable distal pulse usually is an uncommon finding and should not be relied upon to diagnose compartment syndrome. Weakness or paralysis of involved muscles and loss of pulses (because the compartment pressure exceeds the systolic pressure) in the affected limb are late signs of compartment syndrome.

Remember, changes in distal pulses or capillary refill times are not reliable in diagnosing compartment syndrome. Clinical diagnosis is based on the history of injury and physical signs, coupled with a high index of suspicion.

Intracompartmental pressure measurements may be helpful in diagnosing suspected compartment syndrome. Tissue pressures that are greater than 30 to 45 mm Hg suggest decreased capillary blood flow, which may result in increased muscle and nerve damage caused by anoxia. Systemic blood pressure is important: the lower the systemic pressure, the lower the compartment pressure that causes a compartment syndrome. Pressure measurement is indicated in all patients who have an altered response to pain.

Management

All constrictive dressings, casts, and splints applied over the affected extremity must be released. The patient must be carefully monitored and reassessed clinically for the next 30 to 60 minutes. If no significant changes occur, fasciotomy is required. Compartment syndrome is a time-dependent condition. The higher the compartment pressure and the longer it remains elevated, the greater the degree of resulting neuromuscular damage and functional deficit. Delay in performing a fasciotomy may result in myoglobinuria, which may cause decreased renal function. **Surgical consultation for diagnosed or suspected compartment syndrome must be obtained early.**

PITFALL

Compartment syndrome is limb-threatening. Clinical findings must be recognized and surgical consultation obtained early. Remember that in unconscious patients or those with severe hypovolemia, the classic findings of acute compartment syndrome may be masked.

NEUROLOGIC INJURY SECONDARY TO FRACTURE-DISLOCATION

Injury

Fractures and particularly dislocations may cause significant neurologic injury because of the anatomic relationship and proximity of the nerve to the joint—for example, sciatic nerve compression from posterior hip dislocation or axillary nerve injury from anterior shoulder dislocation. Optimal functional outcome is jeopardized unless this injury is recognized and treated early.

Assessment

A thorough examination of the neurologic system is essential in patients with musculoskeletal injury. Determination of neurologic impairment is important, and progressive changes must be documented.

Assessment usually demonstrates a deformity of the extremity. Assessment of nerve function usually requires a cooperative patient. For each significant peripheral nerve, voluntary motor function and sensation must be confirmed systematically (Tables 8-2 and 8-3). Muscle testing must include palpation of the contracting muscle.

In most patients with multiple injuries, it is difficult to initially assess nerve function. However, assessment must be repeated on an ongoing basis, especially after the patient is stabilized. Progression of neurologic findings is indicative of continued nerve compression. The most important aspect of any neurologic assessment is the documentation of progression of neurologic findings. It also is an important aspect of surgical decision making.

Management

The injured extremity should be immobilized in the dislocated position, and surgical consultation obtained immediately. If indicated and if the treating doctor is knowledgeable, a careful reduction of the dislocation may be attempted. After reducing a dislocation, neurologic function should be reevaluated and the limb splinted.

Other Extremity Injuries

Other significant extremity injuries include contusions and lacerations, joint injuries, and fractures.

CONTUSIONS AND LACERATIONS

Simple contusions and/or lacerations should be assessed to rule out vascular and/or neurologic injury. In general, lacerations require debridement and closure. If a laceration extends below the fascial level, it requires operative

TABLE 8-2 ■ Peripheral Nerve Assessment of Upper Extremities

NERVE	MOTOR	SENSATION	INJURY
Ulnar	Index finger abduction	Little finger	Elbow injury
Median distal	Thenar contraction with opposition	Index finger	Wrist dislocation
Median, anterior interosseous	Index tip flexion		Supracondylar fracture of humerus (children)
Musculocutaneous	Elbow flexion	Lateral forearm	Anterior shoulder dislocation
Radial	Thumb, finger metocarpo-phalangeal extension	First dorsal web space	Distal humeral shaft, anterior shoulder dislocation
Axillary	Deltoid	Lateral shoulder	Anterior shoulder dislocation, proximal humerus fractur

TABLE 8-3 ■ Peripheral Nerve Assessment of Lower Extremities

NERVE	MOTOR	SENSATION	INJURY
Femoral	Knee extension	Anterior knee	Pubic rami fractures
Obturator	Hip adduction	Medial thigh	Obturator ring fractures
Posterior tibial	Toe flexion	Sole of foot	Knee dislocation
Superficial peroneal	Ankle eversion	Lateral dorsum of foot	Fibular neck fracture, knee dislocation
Deep peroneal	Ankle/toe dorsiflexion	Dorsal first to second web space	Fibular neck fracture, compartment syndrome
Sciatic nerve	Plantar dorsiflexion	Foot	Posterior hip dislocation
Superior gluteal	Hip abduction		Acetabular fracture
Inferior gluteal	Gluteus maximus hip extension		Acetabular fracture

intervention to more completely debride the wound and assess for damage to underlying structures.

Contusions usually are recognized by pain in the area and decreased function of the extremity. Palpation confirms localized swelling and tenderness. The patient usually cannot use the muscle or experiences decreased function because of pain in the affected extremity. If the patient is seen early, contusions are treated by limiting function of the injured part and applying cold packs.

Small wounds, especially those resulting from crush injuries, may be significant. When a very strong force is applied very slowly over an extremity, significant devascularization and crushing of muscle may occur with only a small skin wound. Crush and degloving injuries can be very subtle and must be suspected based on the mechanism of injury.

The risk of tetanus is increased with wounds that: (1) are more than 6 hours old, (2) are contused and/or abraded,

(3) are more than 1 cm in depth, (4) result from high-velocity missiles, (5) are due to burns or cold, and (6) have significant contamination (especially burn wounds and wounds with denervated or ischemic tissue). ■ See Appendix E: Tetanus Immunization.

JOINT INJURIES

Injury

Joint injuries that are not dislocated (ie, the joint is within its normal anatomic configuration but has sustained significant ligamentous injury) usually are not limb-threatening. However, such joint injuries may decrease the function of the limb.

Assessment

With joint injuries, the patient usually reports some form of abnormal stress to the joint—for example, impact to the anterior tibia that pushed the knee back, impact to the lateral aspect of the leg that resulted in a valgus strain to the knee, or a fall onto an outstretched arm that caused a hyperflexion injury to the elbow.

Physical examination reveals tenderness throughout the affected ligament. A hemarthrosis usually is present unless the joint capsule is disrupted and the bleeding diffuses into the soft tissues. Passive ligamentous testing of the affected joint reveals instability. X-ray examination usually reveals no significant injury. However, some small avulsion fractures from ligamentous insertions or origins may be present radiographically.

Management

Joint injuries should be immobilized. The vascular and neurologic status of the limb distal to the injury should be reassessed. Surgical consultation usually is warranted.

FRACTURES

Injury

Fractures are defined as a break in the continuity of the bone cortex. They may be associated with abnormal motion, some form of soft tissue injury, crepitation, and pain. A fracture can be open or closed.

Assessment

Examination of the extremity demonstrates pain, swelling, deformity, tenderness, crepitation, and abnormal motion at the fracture site. The evaluation for crepitation and abnormal motion at the fracture site may occasionally be necessary to make the diagnosis, but this is painful and may potentially increase soft tissue damage. These diagnostic tests must not be done routinely or repetitively. Usually the swelling, tenderness, and deformity are sufficient to confirm a fracture. It is important to periodically reassess the neurovascular status of a limb, especially if a splint is in place.

X-ray films taken at right angles to one another confirm the history and physical examinations. Depending on the hemodynamic status of the patient, x-ray examination may have to be delayed until the patient is stabilized. X-ray films through the joint above and below the suspected fracture site must be included to exclude occult dislocation and concomitant injury.

Management

Immobilization must include the joint above and below the fracture. After splinting, the neurologic and vascular status of the extremity must be reassessed. Surgical consultation is required for further treatment.

Principles of Immobilization

Splinting of extremity injuries, unless associated with life-threatening injuries, usually can be accomplished during the secondary survey. However, all such injuries must be splinted before a patient is transported. Assess the limb's neurovascular status after applying splints or realigning a fracture.

Specific types of splints can be applied for specific fracture needs. The pneumatic antishock garment (PASG) is not generally recommended as a lower-extremity splint. However, it may be temporarily useful for patients with life-threatening hemorrhage from pelvic injuries or severe lower-extremity injuries with soft tissue injury. Prolonged inflation (>2 hours) of the leg components in patients with hypotension may lead to compartment syndrome.

A long spine board provides a total body splint for patients with multiple injuries who have possible or confirmed unstable spine injuries. However, its hard, unpadded surface may cause pressure sores on the patient's occiput, scapulae, sacrum, and heels. Therefore, as soon as possible, the patient should be moved carefully to an equally supportive padded surface, using a scoop-style stretcher or an appropriate logrolling maneuver to facilitate the transfer. The patient should be fully immobilized, and an adequate number of personnel should be available during this transfer. ■ See Skill Station XI: Spinal Cord Injury: Assessment and Management, and Skill Station XII: Musculoskeletal Trauma: Assessment and Management, Skill XII-B: Principles of Extremity Immobilization.

FEMORAL FRACTURES

Femoral fractures are immobilized temporarily with traction splints (Figure 8-5). The traction splint's force is applied distally at the ankle or through the skin. Proximally, the splint is pushed into the thigh and hip areas by a ring that applies pressure to the buttocks, perineum, and groin. Excessive traction can cause skin damage to the foot, ankle, or perineum. Neurovascular compromise can result from stretching the peripheral nerves. Hip fractures can be similarly immobilized with a traction splint, but are more suit-

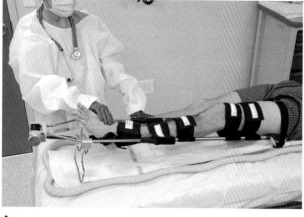

A

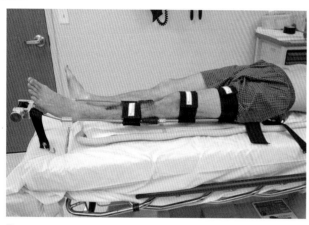

B

■ **Figure 8-5 Traction Splinting.** Proper application of a traction splint includes proper position against the crease of the buttock and sufficient length to apply traction. The straps should be positioned above and below the knee, with the stand extended to suspend the leg. Distal pulses should be evaluated before and after application of the splint **(A)**. It is improper to use the splint without proper placement of the straps and securing traction to the device **(B)**.

ably immobilized with skin traction or a foam boot traction with the knee in slight flexion. A simple method of splinting is to bind the injured leg to the opposite leg. ■ See Skill Station XII: Musculoskeletal Trauma: Assessment and Management, Skill XII-D: Application of a Traction Splint.

KNEE INJURIES

The use of commercially available knee immobilizers or the application of a long-leg plaster splint is very helpful in maintaining comfort and stability. The leg should not be immobilized in complete extension, but should be immobilized with about 10 degrees of flexion to take pressure off the neurovascular structures.

TIBIA FRACTURES

Tibia fractures are best immobilized with a well-padded cardboard or metal gutter long-leg splint. If readily available, plaster splints immobilizing the lower leg, the knee, and the ankle may be used.

ANKLE FRACTURES

Ankle fractures may be immobilized with a pillow splint or padded cardboard splint, thereby avoiding pressure over bony prominences.

UPPER-EXTREMITY AND HAND INJURIES

The hand may be temporarily splinted in an anatomic, functional position, with the wrist slightly dorsiflexed and the fingers gently flexed 45 degrees at the metacarpophalangeal joints. This position usually can be achieved by gently immobilizing the hand over a large roll of gauze and using a short-arm splint.

The forearm and wrist are immobilized flat on padded or pillow splints. The elbow usually is immobilized in a flexed position, either by using padded splints or by direct immobilization with respect to the body using a sling and swath device. The upper arm usually is immobilized by splinting it to the body or applying a sling or swath, which can be augmented by a thoracobrachial bandage. Shoulder injuries are managed by a sling-and-swath device or a Velcro-type of dressing.

Pain Control

Analgesics are generally indicated for joint injuries and fractures. However, the administration of pain medications must be tempered by the patient's clinical situation. The appropriate use of splints significantly decreases the patient's discomfort by controlling the amount of motion that occurs at the injured site.

Patients who do not appear to have significant pain and discomfort from a major fracture may have other associated injuries—for example, intracranial lesions or hypoxia—or may be under the influence of alcohol and/or other drugs.

Effective pain relief usually requires the administration of narcotics, which should be given in small doses intravenously and repeated as needed. Muscle relaxants and sedatives should be administered cautiously in patients with isolated extremity injuries—for example, reduction of a dislocation. Regional nerve blocks have a role in pain relief and the reduction of appropriate fractures. It is essential to assess and document any peripheral nerve injury before administrating a nerve block.

Whenever analgesics, muscle relaxants, or sedatives are administered to an injured patient, the potential exists for respiratory arrest. Consequently, appropriate resuscitative equipment must be immediately available.

Associated Injuries

Certain musculoskeletal injuries, because of their common mechanism of injury, are often associated with second injuries that are not immediately apparent or may be missed (see Table 8-4). Steps to ensure recognition and management of these injuries include:

1. Review the injury history, especially the mechanism of injury, to determine whether another injury is present.

2. Thoroughly reexamine all extremities, placing special emphasis on the hands, wrists, feet, and the joint above and below a fracture or dislocation.

3. Visually examine the patient's dorsum, including the spine and pelvis. Open injuries and closed soft tissue injuries that may be indicative of an unstable injury must be documented.

4. Review the x-rays obtained in the secondary survey to identify subtle injuries that may be associated with more obvious trauma.

Occult Skeletal Injuries

Remember, not all injuries can be diagnosed during the initial assessment and management of injury. Joints or bones that are covered or well padded within muscular areas may contain occult injuries. It can be difficult to identify nondisplaced fractures or joint ligamentous injuries, especially if the patient is unresponsive or there are other severe injuries. It is important to recognize that injuries are commonly discovered days after the injury incident—for example, when the patient is being mobilized. Therefore, is it important to reassess the patient routinely and to relate this possibility to other members of the trauma team and the patient's family.

PITFALL

Despite a thorough examination, occult associated injuries may not be appreciated during the initial evaluation. It is imperative to repeatedly reevaluate the patient to assess for these injuries.

TABLE 8-4 ■ Injuries Associated with Musculoskeletal Injuries

INJURY	MISSED/ASSOCIATED INJURY
Clavicular fracture Scapular fracture Fracture and/or dislocation of shoulder	Major thoracic injury, especially pulmonary contusion and rib fractures
Displaced thoracic spine fracture	Thoracic aortic rupture
Spine fracture	Intraabdominal injury
Fracture/dislocation of elbow	Brachial artery injury Median, ulnar, and radial nerve injury
Major pelvic disruption (motor vehicle occupant)	Abdominal, thoracic, or head injury
Major pelvic disruption (motorcyclist or pedestrian)	Pelvic vascular hemorrhage
Femur fracture	Femoral neck fracture Posterior hip dislocation
Posterior knee dislocation	Femoral fracture Posterior hip dislocation
Knee dislocation or displaced tibial plateau fracture	Popliteal artery and nerve injuries
Calcaneal fracture	Spine injury or fracture Fracture-dislocation of hindfoot Tibial plateau fracture
Open fracture	70% incidence of associated nonskeletal injury

CHAPTER SUMMARY

1 Musculoskeletal injuries, while generally not life-threatening may pose delayed threats to life and limb.

2 The goal of the initial assessment of musculoskeletal trauma is to identify injuries that pose a threat to life and/or limb. Although uncommon, life-threatening musculoskeletal injuries must be properly assessed and managed. Most extremity injuries are appropriately diagnosed and managed during the secondary survey.

3 It is essential to recognize and manage in a timely manner pelvic fractures, arterial injuries, compartment syndrome, open fractures, crush injuries, and fracture-dislocations. Knowledge of the mechanism of injury and history of the injury-producing event enables the doctor to be aware of what associated conditions potentially exist with the injured extremity. Early splinting of fractures and dislocations may prevent serious complications and late sequelae. In addition, an awareness of the patient's tetanus immunization status, particularly in cases of open fractures or significantly contaminated wounds, may prevent serious complications. Armed with the proper knowledge and skills, as outlined in this chapter, the doctor can satisfactorily provide the initial management for most musculoskeletal trauma.

Bibliography

1. Beekley AC, Starnes BW, Sebesta JA. Lessons learned from modern military surgery. *Surg Clin North Am* 2007;87(1):157-84, vii.

2. Bone LB, Johnson KD, Weigelt J, et al. Early versus delayed stabilization of femoral fractures: a prospective, randomized study. *J Bone Joint Surg Am* 1989;71:336-340.

3. Brown CV, Rhee P, Chan L, Evans K, Demetriades D, Velmahos GC. Preventing renal failure in patients with rhabdomyolysis: do bicarbonate and mannitol make a difference? *J Trauma* 2004;56:1191.

4. Browner BD, ed. Controversies and perils. *Techniques Orthop* 1994;9(4):258.

5. Clifford CC. Treating traumatic bleeding in a combat setting. *Mil Med* 2004;169(12 Suppl):8-10, 14.

6. Curet MJ, Schermer CR, Demarest GB, Bieneik EJ, Curet LB. Predictors of outcome in trauma during pregnancy: identification of patients who can be monitored for less than 6 hours. *J Trauma* 2000;49(1):18-24; discussion 24-25.

7. Dalal SA, Burgess AR, Seigel JH, et al. Pelvic fracture in multiple trauma: classification by mechanism is key to pattern of organ injury, resuscitative requirements, and outcome. *J Trauma* 1989;29:981-1000.

8. Elliot GB, Johnstone AJ. Diagnosing acute compartment syndrome. *J Bone Joint Surg Br* 2003;85:625-630

9. Foss NB, Kristensen BB, Bundgaard M, Bak M, Heiring C, Virkelyst C, Hougaard S, Kehlet H. Fascia iliaca compartment blockade for acute pain control in hip fracture patients: a randomized, placebo-controlled trial. *Anesthesiology* 2007;106(4):773-778.

10. Gustilo RB, Anderson JT. Prevention of infection in the treatment of 1025 open fractures of long bones. *J Bone Joint Surg Am* 1976;58:453.

11. Gustilo RB, Mendoza RM, Williams DN. Problems in the management of type III (severe) open fractures: a new classification of type III open fractures. *J Trauma* 1985;24:742.

12. Heetveld MJ, Harris I, Schlaphoff G, Surgrue N. Guidelines for the management of hemodynamically unstable pelvic fracture patients. *Aust NZ J Surg* 2004;74:520-529.

13. Heppenstall RB, Sapega AA, Scott R, et al. The compartment syndrome: an experimental and clinical study of muscular energy metabolism using phosphorus nuclear magnetic resonance spectroscopy. *Clin Orthop* 1988;226:138-155.

14. Ikossi DG, Lazar AA, Morabito D, Fildes J, Knudson MM. Profile of mothers at risk: an analysis of injury and pregnancy loss in 1,195 trauma patients. *J Am Coll Surg* 2005;200(1):49-56.

15. King RB, Filips D, Blitz S, Logsetty S. Evaluation of possible tourniquet systems for use in the Canadian Forces. *J Trauma* 2006;60(5):1061-1071.

16. Klinich KD, Schneider LW, Moore JL, Pearlman MD. Investigations of crashes involving pregnant occupants. *Annu Proc Assoc Adv Automot Med* 2000;44:37-55.

17. Kostler W, Strohm PC, Sudkamp NP. Acute compartment syndrome of the limb. *Injury* 2004;35(12);1221-1227.

18. Koury HI, Peschiera JL, Welling RE. Selective use of pelvic roentgenograms in blunt trauma patients. *J Trauma* 1993;34:236.

19. Lakstein D, Blumenfeld A, Sokolov T, et al. Tourniquets for hemorrhage control on the battlefield: a 4-year accumulated experience. *J Trauma* 2003;54(5 Suppl):S221-S225.

20. Mabry RL. Tourniquet use on the battlefield. *Mil Med* 2006;171(5):352-356.

21. Mattox KL, Goetzl L. Trauma in pregnancy. *Crit Care Med* 2005;33(10 Suppl):S385-S389.

22. Maull KI, Capenhart JE, Cardea JA, et al. Limb loss following MAST application. *J Trauma* 1981;21:60-62.

23. Metz TD, Abbott JT. Uterine trauma in pregnancy after motor vehicle crashes with airbag deployment: A 30-case series. *J Trauma* 2006;61(3):658-661.

24. Moore EE, Ducker TB, Edlich RF, et al., eds. *Early Care of the Injured Patient,* 4th ed. Philadelphia, PA: BC Decker; 1990, chapters 19-24.

25. Ododeh M. The role of reperfusion-induced injury in the pathogenesis of the crush syndrome. *N Engl J Med* 1991;324:1417-1421.

26. Olson SA, Glasgow RR. Acute compartment syndrome in lower extremity musculoskeletal trauma. *J Am Acad Orthop Surg* 2005;13(7):436-444.

27. Shah AJ, Kilcline BA. Trauma in pregnancy. *Emerg Med Clin North Am* 2003;21(3): 615-629.

28. Trafton PG. Orthopaedic emergencies. In: Ho MT, Saunders CE, eds. *Current Emergency Diagnosis and Treatment,* 3rd ed. East Norwalk, CT: Appleton & Lange; 1990.

29. Ulmer T. The clinical diagnosis of compartment syndrome of the lower leg: are clinical findings predictive of the disorder? *J Orthop Trauma* 2002;16(8):572-577.

30. Walters TJ, Mabry RL. Issues related to the use of tourniquets on the battlefield. *Mil Med* 2005;170(9):770-775.

31. Walters TJ, Wenke JC, Kauvar DS, McManus JG, Holcomb JB, Baer DG. Effectiveness of self-applied tourniquets in human volunteers. *Prehosp Emerg Care* 2005;9(4):416-422.

32. Welling DR, Burris DG, Hutton JE, Minken SL, Rich NM. A balanced approach to tourniquet use: lessons learned and re-learned. *J Am Coll Surg* 2006;203(1):106-115.

33. Wolf ME, Alexander BH, Rivara FP, Hickok DE, Maier RV, Starzyk PM. A retrospective cohort study of seatbelt use and pregnancy outcome after a motor vehicle crash. *J Trauma* 1993;34(1):116-119.

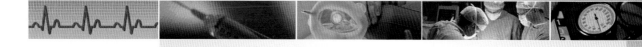

▶▶ Interactive Skill Procedure

Note: **Standard precautions are required when caring for trauma patients.**

A series of x-rays with related scenarios is provided at the conclusion of this section for use during this station in making evaluation and management decisions based on the findings.

The goal of splinting is to prevent further soft tissue injury and control bleeding and pain. Consider the immobilization of fractured extremities with the use of splints as "secondary resuscitation devices" that aid in the control of bleeding.

THE FOLLOWING PROCEDURES ARE INCLUDED IN THIS SKILL STATION:

▶▶ **Skill XII-A:** Physical Examination

▶▶ **Skill XII-B:** Principles of Extremity Immobilization

▶▶ **Skill XII-C:** Realigning a Deformed Extremity

▶▶ **Skill XII-D:** Application of a Traction Splint

▶▶ **Skill XII-E:** Compartment Syndrome: Assessment and Management

▶▶ **Skill XII-F:** Identification and Management of Pelvic Fractures

▶▶ **Skill XII-G:** Identification of Arterial Injury

Performance at this skill station will allow the participant to:

OBJECTIVES

 1 Perform a rapid assessment of the essential components of the musculoskeletal system.

2 Identify life-threatening and limb-threatening injuries of the musculoskeletal system, and institute appropriate initial management of these injuries.

 3 Identify patients who are at risk for compartment syndrome.

 4 Explain the indications for and the value of appropriate splinting of musculoskeletal injuries.

5 Apply standard splints to the extremities, including a traction splint.

6 List the complications associated with the use of splints.

 7 Identify pelvic instability associated with pelvic fracture.

8 Explain the value of the AP pelvic x-ray examination to identify the potential for massive blood loss, and describe the maneuvers that can be used to reduce pelvic volume and control bleeding.

▶ Skill XII-A: Physical Examination

▶▶ LOOK, GENERAL OVERVIEW

External hemorrhage is identified by obvious external bleeding from an extremity, pooling of blood on the stretcher or floor, blood-soaked dressings, and bleeding that occurs during transport to the hospital. The examiner needs to ask about characteristics of the injury incident and prehospital care. Remember, open wounds may not bleed, but may be indicative of nerve injury or an open fracture.

STEP 1. Splint deformed extremities, which are indicative of a fracture or joint injury, before patient transport or as soon as is safely possible.

STEP 2. Assess the color of the extremity. The presence of bruising indicates muscle injury or significant soft tissue injury over bones or joints. These changes may be associated with swelling or hematomas. Vascular impairment may be first identified by a pale distal extremity.

STEP 3. Note the position of the extremity, which can be helpful in determining certain injury patterns. Certain nerve deficits lead to specific positions of the extremity. For example, injury to the radial nerve results in wrist drop, and injury to the peroneal nerve results in foot drop.

STEP 4. Observe spontaneous activity to help determine the severity of injury. Observing whether the patient spontaneously moves an extremity may suggest to the examiner other obvious or occult injuries. An example is a patient with a brain injury who does not follow commands and has no spontaneous lower-extremity movement; this patient could have a thoracic or lumbar fracture.

STEP 5. Note gender and age, which are important clues to potential injuries. Children may sustain growth plate injuries and fractures that may not manifest themselves (eg, buckle fracture). Females are less likely to have urethral injuries than vaginal injuries with a pelvic fracture.

STEP 6. Observe drainage from the urinary catheter. If the urine is bloody or catheter insertion is difficult, the patient may have a pelvic fracture and a urologic injury.

▶▶ FEEL

Life- and limb-threatening injuries are excluded first.

STEP 1. Palpate the pelvis anteriorly and posteriorly to assess for deformity, motion, and/or a gap that indicates a potentially unstable pelvis. The compression-distraction and push-pull tests should be done only once. These tests are dangerous because they can dislodge clots and cause rebleeding.

STEP 2. Palpate pulses in all extremities and document the findings. Any perceived abnormality or difference must be explained. Normal capillary refill (<2 seconds) of the pulp space or nail bed provides a good indication of satisfactory blood flow to the distal parts of the extremity. Loss or diminishment of pulses with normal capillary refill indicates a viable extremity; however, surgical consultation is required. **If an extremity has no pulses and no capillary refill, a surgical emergency exists.** A Doppler device is useful to assess pulses and determine the ankle/arm systolic pressure ratio. Blood pressure is measured at the ankle and on an uninjured arm. The normal ratio exceeds 0.9. If the ratio is below 0.9, a potential injury exists and surgical consultation is required.

STEP 3. Palpate the muscle compartments of all the extremities for compartment syndromes and fractures. This is done by gentle palpation of the muscle and bone. If a fracture is present, the conscious patient reports pain. If the patient is unconscious, only abnormal motion may be felt. A compartment syndrome should be suspected if the muscle compartment is hard, firm, or tender. Compartment syndromes may be associated with fractures.

STEP 4. Assess joint stability by asking the cooperative patient to move the joint through a range of motion. This should not be done if there is an obvious fracture or deformity, or if the patient cannot cooperate. Palpate each joint for tenderness, swelling, and intraarticular fluid. Assess joint stability by applying lateral, medial, and anterior-posterior stress. Any deformed or dislocated joint should be splinted and x-rayed before testing for stability.

STEP 5. Perform a rapid, thorough neurologic examination of the extremities and document the findings. Repeat and record testing as indicated by the patient's clinical condition. Test sensation by light touch and pinprick in each of the extremities. Progression of the neurologic findings indicates a potential problem.

   A. C5—Lateral aspect of the upper arm (also axillary nerve)

B. C6—Palmar aspect of the thumb and index finger (median nerve)

C. C7—Palmar aspect of the long finger

D. C8—Palmar aspect of the little finger (ulnar nerve)

E. T1—Inner aspect of the forearm

F. L3—Inner aspect of the thigh

G. L4—Inner aspect of the lower leg, especially over the medial malleolus

H. L5—Dorsum of the foot between the first and second toes (common peroneal)

I. S1—Lateral aspect of the foot

STEP 6. Perform motor examination of the extremities.

A. Shoulder abduction—Axillary nerve, C5

B. Elbow flexion—Musculocutaneous nerve, C5 and C6

C. Elbow extension—Radial nerve, C6, C7, and C8

D. Hand and wrist—Power grip tests dorsiflexion of the wrist (radial nerve, C6) and flexion of the fingers (median and ulnar nerves, C7 and C8).

E. Finger add/abduction—Ulnar nerve, C8 and T1

F. Lower extremity—Dorsiflexion of the great toe and ankle tests the deep peroneal nerve, L5, and plantar dorsiflexion tests the posterior tibial nerve, S1.

G. Muscle power is graded in the standard form. The motor examination is specific to a variety of voluntary movements of each extremity.
See Chapter 7: Spine and Spinal Cord Trauma.

STEP 7. Assess the deep tendon reflexes.

STEP 8. Assess the patient's back.

▶ Skill XII-B: Principles of Extremity Immobilization

STEP 1. Assess the ABCDEs, and treat life-threatening situations first.

STEP 2. Remove all clothing and completely expose the patient, including the extremities. Remove watches, rings, bracelets, and other potentially constricting devices. Remember to prevent the development of hypothermia.

STEP 3. Assess the neurovascular status of the extremity before applying the splint. Assess for pulses and external hemorrhage, which must be controlled, and perform a motor and sensory examination of the extremity.

STEP 4. Cover any open wounds with sterile dressings.

STEP 5. Select the appropriate size and type of splint for the injured extremity. The device should immobilize the joint above and the joint below the injury site.

STEP 6. Apply padding over bony prominences that will be covered by the splint.

STEP 7. Splint the extremity in the position in which it is found if distal pulses are present in the injured extremity. If distal pulses are absent, one attempt should be made to realign the extremity. Gentle traction should be maintained until the splinting device is secured.

STEP 8. Place the extremity in a splint if normally aligned. If malaligned, the extremity needs to be realigned and then splinted. Do not force realignment of a deformed extremity. If it is not easily realigned, splint the extremity in the position in which it is found.

STEP 9. Obtain orthopedic consultation.

STEP 10. Document the neurovascular status of the extremity before and after every manipulation or splint application.

STEP 11. Administer appropriate tetanus prophylaxis.
See Appendix E: Tetanus Immunization.

▶ Skill XII-C: Realigning a Deformed Extremity

Physical examination determines whether a deformity is from a fracture or a dislocation. The principle of realigning an extremity fracture is to restore length by applying gentle longitudinal traction to correct the residual angulation and then rotational deformities. While maintaining realignment with manual traction, a splint is applied and secured to the extremity by an assistant.

▶▶ **HUMERUS**

STEP 1. Grasp the elbow and manually apply distal traction.

STEP 2. After alignment is obtained, apply a plaster splint and secure the arm to the chest wall with a sling and swath.

▶▶ FOREARM

STEP 1. Manually apply distal traction through the wrist while holding the elbow and applying countertraction.

STEP 2. Secure a splint to the forearm and elevate the injured extremity.

▶▶ FEMUR

STEP 1. Realign the femur by manually applying traction through the ankle if the tibia and fibula are not fractured.

STEP 2. As the muscle spasm is overcome, the leg will straighten and the rotational deformity can be corrected. This maneuver may take several minutes, depending on the size of the patient.

▶▶ TIBIA

STEP 1. Manually apply distal traction at the ankle and countertraction just above the knee, provided that the femur is intact

▶▶ VASCULAR AND NEUROLOGIC DEFICITS

Fractures associated with neurovascular deficits require prompt realignment. Immediate consultation with a surgeon is necessary. If the vascular or neurologic status worsens after realignment and splinting, the splint should be removed and the extremity returned to the position in which blood flow and neurologic status are maximized. The extremity is then immobilized in that position.

▶ Skill XII-D: Application of a Traction Splint

Note: Application of this device requires two people—one person to handle the injured extremity, and the second to apply the splint.

STEP 1. Remove all clothing, including footwear, to expose the extremity.

STEP 2. Apply sterile dressings to open wounds.

STEP 3. Assess the neurovascular status of the extremity.

STEP 4. Cleanse any exposed bone and muscle of dirt and debris before applying traction. Document that the exposed bone fragments were reduced into the soft tissues.

STEP 5. Determine the length of the splint by measuring the uninjured leg. The upper cushioned ring should be placed under the buttocks and adjacent to the ischial tuberosity. The distal end of the splint should extend beyond the ankle by approximately 6 inches (15 cm). The straps on the splint should be positioned to support the thigh and calf.

STEP 6. Align the femur by manually applying traction through the ankle. After realignment is achieved, gently elevate the leg to allow the assistant to slide the splint under the extremity so that the padded portion of the splint rests against the ischial tuberosity.

STEP 7. Reassess the neurovascular status of the distal injured extremity after applying traction.

STEP 8. Position the ankle hitch around the patient's ankle and foot while the assistant maintains manual traction on the leg. The bottom strap should be slightly shorter than, or at least the same length as, the two upper crossing straps.

STEP 9. Attach the ankle hitch to the traction hook while the assistant maintains manual traction and support. Apply traction in increments using the windlass knob until the extremity appears stable, or until pain and muscular spasm are relieved.

STEP 10. Reassess the neurovascular status of the injured extremity. If perfusion of the extremity distal to the injury appears worse after applying traction, gradually release the traction.

STEP 11. Secure the remaining straps.

STEP 12. Frequently reevaluate the neurovascular status of the extremity. Document the neurovascular status after every manipulation of the extremity.

STEP 13. Administer tetanus prophylaxis, as indicated.
◼ See Appendix E: Tetanus Immunization.

▶ Skill XII-E: Compartment Syndrome: Assessment and Management

STEP 1. Consider the following important facts:
- Compartment syndrome can develop insidiously.
- Compartment syndrome can develop in an extremity as the result of compression or crushing forces and without obvious external injury or fracture.
- Frequent reevaluation of the injured extremity is essential.
- The patient who has had hypotension or is unconscious is at increased risk for compartment syndrome.
- Pain is the earliest symptom that heralds the onset of compartment ischemia, especially pain on passive stretch of the involved muscles of the extremity.
- Unconscious or intubated patients cannot communicate the early signs of extremity ischemia.
- Loss of pulses and other classic findings of ischemia occur late, after irreversible damage has occurred.

STEP 2. Palpate the muscular compartments of the extremities, comparing the compartment tension in the injured extremity with that in the noninjured extremity.
- **A.** Asymmetry is a significant finding.
- **B.** Frequent examination for tense muscular compartments is essential.
- **C.** Measurement of compartment pressures is helpful.

STEP 3. Obtain orthopedic or general surgical consultation early.

▶ Skill XII-F: Identification and Management of Pelvic Fractures

STEP 1. Identify the mechanism of injury, which can suggest the possibility of a pelvic fracture—for example, ejection from a motor vehicle, crushing injury, pedestrian-vehicle collision, or motorcycle collision.

STEP 2. Inspect the pelvic area for ecchymosis, perineal or scrotal hematoma, and blood at the urethral meatus.

STEP 3. Inspect the legs for differences in length or asymmetry in rotation of the hips.

STEP 4. Perform a rectal examination, noting the position and mobility of the prostate gland, any palpable fracture, or the presence of gross or occult blood in the stool.

STEP 5. Perform a vaginal examination, noting palpable fractures, the size and consistency of the uterus, or the presence of blood. Remember, females of childbearing age may be pregnant.

STEP 6. If Steps 2 through 5 are abnormal, or if the mechanism of injury suggests a pelvic fracture, obtain an AP x-ray film of the patient's pelvis. (*Note:* The mechanism of injury may suggest the type of fracture.)

STEP 7. If Steps 2 through 5 are normal, palpate the bony pelvis to identify painful areas.

STEP 8. Determine pelvic stability by gently applying anterior-posterior compression and lateral-to-medial compression over the anterosuperior iliac crests. Testing for axial mobility by gently pushing and pulling on the legs will determine stability in a cranial-caudal direction. Immobilize the pelvis properly by using a sheet and/or a commercially available binder (eg, T-pod).

STEP 9. Cautiously insert a urinary catheter, if not contraindicated, or perform retrograde urethrography if a urethral injury is suspected.

STEP 10. Interpret the pelvic x-ray film, giving special consideration to fractures that are frequently associated with significant blood loss—for example, fractures that increase the pelvic volume.
- **A.** Confirm the patient's identification on the film.
- **B.** Systematically evaluate the film for:
  - Width of the symphysis pubis—greater than a 1-cm separation signifies significant posterior pelvic injury.
  - Integrity of the superior and inferior pubic rami bilaterally.
  - Integrity of the acetabula, as well as femoral heads and necks.
  - Symmetry of the ilium and width of the sacroiliac joints.

- Symmetry of the sacral foramina by evaluating the arcuate lines.
- Fracture(s) of the transverse processes of L5.

C. Remember, the bony pelvis is a ring that rarely sustains an injury in only one location. Displacement of ringed structures implies two fracture sites.

D. Remember, fractures that increase the pelvic volume—for example, vertical shear and open-book fractures, are often associated with massive blood loss.

▶▶ TECHNIQUES TO REDUCE BLOOD LOSS FROM PELVIC FRACTURES

STEP 1. Avoid excessive and repeated manipulation of the pelvis.

STEP 2. Internally rotate the lower legs to close an open-book type fracture. Pad bony prominences and tie the rotated legs together. This maneuver can reduce a displaced symphysis, decrease the pelvic volume, and serve as a temporary measure until definitive treatment can be provided.

STEP 3. Apply a pelvic external fixation device (early orthopedic consultation).

STEP 4. Apply skeletal limb traction (early orthopedic consultation).

STEP 5. Embolize pelvic vessels via angiography.

STEP 6. Obtain early surgical and orthopedic consultation to determine priorities.

STEP 7. Place sandbags under each buttock if there is no indication of spinal injury and other techniques to close the pelvis are not available.

STEP 8. Apply a pelvic binder.

STEP 9. Arrange for transfer to a definitive-care facility if local resources are not available to manage this injury.

▶ Skill XII-G: Identification of Arterial Injury

STEP 1. Recognize that ischemia is a limb-threatening and potentially life-threatening condition.

STEP 2. Palpate peripheral pulses bilaterally (dorsalis pedis, anterior tibial, femoral, radial, and brachial) for quality and symmetry.

STEP 3. Document and evaluate any evidence of asymmetry in peripheral pulses.

STEP 4. Reevaluate peripheral pulses frequently, especially if asymmetry is identified. Use Doppler imaging to assess the presence and quality of distal pulses.

STEP 5. Obtain early surgical consultation.

▶ SCENARIOS

SCENARIO XII-1

A 28-year-old man is involved in a head-on motorcycle collision with a car. At the scene, he was combative, his systolic blood pressure was 80 mm Hg, his heart rate 120 beats/min, and his respiratory rate 20 breaths/min. In the ED, his vital signs have returned to normal, and the patient reports pain in his right upper extremity and both lower extremities. His right thigh and left lower extremity are deformed. Prehospital personnel report a large laceration to the left leg, to which they applied a dressing.

SCENARIO XII-2

Scenario A: A 20-year-old woman is found trapped in her automobile. Several hours are required to extricate her because her leg was trapped and twisted beneath the dashboard. In the hospital, she has no hemodynamic abnormalities and is alert. She reports severe pain in her left leg, which is splinted.

Scenario B: A 34-year-old man is shot in the right leg while cleaning his handgun. He is unable to walk because of knee pain and states that his lower extremity is painful, weak, and numb.

SCENARIO XII-3

A 16-year-old boy is thrown approximately 100 feet (33 meters) from the back of a pickup truck. In the ED his skin is cool, and he is lethargic and unresponsive. His systolic blood pressure is 75 mm Hg, his heart rate is 145 beats/min, and his respirations are rapid and shallow. Breath sounds are equal and clear on auscultation. Two large-caliber IVs are initiated, and 2500 mL of warmed crystalloid solution is infused. However, the patient's hemodynamic status does not improve significantly. His blood pressure now is 84/58 mm Hg and his heart rate is 135 beats/min.

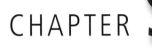

CHAPTER 9 · Thermal Injuries

Upon completion of this topic, the student will be able to identify methods of assessment and outline measures to stabilize, treat, and transfer patients with thermal injuries. Specifically, the doctor will be able to:

OBJECTIVES

 Given a patient with burn injury, estimate the burn size and determine the presence of associated injuries.

 Demonstrate the initial assessment and treatment of patients with thermal injuries.

 Identify special problems encountered in the treatment of patients with thermal injuries, and explain how to resolve them.

 List criteria for the transfer of patients with burns.

Introduction

Thermal injuries are major causes of morbidity and mortality. Attention to the basic principles of initial trauma resuscitation and timely application of simple emergency measures can help to minimize the morbidity and mortality caused by these injuries. These principles include a high index of suspicion for the presence of airway compromise following smoke inhalation, identification and management of associated mechanical injuries, and maintenance of hemodynamic normality with volume resuscitation. The doctor also must take measures to prevent and treat the potential complications of thermal injuries, such as rhabdomyolysis and cardiac dysrhythmias, which are sometimes seen in electrical burns. Temperature control and removal from the injury-provoking environment also are major principles of thermal injury management.

Immediate Lifesaving Measures for Burn Injuries

? What is my first priority?

Lifesaving measures for patients with burn injuries include establishing airway control, stopping the burning process, and establishing intravenous access.

AIRWAY

? How do I identify inhalation injury?

Although the larynx protects the subglottic airway from direct thermal injury, the airway is extremely susceptible to obstruction as a consequence of exposure to heat. Airway

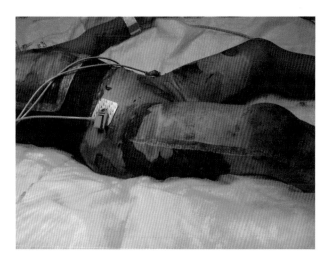

obstruction may not be obvious immediately; however, signs may be present that can warn the examiner of potential airway obstruction. When a patient is admitted to the hospital after sustaining a burn injury, the doctor should be alert to the possibility of airway involvement, identify signs of distress, and initiate supportive measures. Clinical indications of inhalation injury include:

- Face and/or neck burns
- Singeing of the eyebrows and nasal vibrissae
- Carbon deposits and acute inflammatory changes in the oropharynx
- Carbonaceous sputum
- Hoarseness
- History of impaired mentation and/or confinement in a burning environment
- Explosion with burns to head and torso
- Carboxyhemoglobin level greater than 10% in patient who was involved in a fire

Any of the above findings suggests inhalation injury. **Transfer to a burn center is indicated if there is inhalation injury. If the transport time is prolonged, intubation should be performed prior to transport to protect the airway. The symptom of stridor is an indication for immediate endotracheal intubation. Circumferential burns of the neck can lead to swelling of the tissues around the airway. Therefore, early intubation is indicated in this situation.**

STOP THE BURNING PROCESS

All clothing should be removed to stop the burning process; however, do not peel off adherent clothing. Synthetic fabrics can ignite, burn rapidly at high temperatures, and melt into hot residue that continues to burn the patient. Any clothing that was burned by chemicals should be removed carefully. Dry chemical powders should be brushed from the wound, with the individual caring for the patient avoiding direct contact with the chemical, and the involved body-surface areas should be rinsed with copious amounts of tap water. The patient then should be covered with warm, clean, dry linens to prevent hypothermia.

INTRAVENOUS ACCESS

Any patient with burns over more than 20% of the body surface requires fluid resuscitation. After establishing airway patency and identifying and treating immediately life-threatening injuries, intravenous access must be established. Large-caliber (at least #16-gauge) intravenous lines should be introduced immediately in a peripheral vein. If the extent of the burn precludes placement of the catheter through unburned skin, overlying burned skin should not deter placement of the catheter in an accessible vein. The upper extremities are preferable to the lower extremities for venous access because of the high incidence of phlebitis and septic phlebitis when saphenous veins are used for venous access. Begin infusion with an isotonic crystalloid solution. Guidelines for establishing the flow rate are outlined later in this chapter.

Assessment of Patients with Burns

The assessment of patients with burn injuries begins with the patient history and is followed by estimation of the body-surface area burned and the depth of the burn injury.

HISTORY

The injury history is extremely valuable in the treatment of the burn patient. Associated injuries can be sustained while the victim attempts to escape the fire, and injury from explosions can result in internal injuries or fractures (eg, central nervous system, myocardial, pulmonary, and abdominal injuries). It is essential that the time of the burn injury be established. Burns sustained within an enclosed space suggest the potential for inhalation injury.

The history, from the patient or a relative, should include a brief survey of preexisting illnesses (eg, diabetes, hypertension, cardiac, pulmonary, and/or renal disease) and drug therapy, as well as any allergies and drug sensitivities. The patient's tetanus immunization status also should be ascertained.

BODY-SURFACE AREA

> **? How do I estimate burn size and depth?**

The Rule of Nines is a useful and practical guide to determine the extent of the burn (Figure 9-1). The adult body configuration is divided into anatomic regions that represent 9%, or multiples of 9%, of the total body surface. Body-surface area (BSA) differs considerably for children. The infant's or young child's head represents a larger proportion of the surface area, and the lower extremities represent a smaller proportion than an adult's. The percentage of total body surface of the infant's head is twice that of the normal adult. **The palmar surface (including the fingers) of the patient's hand represents approximately 1% of the patient's body surface.** This guideline helps estimate the extent of burns with irregular outlines or distribution.

DEPTH OF BURN

The depth of burn is important in evaluating the severity of the burn, planning for wound care, and predicting functional and cosmetic results.

First-degree burns (eg, sunburn) are characterized by erythema, pain, and the absence of blisters. They are not life-threatening, and generally do not require intravenous fluid replacement. This type of burn is not discussed further in this chapter.

Partial-thickness, or second-degree, burns are characterized by a red or mottled appearance with associated swelling and blister formation (Figure 9-2A). The surface can have a weeping, wet appearance and is painfully hypersensitive, even to air current.

Full-thickness, or third-degree, burns usually appear dark and leathery (Figure 9-2B). The skin also may appear translucent, mottled, or waxy white. The surface is painless and generally dry; it may be red and does not blanch with pressure.

Primary Survey and Resuscitation of Patients with Burns

AIRWAY

A history of confinement in a burning environment or early signs of airway injury on arrival in the emergency department (ED) necessitate evaluation of the airway and definitive management. Pharyngeal thermal injuries can produce marked upper airway edema, and early maintenance of the airway is important. The clinical manifestations of inhalation injury may be subtle, and frequently do not appear in the first 24 hours. If the doctor waits for x-ray evidence of pulmonary injury or change in blood gas determinations, airway edema can preclude intubation, and a surgical airway may be required.

BREATHING

The initial treatment of airway injuries is based on the signs and symptoms, which can result from the following possible injuries:

- Direct thermal injury, producing upper airway edema and/or obstruction

- Inhalation of products of combustion (carbon particles) and toxic fumes, leading to chemical tracheobronchitis, edema, and pneumonia

- Carbon monoxide (CO) poisoning

Always assume CO exposure in patients who were burned in enclosed areas. The diagnosis of CO poisoning is

Pediatric

Adult

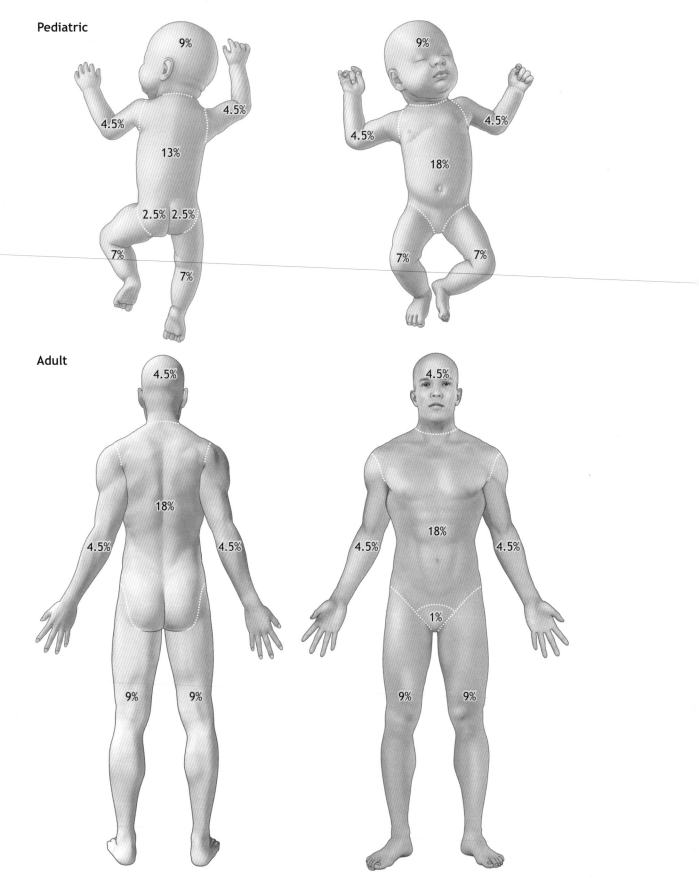

■ **Figure 9-1 Rule of Nines**. This practical guide is used to evaluate the severity of burns and determine fluid management. The adult body is generally divided into surface areas of 9% each and/or fractions or multiples of 9%.

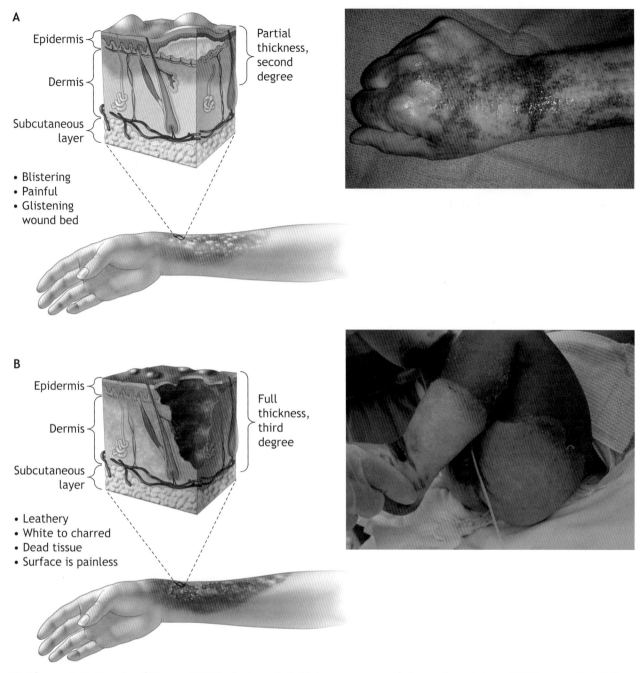

A

Epidermis

Dermis

Subcutaneous layer

Partial thickness, second degree

- Blistering
- Painful
- Glistening wound bed

B

Epidermis

Dermis

Subcutaneous layer

Full thickness, third degree

- Leathery
- White to charred
- Dead tissue
- Surface is painless

■ **Figure 9-2 Depth of Burns. (A)** Shallow partial-thickness or second-degree burn injury. **(B)** Deep partial, full-thickness or third-degree burn injury.

made primarily from a history of exposure and direct measurement of carboxyhemoglobin (HbCO). Patients with CO levels of less than 20% usually have no physical symptoms. Higher CO levels can result in: (1) headache and nausea (20%–30%), (2) confusion (30%–40%), (3) coma (40%–60%), and (4) death (>60%). Cherry-red skin color is rare. Because of the increased affinity of CO for hemoglobin (240 times that of oxygen), it displaces oxygen from the hemoglobin molecule and shifts the oxyhemoglobin dis-

sociation curve to the left. CO dissociates very slowly, and its half-life is 250 minutes (4 hours) while the patient is breathing room air, compared with 40 minutes while breathing 100% oxygen. Therefore, patients in whom CO exposure is suspected should receive high-flow oxygen via a nonrebreathing mask.

Early management of inhalation injury may require endotracheal intubation and mechanical ventilation. Prior to intubation, the patient should be preoxygenated with con-

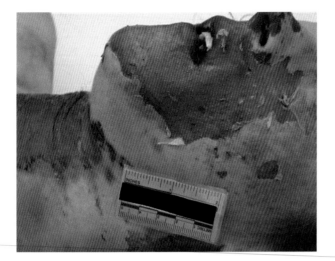

tinuous administration of oxygen. Intubation should be performed early in patients with suspected airway injury. Because there is a high probability of the need for bronchoscopy in burn patients with airway injury, an endotracheal tube of sufficient size should be chosen for a definitive airway. Arterial blood gas determinations should be obtained as a baseline for the evaluation of the patient's pulmonary status. However, measurements of arterial PaO_2 do not reliably predict CO poisoning, because a CO partial pressure of only 1 mm Hg results in a carboxyhemoglobin level of 40% or greater. Therefore, baseline carboxyhemoglobin levels should be obtained, and 100% oxygen should be administered.

If the patient's hemodynamic condition permits and spinal injury has been excluded, elevation of the head and chest by 30 degrees helps to reduce neck and chest wall edema. If a full-thickness burn of the anterior and lateral chest wall leads to severe restriction of the chest wall motion, even in the absence of a circumferential burn, chest wall escharotomy may be required.

CIRCULATING BLOOD VOLUME

❓ What is the rate and type of fluids administered to patients with burns?

Evaluation of circulating blood volume is often difficult in severely burned patients. In addition, these patients may have accompanying injuries that cause hypovolemic shock. Shock should be treated according to resuscitation principles as previously outlined. ◾ See Chapter 3: Shock. Burn resuscitation fluids also should be provided.

Blood pressure measurements can be difficult to obtain and may be unreliable in patients with severe burn injuries, but monitoring of hourly urinary outputs can reliably assess circulating blood volume in the absence of osmotic di-

uresis (eg, glycosuria). Therefore, an indwelling urinary catheter should be inserted. A good rule to follow is to infuse fluids at a rate sufficient to produce 1.0 mL of urine per kilogram of body weight per hour for children who weigh 30 kg or less, and 0.5 to 1.0 mL of urine per kilogram of body weight per hour in adults.

Patients with burns require 2 to 4 mL of Ringer's lactate solution per kilogram of body weight per percent of second-degree and third-degree body-surface burns in the first 24 hours to maintain an adequate circulating blood volume and provide adequate renal perfusion. The calculated fluid volume is then proportioned in the following manner: half the total fluid is provided in the first 8 hours after the burn injury has occurred, and the remaining half is administered in the next 16 hours. **In children who weigh 30 kg or less, the goal is to maintain an average urinary output of 1 mL/kg/hr. In these patients, it is necessary to administer maintenance intravenous fluids containing glucose in addition to the burn formula.**

Resuscitation formulas provide only an estimate of fluid need. Fluid requirement calculations for infusion rates are based on the time from injury, not urinary output from the time fluid resuscitation is initiated. The amount of fluid given should be adjusted according to the individual patient's response—ie, urinary output, vital signs, and general condition. Cardiac dysrhythmias may be the first sign of hypoxia and electrolyte or acid-base abnormalities. Electrocardiography (ECG) should be performed for cardiac rhythm disturbances. Persistent acidemia may be caused by cyanide poisoning. Consultation with a burn center or poison control center should occur if this diagnosis is suspected.

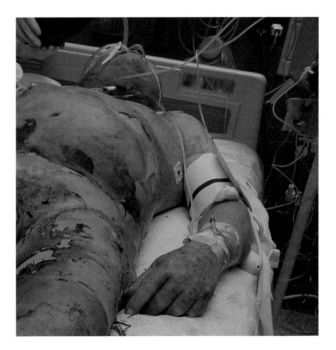

PITFALLS

- Failure to recognize the increased fluid requirement for patients with inhalation injury and those with concomitant blunt or crush trauma and for pediatric burn patients.
- Failure to adjust the fluid administration rate based on a patient's physiologic response.

Secondary Survey and Related Adjuncts

Key aspects of the secondary survey and its related adjuncts include physical examination; documentation; baseline determinations, including blood levels and x-rays; maintenance of peripheral circulation in circumferential extremity burns; gastric tube insertion; narcotics, analgesics, and sedatives; wound care; antibiotics; and tetanus immunization.

PHYSICAL EXAMINATION

In order to plan and direct patient treatment, the doctor must estimate the extent and depth of the burn, assess for associated injuries, and weigh the patient.

DOCUMENTATION

A flow sheet or other report that outlines the patient's treatment should be initiated when the patient is admitted to the ED. This flow sheet should accompany the patient when transferred to the burn unit.

BASELINE DETERMINATIONS FOR PATIENTS WITH MAJOR BURNS

Obtain samples for a complete blood count (CBC), type and crossmatch/screen, carboxyhemoglobin, serum glucose, electrolytes, and pregnancy test in all females of childbearing age. Arterial blood samples also should be obtained for blood gas determinations to include measurement of HbCO.

A chest film also should be obtained, with repeat films as necessary. Other x-rays may be indicated for appraisal of associated injuries.

PERIPHERAL CIRCULATION IN CIRCUMFERENTIAL EXTREMITY BURNS

In order to maintain peripheral circulation in patients with circumferential extremity burns, the doctor should:

1. Remove all jewelry on the patient's extremities.

2. Assess the status of distal circulation, checking for cyanosis, impaired capillary refilling, and progressive neurologic signs, such as paresthesia and deep-tissue pain. Assessment of peripheral pulses in patients with burns is best performed with a Doppler ultrasonic flow meter.

3. Relieve circulatory compromise in a circumferentially burned limb by escharotomy, always with surgical consultation. Escharotomies usually are not needed within the first 6 hours after a burn injury.

4. Although fasciotomy is seldom required, it may be necessary to restore circulation for patients with associated skeletal trauma, crush injury, high-voltage electrical injury, and burns involving tissue beneath the investing fascia.

GASTRIC TUBE INSERTION

Insert a gastric tube and attach it to a suction setup if the patient experiences nausea, vomiting, or abdominal distention, or if burns involve more than 20% of the total BSA. Prior to transfer, it is essential that a gastric tube be inserted and functioning in patients with these symptoms.

NARCOTICS, ANALGESICS, AND SEDATIVES

Severely burned patients may be restless and anxious from hypoxemia or hypovolemia rather than pain. Consequently, hypoxemia and inadequate fluid resuscitation should be managed before administration of narcotic analgesics or sedatives, which can mask the signs of hypoxemia and hypovolemia. Narcotics, analgesics, and sedatives should be administered in small, frequent doses by the intravenous route only.

WOUND CARE

Partial-thickness burns are painful when air currents pass over the burned surface. Gently covering the burn with clean linen relieves the pain and deflects air currents. Do not break blisters or apply an antiseptic agent. Any applied medication must be removed before appropriate antibacterial topical agents can be applied. Application of cold compresses can cause hypothermia. Do *not* apply cold water to a patient with extensive burns (>10% total BSA).

ANTIBIOTICS

Prophylactic antibiotics are not indicated in the early postburn period. Antibiotics should be reserved for the treatment of infection.

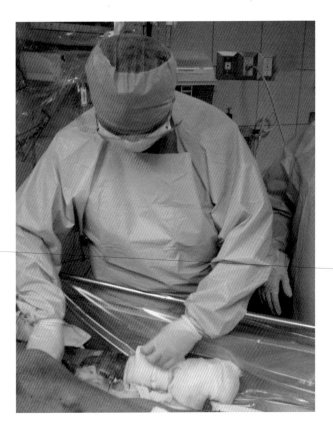

TETANUS

Determination of the patient's tetanus immunization status is very important. ■ See Appendix E: Tetanus Immunization.

Special Burn Requirements

Patients with chemical burns and electrical burns require special considerations in the ED and trauma care settings.

CHEMICAL BURNS

Chemical injury can result from exposure to acids, alkalies, and petroleum products. Alkali burns are generally

PITFALLS

- Failure to recognize development of the compartment syndrome.
- Failure to adequately perform escharotomy.
- Lack of recognition that fasciotomies are seldom necessary.
- Failure to treat CO toxicity.
- Failure to provide adequate pain relief.

more serious than acid burns, because the alkalies penetrate more deeply. Removal of the chemical and immediate attention to wound care are essential. Chemical burns are influenced by the duration of contact, concentration of the chemical, and amount of the agent. Immediately flush away the chemical with large amounts of water, for at least 20 to 30 minutes, using a shower or hose if available (Figure 9-3). Alkali burns require longer irrigation. If dry powder is still present on the skin, brush it away *before* irrigating with water. Neutralizing agents offer no advantage over water lavage, because reaction with the neutralizing agent can itself produce heat and cause further tissue damage. Alkali burns to the eye require continuous irrigation during the first 8 hours after the burn. A small-caliber cannula can be fixed in the palpebral sulcus for irrigation.

ELECTRICAL BURNS

Electrical burns result when a source of electrical power makes contact with a patient's body. Electrical burns frequently are more serious than they appear on the body surface. The body can serve as a volume conductor of electrical energy, and the heat generated results in thermal injury to tissue. Different rates of heat loss from superficial and deep tissues allow for relatively normal overlying skin to coexist with deep-muscle necrosis. Rhabdomyolysis results in myoglobin release, which can cause acute renal failure. Immediate treatment of a patient with a significant electrical burn includes attention to the airway and breathing, establishment of an intravenous line in an uninvolved extremity, electrocardiographic monitoring, and placement of an indwelling catheter. If the urine is dark, assume that hemochromogens are in the urine. Do not wait for laboratory confirmation before instituting therapy for myoglobinuria.

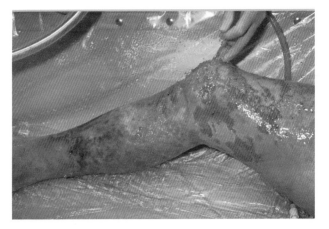

■ **Figure 9-3 Chemical Burn.** Immediately flush away the chemical with large amounts of water, for at least 20 to 30 minutes.

Fluid administration should be increased to ensure a urinary output of 100 mL/hr in adults. If the pigment does not clear with increased fluid administration, 25 g of mannitol should be administered, and 12.5 g of mannitol should be added to subsequent liters of fluid to maintain diuresis. Metabolic acidosis should be corrected by maintaining adequate perfusion and adding sodium bicarbonate to alkalize the urine as necessary and increase the solubility of myoglobin in the urine.

Patient Transfer

❓ *Who do I transfer to a burn center?*

The criteria for transfer must be met and procedures must be followed in the transfer of patients to burn centers.

CRITERIA FOR TRANSFER

The American Burn Association has identified the following types of burn injuries that typically require referral to a burn center:

1. Partial-thickness and full-thickness burns of greater than 10% of the BSA in patients less than 10 years or over 50 years of age

2. Partial-thickness and full-thickness burns on greater than 20% of the BSA in other age groups

3. Partial-thickness and full-thickness burns involving the face, eyes, ears, hands, feet, genitalia, and perineum, as well as those that involve skin overlying major joints

4. Full-thickness burns on greater than 5% of the BSA in any age group

5. Significant electrical burns, including lightning injury (significant volumes of tissue beneath the surface can be injured and result in acute renal failure and other complications)

6. Significant chemical burns

7. Inhalation injury

8. Burn injury in patients with preexisting illness that could complicate treatment, prolong recovery, or affect mortality

9. Any patient with a burn injury who has concomitant trauma poses an increased risk of morbidity or mortality, and may be treated initially in a trauma center until stable before being transferred to a burn center

PITFALLS

- Failure to secure the patient's airway.
- Failure to provide adequate documentation of treatment to the receiving facility.

10. Children with burn injuries who are seen in hospitals without qualified personnel or equipment to manage their care should be transferred to a burn center with these capabilities

11. Burn injury in patients who will require special social and emotional or long-term rehabilitative support, including cases involving suspected child abuse and neglect

TRANSFER PROCEDURES

Transfer of any patient must be coordinated with the burn center doctor. All pertinent information regarding test results, temperature, pulse, fluids administered, and urinary output should be documented on the burn/trauma flow sheet and sent with the patient. Any other information deemed important by the referring or receiving doctor also is sent with the patient.

Cold Injury: Local Tissue Effects

❓ *How does cold affect my patient?*

The severity of cold injury depends on temperature, duration of exposure, environmental conditions, amount of protective clothing, and the patient's general state of health. Lower temperatures, immobilization, prolonged exposure, moisture, the presence of peripheral vascular disease, and open wounds all increase the severity of the injury.

TYPES OF COLD INJURY

❓ *How do I recognize a cold injury?*

Three types of cold injury are seen in trauma patients: frostnip, frostbite, and nonfreezing injury.

Frostnip

Frostnip is the mildest form of cold injury. It is characterized by initial pain, pallor, and numbness of the affected body part. It is reversible with rewarming and does not result in tissue loss, unless the injury is repeated over many years, which causes fat pad loss or atrophy.

Frostbite

Frostbite is due to freezing of tissue with intracellular ice crystal formations, microvascular occlusion, and subsequent tissue anoxia. Some of the tissue damage also can result from reperfusion injury that occurs on rewarming. Similar to thermal burns, frostbite is classified into first-degree, second-degree, third-degree, and fourth-degree according to depth of involvement.

1. First-degree frostbite: Hyperemia and edema without skin necrosis

2. Second-degree frostbite: Large, clear vesicle formation accompanies the hyperemia and edema with partial-thickness skin necrosis

3. Third-degree frostbite: Full-thickness and subcutaneous tissue necrosis occurs, commonly with hemorrhage vesicle formation

4. Fourth-degree frostbite: Full-thickness skin necrosis, including muscle and bone with gangrene

Although the affected body part is typically initially hard, cold, white, and numb, the appearance of the lesion changes frequently during the course of treatment. In addition, the initial treatment regimen is applicable for all degrees of insult, and the initial classification is often not prognostically accurate. Hence, some authorities simply classify frostbite as superficial or deep.

Nonfreezing Injury

Nonfreezing injury is due to microvascular endothelial damage, stasis, and vascular occlusion. Trench foot or cold immersion foot (or hand) describes a nonfreezing injury of the hands or feet, typically in soldiers, sailors, and fishermen, resulting from long-term exposure to wet conditions and temperatures just above freezing (1.6° C to 10° C, or 35° F to 50° F). Although the entire foot can appear black, deep-tissue destruction may not be present. Alternating arterial vasospasm and vasodilation occur, with the affected tissue first cold and numb, and then progressing to hyperemia in 24 to 48 hours. With hyperemia comes intense, painful burning and dysesthesia, as well as tissue damage characterized by edema, blistering, redness, ecchymosis, and ulcerations. Complications of local infection, cellulitis, lymphangitis, and gangrene can occur. Proper attention to foot hygiene can prevent the occurrence of most such injuries.

Chilblain, or pernio, is primarily a dermatologic manifestation of chronic, repetitive, damp cold exposure, or long-term, dry cold exposure, as might occur in mountain climbers. It typically occurs on the face, anterior tibial muscle surface, and dorsum of the hands and feet, which are areas that are poorly protected or chronically exposed to the environment. It is characterized by pruritic, red-purple skin lesions (papules, macules, plaques, or nodules). With continued exposure, ulcerative or hemorrhagic lesions appear and progress to scarring, fibrosis, or atrophy, with itching replaced by tenderness and pain. This condition is more annoying and chronic than destructive. Careful protection from further exposure and the use of antiadrenergics or calcium-channel blockers are often helpful.

MANAGEMENT OF FROSTBITE AND NONFREEZING COLD INJURIES

❓ *How do I treat local cold injuries?*

Treatment should be immediate to decrease the duration of tissue freezing, although rewarming should not be undertaken if there is the risk of refreezing. Constricting, damp clothing should be replaced by warm blankets, and the patient should be given hot fluids by mouth, if he or she is able to drink.

Place the injured part in circulating water at a constant 40° C (104° F) until pink color and perfusion return (usually within 20 to 30 minutes). This is best accomplished in an inpatient setting in a large tank, such as a whirlpool tank. Avoid dry heat, and do not rub or massage the area. Rewarming can be extremely painful, and adequate analgesics (intravenous narcotics) are essential. Cardiac monitoring during rewarming is advised.

Local Wound Care of Frostbite

The goal of wound care for frostbite is to preserve damaged tissue by preventing infection, avoiding opening uninfected vesicles, and elevating the injured area, which is left open to air. The affected tissue should be protected by a tent or cradle, and pressure spots should be avoided.

Only rarely is fluid loss massive enough to require resuscitation with intravenous fluids, although patients may be dehydrated. Tetanus prophylaxis depends on the patient's tetanus immunization status. Systemic antibiotics are reserved for identified infections. The wounds should be kept clean, and uninfected blebs left intact for 7 to 10 days to provide a sterile biologic dressing to protect underlying epithelialization. Tobacco, nicotine, and other vasoconstrictive agents must be withheld. Weight bearing is prohibited until edema is resolved.

Numerous adjuvants have been attempted in an effort to restore blood supply to cold-injured tissue. Unfortunately, most are ineffective. Sympathetic blockade (sympathectomy, drugs) and vasodilating agents have generally not proven helpful in altering the natural history of the acute cold injury. Heparin and hyperbaric oxygen also have failed to demonstrate substantial treatment benefit. Low-molecular-weight dextran has shown some benefit during the re-

PITFALLS

- Failure to rapidly rewarm the affected area.
- Overzealous debridement of tissue of questionable viability.

warming phase in animal models. Thrombolytic agents have also shown some promise.

With all cold injuries, estimations of depth of injury and extent of tissue damage are not usually accurate until demarcation is evident. This often requires several weeks or months of observation. Earlier surgical debridement or amputation is seldom necessary, unless infection with sepsis occurs.

Cold Injury: Systemic Hypothermia

Hypothermia is defined as a core body temperature below 35° C (95° F). In the absence of concomitant traumatic injury, hypothermia may be classified as mild (35° C to 32° C, or 95° F to 89.6° F), moderate (32° C to 30° C, or 89.6° F to 86° F), or severe (below 30° C, or 86° F). This drop in core temperature can be rapid, as in immersion in near-freezing water, or slow, as in exposure to more temperate environments.

The elderly are particularly susceptible to hypothermia because of their impaired ability to increase heat production and decrease heat loss by vasoconstriction. Children also are more susceptible because of their relative increased BSA and limited energy sources. Trauma patients also are susceptible to hypothermia, and *any* degree of hypothermia in trauma patients can be detrimental. In trauma pa-

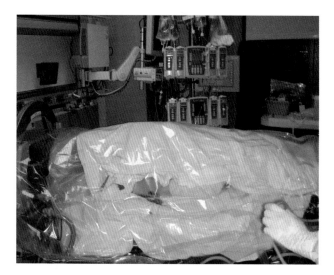

tients, hypothermia should be considered to be any core temperature below 36° C (96.8° F), and severe hypothermia is any core temperature below 32° C (89.6° F). Hypothermia is common in the severely injured, but further loss of core temperature can be limited with the administration of *only* warmed intravenous fluids and blood, judicious exposure of the patient, and maintenance of a warm environment.

Because determination of the core temperature, preferably esophageal, is essential for the diagnosis of systemic hypothermia, special thermometers capable of registering low temperatures are required.

SIGNS

In addition to a decrease in core temperature, a depressed level of consciousness is the most common feature of hypothermia. The patient is cold to the touch and appears gray and cyanotic. Vital signs, including pulse rate, respiratory rate, and blood pressure, are all variable, and the absence of respiratory or cardiac activity is not uncommon in patients who eventually recover. Because of severe depression of the respiratory rate and heart rate, signs of respiratory and cardiac activity are easily missed unless careful assessment is conducted.

MANAGEMENT

? *How do I treat a systemic cold injury?*

Immediate attention is devoted to the ABCDEs, including the initiation of cardiopulmonary resuscitation (CPR) and establishment of intravenous access if the patient is in cardiopulmonary arrest. Care must be taken to identify the presence of an organized cardiac rhythm; if one exists, sufficient circulation in patients with markedly reduced metabolism is likely present, and vigorous chest compressions can convert this rhythm to fibrillation. In the absence of an organized rhythm, CPR should be instituted and continued until the patient is rewarmed or there are other indications to discontinue CPR. However, the exact role of CPR as an adjunct to rewarming remains controversial.

Prevent heat loss by removing the patient from the cold environment and replacing wet, cold clothing with warm blankets. Administer oxygen via a bag-reservoir device. The patient should be treated in a critical care setting whenever possible. Cardiac monitoring is required. A careful search for associated disorders—such as diabetes, sepsis, and drug or alcohol ingestion—or occult injuries should be conducted, and the disorders should be treated promptly. Blood should be drawn for CBC, electrolytes, blood glucose, alcohol, toxins screen, creatinine, amylase, and blood cultures. Abnormalities should be treated accordingly; for example, hypoglycemia requires intravenous glucose administration.

Determination of death can be very difficult in patients with hypothermia. Patients who appear to have suffered a cardiac arrest or death as a result of hypothermia should not be pronounced dead until they have been rewarmed. **Remember the axiom: You are not dead until you are warm and dead!** An exception to this rule is the patient with hypothermia who has sustained an anoxic event while still normothermic, who has no pulse or respiration, and who has a serum potassium level greater than 10 mmol/L.

The appropriate rewarming technique depends on the patient's temperature and his or her response to simpler measures, as well as the presence or absence of concomitant injuries. For example, treat mild and moderate exposure hypothermia with passive external rewarming in a warm room using warm blankets and clothing and warmed intravenous fluids. Severe hypothermia may require active core rewarming methods, which may include invasive surgical rewarming techniques such as peritoneal lavage, thoracic/pleural lavage, arteriovenous rewarming, and cardiopulmonary bypass, all of which are best accomplished in a critical care setting.

Cardiac output falls in proportion to the degree of hypothermia, and cardiac irritability begins at about 33° C (91.4° F). Ventricular fibrillation becomes increasingly common as the temperature falls below 28° C (82.4° F), and at temperatures below 25° C (77° F) asystole can occur. Cardiac drugs and defibrillation are not usually effective in the presence of acidosis, hypoxia, and hypothermia. In general, these treatment methods should be postponed until the patient is warmed to at least 28° C (82.4° F). Bretylium tosylate is the only dysrhythmia agent known to be effective; lidocaine is ineffective in patients with hypothermia who have ventricular fibrillation. Dopamine is the single inotropic agent that has some degree of action in patients with hypothermia. Administer 100% oxygen while the patient is being rewarmed. Arterial blood gases are probably best interpreted "uncorrected"—that is, the blood warmed to 37° C (98.6° F), with the values used as guides to administering sodium bicarbonate and adjusting ventilation parameters during rewarming and resuscitation. Attempts to actively rewarm the patient should not delay transfer to a critical care setting.

PITFALL

Failure to adequately rewarm patients.

CHAPTER SUMMARY

1 The Rule of Nines is a useful and practical guide to determine the extent of the burn. The adult body configuration is divided into anatomic regions that represent 9%, or multiples of 9%, of the total body surface. Body-surface area differs considerably for children. The infant's or young child's head represents a larger proportion of the surface area, and the lower extremities represent a smaller proportion than an adult's. This guideline helps estimate the extent of burns with irregular outlines or distribution. Associated injuries can be sustained while the victim attempts to escape the fire, and injury from explosions can result in internal injuries or fractures (eg, central nervous system, myocardial, pulmonary, and abdominal injuries).

2 Immediate lifesaving measures for patients with burn injury include the recognition of inhalation injury and subsequent endotracheal intubation, and the rapid institution of intravenous fluid therapy. All clothing should be removed rapidly. Early stabilization and treatment of the burn patient include identifying the extent and depth of the burn, establishing fluid guidelines according to the patient's weight, initiating a patient-care flow sheet, obtaining baseline laboratory and x-ray studies, maintaining peripheral circulation in circumferential burns by performing an escharotomy if necessary, and identifying which burn patients require transfer to a burn unit or center.

Diagnose the cause and severity of cold injury by obtaining an adequate history and noting the physical findings, as well as measuring the core temperature using a low-temperature range thermometer (esophageal temperature probe is preferred). The patient should be removed from the cold environment immediately, and vital signs should be monitored and supported continuously. Rewarming techniques should be applied as soon as possible. The patient with hypothermia should not be considered dead until rewarming has occurred. Early management of cold-injured patients includes: adhering to the ABCDEs of resuscitation, identifying the type and extent of cold injury, measuring the patient's core temperature, initiating a patient-care flow sheet, initiating rapid rewarming techniques, and determining the patient's life or death status after rewarming.

3 Attention must be paid to special problems unique to thermal injuries. Carbon monoxide poisoning should be suspected and identified. Circumferential burns may require escarotomy. Chemical burns require immediate removal of clothing to prevent further injury and copious irrigation. Electrical burns may be associated with extensive occult myonecrosis. Patients sustaining thermal injury are at risk for hypothermia. Judicious analgesia should not be overlooked.

4 The American Burn Association has identified the following types of burn injuries that typically require referral to a burn center: (1) Partial-thickness and full-thickness burns on greater than 10% of the total BSA in patients less than 10 years or over 50 years of age; (2) partial-thickness and full-thickness burns on greater than 20% of the BSA in other age groups; (3) partial-thickness and full-thickness burns involving the face, eyes, ears, hands, feet, genitalia, and perineum, as well as those that involve skin overlying major joints; (4) full-thickness burns on greater than 5% of the BSA in any age group; (5) significant electrical burns, including lightning injury (significant volumes of tissue beneath the surface can be injured and result in acute renal failure and other complications); (6) significant chemical burns; (7) inhalation injury; (8) burn injury in patients with preexisting illness that could complicate treatment, prolong recovery, or affect mortality; (9) any patient with a burn injury who has concomitant trauma poses an increased risk of morbidity or mortality, and may be treated initially in a trauma center until stable before transfer to a burn center; (10) children with burn injuries who are seen in hospitals without qualified personnel or equipment to manage their care should be transferred to a burn center with these capabilities; (11) burn injury in patients who will require special social and emotional or long-term rehabilitative support, including cases involving suspected child abuse and neglect.

BIBLIOGRAPHY

1. Amy BW, McManus WF, Goodwin CW Jr, et al. Lightning injury with survival in five patients. *JAMA* 1985;253:243-245.

2. Britt LD, Dascombe WH, Rodriguez A. New horizons in management of hypothermia and frostbite injury. *Surg Clin North Am* 1991;71(2):345-370.

3. Cioffi WG, Graves TA, McManus WF, et al. High frequency percussive ventilation in patients with inhalation injury. *J Trauma* 1989;29:350-354.

4. Danzl D, Pozos R, Auerbach P, et al. Multicenter hypothermia survey. *Ann Emerg Med* 1987;16:1042-1055.

5. Demling HR. Burn care in the immediate resuscitation period. Section III, Thermal injury. In: Wilmor DW, ed. *Scientific American Surgery.* New York: Scientific American; 1998.

6. Edlich R, Change D, Birk K, et al. Cold injuries. *Compr Ther* 1989;15(9):13-21.

7. Gentilello LM, Cobean RA, Offner PJ, et al. Continuous arteriovenous rewarming: rapid reversal of hypothermia in critically ill patients. *J Trauma* 1992;32(3):316-327.

8. Gentilello LM, Jurkovich GJ, Moujaes S. Hypothermia and injury: thermodynamic principles of prevention and treatment. In: Levine B, ed. *Perspectives in Surgery.* St. Louis: Quality Medical; 1991.

9. Graves TA, Cioffi WG, McManus WF, et al. Fluid resuscitation of infants and children with massive thermal injury. *J Trauma* 1988;28:1656-1659.

10. Gunning K, ed.. *Burns Trauma Handbook.* 5th ed. Liverpool, UK: Liverpool Hospital Department of Trauma Services; 1994.

11. Halebian P, Robinson N, Barie P, et al. Whole body oxygen utilization during carbon monoxide poisoning and isocapneic nitrogen hypoxia. *J Trauma* 1986;26:110-117.

12. Haponik EF, Munster AM, eds. *Respiratory Injury: Smoke Inhalation and Burns.* New York: McGraw-Hill; 1990.

13. Jacob J, Weisman M, Rosenblatt S, et al. Chronic pernio: a historical perspective of cold-induced vascular disease. *Arch Intern Med* 1986;146:1589-1592.

14. Jurkovich GJ. Hypothermia in the trauma patient. In: Maull KI, Cleveland HC, Strauch GO, et al., eds. *Advances in Trauma.* Vol. 4. Chicago: Yearbook; 1989:11-140.

15. Jurkovich GJ, Greiser W, Luterman A, et al. Hypothermia in trauma victims: an ominous predictor of survival. *J Trauma* 1987;27:1019-1024.

16. Lund T, Goodwin CW, McManus WF, et al. Upper airway sequelae in burn patients requiring endotracheal intubation or tracheostomy. *Ann Surg* 1985;201:374-382.

17. Millard LG, Rowell NR. Chilblain lupus erythematosus (Hutchinson): a clinical and laboratory study of 17 patients. *Br J Dermatol* 1978;98(5):497-506.

18. Mills WJ Jr. Summary of treatment of the cold injured patient: frostbite [1983 classic article]. *Ala Med* 1993;35(1):61-66.

19. Moss J. Accidental severe hypothermia. *Surg Gynecol Obstet* 1986;162:501-513.

20. Mozingo DW, Smith AA, McManus WF, et al. Chemical burns. *J Trauma* 1988;28:642-647.

21. O'Malley J, Mills W, Kappes B, et al. Frostbite: general and specific treatment, the Alaskan method. *Ala Med* 1993;27(1):pull-out.

22. Perry RJ, Moore CA, et al. Determining the approximate area of burn: an inconsistency investigated and reevaluated. *BMJ* 1996;312:1338.

23. Pruitt BA Jr. The burn patient: I. Initial care. *Curr Probl Surg* 1979;16(4):1-55.

24. Pruitt BA Jr. The burn patient: II. Later care and complications of thermal injury. *Curr Probl Surg* 1979;16(5):1-95.

25. Reed R, Bracey A, Hudson J, et al. Hypothermia and blood coagulation: dissociation between enzyme activity and clotting factor levels. *Circ Shock* 1990;32:141-152.

26. Rustin M, Newton J, Smith N, et al. The treatment of chilblains with nifedipine: the results of a pilot study, a double-blind placebo-controlled randomized study and a long-term open trial. *Br J Dermatol* 1989;120:267-275.

27. Saffle JR, Crandall A, Warden GD. Cataracts: a long-term complication of electrical injury. *J Trauma* 1985;25:17-21.

28. Schaller M, Fischer A, Perret C. Hyperkalemia: a prognostic factor during acute severe hypothermia. *JAMA* 1990;264:1842-1845.

29. Sheehy TW, Navari RM. Hypothermia. *Ala J Med Sci* 1984;21(4):374-381.

30. Stratta RJ, Saffle JR, Kravitz M, et al. Management of tar and asphalt injuries. *Am J Surg* 1983;146:766-769.

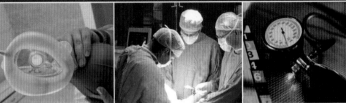

CHAPTER **10** Pediatric Trauma

Upon completion of this topic, the student will demonstrate the ability to apply the principles of trauma care to treatment of acutely injured pediatric patients. Specifically, the doctor will be able to:

OBJECTIVES

1 Identify the unique characteristics of the child as a trauma patient, including types of injury, patterns of injury, anatomic and physiologic differences in children as compared with adults, and long-term effects of injury.

2 Describe the primary management of critical injuries in children, including related issues unique to pediatric patients, emphasizing the anatomic and physiologic differences as compared with adults and their impact on resuscitation:

Airway with cervical spine control

Breathing with recognition and management of immediately life-threatening chest injuries

Circulation with bleeding control and shock recognition and management

Disability with recognition and initial management of altered mental status and intracranial mass lesions

Exposure with maintenance of body heat

Central nervous system and cervical spine injuries

Chest and abdominal injuries

Musculoskeletal injuries

Fluid and medication dosages

Psychological and family support

3 Identify the injury patterns associated with child abuse, and describe the elements that lead to the suspicion of child abuse.

Introduction

Injury continues to be the most common cause of death and disability in childhood. Each year, more than 10 million children in the United States require emergency department care for the treatment of injuries, representing nearly 1 of every 6 children. And each year more than 10,000 children in the United States die from serious injury. Injury morbidity and mortality surpass all major diseases in children and young adults, making injury the most serious public health and health care problem in this population. Because failure to secure the airway, support the breathing, and recognize and respond to intraabdominal and intracranial hemorrhage are known to be the leading causes of unsuccessful resuscitation in severe pediatric trauma, application of ATLS® principles to the care of the injured child can have a significant impact on ultimate survival.

Types and Patterns of Injury

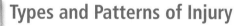

? *What types of injuries do children sustain?*

Motor vehicle-associated injuries are the most common cause of deaths in children of all ages, whether the child is an occupant, pedestrian, or cyclist. Deaths due to drowning, house fires, homicides, and falls follow in de-

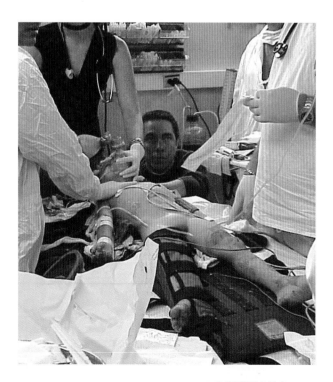

scending order. Child battering—that is, physical abuse—accounts for the great majority of homicides in infants, whereas firearm injuries account for the majority of homicides in children and adolescents. Falls account for the majority of all pediatric injuries, but infrequently result in death.

Blunt mechanisms of injury and children's physical characteristics result in multisystem injury being the rule rather than the exception (Table 10-1). Penetrating injuries have increased in childhood and adolescence in many large cities. Therefore, it should be presumed that all organ systems may be injured until proven otherwise. **Although the condition of the majority of injured children will not deteriorate, and most injured children have no hemodynamic abnormalities, the fact remains that some children with multisystem injuries will have rapid deterioration and serious complications will develop. Therefore, such patients should be transferred early to a facility capable of treating children with multisystem injuries.** The recently revised Triage Decision Scheme and Pediatric Trauma Score are both useful tools for the early identification of pediatric patients with multisystem injuries. See Triage Decision Scheme (Figure 1-1, page 3) and Pediatric Trauma Score (Table C-2, page 291).

Unique Characteristics of Pediatric Patients

? *What aspects of childhood anatomy do I need to consider?*

The priorities of assessment and management of injuries in children are the same as in the adult. However, the unique anatomic and physiologic characteristics of pediatric patients combine with the different mechanisms of injury to produce distinct patterns of injury. For example, most serious pediatric trauma is blunt trauma that involves the brain. As a result, apnea, hypoventilation, and hypoxia occur five times more often than hypovolemia with hypotension in seriously injured children. Therefore, treatment protocols for pediatric trauma patients emphasize aggressive management of the airway and breathing.

SIZE AND SHAPE

Because of the smaller body mass of children, the energy imparted from, for example, fenders, bumpers, and falls results in a greater force applied per unit of body area. This more intense energy is transmitted to a body that has less fat, less connective tissue, and close proximity of multiple organs. This results in the high frequency of multiple injuries seen in the pediatric population. In addition, the head

TABLE 10-1 ■ Common Mechanisms of Injury and Associated Patterns of Injury in Pediatric Patients	
MECHANISM OF INJURY	**COMMON PATTERNS OF INJURY**
Pedestrian struck	• Low speed: Lower extremity fractures • High speed: Multiple trauma, head and neck injuries, lower extremity fractures
Automobile occupant	• Unrestrained: Multiple trauma, head and neck injuries, scalp and facial lacerations • Restrained: Chest and abdomen injuries, lower spine fractures
Fall from a height	• Low: Upper extremity fractures • Medium: Head and neck injuries, upper and lower extremity fractures • High: Multiple trauma, head and neck injuries, upper and lower extremity fractures
Fall from a bicycle	• Without helmet: Head and neck lacerations, scalp and facial lacerations, upper extremity fractures • With helmet: Upper extremity fractures • Striking handlebar: Internal abdominal injuries

is proportionately larger in young children, resulting in a higher frequency of blunt brain injuries in this age group.

SKELETON

The child's skeleton is incompletely calcified, contains multiple active growth centers, and is more pliable. For these reasons, internal organ damage is often noted without overlying bony fracture. For example, rib fractures in children are uncommon, but pulmonary contusion is not. Other soft tissues of the thorax, the heart, and mediastinal structures also may sustain significant damage without evidence of bony injury. The identification of skull or rib fractures in a child suggests the transfer of a massive amount of energy, and underlying organ injuries, such as traumatic brain injury and pulmonary contusion, should be suspected.

SURFACE AREA

The ratio of a child's body surface area to body volume is highest at birth and diminishes as the child matures. As a result, thermal energy loss is a significant stress factor in the child. Hypothermia may develop quickly and complicate the treatment of the pediatric patient with hypotension.

PSYCHOLOGICAL STATUS

There may be significant psychological ramifications of injuries in children. In very young children, emotional instability frequently leads to a regressive psychological behavior when stress, pain, and other perceived threats intervene in the child's environment. The child's ability to interact with unfamiliar individuals in strange and difficult situations is limited, making history taking and cooperative manipula-

tion, especially if it is painful, extremely difficult. The doctor who understands these characteristics and is willing to cajole and soothe an injured child is more likely to establish a good rapport. Although this rapport facilitates comprehensive assessment of the child's psychological and physical injuries, the presence of parents or guardians during evaluation and treatment, including resuscitation, does not present a hindrance, and may provide the treating doctor with even greater help during early care of the pediatric trauma patient by minimizing the injured child's natural fears and anxieties.

LONG-TERM EFFECTS

A major consideration in treating injured children is the effect that injury can have on their subsequent growth and development. Unlike the adult, the child must not only recover from the effects of the traumatic event, but also must continue the normal process of growth and development. The physiologic and psychological effects of injury on this process should not be underestimated, particularly in cases involving long-term function, growth deformity, or subsequent abnormal development. Children who sustain even a minor injury may have prolonged disability in cerebral function, psychological adjustment, or organ system disability.

Some evidence suggests that as many as 60% of children who sustain severe multisystem trauma have residual personality changes at 1 year after hospital discharge, and 50% show cognitive and physical handicaps. Social, affective, and learning disabilities are present in half of seriously injured children. In addition, childhood injuries have a significant impact on the family, with personality and emotional disturbances found in two-thirds of uninjured

PITFALLS

- The unique anatomic and physiologic characteristics of children occasionally lead to pitfalls in their treatment.
- The small size of the endotracheal tube promotes obstruction from inspissated secretions.
- Uncuffed tubes may be dislodged, especially during patient movement or transportation.
- The necessity of frequent reassessment cannot be overemphasized.
- The same prudent attention to all tubes and catheters used for resuscitation and stabilization is essential.

siblings. Frequently, a child's injuries impose a strain on the parents' marital relationship, including financial and sometimes employment hardships.

Trauma may affect not only the child's survival, but also the quality of the child's life for years to come. Bony and solid visceral injuries are cases in point:

- Injuries through growth centers may result in growth abnormalities of the injured bone. If the injured bone is a femur, a leg length discrepancy may result, causing a lifelong disability in running and walking. If the fracture is through the growth center of one thoracic vertebra (or more), the result may be scoliosis, kyphosis, or even gibbus.

- Massive disruption of a child's spleen may require a splenectomy. The loss of the spleen predisposes the child to a lifelong risk of overwhelming post-splenectomy sepsis and death.

Nevertheless, the long-term quality of life for children with disabilities is surprisingly robust, given the fact that disabled children in many cases suffer lifelong physical handicaps. Most such patients report a good to excellent quality of life, and most find gainful employment, justifying aggressive resuscitation attempts, even for pediatric patients whose initial physiologic status, eg, Glasgow Coma Scale (GCS) score, might suggest otherwise.

EQUIPMENT

Immediately available equipment of the appropriate sizes is essential for the successful initial treatment of injured children (Table 10-2). A length-based resuscitation tape, such as the Broselow™ Pediatric Emergency Tape, is an ideal adjunct for the rapid determination of weight based on length for appropriate fluid volumes, drug doses, and equipment size. ■ See Skill Station IV: Shock Assessment and Management, Skill IV-F: Broselow™ Pediatric Emergency Tape.

Airway: Evaluation and Management

? How do I apply ATLS principles to the treatment of children?

The "A" of the ABCDEs of initial assessment is the same in the child as it is in the adult. Establishing a patent airway to provide adequate tissue oxygenation is the first objective. The inability to establish and/or maintain a patent airway with the associated lack of oxygenation and ventilation is the most common cause of cardiac arrest in children. Therefore, the child's airway is the first priority.

ANATOMY

The smaller the child, the greater is the disproportion between the size of the cranium and the midface. This leads to a propensity for the posterior pharynx to buckle anteriorly as a result of passive flexion of the cervical spine caused by the large occiput. Avoiding passive flexion of the cervical spine requires that the plane of the midface be kept parallel to the spine board in a neutral position, rather than in the "sniffing position" (Figure 10-1A). Placement of a 1-inch-thick layer of padding beneath the infant's or toddler's entire torso will preserve neutral alignment of the spinal column (Figure 10-1B).

The soft tissues in an infant's oropharynx (ie, tongue and tonsils) are relatively large compared with those in the oral cavity, which may make visualization of the larynx difficult. A child's larynx is funnel-shaped, allowing secretions to accumulate in the retropharyngeal area. It is also more cephalad and anterior in the neck, and the vocal cords have a slightly more anterocaudal angle. The vocal cords are frequently more difficult to visualize when the child's head is in the normal, supine, anatomical position during intubation than when it is in the neutral position required for optimal cervical spine protection. The infant's trachea is approximately 5 cm long and grows to 7 cm by about 18 months. Failure to appreciate this short length may result in intubation of the right mainstem bronchus, inadequate ventilation, accidental tube dislodgment, and/or mechanical barotrauma.

MANAGEMENT

In a spontaneously breathing child with a partially obstructed airway, the airway should be optimized by keeping the plane of the face parallel to the plane of the stretcher or gurney, while maintaining neutral alignment of the cervical spine. The jaw-thrust maneuver combined with bimanual in-line spinal immobilization is used to open the airway. After the mouth and oropharynx are cleared of secretions or debris, supplemental oxygen is administered. If the patient is unconscious, mechanical methods of maintaining

TABLE 10-2 ■ Pediatric Equipment[1]

AGE AND WEIGHT	AIRWAY AND BREATHING								CIRCULATION			SUPPLEMENTAL EQUIPMENT				
	O₂ MASK	ORAL AIRWAY	BAG-VALVE	LARYN-GOSCOPE	ET TUBE	STYLET	SUCTION		BP CUFF	IV CATHETER[2]		OG/NG TUBE	CHEST TUBE	URINARY CATHETER	CERVICAL COLLAR
Premie 3 kg	Premie, newborn	Infant	Infant	0 straight	2.5–3.0 no cuff	6 Fr	6–8 Fr		Premie, newborn	22–24 ga		8 Fr	10–14 Fr	5 Fr feeding	—
0–6 mos 3.5 kg	Newborn	Infant, small	Infant	1 straight	3.0–3.5 no cuff	6 Fr	8 Fr		Newborn, infant	22 ga		10 Fr	12–18 Fr	6 Fr or 5–8 Fr feeding	—
6–12 mos 7 kg	Pediatric	Small	Pediatric	1 straight	3.5–4.0 no cuff	6 Fr	8–10 Fr		Infant, child	22 ga		12 Fr	14–20 Fr	8 Fr	Small
1–3 yr 10–12 kg	Pediatric	Small	Pediatric	1 straight	4.0–4.5 no cuff	6 Fr	10 Fr		Child	20–22 ga		12 Fr	14–24 Fr	10 Fr	Small
4–7 yr 16–18 kg	Pediatric	Medium	Pediatric	2 straight or curved	5.0–5.5 no cuff	14 Fr	14 Fr		Child	20 ga		12 Fr	20–28 Fr	10–12 Fr	Small
8–10 yr 24–30 kg	Adult	Medium, large	Pediatric, adult	2–3 straight or curved	5.5–6.5 cuffed	14 Fr	14 Fr		Child, adult	18–20 ga		14 Fr	28–38 Fr	12 Fr	Medium

[1]Use of a length-based resuscitation tape, such as a Broselow™ Pediatric Emergency Tape, is preferred.
[2]The largest IV catheter that can readily be inserted with reasonable certainty of success is preferred.

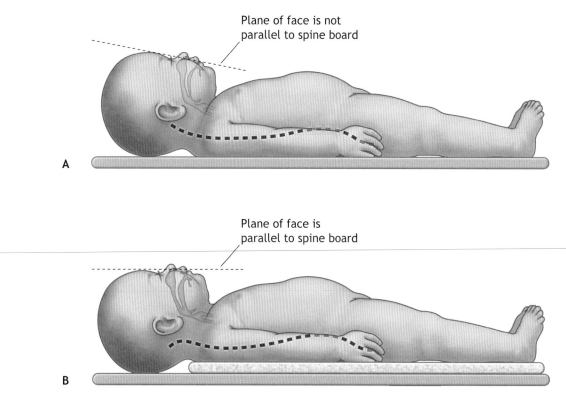

Plane of face is not
parallel to spine board

A

Plane of face is
parallel to spine board

B

■ **Figure 10-1 (A)** Improper positioning of a child to maintain a patent airway. The disproportion between the size of a child's cranium and the midface leads to a propensity for the posterior pharynx to buckle anteriorly. The large occiput causes passive flexion of the cervical spine. **(B)** Proper positioning of a child to maintain a patient airway. Avoid passive flexion of the cervical spine by keeping the plane of the midface parallel to the spine board in a neutral position, rather than in the "sniffing position." Placement of a one-inch-thick layer of padding beneath a child's entire torso will preserve neutral alignment of the spinal column.

the airway may be necessary. **Before attempts are made to mechanically establish an airway, the child should be fully preoxygenated.**

Oral Airway

An oral airway should only be inserted if a child is unconscious, since vomiting is likely if the gag reflex is intact. The practice of inserting the airway backward and rotating it 180 degrees is not recommended for children, as trauma with resultant hemorrhage into soft tissue structures of the oropharynx may occur. The oral airway should be gently inserted directly into the oropharynx. The use of a tongue blade to depress the tongue may be helpful.

Orotracheal Intubation

Endotracheal intubation is indicated for injured children in a variety of situations—for example, a child with severe brain injury who requires controlled ventilation, a child in whom an airway cannot be maintained, a child who exhibits signs of ventilatory failure, and a child who has suffered significant hypovolemia who has a depressed sensorium or requires operative intervention.

Orotracheal intubation is the most reliable means of establishing an airway and administering ventilation to a child. Uncuffed tubes—of appropriate size, to avoid subglottic edema, ulceration, and disruption of the infant's or child's fragile airway—should be used initially. The smallest area of the young child's airway is at the cricoid ring, which forms a natural seal with the endotracheal tube. Therefore, cuffed endotracheal tubes are uncommonly used in children under the age of 9 years who are acutely injured. A simple technique to gauge the size of the endotracheal tube needed is to approximate the diameter of the child's external nares or the tip of the child's small finger to the tube diameter. A length-based pediatric resuscitation tape, such as the Broselow™ Pediatric Emergency Tape, also lists appropriate tube sizes for endotracheal intubation. However, be sure to have tubes readily available that are one size larger and one size smaller than the predicted size. If a stylet is used to facilitate endotracheal intubation, be sure that the tip does not extend beyond the end of the tube.

Most trauma centers use a protocol for emergency intubation, referred to as drug-assisted intubation (DAI), previously known as rapid sequence intubation (RSI). Careful attention must be paid to the child's weight, vital signs (pulse and blood pressure), and level of consciousness to determine which branch of the algorithm to use (Figure 10-2).

Preoxygenation should be administered in children who require an endotracheal tube for airway control. Infants and children have a more pronounced vagal response to endotracheal intubation than adults. Such responses may be caused by hypoxia, vagal stimulation during laryngoscopy, or pharmacologic agents, and they can be minimized by atropine pretreatment. Atropine also dries oral secretions, permitting easier visualization of landmarks for intubation. The dose of atropine is 0.1 to 0.5 mg given at least 1 to 2 minutes before intubation. Appropriate drugs for intubation include etomidate (0.3 mg/kg) or midazolam (0.3 mg/kg) in the children with normovolemia or etomidate (0.1 mg/kg) or midazolam (0.1 mg/kg) in children with hypovolemia. The specific antidote for midazolam is flumazenil, which should be immediately available.

After sedation, cricoid pressure is maintained to help avoid aspiration of gastric contents. This is followed by temporary chemical paralysis with one of two agents. **Ideally, a short-acting, depolarizing, neuromuscular blocking (chemical paralytic) agent should be used, such as succinylcholine (2 mg/kg in children <10 kg; 1 mg/kg in children >10 kg).** Succinylcholine has a rapid onset, a short duration of action, and may be the safest drug of choice (unless the patient has a previously known spinal cord injury). **If a longer period of paralysis is needed—for example, in a child who needs a computed tomographic (CT) scan for further evaluation—a longer-acting, nondepolarizing, neuromuscular blocking agent, such as vecuronium (0.2 mg/kg) or rocuronium (0.6 mg/kg), may be indicated.**

After the endotracheal tube is inserted, its position must be assessed clinically (see below) and, if correct, the tube carefully secured. Cricoid pressure then may be released. If it is not possible to place the endotracheal tube after the child is chemically paralyzed, the child must receive ventilation with 100% oxygen administered with a self-inflating bag-mask device until a definitive airway is secured.

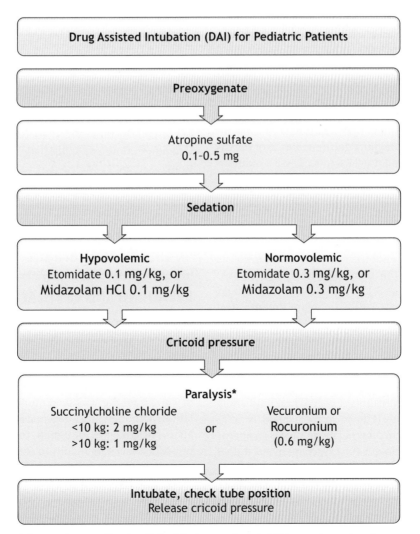

* Proceed according to clinical judgement and skill/experience level.

■ **Figure 10-2 Algorithm for Drug-Assisted Intubation (DAI) in Pediatric Patients.**

Orotracheal intubation under direct vision with adequate immobilization and protection of the cervical spine is the preferred method of obtaining initial airway control. Nasotracheal intubation should not be performed in children under the age of 9 years, as it requires blind passage around a relatively acute angle in the nasopharynx toward the anterosuperiorly located glottis, making intubation by this route difficult. The potential for penetrating the child's cranial vault or damaging the more prominent nasopharyngeal (adenoidal) soft tissues and causing hemorrhage also makes using the nasotracheal route for airway control ill-advised.

Once past the glottic opening, the endotracheal tube should be positioned 2 to 3 cm below the level of the vocal cords and carefully secured in place. Primary confirmation techniques, such as auscultation of both hemithoraces in the axillae, should then be performed to ensure that right mainstem bronchial intubation has not occurred and that both sides of the chest are being adequately ventilated. A secondary confirmation device, such as a real-time capnograph, a colorimetric end-tidal carbon dioxide ($ETCO_2$) detector, or an esophageal detector device (EDD), should then be used to document tracheal intubation and a chest x-ray film obtained to accurately identify the position of the endotracheal tube.

Because of the short length of the trachea in young children (5 cm in infants, 7 cm in toddlers), any movement of the head may result in displacement of the endotracheal tube, inadvertent extubation, right mainstem bronchial intubation, or vigorous coughing due to irritation of the carina by the tip of the endotracheal tube. These conditions may not be recognized clinically until significant deterioration has occurred. Thus, breath sounds should be evaluated periodically to ensure that the tube remains in the appropriate position and to identify the possibility of evolving ventilatory dysfunction. If there is any doubt about correct placement of the endotracheal tube that cannot be resolved expeditiously, the tube should be removed and replaced immediately. ◾ See Skill Station II: Airway and Ventilatory Management, Skill II-G: Infant Endotracheal Intubation.

Cricothyroidotomy

When airway maintenance and control cannot be accomplished by bag-mask ventilation or orotracheal intubation, needle cricothyroidotomy is the preferred method. Needle-jet insufflation via the cricothyroid membrane is an appropriate, temporizing technique for oxygenation, but it does not provide adequate ventilation, and progressive hypercarbia may occur. ◾ See Chapter 2: Airway and Ventilatory Management and Skill Station III: Cricothyroidotomy, Skill III-A: Needle Cricothyroidotomy.

Surgical cricothyroidotomy is rarely indicated for infants or small children. It can be performed in older children in whom the cricothyroid membrane is easily palpable (usually by the age of 12 years). ◾ See Skill Station III: Cricothyroidotomy, Skill III-B: Surgical Cricothyroidotomy.

PITFALL

Unrecognized inadvertent dislodgment of the endotracheal tube—which most often occurs as the patient is transferred from an ambulance stretcher to a hospital gurney in the emergency department, or from gurney to gantry, and vice versa, in the CT suite—is likely the most common cause of sudden deterioration in the intubated pediatric patient, emphasizing the need for use of transport monitors whenever a child must be transferred from one care environment to another. Desaturation may also result from obstruction of the endotracheal tube by clotted blood or inspissated secretions, worsening of tension pneumothorax with positive-pressure ventilation (particularly if diagnostic findings were absent on initial evaluation), and equipment failure—either kinking of the softer, narrower endotracheal tubes used in children or an empty oxygen tank. Use of the mnemonic, "Don't be a DOPE," (D for dislodgment, O for obstruction, P for pneumothorax, E for equipment failure) may help to remind the treating doctor of the most likely calamities when the condition of an intubated child begins to deteriorate.

Breathing: Evaluation and Management

BREATHING AND VENTILATION

The respiratory rate in children decreases with age. An infant breathes 30 to 40 times per minute, whereas an older child breathes 15 to 20 times per minute. Normal, spontaneous tidal volumes vary from 6 to 8 mL/kg for infants and children, although slightly larger tidal volumes of 7 to 10 mL/kg may be required during assisted ventilation. Although most bag-mask devices used with pediatric patients are designed to limit the amount of pressure exerted manually on the child's airway, excessive volume or pressure during assisted ventilation substantially increases the potential for iatrogenic barotrauma because of the fragile nature of the immature tracheobronchial tree and alveoli.

Hypoxia is the most common cause of cardiac arrest in the child. However, before cardiac arrest occurs, hypoventilation causes respiratory acidosis, which is the most common acid/base abnormality encountered during the resuscitation of injured children. With adequate ventilation and perfusion, a child should be able to maintain a relatively normal pH. **In the absence of adequate ventilation and perfusion, attempting to correct an acidosis with sodium bicarbonate results in further hypercarbia and worsened acidosis.**

NEEDLE AND TUBE THORACOSTOMY

Injuries that disrupt pleural apposition—for example, hemothorax, pneumothorax, and hemopneumothorax, have similar physiologic consequences in children and adults. These injuries are managed with pleural decompression, preceded in the case of tension pneumothorax by needle decompression just over the top of the third rib on the midclavicular line. Care should be taken during this procedure to avoid using 14- to 18-gauge over-the-needle catheters in infants and small children, since the longer needle length may cause, rather than cure, a tension pneumothorax. Chest tubes will need to be small (see Table 10-3) and are placed into the thoracic cavity by tunneling the tube over the rib above the skin incision site, and directing it superiorly and posteriorly along the inside of the chest wall. Tunneling is especially important in children because of the thinner chest wall. The site of chest tube insertion is the same in children as in adults: the fifth intercostal space, just anterior to the midaxillary line. ◾ See Chapter 4: Thoracic Trauma, and Skill Station VII: Chest Trauma Management.

Circulation and Shock: Evaluation and Management

? What physiologic differences will have an impact on my treatment of pediatric trauma patients?

Key factors in the evaluation and management of circulation in pediatric trauma patients include recognition of circulatory compromise, fluid resuscitation, blood replacement, venous access, urine output, and thermoregulation.

RECOGNITION

Injuries in children may result in significant blood loss. A child's increased physiologic reserve allows for maintenance of systolic blood pressure in the normal range, even in the presence of shock (Figure 10-3). Up to a 30% diminution in circulating blood volume may be required to manifest a decrease in the child's systolic blood pressure. This may be misleading to medical professionals who are not familiar with the subtle physiologic changes manifested by children in hypovolemic shock. Tachycardia and poor skin perfusion often are the only keys to early recognition of hypovolemia and the early initiation of appropriate crystalloid fluid resuscitation. **Early assessment by a surgeon is essential to the appropriate treatment of injured children.**

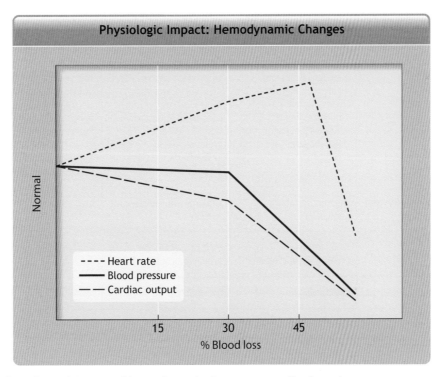

■ **Figure 10-3** Physiological impact of hemodynamic changes on pediatric patients.

Although a child's primary response to hypovolemia is tachycardia, this sign also may be caused by pain, fear, and psychological stress. Other more subtle signs of blood loss in children include progressive weakening of peripheral pulses, a narrowing of pulse pressure to less than 20 mm Hg, skin mottling (which substitutes for clammy skin in infants and young children), cool extremities compared with the torso skin, and a decrease in the level of consciousness with a dulled response to pain. A decrease in blood pressure and other indices of inadequate organ perfusion, such as urinary output, should be monitored closely, but generally develop later. Changes in vital organ function are outlined in Table 10-3.

The mean normal systolic blood pressure for children is 90 mm Hg plus twice the child's age in years, and the diastolic pressure should be two-thirds of the systolic blood pressure. The lower limit of normal systolic blood pressure in children is 70 mm Hg plus twice the age in years. (Normal vital functions by age group are listed in Table 10-4.) Hypotension in a child represents a state of decompensated shock and indicates severe blood loss of greater than 45% of the circulating blood volume. Tachycardia changing to bradycardia often accompanies this hypotension, and this change may occur suddenly in infants. These physiologic changes must be treated by a rapid infusion of both isotonic crystalloid and blood.

FLUID RESUSCITATION

The goal of fluid resuscitation is to rapidly replace the circulating volume. A child's blood volume can be estimated at 80 mL/kg. When shock is suspected, a bolus of 20 mL/kg of warmed isotonic crystalloid solution is needed. If it were to remain in the vascular space, this would represent 25% of the child's blood volume. The 3-for-1 rule applies to the pediatric patient as well as to the adult patient. Because the goal is to replace the lost intravascular volume, it may be necessary to give three boluses of 20 mL/kg, or a total of 60 mL/kg, to achieve a replacement of the lost 25%. ◾ See Chapter 3: Shock. When starting the third 20 mL/kg bolus, the use of packed red blood cells (PRBCs) should be considered. PRBCs are administered as a bolus of 10 mL/kg.

Fluid resuscitation in the child is based on the child's weight. It is often very difficult for emergency department (ED) personnel to estimate the weight of a child, particularly if these personnel do not treat many children. The simplest and quickest method of determining the child's weight to accurately calculate fluid volumes and drug dosages is to use a length-based resuscitation tape, such as the Broselow™ Pediatric Emergency Tape. This tool rapidly provides the child's approximate weight, respiratory rate, fluid resuscitation volume, and a variety of drug dosages.

TABLE 10-3 ■ Systemic Responses to Blood Loss in Pediatric Patients

SYSTEM	MILD BLOOD VOLUME LOSS (<30%)	MODERATE BLOOD VOLUME LOSS (30%-45%)	SEVERE BLOOD VOLUME LOSS (>45%)
Cardiovascular	Increased heart rate; weak, thready peripheral pulses; normal systolic blood pressure (80-90 + 2 x age in years); normal pulse pressure	Markedly increased heart rate; weak, thready central pulses; absent peripheral pulses; low normal systolic blood pressure (70-80 + 2 x age in years); narrowed pulse pressure	Tachycardia followed by bradycardia; very weak or absent central pulses; absent peripheral pulses; hypotension (<70 + 2 x age in years); widened pulse pressure (or undetectable diastolic blood pressure)
Central Nervous System	Anxious; irritable; confused	Lethargic; dulled response to pain[1]	Comatose
Skin	Cool, mottled; prolonged capillary refill	Cyanotic; markedly prolonged capillary refill	Pale and cold
Urine Output[2]	Low to very low	Minimal	None

[1]The child's dulled response to pain with this degree of blood loss (30%-45%) may be indicated by a decreased response to IV catheter insertion.

[2]After initial decompression by urinary catheter. Low normal is 2 ml/kg/hr (infant), 1.5 ml/kg/hr (younger child), 1 ml/kg/hr (older child), and 0.5 ml/hg/hr (adolescent). IV contrast can falsely elevate urinary output.

TABLE 10-4 ■ Vital Functions					
AGE GROUP	WEIGHT RANGE (IN KG)	HEART RATE (BEATS/MIN)	BLOOD PRESSURE (MM HG)	RESPIRATORY RATE (BREATHS/MIN)	URINARY OUTPUT (ML/KG/HR)
Infant 0–12 mo	0–10	<160	>60	<60	2.0
Toddler 1–2 yr	10–14	<150	>70	<40	1.5
Preschool 3–5 yr	14–18	<140	>75	<35	1.0
School age 6–12 yr	18–36	<120	>80	<30	1.0
Adolescent 13 yr	36–70	<100	>90	<30	0.5

Injured children should be monitored carefully for response to fluid resuscitation and adequacy of organ perfusion. A return toward hemodynamic normality is indicated by:

- Slowing of the heart rate toward normal (with improvement of other physiologic signs; this response is age-dependent)
- Clearing of the sensorium
- Return of peripheral pulses
- Return of normal skin color
- Increased warmth of extremities
- Increased systolic blood pressure (normal is approximately 90 mm Hg plus twice the age in years)
- Increased pulse pressure (>20 mm Hg)
- Urinary output of 1 to 2 mL/kg/hour (age-dependent)

Children generally have one of four responses to fluid resuscitation. The condition of most children will be stabilized by the use of crystalloid fluid only; blood will not be required; this group is considered "responders." Some children respond to crystalloid and blood resuscitation (also "responders"). In some children there is an initial response to crystalloid fluid and blood, but then deterioration occurs; this group is termed "transient responders." Other children do not respond at all to crystalloid fluid and blood infusion; this group is referred to as "nonresponders." The two latter groups of children (transient responders and nonresponders) are candidates for prompt infusion of additional blood and consideration for operation.

The resuscitation flow diagram is a useful aid in the initial treatment of injured children (Figure 10-4).

BLOOD REPLACEMENT

Failure to improve hemodynamic abnormalities following the first bolus of resuscitation fluid raises the suspicion of continuing hemorrhage, prompts the need for administration of a second and perhaps a third 20-mL/kg bolus of isotonic crystalloid fluid, and requires the prompt involvement of a surgeon. When starting the third bolus of isotonic crystalloid fluid or if the child's condition deteriorates, consideration must be given to the use of 10 mL/kg of type-specific or O-negative warmed PRBCs.

VENOUS ACCESS

Severe hypovolemic shock usually occurs as the result of disruption of intrathoracic or intraabdominal organs or blood vessels. Venous access is preferably established by a peripheral percutaneous route. If percutaneous access is unsuccessful after two attempts, consideration should be given to intraosseous infusion via a bone marrow needle (18 gauge in infants, 15 gauge in young children) or insertion of a femoral venous line using the Seldinger technique or a through-the-needle catheter of appropriate size. If these procedures fail, a doctor with skill and expertise can safely perform direct venous cutdown. However, this should be done only as a last resort, since venous cutdown can rarely be performed in less than 10 minutes, even in experienced hands, whereas an intraosseous needle can reliably be placed in the bone marrow cavity in less than 1 minute, even by providers with limited skill and expertise. ■ See Skill Station IV: Shock Assessment and Management.

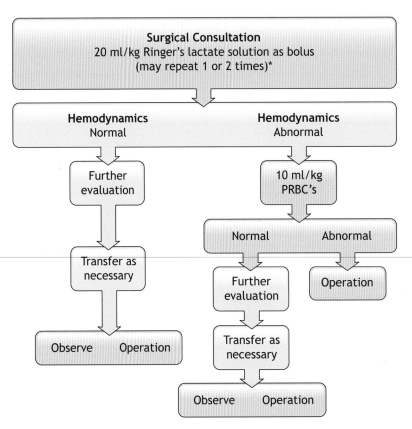

■ Figure 10-4 Resuscitation Flow Diagram for Pediatric Patients with normal and abnormal hemodynamics.
*Additional fluid resuscitation is guided by response to initial bolus.

The preferred sites for venous access in children are:

- Percutaneous peripheral (two attempts)—Antecubital fossa(e), saphenous vein(s) at the ankle

- Intraosseous placement—Anterior tibial bone marrow

- Percutaneous placement—Femoral vein(s)

- Percutaneous placement—External jugular vein(s) (should be reserved for pediatric experts; do not use if there is airway compromise, or a cervical collar is applied)

- Venous cutdown—Saphenous vein(s) at the ankle

Intravenous access in children with hypovolemia who are younger than 6 years of age is a perplexing and challenging problem, even in the most experienced hands. Intraosseous infusion, cannulating the marrow cavity of a long bone in an uninjured extremity, is an appropriate emergency access procedure. The intraosseous route is safe and efficacious, and requires far less time than does venous cutdown. However, intraosseous infusion should be discontinued when suitable peripheral venous access has been established.

Indications for intraosseous infusion are limited to children for whom venous access is impossible because of circulatory collapse or for whom two attempts at percutaneous

peripheral venous cannulation have failed. Complications of this procedure include cellulitis, osteomyelitis, compartment syndrome, and iatrogenic fracture. The preferred site for intraosseous cannulation is the proximal tibia, below the level of the tibial tuberosity. If the tibia is fractured, the needle may be inserted into the distal femur, although the contralateral proximal tibia is preferred, if uninjured. Intraosseous cannulation should not be performed distal to a fracture site.

URINE OUTPUT

Urine output varies with age. Output for infants up to 1 year of age is 2 mL/kg/hr, for younger children 1.5 mL/kg/hr, and for older children 1 mL/kg/hr. The lower limit of urinary output does not achieve the normal adult value of 0.5 mL/kg/hr until the adolescent has stopped growing. (See Table 10-4.)

Urine output combined with urine specific gravity is an excellent method of determining the adequacy of volume resuscitation. Once the circulating blood volume has been restored, the urinary output should return to normal. Insertion of a urinary catheter facilitates accurate measurement of the child's urinary output. A straight catheter, rather than one with a balloon, may be used in children who weigh less than 15 kg, although urinary catheters with balloons are now available with a diameter as small as 6 French. Catheters

PITFALL

The ability of a child's body to compensate in the early phases of blood loss may create an illusion of hemodynamic normality, resulting in inadequate fluid resuscitation and rapid deterioration, which is often precipitous.

containing temperature probes are available for children who need intensive care.

THERMOREGULATION

The high ratio of body surface area to body mass in children increases heat exchange with the environment and directly affects the body's ability to regulate core temperature. Thin skin and the lack of substantial subcutaneous tissue contribute to increased evaporative heat loss and caloric expenditure. Hypothermia may render the child's injuries refractory to treatment, prolong coagulation times, and adversely affect central nervous system (CNS) function. While the child is exposed during the initial survey and resuscitation phase, overhead heat lamps, heaters, or thermal blankets may be necessary to preserve body heat. It is advisable to warm the room as well as the intravenous fluids, blood products, and inhaled gases.

Chest Trauma

Eight percent of all injuries in children involve the chest. Chest injury also serves as a marker for other organ system injury, since more than two-thirds of children with chest injury will have multiple injuries. The mechanism of injury and the anatomy of the child's chest are directly responsible for the spectrum of injuries seen.

The vast majority of chest injuries in childhood are due to blunt mechanisms, caused principally by motor vehicles. The pliability, or compliance, of a child's chest wall allows impacting forces to be transmitted to the underlying pulmonary parenchyma, causing pulmonary contusion. Rib fractures and mediastinal injuries are not common, but if present, they indicate a severe impacting force. The specific injuries caused by thoracic trauma in children are similar to those encountered in adults, although the frequencies of these injuries are somewhat different.

Mobility of mediastinal structures makes the child more susceptible to tension pneumothorax. Diaphragmatic rupture, aortic transection, major tracheobronchial tears, flail chest, and cardiac contusions are rarely encountered in childhood. When identified, treatment for these injuries is the same as in the adult. Significant injuries rarely occur

alone and are frequently a component of major multisystem injury. Most pediatric thoracic injuries can be successfully managed using an appropriate combination of supportive care and tube thoracostomy. Thoracotomy is not generally needed in children.

The incidence of penetrating thoracic injury increases after 10 years of age. Penetrating trauma to the chest in children is managed the same way as in adults. See Chapter 4: Thoracic Trauma, and Skill Station VII: Chest Trauma Management.

Abdominal Trauma

Most pediatric abdominal injuries occur as the result of blunt trauma, primarily involving motor vehicles and falls. Serious intra-abdominal injuries warrant prompt involvement by a surgeon, and hypotensive children who sustain penetrating abdominal trauma require prompt operative intervention.

ASSESSMENT

Conscious infants and young children are generally frightened by the events preceding admission to the ED, which may affect the abdominal examination. While talking quietly and calmly to the child, ask questions about the presence of abdominal pain and gently assess the tone of the abdominal musculature. Deep, painful palpation of the abdomen should be avoided at the onset of the examination to prevent voluntary guarding that may confuse the abdominal findings. Almost all infants and young children who are stressed and crying will swallow large amounts of air. If the upper abdomen is distended on examination, inserting a gastric tube to decompress the stomach should be a part of the resuscitation phase. Orogastric tube decompression is preferred in infants. Tenseness of the abdominal wall often decreases as gastric distention is relieved, allowing for more careful and reliable evaluation. The presence of shoulder- or lap-belt marks increases the likelihood that abdominal injuries are present.

Abdominal examination in unconscious patients does not vary greatly with age. Decompression of the urinary bladder also facilitates abdominal evaluation. Since gastric dilation and a distended urinary bladder may both cause abdominal tenderness, abdominal tenderness must be interpreted with caution, unless these organs have been fully decompressed.

DIAGNOSTIC ADJUNCTS

Diagnostic adjuncts for assessment of abdominal trauma include computed tomography, focused assessment sonography in trauma, and diagnostic peritoneal lavage.

Computed Tomography

The advent of helical CT scanning allows for extremely rapid and precise identification of injuries. CT scanning is often used to evaluate the abdomen of children who have sustained blunt trauma and have no hemodynamic abnormalities. **CT scanning should be immediately available, performed early, and must not delay further treatment.** The identification of intraabdominal injuries by CT scan in pediatric patients with no hemodynamic abnormalities can allow for nonoperative management by the surgeon. Early involvement of the surgeon is essential to establish a baseline that will allow the surgeon to determine whether, and when, operation is indicated.

Injured children who require CT scanning as an adjunctive study often require sedation to prevent movement during the scanning process. Thus, an injured child requiring resuscitation or sedation who undergoes CT scan should be accompanied by a doctor skilled in pediatric airway management and pediatric vascular access. CT should routinely be performed with contrast agents according to local practice.

Focused Assessment Sonography in Trauma

The utility of FAST in managing pediatric patients remains uncertain. Although comparatively few studies on the efficacy of ultrasound in children with abdominal injury have been reported, its use as an extension of the abdominal examination in injured children is rapidly evolving, and it has the advantage that imaging may be repeated. Focused assessment sonography in trauma (FAST) can identify even small amounts of intraabdominal blood in pediatric trauma patients, a finding that is unlikely to be associated with significant injury. If large amounts of intraabdominal blood are found, significant injury is more likely to be present. However, even in these patients, operative management is indicated not by the amount of intraperitoneal blood, but by hemodynamic abnormality and its response to treatment. FAST is not consistently able to identify isolated intraparenchymal injuries, which account for up to one-third of solid organ injuries in children.

Diagnostic Peritoneal Lavage

Diagnostic peritoneal lavage (DPL) may be used to detect intraabdominal bleeding in children with hemodynamic abnormalities who cannot be safely transported to the CT scanner, or when CT and FAST are not readily available. However, although DPL continues to be used for screening by some experts, CT is now considered the preferred diagnostic study in most injured children, since most such patients have self-limited intraabdominal injuries and no hemodynamic abnormalities. Moreover, FAST is a more rapid and less invasive means of detecting significant intraabdominal hemorrhage as compared with DPL. In addition, most patients with significant intraabdominal bleeding will have hemodynamic abnormalities, and with few exceptions, should undergo emergency laparotomy.

As in adults, warmed crystalloid solution in volumes of 10 mL/kg (up to 1000 mL) is used for DPL. Because a child's abdominal wall is relatively thin compared with that of an adult, uncontrolled penetration of the peritoneal cavity may produce iatrogenic injury to the abdominal contents, even when an open technique is used. DPL has utility in diagnosing injuries to intraabdominal viscera only; retroperitoneal organs cannot be evaluated reliably by this technique.

The interpretation of a positive lavage is the same in both children and adults. Aspiration of blood on catheter insertion or more than 100,000 red cells per cubic millimeter in the lavage effluent is considered a positive finding. Although the definition of a positive peritoneal lavage is the same for children and adults, the presence of blood in the peritoneum does not in and of itself mandate laparotomy in a child who responds to resuscitation. The presence of leukocytosis, feces, vegetable fibers, and/or bile in the lavage effluent mandates laparotomy.

Only the surgeon who will care for the child should perform the DPL, because DPL may interfere with subsequent abdominal examinations upon which the decision to operate may in part be based.

NONOPERATIVE MANAGEMENT

Selective, nonoperative management of blunt abdominal injuries in children is performed in many trauma centers, especially those with pediatric capabilities. The presence of intraperitoneal blood on CT, FAST, or DPL does not necessarily mandate a laparotomy. It has been well demonstrated that bleeding from an injured spleen, liver, or kidney generally is self-limited. Therefore, a CT, FAST, or DPL that is positive for blood alone does not mandate a laparotomy in a child with initial abnormal hemodynamics that are readily normalized by fluid resuscitation. **If the child's condition cannot be normalized hemodynamically and if the diagnostic procedure performed is positive for blood, a prompt laparotomy to control hemorrhage is indicated.**

When nonoperative management is selected, these children *must* be treated in a facility that offers pediatric intensive care capabilities and under the supervision of a qualified surgeon with a special interest in and commitment to the care of injured children. Intensive care must include continuous pediatric nursing staff coverage, continuous monitoring of vital signs, and *immediate* availability of surgical personnel and operating room resources.

The chief indication for operative management in children who continue to have no hemodynamic abnormalities is a transfusion requirement that exceeds one-half the child's blood volume, or 40 mL/kg, during the first 24 hours after injury. In most children who require operation for solid organ injury, the need presents itself early, within 6 to 12 hours.

Frequent, repeated examinations by the surgeon are necessary to adequately assess the evolving status of the child.

Nonoperative management of confirmed abdominal visceral injuries is a surgical decision made by surgeons, just as is the decision to operate. Therefore, the surgeon must supervise the treatment of pediatric trauma patients.

SPECIFIC VISCERAL INJURIES

A number of abdominal visceral injuries are more common in children than in adults. Duodenal hematoma results from a combination of thinner abdominal musculature and a mechanism of injury such as a bicycle handlebar or an elbow striking the child in the right upper quadrant. This injury also may be caused by child abuse. It is most often treated nonoperatively with nasogastric suction and parenteral nutrition.

Blunt pancreatic injuries occur from similar mechanisms, with their treatment dependent on the extent of injury. Small bowel perforations at or near the ligament of Treitz are more common in children than in adults, as are mesenteric, small bowel avulsion injuries. These particular injuries are often diagnosed late because of the vague early symptoms and the potential for late perforation.

Children who are restrained by a lap belt are at particular risk for enteric disruption, especially if they have a lap-belt mark on the abdominal wall or sustain a flexion-distraction (Chance) fracture of the lumbar spine. Any patient with this mechanism of injury and these findings should be presumed to have a high likelihood of injury to the gastrointestinal tract until proven otherwise. **Rupture of a hollow viscus requires early operative intervention.**

Bladder rupture is also more common in children than in adults, because of the shallow depth of the child's pelvis. Penetrating injuries of the perineum, or straddle injuries, may occur with falls onto a prominent object, and may result in intraperitoneal injuries because of the proximity of the peritoneum to the perineum.

A child's spleen, liver, and kidneys are frequently disrupted in the face of a blunt force. It is uncommon for these injuries to require operative repair. It is not uncommon for

a child with hemodynamic abnormalities to present to the ED and receive rapid crystalloid fluid resuscitation, with return to hemodynamic normality. When an injury to the liver, spleen, or kidney is suspected, the child should undergo a CT scan. A child with grade II or higher injuries to these organs is often admitted to the pediatric transitional or intensive care unit for continuous monitoring. Delayed hemorrhage from splenic rupture usually does not occur. The presence of a splenic blush on CT with intravenous contrast does not mandate exploration. The decision to operate continues to be based on the amount of blood lost as well as abnormal physiologic parameters.

Head Trauma

The information provided in Chapter 6: Head Trauma, also applies to pediatric patients. This section emphasizes additional points specific to children.

Most head injuries in the pediatric population are the result of motor vehicle crashes, bicycle crashes, and falls. Analysis of national pediatric trauma data repositories indicate that an understanding of the interaction between the CNS and extracranial injuries is imperative, because hypotension and hypoxia from associated injuries have an adverse effect on the outcome from intracranial injury. Lack of attention to the ABCDEs and associated injuries significantly increases mortality from head injury. As in adults, hypotension is infrequently caused by head injury alone, and other explanations for this finding should be investigated aggressively.

The brain of the child is anatomically different from that of the adult. It doubles in size in the first 6 months of life and achieves 80% of the adult brain size by 2 years of age. There is increased water content of the brain up to 2 years of age. Neuronal plasticity is evident after birth and includes incomplete neuronal synapse formation and arborization, incomplete myelinization, and a vast number of neurochemical changes. The subarachnoid space is relatively smaller, and hence offers less protection to the brain because there is less buoyancy. Thus, head momentum is more likely to impart parenchymal structural damage. Normal cerebral blood flow increases progressively to nearly twice that of adult levels by the age of 5 years, and then decreases. This accounts in part for children's severe susceptibility to cerebral hypoxia.

ASSESSMENT

Children and adults may differ in their response to head trauma, which may influence the evaluation of the injured child. The principal differences include:

1. The outcome in children who suffer severe brain injury is better than that in adults. However, the out-

---

PITFALL

Delays in the recognition of abdominal hollow viscus injury are possible, especially when the decision is made to manage solid organ injury nonoperatively. Such an approach to the management of these injuries in children must be accompanied by an attitude of anticipation, frequent reevaluation, and preparation for immediate surgical intervention. These children should all be treated by a surgeon in a facility equipped to handle any contingencies in an expeditious manner.

come in children younger than 3 years of age is worse than a similar injury in an older child. Children are particularly susceptible to the effects of the secondary brain injury that may be produced by hypovolemia, with attendant reductions in cerebral perfusion, hypoxia, seizures, or hyperthermia. The effect of the combination of hypovolemia and hypoxia on the injured brain is devastating, but hypotension from hypovolemia is the worst single risk factor. **Adequate and rapid restoration of an appropriate circulating blood volume and avoidance of hypoxia are mandatory.**

2. Although it is an infrequent occurrence, hypotension may occur in small infants as the result of blood loss into either the subgaleal or epidural space. This hypovolemia, due to intracranial injury, occurs because of open cranial sutures and fontanelles in infants. Treatment is directed toward appropriate volume restoration, as is appropriate for blood loss from other body regions.

3. The young child with an open fontanelle and mobile cranial sutures has more tolerance for an expanding intracranial mass lesion or brain swelling. Signs of these conditions may be hidden until rapid decompensation occurs. **Therefore, an infant who is not in a coma but who has bulging fontanelles or suture diastases should be treated as having a more severe injury.** Early neurosurgical consultation is essential.

4. Vomiting and even amnesia are common after brain injury in children and do not necessarily imply increased intracranial pressure. However, persistent vomiting or vomiting that becomes more frequent is a concern and mandates CT of the head. Gastric decompression is essential, because of the risk of aspiration.

5. Impact seizures—that is, seizures that occur shortly after brain injury—are more common in children and are usually self-limited. All seizure activity requires investigation by CT of the head.

6. Children tend to have fewer focal mass lesions than do adults, but elevated intracranial pressure due to brain swelling is more common. Rapid restoration of normal circulating blood volume is necessary. Some practitioners fear that restoration of a child's circulating blood volume places the child at greater risk for worsening of the existing head injury. However, the opposite is true. If hypovolemia is not corrected promptly, the outcome from head injury is made worse because of secondary brain injury. Emergency CT is vital to identify children who require emergency operation.

7. The GCS is useful when applied to the pediatric age group. However, the verbal score component must be modified for children younger than 4 years (Table 10-5). ◾ Also see Appendix C: Trauma Scores: Revised and Pediatric.

8. Because increased intracranial pressure frequently develops in children, neurosurgical consultation to consider intracranial pressure monitoring should be obtained *early* in the course of resuscitation for children with:

   • A GCS score of 8 or less, or motor scores of 1 or 2

   • Multiple injuries associated with brain injury that require major volume resuscitation, immediate lifesaving thoracic or abdominal surgery, or for which stabilization and assessment is prolonged

   • A CT scan of the brain that demonstrates evidence of brain hemorrhage, cerebral swelling, or transtentorial or cerebellar herniation

9. Medication dosages must be adjusted as dictated by the child's size and in consultation with a neurosurgeon. Drugs often used in children with head injuries include:

   • Phenobarbital, 10 to 20 mg/kg/dose

   • Diazepam, 0.1 to 0.2 mg/kg/dose; slow IV bolus

   • Phenytoin or fosphenytoin, 15 to 20 mg/kg, administered at 0.5 to 1.5 mL/kg/min as a loading dose, then 4 to 7 mg/kg/day for maintenance

   • Mannitol, 0.5 to 1.0 g/kg (rarely required); diuresis with the use of mannitol or furosemide may worsen hypovolemia and should be withheld early in the resuscitation of children with head injury unless there are incontrovertible signs of transtentorial herniation

TABLE 10-5 ◾ Pediatric Verbal Score

VERBAL RESPONSE	V-SCORE
Appropriate words or social smile, fixes and follows	5
Cries, but consolable	4
Persistently irritable	3
Restless, agitated	2
None	1

MANAGEMENT

Management of traumatic brain injury in children involves:

1. Rapid, early assessment and management of the ABCDEs

2. Appropriate neurosurgical involvement from the beginning of treatment

3. Appropriate sequential assessment and management of the brain injury with attention directed toward the prevention of secondary brain injury—that is, hypoxia and hypoperfusion. Early endotracheal intubation with adequate oxygenation and ventilation are indicated to avoid progressive CNS damage. Attempts to orally intubate the trachea in an uncooperative, child with a brain injury may be difficult and actually increase intracranial pressure. In the hands of doctors who have considered the risks and benefits of intubating such children, pharmacologic sedation and neuromuscular blockade may be used to facilitate intubation.

4. Continuous reassessment of all parameters ■ See Skill Station IX: Head and Neck Trauma: Assessment and Management.

Spinal Cord Injury

The information provided in Chapter 7: Spine and Spinal Cord Trauma also applies to pediatric patients. This section emphasizes points specific to pediatric spinal injury.

Spinal cord injury in children is fortunately uncommon—only 5% of spinal cord injuries occur in the pediatric age group. For children younger than 10 years of age, motor vehicle crashes most commonly produce these injuries. For children aged 10 to 14 years, motor vehicles and sporting activities account for an equal number of spinal injuries.

ANATOMIC DIFFERENCES

The anatomic differences in children to be considered with regard to spinal injury include:

1. Interspinous ligaments and joint capsules are more flexible.

2. Vertebral bodies are wedged anteriorly and tend to slide forward with flexion.

3. The facet joints are flat.

4. The child has a relatively large head compared with the neck. Therefore, the angular momentum forces applied to the upper neck are relatively greater than in the adult.

RADIOLOGIC CONSIDERATIONS

Pseudosubluxation frequently complicates the radiographic evaluation of a child's cervical spine. About 40% of children younger than 7 years of age show anterior displacement of C2 on C3, and 20% of children up to 16 years exhibit this phenomenon. This radiographic finding is seen less commonly at C3 to C4. More than 3 mm of movement may be seen when these joints are studied by flexion and extension maneuvers.

When subluxation is seen on a lateral cervical spine x-ray, the doctor must ascertain whether this is a pseudosubluxation or a true cervical spine injury. Pseudosubluxation of the cervical vertebrae is made more pronounced by the flexion of the cervical spine that occurs when a child lies supine on a hard surface. To correct this radiographic anomaly, place the child's head in a neutral position by placing a 1-inch-thick layer of padding beneath the entire body from shoulders to hips, but not the head, and repeat the x-ray. (See Figure 10-2.) Cervical spine injury usually can be identified from neurologic examination findings and by detection of an area of soft tissue swelling, muscle spasm, or a step-off deformity on careful palpation of the posterior cervical spine.

An increased distance between the dens and the anterior arch of C1 occurs in approximately 20% of young children. Gaps exceeding the upper limit of normal for the adult population are seen frequently.

Skeletal growth centers can resemble fractures. Basilar odontoid synchondrosis appears as a radiolucent area at the base of the dens, especially in children younger than 5 years. Apical odontoid epiphyses appear as separations on the odontoid x-ray and are usually seen between the ages of 5 and 11 years. The growth center of the spinous process can resemble fractures of the tip of the spinous process.

Children may sustain "spinal cord injury without radiographic abnormalities" (SCIWORA) more commonly than adults. A normal cervical spine series may be found in up to two-thirds of children who have suffered spinal cord injury. Thus, if spinal cord injury is suspected, based on history or the results of the neurologic examination, normal spine x-ray examination does not exclude significant spinal cord injury. **When in doubt about the integrity of the cervical spine or spinal cord, assume that an unstable injury exists, maintain immobilization of the child's head and neck, and obtain appropriate consultation.**

Spinal cord injury in children is treated in the same way as spinal cord injuries in adults. Consultation with a neurosurgeon should be obtained early. ■ See Chapter 7: Spine and Spinal Cord Trauma, Skill Station X: X-Ray Identification of Spine Injuries, and Skill Station XI: Spinal Cord Injury: Assessment and Management.

Musculoskeletal Trauma

The initial priorities in the management of skeletal trauma in the child are similar to those for the adult, with additional concerns about potential injury to the growth plate. See Chapter 8: Musculoskeletal Trauma.

HISTORY

History is of vital importance. In younger children, x-ray diagnosis of fractures and dislocations is difficult because of the lack of mineralization around the epiphysis and the presence of a physis (growth plate). Information about the magnitude, mechanism, and time of the injury facilitates better correlation of the physical and x-ray findings. Radiographic evidence of fractures of differing ages should alert the doctor to possible child abuse, as should lower-extremity fractures in children who are too young to walk.

BLOOD LOSS

Blood loss associated with long-bone and pelvic fractures is proportionately more in children than in adults. Blood loss related to an isolated closed femur fracture that is treated appropriately is associated with an average fall in hematocrit of 4 points, which is not enough to cause shock. Hemodynamic instability in the presence of an isolated femur fracture should prompt evaluation for other sources of blood loss, which usually will be found within the abdomen.

SPECIAL CONSIDERATIONS OF THE IMMATURE SKELETON

Bones lengthen as new bone is laid down by the physis near the articular surfaces. Injuries to, or adjacent to, this area be-fore the physis has closed may potentially retard the normal growth or alter the development of the bone in an abnormal way. Crush injuries to the physis, which are often difficult to recognize radiographically, have the worst prognosis.

The immature, pliable nature of bones in children may lead to a so-called greenstick fracture. Such fractures are incomplete, with angulation maintained by cortical splinters on the concave surface. The torus, or "buckle," fracture, seen in small children, involves angulation due to cortical impaction with a radiolucent fracture line. Both types of fractures may suggest abuse in patients with vague, inconsistent, or conflicting histories. Supracondylar fractures at the elbow or knee have a high propensity for vascular injury as well as injury to the growth plate.

PRINCIPLES OF IMMOBILIZATION

Simple splinting of fractured extremities in children usually is sufficient until definitive orthopedic evaluation can be performed. Injured extremities with evidence of vascular compromise require emergency evaluation to prevent the adverse sequelae of ischemia. A single attempt to reduce the fracture to restore blood flow is appropriate, followed by simple splinting or traction splinting of the femur. See Skill Station XII: Musculoskeletal Trauma: Assessment and Management.

The Battered, Abused Child

? *How do I recognize abuse injuries?*

Any child who sustains an intentional injury as the result of acts by parents, guardians, or acquaintances is considered to be a battered, abused child. Homicide is the most common cause of injury death in the first year of life. Therefore, a history and careful evaluation of the child in whom abuse is suspected is critically important to prevent eventual death, especially in children who are younger than 1 year of age. A doctor should suspect abuse if:

1. A discrepancy exists between the history and the degree of physical injury—for example, a young child loses consciousness after falling from a bed or sofa, fractures an extremity during play with siblings or other children, or sustains a lower-extremity fracture but is too young to walk.

2. A prolonged interval has passed between the time of the injury and presentation for medical care.

3. The history includes repeated trauma, treated in the same or different EDs.

4. The history of injury changes or is different between parents or guardians.

PITFALLS

- Many orthopedic injuries in children produce only subtle symptoms, and positive findings on physical examination are difficult to detect.
- Any evidence of unusual behavior—for example, a child who refuses to use an arm or bear weight on an extremity, must be carefully evaluated for the possibility of an occult bony or soft tissue injury.
- The parents are often the ones who note behavior that is out of the ordinary for their child.
- The doctor must remember the potential for child abuse. The history of the injury event should be viewed suspiciously when the findings do not corroborate the parent's story.

5. There is a history of hospital or doctor "shopping."

6. Parents respond inappropriately to or do not comply with medical advice—for example, leaving a child unattended in the emergency facility.

The following findings, on careful physical examination, should suggest child abuse and indicate more intensive investigation:

1. Multicolored bruises (bruises in different stages of healing)

2. Evidence of frequent previous injuries, typified by old scars or healed fractures on x-ray examination

3. Perioral injuries

4. Injuries to the genital or perianal area

5. Fractures of long bones in children younger than 3 years of age

6. Ruptured internal viscera without antecedent major blunt trauma

7. Multiple subdural hematomas, especially without a fresh skull fracture

8. Retinal hemorrhages

9. Bizarre injuries, such as bites, cigarette burns, or rope marks

10. Sharply demarcated second- and third-degree burns in unusual areas

In many nations, doctors are bound by law to report incidents of child abuse to governmental authorities, even cases in which abuse is only suspected. Abused children are at increased risk for fatal injuries, and no one is served by failing to report. The system protects doctors from legal liability for identifying confirmed or even suspicious cases of abuse. Although the reporting procedures may vary, it is most commonly handled through local social service agencies or the state's health and human services department. The process of reporting child abuse assumes greater importance when one realizes that 50% of abused children who die or are dead on arrival at the hospital were victims of previous episodes of abuse that went unreported or were not taken seriously.

Prevention

The greatest pitfall related to pediatric trauma is failure to have prevented the child's injuries in the first place. Up to 80% of childhood injuries could have been prevented by the application of simple strategies in the home and the community. The ABCDEs of injury prevention have been described, and warrant special attention in a population among whom the lifetime benefits of successful injury prevention are self-evident (Box 10-1). Not only is the social and familial disruption associated with childhood injury avoided, but for every dollar invested in injury prevention, four dollars are saved in hospital care.

Box 10-1
ABCDEs of Injury Prevention

- **Analyze injury data**
  —Local injury surveillance

- **Build local coalitions**
  —Hospital community partnerships

- **Communicate the problem**
  —Injuries are preventable

- **Develop prevention activities**
  —Create safer environments

- **Evaluate the interventions**
  —Ongoing injury surveillance

Source: Pressley J, Barlow B, Durkin M, Jacko SA, Roca-Dominguez D, Johnson L. A national program for injury prevention in children and adolescents: the Injury Free Coalition for Kids. *J Urban Health* 2005;82:389-402.

CHAPTER SUMMARY

 1 Unique characteristics of children include important differences in anatomy, body surface area, chest wall compliance, and skeletal anatomy. Normal vital signs vary significantly with age.

2 Initial assessment and management of severely injured children is guided by the ABCDE approach. Early involvement of a general surgeon or pediatric surgeon is imperative in the management of injuries in a child. Nonoperative management of abdominal visceral injuries should be performed only by surgeons in facilities equipped to handle any contingency in an expeditious manner.

3 Child abuse should be suspected if suggested by suspicious findings on history or physical examination. These include discrepant history, delayed presentation, frequent prior injuries, and perineal injuries.

Bibliography

1. Carney NA, Chesnut R, Kochanek PM, et al. Guidelines for the acute medical management of severe traumatic brain injury in infants, children, and adolescents. *J Trauma* 2003;54:S235-S310.

2. Chesnut RM, Marshall LF, et al, The role of secondary brain injury in determining outcome from severe head injury. *J Trauma* 1993;43:216-222.

3. Cloutier DR, Baird TB, Gormley P, McCarten KM, Bussey JG, Luks FI. Pediatric splenic injuries with a contrast blush: successful nonoperative management without angiography and embolization. *J Pediatr Surg* 2004;39(6):969-971.

4. Cooper A, Barlow B, DiScala C, et al. Mortality and truncal injury: the pediatric perspective. *J Pediatr Surg* 1994;29:33.

5. Cooper A, Barlow B, DiScala C. Vital signs and trauma mortality: the pediatric perspective. *Pediatr Emerg Care* 2000;16:66.

6. Corbett SW, Andrews HG, Baker EM, Jones WG. ED evaluation of the pediatric trauma patient by ultrasonography. *Am J Emerg Med* 2000;18(3):244-249.

7. DiScala C, Sage R, Li G, et al. Child abuse and unintentional injuries. *Arch Pediatr Adolesc Med* 2000;154:16-22.

8. Emery KH, McAneney CM, Racadio JM, Johnson ND, Evora DK, Garcia VF. Absent peritoneal fluid on screening trauma ultrasonography in children: a prospective comparison with computed tomography. *J Pediatr Surg* 2001;36(4):565-569.

9. Gerardi MJ, Sacchett AD, Cantor RM, et al. Rapid-sequence intubation of the pediatric patient. *Ann Emerg Med* 1996;28:55-74.

10. Hannan E, Meaker P, Fawell L, et al. Predicting inpatient mortality for pediatric blunt trauma patients: a better alternative. *J Pediatr Surg* 2000;35:155-159.

11. Harris BH, Schwaitzberg SD, Seman TM, et al. The hidden morbidity of pediatric trauma. *J Pediatr Surg* 1989;24:103-106.

12. Herzenberg JE, Hensinger RN, Dedrick DE, et al. Emergency transport and positioning of young children who have an injury of the cervical spine. *J Bone Joint Surg Am* 1989;71:15-22.

13. Holmes JF, Brant WE, Bond WF, Sokolove PE, Kuppermann N. Emergency department ultrasonography in the evaluation of hypotensive and normotensive children with blunt abdominal trauma. *J Pediatr Surg* 2001;36(7):968-973.

14. Holmes JF, London KL, Brant WE, Kuppermann N. Isolated intraperitoneal fluid on abdominal computed tomography in children with blunt trauma. *Acad Emerg Med* 2000;7(4): 335-341.

15. Lutz N, Nance ML, Kallan MJ, Arbogast KB, Durbin DR, Winston FK. Incidence and clinical significance of abdominal wall bruising in restrained children involved in motor vehicle crashes. *J Pediatr Surg* 2004;39(6):972-975.

16. Mutabagani KH, Coley BD, Zumberge N, et al. Preliminary experience with focused abdominal sonography for trauma (FAST) in children: is it useful? *J Pediatr Surg* 1999;34:48-54.

17. National Safety Council. *Injury Facts*. Itasca, IL: National Safety Council; 2007.

18. Paddock HN, Tepas JJ, Ramenofsky ML. Management of blunt pediatric hepatic and splenic injury: similar process, different outcome. *Am Surg* 2004;70:1068-1072.

19. Patel JC, Tepas JJ. The efficacy of focused abdominal sonography for trauma (FAST) as a screening tool in the assessment of injured children. *J Pediatr Surg* 1999;34:44-47.

20. Pershad J, Gilmore B. Serial bedside emergency ultrasound in a case of pediatric blunt abdominal trauma with severe abdominal pain. *Pediatr Emerg Care* 2000;16(5):375-376.

21. Pigula FA, Wald SL, Shackford SR, et al. The effect of hypotension and hypoxia on children with severe head injuries. *J Pediatr Surg* 1993;28:310-316.

22. Pressley J, Barlow B, Durkin M, Jacko SA, Roca-Dominguez D, Johnson L. A national program for injury prevention in children and adolescents: the Injury Free Coalition for Kids. *J Urban Health* 2005;82:389-402.

23. Rathaus V, Zissin R, Werner M, et al. Minimal pelvic fluid in blunt abdominal trauma in children: the significance of this sonographic finding. *J Pediatr Surg* 2001;36(9):1387-1389.

24. Rogers CG, Knight V, MacUra KJ. High-grade renal injuries in children—is conservative management possible? *Urology* 2004;64:574-9.

25. Schwaitzberg SD, Bergman KS, Harris BW. A pediatric trauma model of continuous hemorrhage. *J Pediatr Surg* 1988;23:605-609.

26. Soudack M, Epelman M, Maor R, et al. Experience with focused abdominal sonography for trauma (FAST) in 313 pediatric patients. *J Clin Ultrasound* 2004;32(2):53-61.

27. Soundappan SV, Holland AJ, Cass DT, Lam A. Diagnostic accuracy of surgeon-performed focused abdominal sonography (FAST) in blunt paediatric trauma. *Injury* 2005;36(8):970-975.

28. Stylianos S. Compliance with evidence-based guidelines in children with isolated spleen or liver injury: a prospective study. *J Pediatr Surg* 2002;37:453-456.

29. Suthers SE, Albrecht R, Foley D, et al. Surgeon-directed ultrasound for trauma is a predictor of intra-abdominal injury in children. *Am Surg* 2004;70(2):164-167; discussion 167-168.

30. Tepas JJ, DiScala C, Ramenofsky ML, et al. Mortality and head injury: the pediatric perspective. *J Pediatr Surg* 1990;25:92-96.

31. Tepas JJ, Ramenofsky ML, Mollitt DL, et al. The Pediatric Trauma Score as a predictor of injury severity: an objective assessment. *J Trauma* 1988;28:425-429.

32. van der Sluis CK, Kingma J, Eisma WH, ten Duis HJ. Pediatric polytrauma: short-term and long-term outcomes. *J Trauma* 1997;43(3):501-506.

CHAPTER **11** Geriatric Trauma

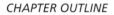

Upon completion of this topic, the student will demonstrate the ability to apply the principles of trauma care to acutely injured geriatric patients. Specifically, the doctor will be able to:

OBJECTIVES

1 Identify the unique characteristics of elderly trauma patients, including common types of injury, patterns of injury, and their anatomic and physiologic differences.

2 Describe the primary management of critical injuries in geriatric patients, including related issues unique to geriatric patients, emphasizing the anatomic and physiologic differences from younger patients and their impact on resuscitation.

   Airway management

   Breathing and ventilation

   Shock, fluid, and electrolyte management

   Central nervous system and cervical spine injuries

3 Identify common causes and signs of elder abuse, and formulate a strategy for managing situations of elder abuse.

Introduction

Globally, human populations continue to age at an impressive rate. Between 1900 and 1992, the number of individuals aged 65 and above increased from 1% (15 million) to 6% (342 million) of the world's population. By the year 2050, these figures will have risen to 20%, or 2.5 billion. At that time, it is projected that the elderly will represent 25% of the population in the United States. The rapid growth of the senior population has already had a significant economic impact because of their unique medical requirements and the fact that seniors consume more than one-third of the country's health care resources. Currently, trauma is the seventh leading cause of death in the elderly, surpassed only by heart disease, cancer, chronic obstructive pulmonary disease, stroke, diabetes, and pneumonia.

Types and Patterns of Injury

? *What are the unique characteristics of geriatric trauma?*

Although patients aged 65 and older are less likely to be injured than are younger individuals, older patients are more likely to have a fatal outcome from their injuries. However, more than 80% of the injured can return to their preexist-

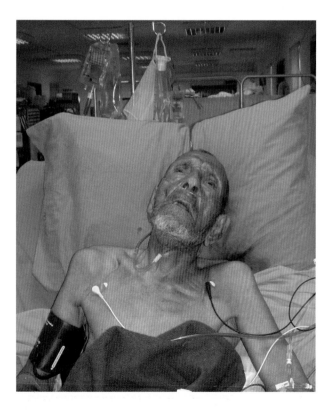

ing level of independent living after aggressive resuscitation and follow-up care. Despite this, in the United States in 1997 more than 36,000 elderly patients died from injuries, accounting for 25% of all injury fatalities. This high mortality rate likely reflects the decreased physical reserves of the elderly due to the changes of aging, the comorbidities that develop, and a lack of understanding of their needs by many health-care providers. Figure 11-1 illustrates the effects of aging on organ systems, and Box 11-1 outlines the impact of preexisting disease on trauma outcome. Milzman et al. reported that preexisting disease was more common in the older age group (mean age, 49.2) than in the younger age group (mean age, 30.0), and the mortality rate was three times greater in the older patients with preexisting disease (9.2% vs 3.2%).

The three leading causes of death due to injury among the elderly in the United States are falls, motor vehicle crashes, and burns. Falls, which are the most common cause of unintentional injury and death among the elderly, account for 40% of the deaths in this age group. Both the incidence of falls and the severity of complications rise with age, and large numbers of emergency department visits and subsequent hospital admissions occur as a result of falls. Although fall-related injury rates are higher in older adults, the majority do not result in serious injury. Only 5% to 15% of falls in community-dwelling older adults cause serious injuries, including head trauma, fractures, dislocation, and serious soft tissue injury.

The accumulated effects of the aging process and environmental hazards most frequently cause falls. Changes in the central nervous and musculoskeletal systems make older people more stiff and less coordinated than younger adults, and older people may have an unsteady gait. Visual, hearing, and memory impairments place older adults at high risk for hazards that can cause falls. Falls resulting from dizziness or vertigo are extremely common. Finally, drugs—including alcohol—cause or contribute to many falls. **Seemingly minor mechanisms of injury can produce serious injury and complications because of the effect of multiple medications, especially anticoagulants.**

Annually in the United States, more than 4000 elderly people are killed in motor vehicle crashes, either as drivers or passengers. In addition, 2000 elderly people are killed as pedestrians when struck by motor vehicles. The effects of the aging process are a major influence on the incidence of injury and death. Often, the elderly have diminished visual and auditory acuity. Daylight acuity, glare resistance, and night vision decrease markedly with age. Medical conditions and their treatments may alter attention and consciousness. Because of the onset of senile changes in the brain, judgment may be altered. **Finally, there often is decreased ability to implement appropriate actions because of impairment from medical conditions, including severe arthritis, osteoporosis, emphysema, heart disease, and decreased muscle mass.**

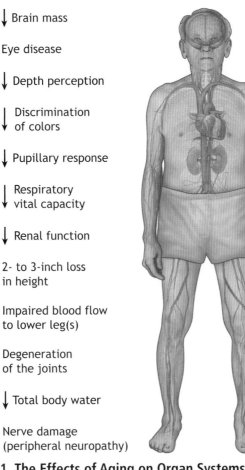

↓ Brain mass

Eye disease

↓ Depth perception

↓ Discrimination of colors

↓ Pupillary response

↓ Respiratory vital capacity

↓ Renal function

2- to 3-inch loss in height

Impaired blood flow to lower leg(s)

Degeneration of the joints

↓ Total body water

Nerve damage (peripheral neuropathy)

Stroke

Diminished hearing

↓ Sense of smell and taste

↓ Saliva production

↓ Esophageal activity

↓ Cardiac stroke volume and rate

Heart disease and high blood pressure

Kidney disease

↓ Gastric secretions

↓ Number of body cells

↓ Elasticity of skin Thinning of epidermis

↓ 15%-30% body fat

■ **Figure 11-1 The Effects of Aging on Organ Systems.**

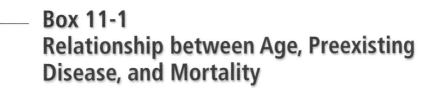

Box 11-1
Relationship between Age, Preexisting Disease, and Mortality

- Mean age of patients with preexisting disease: 49.2

- Mean age of patients without preexisting disease: 30.6

- Mortality rate for older patients with preexisting disease: 9.2%

- Mortality rate for younger patients without preexisting disease: 3.2%

Source: Milzman DP, Boulanger BR, Rodriguez A, et al. Pre-existing disease in trauma patients: a predictor of fate independent of age and injury severity score. *J Trauma* 1992;31:236-244.

Thermal injury is the third leading cause of death due to injury in the elderly, accounting for almost 2000 deaths annually. One-third of these individuals are fatally injured while under the influence of alcohol, while smoking in bed, or when exposed to heat and toxic products of combustion while caught in a building fire. Of the remainder, the majority sustain injury and death because of their clothing being ignited or because of prolonged contact with hot substances. As with falls, factors associated with degenerative disease and physical impairment appear to contribute substantially to the rate of thermal injury in the elderly. Elderly persons who come into contact with hot surfaces or liquids or are exposed to fire often are not able to remove themselves until after extensive injury occurs. Finally, preexisting cardiovascular, respiratory, and renal diseases often make it impossible for the injured person to overcome serious but potentially survivable burns.

Airway

How do I apply ATLS airway principles to the treatment of elderly patients?

The "A" of the ABCDE mnemonic of the primary survey is the same in the elderly as for any other trauma patient. **Establishing and then maintaining a patent airway to provide adequate tissue oxygenation is the first objective.** Supplemental oxygen should be administered as soon as possible, even in the presence of chronic pulmonary disease. Because of the elderly patient's likely limitation in cardiopulmonary reserve, early intubation of the injured elder should be considered for those presenting in shock. Early intubation also should be considered for those with chest wall injury or alteration in the level of consciousness.

Features that affect management of the airway in the elderly include dentition, nasopharyngeal fragility, macroglossia (enlargement of tongue), microstomia (small oral aperture), and cervical arthritis. A lack of teeth can interfere with achieving a proper seal on a face mask. **Consequently, whereas broken dentures should be removed, intact well-fitted dentures are often best left in place until after airway control is achieved.** Care must be taken when placing nasogastric and nasotracheal tubes because of nasopharyngeal tissue friability, especially around the turbinates. Profuse bleeding can ensue, complicating an already dangerous situation. The oral cavity may be compromised by either macroglossia, associated with amyloidosis or acromegaly, or microstomia, such as the constricted, birdlike mouth of progressive systemic sclerosis. **Finally, arthritis can affect the temporomandibular joints and the cervical spine, making endotracheal intubation more difficult and increasing the risk of spinal cord injury with manipulation of the osteoarthritic spine.** Degenerative changes and calcification in laryngeal cartilage place the elderly population at increased risk of injury from minor blows to the neck.

The principles of airway management remain the same, with endotracheal intubation as the preferred method for definitive airway control. If acute airway obstruction exists or the vocal cords cannot be visualized, surgical cricothyroidotomy should be performed. ◼ See Chapter 2: Airway and Ventilatory Management, and Skill Station III: Cricothyroidotomy, Skill III-B: Surgical Cricothyroidotomy.

Breathing and Ventilation

Many of the changes that occur in the airway and lungs of elderly patients are difficult to ascribe purely to the process of aging and may be the result of chronic exposure to toxic agents such as tobacco smoke and other environmental toxins throughout life. **The loss of respiratory reserve, due to the effects of aging and chronic diseases (eg, chronic bronchitis and emphysema), makes careful monitoring of the geriatric patient's respiratory system imperative.** Administration of supplemental oxygen is mandatory, although caution should be exercised with its use because some elderly patients rely on a hypoxic drive to maintain ventilation. Oxygen administration can result in loss of this hypoxic drive, causing CO_2 retention and respiratory acidosis. In the acute trauma situation, however, hypoxemia should be corrected by administering oxygen while accepting the risk of hypercarbia. In these situations, if respiratory failure is imminent, intubation and mechanical ventilation is necessary

Chest injuries occur in patients of all ages with similar frequency, but the mortality rate for elderly patients is higher. Chest wall injury with rib fractures or pulmonary contusions are common and not well tolerated. Simple pneumothorax and hemothorax also are poorly tolerated. Respiratory failure may result from the increased work of breathing combined with a decreased energy reserve. Adequate pain control and vigorous pulmonary toilet are essential for a satisfactory outcome. Pulmonary complications—such as atelectasis, pneumonia, and pulmonary edema—occur in the elderly with great frequency. Marginal cardiopulmonary reserve coupled with overzealous crystalloid infusion increases the potential for pulmonary edema and worsening of pulmonary contusions. Admission to the hospital usually is necessary even with apparently minor injuries.

PITFALLS

- Failure to recognize indications for early intubation.
- Undue manipulation of the osteoarthritic cervical spine, leading to cord injury.
- Failure to recognize the serious effects of rib fractures and lung contusion, which may require mechanical ventilation.

Circulation

CHANGES WITH AGING

As the heart ages, there is progressive loss of function. By the age of 65 years, nearly 50% of the population has coronary artery stenosis. The cardiac index falls off linearly with age, and the maximal heart rate also begins to decrease from about 40 years of age. The formula for maximal heart rate is 220 minus the individual's age in years. Although the resting heart rate varies little, the maximum tachycardic response decreases with age.

The cause of this diminution of function is multifaceted. With aging, total blood volume decreases and circulation time increases. There is increasing myocardial stiffness, slowed electrophysiologic conduction, and loss of myocardial cell mass. The response to endogenous catecholamine release with stress is also different, which is likely related to a reduction in responsiveness of the cellular membrane receptor. These changes predispose the aged heart to reentry dysrhythmias. In addition, diastolic dysfunction makes the heart more dependent on atrial filling to increase cardiac output.

In addition, the kidney loses mass rapidly after the age of 50 years. This loss involves entire nephron units and is accompanied by a decrement in the glomerular filtration rate and renal blood flow. Levels of serum creatinine usually remain within normal limits, presumably because of a reduction in creatinine production by muscles. The aged kidney is less able to resorb sodium and excrete potassium or hydrogen ions. The maximum concentration ability of the kidney of an octogenarian is only 850 mOsm/kg, which is 70% of the ability of a 30-year-old kidney. A decrease in the production of, and responsiveness of the kidney to, renin and angiotensin occurs with age. As a result, creatinine clearance in the elderly is markedly reduced, and the aged kidney is more susceptible to injury from hypovolemia, medications, and other nephrotoxins.

EVALUATION AND MANAGEMENT

A common pitfall in the evaluation of geriatric trauma patients is the mistaken impression that "normal" blood pressure and heart rate indicate normovolemia. Early monitoring of the cardiovascular system must be instituted. Blood pressure generally increases with age. Thus, a systolic blood pressure of 120 mm Hg can represent hypotension in an elderly patient whose normal preinjury systolic blood pressure was 170 to 180 mm Hg. A significant loss of blood volume can be masked by the absence of early tachycardia. The onset of hypotension also may be delayed. In addition, the chronic high afterload state induced by elevated peripheral vascular resistance can limit cardiac output and ultimately cerebral, renal, coronary, and peripheral oxygen delivery.

Geriatric patients have a limited physiologic reserve and may have difficulty generating an adequate response to injury. **Severely injured elderly patients with hypotension and metabolic acidosis almost always die, especially if they have sustained brain injury.** Fluid requirements—once corrected for the lesser, lean body mass—are similar to those of younger patients. **Elderly patients with hypertension who are on chronic diuretic therapy may have a chronically contracted vascular volume and a serum potassium deficit; therefore careful monitoring of the administration of crystalloid solutions is important, to prevent electrolyte disorders.**

Isotonic electrolyte solutions are used for initial resuscitation. Initially, 1 or 2 L are administered rapidly while observing the patient's physiologic response. Further decisions with respect to fluid resuscitation are predicated on this observed response. ◼ See Chapter 3: Shock.

The optimal hemoglobin level for an injured elderly patient is a point of controversy. Many authors suggest that, in people over the age of 65 years, hemoglobin concentrations of over 10 g/dL should be maintained to maximize oxygen-carrying capacity and delivery. **However, indiscriminate blood transfusion should be avoided because of the attendant risk of bloodborne infections, its known impairment of the immune host response and its resulting complications, and the effect of the high hematocrit on blood viscosity, which can adversely affect myocardial function. Early recognition and correction of coagulation defects is crucial, including reversal of drug-induced anticoagulation.**

Because elderly patients may have significant limitation in cardiac reserve, a rapid and complete assessment for all sources of blood loss is necessary. The focused assessment sonography in trauma (FAST) examination is a rapid means of determining the presence of abnormal intraabdominal fluid collections. When this is unavailable, diagnostic peritoneal lavage (DPL) may be of use. There is at present little role for nonoperative management of blunt abdominal solid viscus injuries in elderly patients. **The risk of nonoperative management may be greater than the risk of an early operation.**

The retroperitoneum is an often-unrecognized source of blood loss. Exsanguinating retroperitoneal hemorrhage may develop in elderly patients after relatively minor pelvic or hip fractures. A patient with pelvic, hip, or lumbar vertebral fractures who demonstrates continuing blood loss without a specific source, especially after a negative DPL or FAST examination, should have prompt angiography and attempted control with transcatheter embolization.

The process of aging and superimposed disease states make close monitoring mandatory, especially in cases of injury with acute intravascular volume loss and shock. The mortality rate in patients who on initial assessment appear to be uninjured or to have only minor injuries can be significant (up to 44%). Approximately 33% of elderly patients do not die from direct consequences of their injury, but from "inexplicable" sequential organ failure, which may reflect early, unsuspected states of hypoperfusion. Failure to recognize inadequate oxygen delivery creates an oxygen

PITFALLS

- Equating normal blood pressure with normovolemia.
- Failure to recognize metabolic acidosis as a predictor of mortality.
- Failure to institute early hemodynamic monitoring.
- Failure to recognize the effects of indiscriminate blood transfusion.

deficit from which the geriatric patient is not able to recover. Because of associated coronary artery disease, hypotension from hypovolemia frequently results in impaired cardiac performance from myocardial ischemia. Thus, hypovolemic and cardiogenic shock may coexist. Early and aggressive invasive monitoring, perhaps with a pulmonary artery catheter, may be beneficial. Hemodynamic resuscitation may require the use of inotropes after volume restoration in these patients. Thus, prompt transfer to a trauma center may be lifesaving.

Disability: Brain and Spinal Cord Injuries

CHANGES WITH AGING

Brain weight decreases about 10% by 70 years of age, with progressive loss of neurons, resulting in cerebral atrophy. This loss is replaced by cerebrospinal fluid. Concomitantly, the dura becomes tightly adherent to the skull. **Although the increased space created around the brain may serve to protect it from contusion, it also causes stretching of the parasagittal bridging veins, making them more prone to rupture on impact.** This loss of brain volume also allows for more brain movement in response to angular acceleration/deceleration. Significant amounts of blood can collect around the brain of an elderly individual before overt symptoms become apparent.

Cerebral blood flow is reduced by 20% by the age of 70 years. This is further reduced if atheromatous debris occludes conducting arteries. Peripheral conduction velocity slows as a result of demyelinization. Reduced acquisition or retention of information can cause clinically subtle changes in mental status. Visual and auditory acuity declines, vibratory and position sensation is impaired, and reaction time increases. In addition to complicating the evaluation process of injured elderly patients, these changes place the individual at greater risk for injury. Finally, preexisting medical conditions or their treatment may be a cause of confusion in the elderly.

In the spine, the most dramatic changes occur in the intervertebral disks. Loss of water and proteins affects the shape and compressibility of the disks. These changes shift the loads on the vertebral column to the facets, ligaments, and paraspinal muscles and contribute to degeneration of the facet joints and development of spinal stenosis. Progressively, these alterations place the spine and spinal cord at increased risk for injury. This risk is increased in the presence of osteoporosis, whether or not it is apparent radiographically. Finally, osteoarthritis may cause diffuse canal stenosis, segmental immobility, and kyphotic deformity, which are most severe in the cervical region (Figure 11-2).

EVALUATION AND MANAGEMENT

Elderly patients with brain injury have fewer severe cerebral contusions than do younger patients. However, the elderly have a higher incidence of subdural and intraparenchymal hematoma. Subdural hematomas are nearly three times as frequent in elderly as in younger patients, perhaps in part because elderly individuals are more likely to be taking anticoagulant medications for cardiac or cerebral disease. Subdural hematomas may produce a rather gradual onset of neurologic decline, especially in elderly patients. In fact, chronic subdural hematomas resulting from an earlier fall may be the cause of the fall for which the patient is currently being examined. CT scans of the head provide rapid, accurate, and detailed information on structural damage to the brain, skull, and supporting elements. Liberal use of this ex-

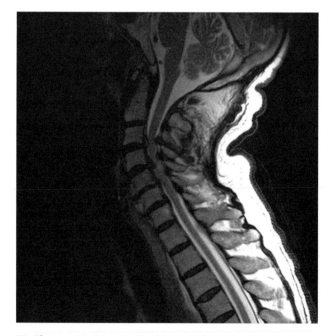

■ **Figure 11-2** A sagittal T$_2$-weighted image shows severe multilevel degenerative changes affecting disk spaces and posterior elements, associated with severe central canal stenosis, cord compression and small foci of myelomalacia at the C4-C5 level.

amination method is encouraged in elderly patients with brain injury. ◼ See Chapter 6: Head Trauma.

Cervical spine injuries appear to be more common in elderly trauma patients, although they may be more occult and particularly difficult to diagnose if osteoporosis and osteoarthritis are present. Severe osteophytic disease makes diagnosis of fracture challenging. Degeneration of intervertebral ligaments can increase the degree of intervertebral subluxation that is physiologic. Preexisting canal stenosis due to anterior osteophytes and posterior ligamentous hypertrophy increases the risk for central and anterior cord syndromes. These injuries often result from relatively mild extension injuries after falls or rear-end motor vehicle crashes. Magnetic resonance imaging (MRI) is particularly useful for diagnosing these injuries. ◼ See Chapter 7: Spine and Spinal Cord Trauma.

Exposure and Environment

The skin and connective tissues of elderly individuals undergo extensive changes, including a decrease in cell numbers, loss of strength, and impaired function. The epidermal keratinocytes lose a significant proportion of their proliferative ability with aging. The dermis loses as much as 20% of its thickness, undergoes a significant loss of vascularity, and has a marked decrease in the number of mast cells. **These changes result in the loss of thermal regulatory ability, decreased barrier function against bacterial invasion, and significant impairment to wound healing.**

Injured elderly patients must be protected from hypothermia. **Hypothermia not attributable to shock or exposure should alert the physician to the possibility of occult disease—in particular, sepsis, endocrine disease, or drug ingestion.**

The potential for invasive bacterial infection through injured skin must be recognized. Appropriate care, including assessing tetanus immunization status to prevent infection, must be instituted early. ◼ See Appendix E: Tetanus Immunization.

Other Systems

Other systems that warrant special attention with regard to the treatment of elderly trauma patients include the musculoskeletal system, nutrition and metabolism, and the immune system.

MUSCULOSKELETAL SYSTEM

Disorders of the musculoskeletal system are the most common presenting symptom of the middle-aged and elderly population. These disorders are the most likely cause of restrictions in an individual's daily life and are the key components of the loss of independence. Aging results in the stiffening of ligaments, cartilage, intervertebral disks, and joint capsules. Deterioration of tendons, ligaments, and joint capsules leads to an increased risk of injury, spontaneous rupture, and decreased joint stability. The risk of injury increases not only for the musculoskeletal system, but also for the adjacent soft tissues.

Aging causes a general decline in responsiveness to many anabolic hormones and an absolute reduction in the levels of growth hormones. After the age of 25 years, muscle mass decreases by 4% every 10 years. After the age of 50 years, the rate is 10% per decade unless the levels of growth factors are low, in which case the rate of decrease approaches 35%. This is manifested by a reduction in the size and total number of muscle cells. The decrease in muscle mass is directly correlated to the decrease in strength seen with the aging process.

Osteoporosis results in a decrease of histologic normal bone with a consequent loss of strength and resistance to fractures. This disorder is endemic in the elderly population, clinically affecting almost 50% of these individuals. The causes of osteoporosis include loss of estrogen hormones, loss of body mass, decreasing levels of physical activity, and inadequate consumption and inefficient use of calcium.

The consequences of these changes on the musculoskeletal system are frequently disabling and at times devastating. Injuries to ligaments and tendons affect joints and adjacent soft tissues. Osteoporosis contributes to the occurrence of spontaneous vertebral compression fractures and to the high incidence of hip fractures in the elderly. The yearly incidence approaches 1% for men and 2% for women over the age of 85 years. The ease with which fractures occur in the elderly patient magnifies the effect of force applied during injury in these patients.

Elderly individuals are particularly susceptible to fractures of the long bones, with attendant disability and associated pulmonary morbidity and mortality. Early stabilization of these fractures may decrease this risk, provided the patient is in an optimal hemodynamic state. Resuscitation should be targeted at normalizing tissue perfusion as early as possible and before fracture fixation is performed.

The most common locations of fractures in elderly patients are the proximal femur, hip, humerus, and wrist. Patients report pain in the area of the greater trochanter or anterior pelvis. In general, these individuals are unable to walk. Isolated hip fractures do not usually cause class III or IV shock. Neurovascular integrity should be assessed and compared with that of the opposite extremity.

Fractures of the humerus usually are caused by falls on an outstretched extremity. The resulting injury is a fracture of the surgical neck of the humerus. Usually, there is pain and tenderness in the shoulder or upper humerus area. Of major importance in the evaluation of these patients is the determination of whether the fracture is impacted or nonimpacted. Impacted fractures demonstrate no false motion of the humerus when the shoulder is rotated gently from a flexed elbow. Patients with nonimpacted fractures generally experience pain on movement of the arm. These latter fractures require hospitalization for orthopedic consultation and often operation.

Colles' fracture results from a fall on the outstretched, dorsiflexed hand, causing a metaphyseal fracture of the distal radius. The classic finding of a fracture at the base of the ulna styloid process occurs in 69% of cases. Evaluation should include careful testing of the median nerve and motor function of the finger flexors. The wrist should be examined radiographically, and all of the carpal bones should be visualized to exclude a more complex injury.

The aim of treatment for musculoskeletal injuries should be to undertake the least invasive, most definitive procedure that will permit early mobilization. Prolonged inactivity and disease often limit the ultimate functional outcome and impact survival.

NUTRITION AND METABOLISM

Caloric needs decline with age, as lean body mass and metabolic rate gradually decrease. Protein requirements actually may increase as a result of inefficient utilization. There is a widespread occurrence of chronically inadequate nutrition among the elderly, and poor nutritional status contributes to a significantly increased complication rate. **Early and adequate nutritional support of injured elderly patients is a cornerstone of successful trauma care.**

IMMUNE SYSTEM AND INFECTIONS

Mortality from most diseases increases with age. Why this is true is uncertain, but the loss of competence of the immune system with age certainly plays a role. Thymic tissue is less than 15% of its maximum by 50 years of age. Liver and spleen size also decrease. With aging, cell-mediated and humoral immune response to foreign antigens is decreased, whereas the response to autologous antigens is increased. It is not clear whether aging alters granulocyte function, but chronic diseases of the elderly, such as diabetes mellitus, may do so. As a consequence, elderly persons have an impaired ability to respond to bacteria and viruses, a reduced ability

to respond to vaccination, and a lack of reliable response to skin antigen testing. Clinically, elderly individuals are less able to tolerate infection and more prone to multiple organ system failure. The absence of fever, leukocytosis, and other manifestations of the inflammatory response may be due to poor immune function.

Special Circumstances

What are the special issues to consider in treating geriatric trauma patients?

Special circumstances that require consideration in the treatment of elderly trauma patients include medications, elder abuse, and end-of-life decisions.

MEDICATIONS

Concomitant disease may require the use of medications, and elderly patients are often already taking many pharmacologic agents. **Drug interactions are frequently encountered, and side effects are much more common because of the very narrow therapeutic range in the elderly.** Adverse reactions to some medications may even contribute to the injury-producing event. **ß-adrenergic blocking agents may limit chronotropic activity, and calcium-channel blockers may prevent peripheral vasoconstriction and contribute to hypotension.** Nonsteroidal antiinflammatory agents may contribute to blood loss because of their adverse effects on platelet

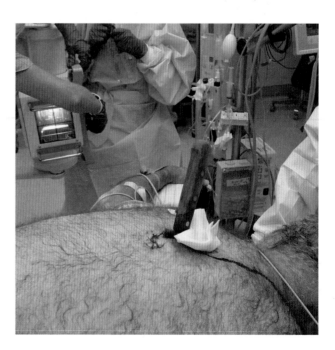

PITFALLS

- Failure to recognize that minimal trauma may result in fractures and serious disability.
- Poor hemodynamic reserve combined with underestimation of blood loss from fractures may be lethal.

function. Steroids and other drugs may further reduce the inflammatory and immune response. Long-term anticoagulant use may increase blood loss, and long-term diuretic use may render elderly patients dehydrated, leading to total body deficits of potassium and sodium. Hypoglycemic agents not only may contribute to the injury event itself but also may make control of serum glucose difficult if their use is unrecognized. **Psychotropic medications, commonly prescribed for elderly patients, may mask injuries or become problematic if discontinued abruptly.** Changes in central nervous system (CNS) function resulting from the use of these medications also may contribute to the injury. Finally, elderly individuals frequently neglect to keep their tetanus immunization current.

Pain relief in injured elderly trauma patients should not be neglected after resuscitation. Morphine is safe and effective and should be given in small, titrated (0.5 to 1.0 mg) intravenous doses. Antiemetic agents should be given with caution to avoid extrapyramidal effects. Finally, nephrotoxic drugs (eg, antibiotics and radiographic dyes) must be given in doses that reflect the elderly patient's decreased renal function, contracted intravascular volume, and other comorbid conditions.

ELDER ABUSE

When evaluating an injured elderly patient, consider that the injury may have been inflicted intentionally. Abuse of elderly individuals may be as common as child abuse. Abuse is defined as any willful infliction of injury, unreasonable confinement, intimidation, or cruel punishment that results in physical harm, pain, mental anguish, or other willful deprivation by a caretaker.

Elder abuse can be classified into six categories:

- Physical abuse
- Sexual abuse
- Neglect
- Psychological abuse
- Financial and material exploitation
- Violation of rights

Often several types of abuse occur simultaneously. Multifaceted in cause, elder abuse often is not recognized and is underreported. Many cases of abused elderly persons involve only subtle signs (eg, poor hygiene and dehydration) and have great potential to go undetected. Physical abuse occurs in up to 14% of elder trauma, resulting in a higher mortality than in younger patients.

Physical findings suggesting elder abuse include:

- Contusions affecting the inner arms, inner thighs, palms, soles, scalp, ear (pinna), mastoid area, buttocks, various planes of the body, or multiple and clustered contusions
- Abrasions to the axillary area (from restraints) or the wrist and ankles (from ligatures)
- Nasal bridge and temple injury (eyeglasses)
- Periorbital ecchymoses
- Oral injury
- Unusual alopecia pattern
- Untreated decubitus ulcers or ulcers in nonlumbar/sacral areas
- Untreated fractures
- Fractures not involving the hip, humerus, or vertebra
- Injuries in various stages of evolution
- Injuries to the eyes or nose
- Contact burns and scalds
- Scalp hemorrhage or hematoma

The presence of these findings should prompt a detailed history, which may be at variance with the physical findings and may uncover a significant delay in seeking treatment. These findings should prompt reporting and further investigation to confirm elder abuse. If present, appropriate action should be taken, including removal of the elderly patient from the abusive situation. The 2004 report of the National Center on Elder Abuse stated that 8.3 cases of abuse are reported for every 1000 elder Americans, and several studies have reported that only one of 13 or 14 cases of elder abuse is ever reported. This statistic applies even though every state in United States mandates reporting of elder abuse. A multidisciplinary approach is required.

END-OF-LIFE DECISIONS

Many elderly patients return to their preinjury level of function and independence after recovering from injury. **Age significantly increases mortality from injury, but more aggressive care, especially early in the evaluation and resuscitation of elderly trauma patients, has been shown to improve survival.** Attempts to identify which elderly trauma patients are at greatest risk for mortality have not found much utility in clinical practice.

PITFALLS

- Failure to take a drug history or note its impact on hemodynamics and CNS findings.
- Failure to titrate drug dosage, leading to increased incidence of side effects.

Certainly there are circumstances in which the doctor and patient, or family member(s), may choose to forgo life-saving measures and provide only supportive care. This decision is particularly clear in the case of elderly patients who have sustained extensive burns and when survival from the injuries sustained is unprecedented. In other circumstances, it can be more difficult to predict patient outcome or to be dogmatic about therapy. In many situations, the doctor confronts poorly defined probabilities. **The trauma team should always seek the existence of a living will, advance directives, or similar legal documents.** Although no absolute ethical guidelines can be given, the following observations may be helpful:

- The patient's right to self-determination is paramount.

- Medical intervention is appropriate only when it is in the patient's best interests.

- Medical therapy is appropriate only when its likely benefits outweigh its likely adverse consequences.

The ethical issue of appropriateness of care in an environment of declining hospital resources and restrictions on finances is more challenging.

CHAPTER SUMMARY

The number of elderly persons is increasing globally. Although the elderly are less likely to be injured than younger people, the mortality rate for the elderly population is higher. Many geriatric trauma patients can be returned to their preinjury medical status and independence. Knowledge of the changes that occur with aging, an appreciation of the injury patterns seen in the elderly, and an understanding of the need for aggressive resuscitation and monitoring of injured geriatric patients are necessary for improved outcome.

Increased awareness of elder abuse, including the patterns of injury, is necessary so that reporting can be improved. This should lead to earlier diagnosis and improved treatment of elderly injured patients.

1. Anatomic and physiologic changes in the elderly are associated with increased morbidity and mortality following trauma. Comorbidity increases with age. Frequent use of medications including beta-blockers and anticoagulants complicate assessment and management.

2. Treatment of the geriatric trauma patient follows the same pattern as that for younger patients, but caution and a high index of suspicion for injuries specific to this age group are required for optimal treatment. Comorbidities and medications may not only cause but also complicate injuries in the elderly. Careful volume resuscitation with close hemodynamic monitoring should guide treatment.

3. Consider the possibility of elder abuse and take appropriate action when assessing the geriatric trauma patient.

BIBLIOGRAPHY

1. Alexander BH, Rivara FP, Wolf ME. The cost and frequency of hospitalization for fall-related injuries in older adults. *Am J Public Health* 1992;82:1020-1023.

2. Allen JE, Schwab CW. Blunt chest trauma in the elderly. *Am Surg* 1985;51:697-700.

3. Bouchard JA, Barei D, Cayer D, et al. Outcome of femoral shaft fractures in the elderly. *Clin Orthop* 1996;332:105-109.

4. Burdge JJ, Katz B, Edwards R, et al. Surgical treatment of burns in elderly patients. *J Trauma* 1988;28:214-217.

5. Clayton MC, Solem LB, Ahrenholtz DH. Pulmonary failure in geriatric patients with burns: the need for diagnostic-related group modifier. *J Burn Care Rehab* 1995;16:451-454.

6. Collins KM. Elder maltreatment—a review. *Arch Pathol Lab* 2006;130:1290-1296.

7. Collins KA, Bennett AT, Hanzlick R. Elder abuse and neglect. *Arch Intern Med* 2000;160:1567-1568.

8. Corwin HL, Gettinger A, Pearl RG, et al. The CRIT study: anemia and blood transfusion in the critically ill—current clinical practice in the United States. *Crit Care Med* 2004;32:39.

9. Council Report. Decisions near the end of life. *JAMA* 1992;267:2229-2233.

10. Curreri PW, Luterman A, Braun DW Jr, et al. Brain injury: analysis of survival and hospitalization time for 937 patients. *Ann Surg* 1980;192:472-478.

11. DeGoede KM, Ashton-Miller JA, Schultz AB. Fall-related upper body injuries in the older adult: a review of the biochemical issues. *J Biomech* 2003;36:1043-1053.

12. De Laet CE, Pols HA. Fractures in the elderly: epidemiology and demography. *Baillieres Best Pract Res Clin Endocrinol Metab* 2004;14:171-179.

13. Demarest GB, Osler TM, Clevenger FW. Injuries in the elderly: evaluation and initial response. *Geriatrics* 1990;45(8):36-38, 41-42.

14. DeMaria EJ, Kenney PR, Merriam MA, et al. Aggressive trauma care benefits the elderly. *J Trauma* 1987;27:1200-1206.

15. DeMaria EJ, Merriam MA, Casanova LA, et al. Do DRG payments adequately reimburse the costs of trauma care in geriatric patients? *J Trauma* 1989;28:1244-1249.

16. Finelli FC, Jonsson J, Champion HR, et al. A case control study for major trauma in geriatric patients. *J Trauma* 1989;29:541-548.

17. Gakuu LN, Kabetu CE. An overview on management of the traumatised elderly patient. *East Afr Med J* 1997;74:618-621.

18. Gubler KD, Maier RV, Davis R, et al. Trauma recidivism in the elderly. *J Trauma* 1996;41(6):952-956.

19. Hebert PC, Wells G, Blajchman MA, et al. A multicenter, randomized, controlled clinical trial of transfusion requirements in critical care. *N Engl J Med* 1999;340:409.

20. Hebert PC, Yetisir E, Martin C, et al. Is a low transfusion threshold safe in critically ill patients with cardiovascular diseases? *Crit Care Med* 2001;29:227.

21. Horan MA, Clague JE. Injury in the aging: recovery and rehabilitation. *Br Med Bull* 1999;55:895-909.

22. Horst HM, Obeid FJ, Sorensen VJ, et al: Factors influencing survival of elderly trauma patients. *Crit Care Med* 1986;14:681-684.

23. Kanis JA. The incidence of hip fracture in Europe. *Osteoporosis Int* 1993;3(suppl 1):10-15.

24. Koepsell TD, Wolf ME, McCloskey L, et al. Medical conditions and motor vehicle collisions in older adults. *J Am Geriatr Soc* 1994;42:695-700.

25. Lachs MS, Pillemer K. Abuse and neglect of elderly persons. *N Engl J Med* 1995;332:437-443.

26. Mackenzie EJ, Morris JA, Edelstein SL. Effect of pre-existing disease on length of stay in trauma patients. *J Trauma* 1989;29:757-764.

27. Mackenzie EJ, Morris JA, Smith GS, et al. Acute hospital costs of trauma in the United States: implications for regionalized systems of care. *J Trauma* 1990;30:1096-1101.

28. Manton DK, Vaupel JW. Survival after the age of 80 in the United States, Sweden, France, England, and Japan. *N Engl J Med* 1995;333:1232-1235.

29. McMahon DJ, Schwab CW, Kauder DR. Comorbidity and the elderly trauma patient. *World J Surg* 1996;20:1113-1119.

30. Milzman DP, Boulanger BR, Rodriguez A, et al. Pre-existing disease in trauma patients: a predictor of fate independent of age and injury severity score. *J Trauma* 1992;31:236-244.

31. Morris JA, Auerbach PS, Marshall GA, et al. The Trauma Score as a triage tool in the prehospital setting. *JAMA* 1986;256:1319-1325.

32. Morris JA, Mackenzie EJ, Edelstein SL: The effect of pre-existing conditions on mortality in trauma patients. *JAMA* 1990;263:1942-1946.

33. Oreskovich MR, Howard JD, Copass MK, et al. Geriatric trauma: Injury patterns and outcome. *J Trauma* 1984;24:565-572.

34. Osler T, Hales K, Baack B, et al. Trauma in the elderly. *Am J Surg* 1988;156:537-543.

35. Pennings JL, Bachulis BL, Simons CT, et al. Survival after severe brain injury in the aged. *Arch Surg* 1993;128:787-794.

36. Phillips S, Rond PC, Kelly SM, et al. The failure of triage criteria to identify geriatric patients with trauma: results from the Florida trauma triage study. *J Trauma* 1996;40:278-283.

37. Riggs JE. Mortality from accidental falls among the elderly in the United States, 1962-1988: demonstrating the impact of improved trauma management. *J Trauma* 1993;35:212-219.

38. Rowe JW. Health care myths at the end of life. *Bull Am Coll Surg* 1996;81:11-18.

39. Scalea TM, Simon HM, Duncan AO, et al. Geriatric blunt multiple trauma: Improved survival with early invasive monitoring. *J Trauma* 1990;30:129-134.

40. Schwab CW, Kauder DR. Trauma in the geriatric patient. *Arch Surg* 1992;127:701-706.

41. Shabot MM, Johnson CL. Outcome from critical care in the "oldest old" trauma patients. *J Trauma* 1995;39:254-259.

42. Smith DP, Enderson BL, Maull KI. Trauma in the elderly: determinants of outcomes. *South Med J* 1990;83:171-177.

43. Timberlake GA. Elder abuse. In: Kaufman HH, ed. *The Physician's Perspective on Medical Law.* Park Ridge, IL: American Association of Neurological Surgeons; 1997.

44. van Aalst JA, Morris JA, Yates HK, et al. Severely injured geriatric patients return to independent living: a study of factors influencing function and independence. *J Trauma* 1991;31:1096-1101; 1101-1102.

45. van der Sluis CK, Klasen HJ, Eisma WH, et al. Major trauma in young and old: what is the difference? *J Trauma* 1996;40:78-82.

46. Wardle TD. Co-morbid factors in trauma patients. *Br Med Bull* 1999;55:744-756.

47. Zietlow SP, Capizzi PJ, Bannon MP, et al. Multisystem geriatric trauma. *J Trauma* 1994;37:985-988.

CHAPTER **12** **Trauma in Women**

Upon completion of this topic, the student will demonstrate the ability to initially assess and treat a pregnant trauma patient and her fetus. Specifically, the doctor will be able to:

OBJECTIVES

1 Describe the anatomic and physiologic alterations of pregnancy, including their effects on patient treatment.

2 Identify common mechanisms of injury to the pregnant patient and her fetus.

3 Outline the treatment priorities and assessment methods for both patients (mother and fetus).

4 Identify the indications for operative intervention that are unique to injured pregnant patients.

5 Explain the potential for isoimmunization and the need for immunoglobulin therapy in pregnant trauma patients.

6 Identify patterns of domestic violence.

Introduction

Any female patient between the ages of 10 and 50 years can be pregnant. Pregnancy causes major physiologic changes and altered anatomic relationships involving nearly every organ system of the body. These changes of structure and function can influence the evaluation of injured pregnant patients by altering the signs and symptoms of injury, the approach and responses to resuscitation, and the results of diagnostic tests. Pregnancy also can affect the patterns and severity of injury. The doctor attending a pregnant trauma patient must remember that there are two patients: mother and fetus. Nevertheless, initial treatment priorities for an injured pregnant patient remain the same as for the nonpregnant patient. **The best initial treatment for the fetus is the provision of optimal resuscitation of the mother and early assessment of the fetus.** Monitoring and evaluation techniques should allow assessment of the mother and the fetus. If x-ray examination is indicated during critical management, it should not be withheld because of the pregnancy. **A qualified surgeon and an obstetrician should be consulted early in the evaluation of pregnant trauma patients.**

Anatomic and Physiologic Alterations of Pregnancy

? *What changes occur with pregnancy?*

An understanding of the anatomic and physiologic alterations of pregnancy, as well as of the physiologic relationship between a pregnant patient and her fetus, is essential to serve the best interests of both patients. Such alterations include differences in anatomy, blood volume and composition, and hemodynamics, as well as changes in the respiratory, gastrointestinal, urinary, endocrine, musculoskeletal, and neurologic systems.

ANATOMIC DIFFERENCES

The uterus remains an intrapelvic organ until approximately the 12th week of gestation, when it begins to rise out of the pelvis. By 20 weeks, the uterus is at the umbilicus, and at 34 to 36 weeks, it reaches the costal margin (Figure 12-1). During the last 2 weeks of gestation, the fundus frequently descends as the fetal head engages the pelvis. As the uterus enlarges, the bowel is pushed cephalad, so that the bowel lies

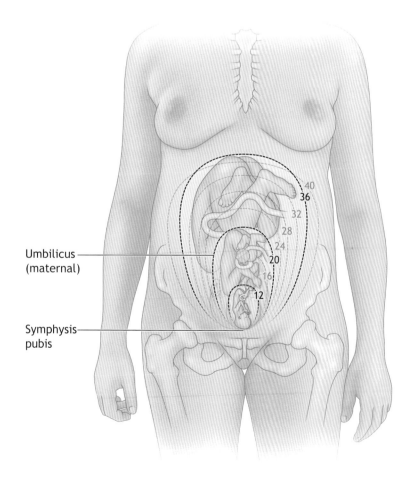

Umbilicus (maternal)

Symphysis pubis

■ **Figure 12-1 Changes in Fundal Height in Pregnancy.** As the uterus enlarges, the bowel is pushed cephalad, so that it lies mostly in the upper abdomen. As a result, the bowel is somewhat protected in blunt abdominal trauma, whereas the uterus and its contents (fetus and placenta) become more vulnerable.

mostly in the upper abdomen. As a result, the bowel is somewhat protected in blunt abdominal trauma, whereas the uterus and its contents (fetus and placenta) become more vulnerable. However, penetrating trauma to the upper abdomen during late gestation may result in complex intestinal injury because of this cephalad displacement.

During the first trimester, the uterus is a thick-walled structure of limited size, confined within the bony pelvis. During the second trimester, it enlarges beyond its protected intrapelvic location, but the small fetus remains mobile and cushioned by a generous amount of amniotic fluid. The amniotic fluid may cause amniotic fluid embolism and disseminated intravascular coagulation following trauma if the fluid gains access to the maternal intravascular space. By the third trimester, the uterus is large and thin-walled. In the vertex presentation, the fetal head is usually within the pelvis, with the remainder of the fetus exposed above the pelvic brim (Figure 12-2). Pelvic fracture(s) in late gestation may result in skull fracture or serious intracranial injury to the fetus. Unlike the elastic myometrium, the placenta has little elasticity. This lack of placental elastic tissue results in vulnerability to shear forces at the uteroplacental interface, which may lead to abruptio placentae. The placental vasculature is maximally dilated throughout gestation, yet it is exquisitely sensitive to catecholamine stimulation. **An abrupt decrease in maternal intravascular volume can result in a profound increase in uterine vascular resistance, reducing fetal oxygenation despite reasonably normal maternal vital signs.**

BLOOD VOLUME AND COMPOSITION

Plasma volume increases steadily throughout pregnancy and plateaus at 34 weeks of gestation. A smaller increase in red-blood-cell (RBC) volume occurs, resulting in a decreased hematocrit (physiologic anemia of pregnancy). In late pregnancy, a hematocrit of 31% to 35% is normal. Otherwise healthy pregnant patients can lose 1200 to 1500 mL of their blood volume before exhibiting signs and symptoms of hypovolemia. However, this amount of hemorrhage may be reflected by fetal distress evidenced by an abnormal fetal heart rate.

The white-blood-cell (WBC) count increases during pregnancy. It is not unusual to see WBC counts of 15,000/mm³ during pregnancy or as high as 25,000/mm³ during labor. Levels of serum fibrinogen and other clotting factors are mildly elevated. Prothrombin and partial thromboplastin times may be shortened, but bleeding and clotting times are unchanged. The serum albumin level falls to 2.2 to 2.8 g/dL during pregnancy, causing a drop in serum protein levels by approximately 1.0 g/dL. Serum osmolarity remains at about 280 mOsm/L throughout pregnancy. Table 12-1 outlines normal laboratory values during pregnancy.

HEMODYNAMICS

Important hemodynamic factors to consider in pregnant trauma patients include cardiac output, heart rate, blood

TABLE 12-1 ■ Normal Laboratory Values during Pregnancy

Hematocrit	32%–42%
WBC count	5000–12,000 / L
Arterial pH	7.40–7.45
Bicarbonate	17–22 mEq/L
PaCO₂	25–30 mm Hg (3.3–4 kPa)

pressure, venous pressure, and electrocardiographic changes.

Cardiac Output

After the 10th week of pregnancy, cardiac output can be increased by 1.0 to 1.5 L/min because of the increase in plasma volume and decrease in vascular resistance of the uterus and placenta, which receive 20% of the patient's cardiac output during the third trimester of pregnancy. This increased output may be greatly influenced by the mother's position during the second half of pregnancy. In the supine position, vena cava compression can decrease cardiac output by 30% because of decreased venous return from the lower extremities.

Heart Rate

Heart rate increases gradually, by 10 to 15 beats/min, during pregnancy, reaching a maximum rate by the third trimester. This change in heart rate must be considered when interpreting the tachycardic response to hypovolemia.

Blood Pressure

Pregnancy results in a 5 to 15 mm Hg fall in systolic and diastolic pressures during the second trimester. Blood pressure returns to near-normal levels at term. Some pregnant women exhibit hypotension when placed in the supine position (supine hypotensive syndrome), caused by compression of the inferior vena cava. This hypotension is corrected by relieving uterine pressure on the inferior vena cava, as described later in this chapter. The normal changes in blood pressure, pulse, hemoglobin, and hematocrit during pregnancy must be interpreted carefully in pregnant trauma patients.

Venous Pressure

The resting central venous pressure (CVP) is variable with pregnancy, but the response to volume is the same as in the nonpregnant state. Venous hypertension in the lower extremities is present during the third trimester.

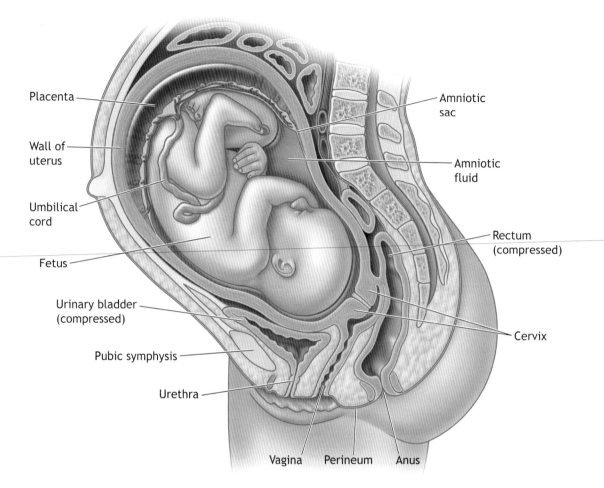

Placenta

Wall of uterus

Umbilical cord

Fetus

Urinary bladder (compressed)

Pubic symphysis

Urethra

Amniotic sac

Amniotic fluid

Rectum (compressed)

Cervix

Vagina   Perineum   Anus

■ **Figure 12-2 Full-Term Fetus in Vertex Presentation.** Note the displacement and compression of the abdominal viscera. Most of the viscera would be displaced cephalad. You cannot see them in this picture.

Electrocardiographic Changes

The axis may shift leftward by approximately 15 degrees. Flattened or inverted T waves in leads III and AVF and the precordial leads may be normal. Ectopic beats are increased during pregnancy.

RESPIRATORY SYSTEM

Minute ventilation increases primarily as a result of an increase in tidal volume because of increased levels of progesterone during pregnancy. Hypocapnia (Paco₂ of 30 mm Hg) is therefore common in late pregnancy. **A Paco₂ of 35 to 40 mm Hg may indicate impending respiratory failure during pregnancy.** Although the forced vital capacity fluctuates slightly during pregnancy, it is largely maintained throughout pregnancy by equal and opposite changes in inspiratory capacity (which increases) and residual volume (which decreases). Anatomic alterations in the thoracic cavity appear to account for the decreased residual volume that is associated with diaphragmatic elevation with increased lung markings and prominence of the pulmonary

vessels seen on chest x-ray examination. Oxygen consumption is increased during pregnancy. Therefore, it is important to maintain and ensure adequate arterial oxygenation during the resuscitation of the injured pregnant patient.

GASTROINTESTINAL SYSTEM

Gastric emptying time is prolonged during pregnancy, and doctors should always assume that the stomach of a pregnant patient is full. Therefore, early gastric tube decompression is particularly important to avoid the aspiration of gastric contents. The intestines are relocated to the upper part of the abdomen and may be shielded by the uterus. The position of the patient's spleen and liver are essentially unchanged by pregnancy.

URINARY SYSTEM

The glomerular filtration rate and renal blood flow increase during pregnancy, whereas levels of creatinine and serum urea nitrogen fall to approximately half of normal prepreg-

PITFALLS

- Not understanding the anatomic changes that occur during pregnancy
- Not recognizing that a normal $PaCO_2$ may indicate impending respiratory failure during pregnancy
- Mistaking eclampsia for head injury

TABLE 12-2 ■ Incidence of Various Types of Blunt Trauma in Pregnancy

TYPE OF BLUNT TRAUMA	TOTAL NUMBER	PERCENTAGE
Motor vehicle accidents/pedestrians	1098	59.6
Falls	411	22.3
Direct assaults	308	16.7
Other	24	0.1

Source: Shah AJ, Kilcline BA. Trauma in pregnancy. *Emerg Med Clin N Am* 2003;21:615-29.

nancy levels. Glycosuria is common during pregnancy. There is a physiologic dilatation of the renal calices, pelves, and ureters outside of the pelvis, which may persist for several weeks following pregnancy. Because of frequent dextrorotation of the uterus, the right renal collection system is often more dilated than the left.

ENDOCRINE SYSTEM

The pituitary gland increases in size and weight by 30% to 50% during pregnancy. Shock can cause necrosis of the anterior pituitary gland, resulting in pituitary insufficiency.

MUSCULOSKELETAL SYSTEM

The symphysis pubis widens to 4 to 8 mm, and the sacroiliac joint spaces increase by the seventh month of gestation. These factors must be considered in interpreting x-ray films of the pelvis.

NEUROLOGIC SYSTEM

Eclampsia is a complication of late pregnancy that can mimic head injury. It should be considered if seizures occur with associated hypertension, hyperreflexia, proteinuria, and peripheral edema. Expert neurologic and obstetric consultation frequently is helpful in differentiating between eclampsia and other causes of seizures.

Mechanisms of Injury

? *What are the unique risks of pregnancy?*

Most mechanisms of injury are similar to those sustained by nonpregnant patients, but certain differences must be recognized in pregnant patients who sustain blunt or penetrating injury.

BLUNT INJURY

The incidence of various types of blunt trauma in pregnancy is outlined in Table 12-2. The abdominal wall, uterine myometrium, and amniotic fluid act as buffers to direct fetal in-

jury from blunt trauma. Nonetheless, fetal injuries may occur when the abdominal wall strikes an object, such as the dashboard or steering wheel, or when a pregnant patient is struck by a blunt instrument. Indirect injury to the fetus may occur from rapid compression, deceleration, the contrecoup effect, or a shearing force resulting in abruptio placentae.

Compared with restrained pregnant women involved in collisions, unrestrained pregnant women have a higher risk of premature delivery and fetal death. The type of restraint system affects the frequency of uterine rupture and fetal death. The use of a lap belt alone allows forward flexion and uterine compression with possible uterine rupture or abruptio placentae. A lap belt worn too high over the uterus may produce uterine rupture because of the transmission of direct force to the uterus on impact. The use of shoulder restraints in conjunction with the lap belt reduces the likelihood of direct and indirect fetal injury, presumably because of the greater surface area over which the deceleration force is dissipated, as well as the prevention of forward flexion of the mother over the gravid uterus. Therefore, determination of the type of restraint device worn by the pregnant patient, if any, is important in the overall assessment. There does not appear to be any increase in pregnancy-specific risks from the deployment of airbags in motor vehicles.

PENETRATING INJURY

As the gravid uterus increases in size, the other viscera are relatively protected from penetrating injury, whereas the likelihood of uterine injury increases. The dense uterine musculature in early pregnancy can absorb a great amount of energy from penetrating missiles, decreasing missile velocity and lessening the likelihood of injury to other viscera. The amniotic fluid and conceptus also absorb energy and contribute to slowing of the penetrating missile. The result-ing low incidence of associated maternal visceral injuries ac-counts for the generally excellent maternal outcome in the penetrating wounds of the gravid uterus. However, the fetus generally fares poorly when there is a penetrating injury to the uterus.

Severity of Injury

The severity of maternal injuries determines maternal and fetal outcome. Therefore, treatment methods also depend on the severity of maternal injuries. All pregnant patients with major injuries require admission to a facility with trauma and obstetric capabilities, since there is an increased maternal and fetal mortality rate in this group of patients. Eighty percent of pregnant women who survive hemor-rhagic shock will experience fetal death. Even the pregnant patient with minor injuries should be carefully observed, since occasionally even minor injuries are associated with abruptio placentae and fetal loss. Direct fetal injuries usually occur in late pregnancy and are typically associated with serious maternal trauma.

Assessment and Treatment

❓ *How do I evaluate and treat two patients?*

For optimal outcome of mother and fetus, it is recommended that doctors assess and resuscitate the mother first, and then assess the fetus before conducting a secondary survey of the mother.

PRIMARY SURVEY AND RESUSCITATION

Mother

Ensure a patent airway, adequate ventilation and oxygena-tion, and effective circulatory volume. If ventilatory support is required, intubation is appropriate for the pregnant pa-tient, and consideration should be given to hyperventilating her. ◼ See Chapter 2: Airway and Ventilatory Management.

Uterine compression of the vena cava may reduce ve-nous return to the heart, thereby decreasing cardiac output and aggravating the shock state. **The uterus should be dis-placed manually to the left side to relieve pressure on the in-ferior vena cava.** If the patient requires immobilization in a supine position, the patient or spine board can be logrolled 4 to 6 inches (or 15 degrees) to the left and supported with a bolstering device, thus maintaining spinal precautions and decompressing the vena cava (Figure 12-3).

Because of their increased intravascular volume, preg-nant patients can lose a significant amount of blood before

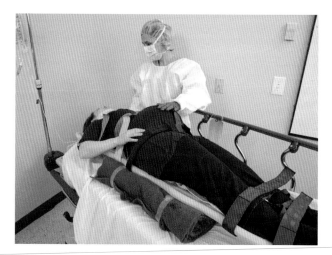

◼ **Figure 12-3 Proper Immobilization of a Preg-nant Patient.** If the patient requires immobilization in a supine position, the patient or spine board can be logrolled 4 to 6 inches (or 15 degrees) to the left and supported with a bolstering device, thus maintaining spinal precautions and decompressing the vena cava.

tachycardia, hypotension, and other signs of hypovolemia occur. Thus, the fetus may be in distress and the placenta de-prived of vital perfusion while the mother's condition and vital signs appear stable. Crystalloid fluid resuscitation and early type-specific blood administration are indicated to support the physiologic hypervolemia of pregnancy. Do not admin-ister vasopressors to restore maternal blood pressure, be-cause these agents further reduce uterine blood flow, resulting in fetal hypoxia. As intravenous lines are started, blood samples should be drawn for appropriate laboratory analyses, including type and crossmatch, toxicology studies, and fibrinogen levels.

Fetus

The abdominal examination during pregnancy is critically important, as rapid identification of serious maternal in-juries and fetal well-being depend on a thorough evaluation. The main cause of fetal death is maternal shock and mater-nal death. The second most common cause of fetal death is placental abruption. Abruptio placentae is suggested by vaginal bleeding (70% of cases), uterine tenderness, frequent uterine contractions, uterine tetany, and uterine irritability (uterus contracts when touched). In 30% of abruptions fol-lowing trauma, vaginal bleeding may not occur. Uterine ul-trasonography may demonstrate the lesion, but the test is not definitive. Late in pregnancy, abruption may occur fol-lowing relatively minor injuries.

Uterine rupture, a rare injury, is suggested by findings of abdominal tenderness, guarding, rigidity, or rebound ten-derness, especially if there is profound shock. Frequently, peritoneal signs are difficult to appreciate in advanced ges-tation because of expansion and attenuation of the abdom-inal wall musculature. Other abnormal findings suggestive of uterine rupture include abnormal fetal lie (eg, oblique or transverse lie), easy palpation of fetal parts because of their extrauterine location, and inability to readily palpate the uterine fundus when there is fundal rupture. X-ray evidence of rupture includes extended fetal extremities, abnormal fetal position, and free intraperitoneal air. Operative exploration may be necessary to diagnose uterine rupture.

In most cases of either abruptio placentae or uterine rupture, the patient reports abdominal pain or cramping. Signs of hypovolemia can accompany each of these injuries.

Initial fetal heart tones can be auscultated with Doppler ultrasound at 10 weeks of gestation. Continuous fetal monitoring should be performed beyond 20 to 24 weeks of gestation. Patients with no risk factors for fetal loss should have continuous monitoring for 6 hours, whereas patients with risk factors for fetal loss or placental abruption should be monitored for 24 hours. The risk factors are maternal heart rate >110, an Injury Severity Score >9, evidence of placental abruption, fetal heart rate >160 or <120, ejection during a motor vehicle accident, and motorcycle or pedestrian collisions.

ADJUNCTS TO PRIMARY SURVEY AND RESUSCITATION

Mother

If possible, the patient should be monitored on her left side after physical examination. Monitoring of the CVP response to fluid challenge may be valuable in maintaining the relative hypervolemia required in pregnancy. Monitoring should include pulse oximetry and arterial blood gas determinations. Remember, maternal bicarbonate is normally low during pregnancy.

Fetus

Obstetric consultation should be obtained, since fetal distress can occur at any time and without warning. Fetal heart rate is a sensitive indicator of both maternal blood volume status and fetal well-being. Fetal heart tones should be monitored in every injured pregnant woman. Intermittent and repeated Doppler examination can be used to detect fetal heart tones after 10 weeks of gestation. Continuous fetal monitoring with a cardiac tocodynamometer is useful after 20 to 24 weeks of gestation. The normal range for fetal heart rate is 120 to 160 beats/min. An abnormal fetal heart rate, repetitive decelerations, absence of accelerations or beat-to-beat variability, and frequent uterine activity can be signs of impending maternal and/or fetal decompensation (eg, hypoxia and/or acidosis) and should prompt immediate obstetric consultation.

Indicated radiographic studies should be performed, because the benefits certainly outweigh the potential risk to the fetus. However, unnecessary duplication of films should be avoided.

SECONDARY ASSESSMENT

The maternal secondary survey should follow the same pattern as for nonpregnant patients. ◾ See Chapter 1: Initial

Assessment and Management. Indications for abdominal computed tomography, focused assessment sonography in trauma, and diagnostic peritoneal lavage (DPL) are the same. However, if DPL is performed, the catheter should be placed above the umbilicus using the open technique. Pay careful attention to the presence of uterine contractions suggesting early labor or tetanic contractions suggesting placental abruption. Evaluation of the perineum should include a formal pelvic examination, ideally performed by a doctor skilled in obstetric care. The presence of amniotic fluid in the vagina, evidenced by a pH of 7 to 7.5, suggests ruptured chorioamnionic membranes. Cervical effacement and dilation, fetal presentation, and the relationship of the fetal presenting part to the ischial spines should be noted. Because vaginal bleeding in the third trimester may indicate disruption of the placenta and impending death of the fetus, a vaginal examination is vital. Repeated vaginal examinations should be avoided. The decision regarding an emergency cesarean section should be made with advice from an obstetrician.

Admission to the hospital is mandatory in the presence of vaginal bleeding, uterine irritability, abdominal tenderness, pain or cramping, evidence of hypovolemia, changes in or absence of fetal heart tones, or leakage of amniotic fluid. Care should be provided at a facility with appropriate fetal and maternal monitoring and treatment capabilities. **The fetus may be in jeopardy even with apparently minor maternal injury.**

DEFINITIVE CARE

Obstetric consultation should be obtained whenever specific uterine problems exist or are suspected. With extensive placental separation or amniotic fluid embolization, widespread intravascular clotting may develop, causing depletion of fibrinogen (<250 mg/dL), other clotting factors, and platelets. This consumptive coagulopathy can emerge rapidly. In the presence of life-threatening amniotic fluid embolism and/or disseminated intravascular coagulation, uterine evacuation should be accomplished on an urgent basis, along with replacement of platelets, fibrinogen, and other clotting factors if necessary.

Consequences of fetomaternal hemorrhage include not only fetal anemia and death, but also isoimmunization if the mother is Rh-negative. Because as little as 0.01 mL of Rh-positive blood will sensitize 70% of Rh-negative patients, the presence of fetomaternal hemorrhage in an Rh-negative mother should warrant Rh immunoglobulin therapy. Although a positive Kleihauer-Betke test (a maternal blood smear allowing detection of fetal RBCs in the maternal circulation) indicates fetomaternal hemorrhage, a negative test does not exclude minor degrees of fetomaternal hemorrhage that are capable of sensitizing the Rh-negative mother. **All pregnant Rh-negative trauma patients should receive Rh immunoglobulin therapy unless the injury is remote from the uterus (eg, isolated distal extremity injury).** Im-

PITFALLS

- Failure to recognize the need to displace the uterus to the left side in a hypotensive pregnant patient.
- Failure to recognize need for Rh immunoglobulin therapy in an Rh-negative mother.

munoglobulin therapy should be instituted within 72 hours of injury.

The large, engorged pelvic vessels that surround the gravid uterus can contribute to massive retroperitoneal bleeding after blunt trauma with associated pelvic fractures. **Initial management is directed at resuscitation and stabilization of the pregnant patient because the fetal life at this point is totally dependent on the mother's condition. Fetal monitoring should be maintained after satisfactory resuscitation and stabilization of the mother. The presence of two patients (mother and fetus) and the potential for multiple injuries emphasize the importance of a surgeon working in concert with an obstetric consultant.**

Perimortem Cesarean Section

There are few data to support perimortem cesarean section in pregnant trauma patients who experience hypovolemic cardiac arrest. Remember, fetal distress can be present when the mother has no hemodynamic abnormalities, and progressive maternal instability compromises fetal survival. At the time of maternal hypovolemic cardiac arrest, the fetus already has suffered prolonged hypoxia. For other causes of maternal cardiac arrest, perimortem cesarean section occasionally may be successful if performed within 4 to 5 minutes of the arrest.

Domestic Violence

❓ How do I recognize domestic violence?

Domestic violence is a major cause of injury to women during cohabitation, marriage, and pregnancy regardless of ethnic background, cultural influences, or socioeconomic status. Seventeen percent of injured pregnant patients experience trauma inflicted by another person, and 60% of these patients experience repeated episodes of domestic violence. According to estimates from the U.S. Department of Justice, 2 million to 4 million incidents of domestic violence occur per year and almost half of all women over their lifetimes are abused in some manner. As with child abuse, this information must be identified and documented. These attacks can result in death and disability. They also represent an increasing number of emergency department (ED) visits.

Indicators that suggest the presence of domestic violence include:

- Injuries inconsistent with the stated history
- Diminished self-image, depression, or suicide attempts
- Self-abuse
- Frequent ED or doctor's office visits
- Symptoms suggestive of substance abuse
- Self-blame for injuries
- Partner insists on being present for interview and examination and monopolizes discussion

These indicators raise the suspicion of the potential for domestic violence and should serve to initiate further investigation. The three questions in Box 12-1, when asked in a nonjudgmental manner and without the patient's partner being present, can identify 65% to 70% of domestic violence victims. Suspected cases of domestic violence should be handled through local social service agencies or the state health and human services department.

Box 12-1
Partner Violence Screen

1 Have you been kicked, hit, punched, or otherwise hurt by someone within the past year? If so, by whom?

2 Do you feel safe in your current relationship?

3 Is there a partner from a previous relationship who is making you feel unsafe now?

Reprinted with permission from Feldhaus KM, Koziol-McLain J, Amsbury HL, et al. Accuracy of 3 brief screening questions for detecting partner violence in the emergency department. *JAMA* 1997; 277:1357-1361.

CHAPTER SUMMARY

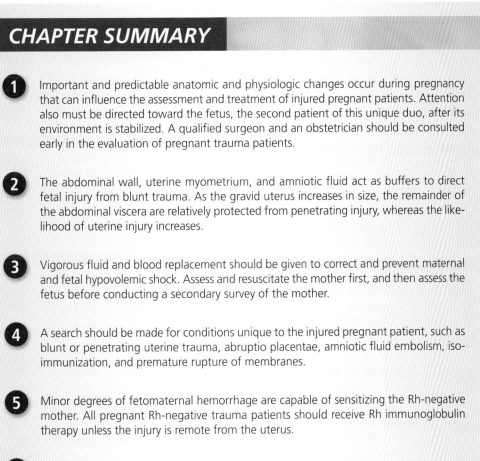

1 Important and predictable anatomic and physiologic changes occur during pregnancy that can influence the assessment and treatment of injured pregnant patients. Attention also must be directed toward the fetus, the second patient of this unique duo, after its environment is stabilized. A qualified surgeon and an obstetrician should be consulted early in the evaluation of pregnant trauma patients.

2 The abdominal wall, uterine myometrium, and amniotic fluid act as buffers to direct fetal injury from blunt trauma. As the gravid uterus increases in size, the remainder of the abdominal viscera are relatively protected from penetrating injury, whereas the likelihood of uterine injury increases.

3 Vigorous fluid and blood replacement should be given to correct and prevent maternal and fetal hypovolemic shock. Assess and resuscitate the mother first, and then assess the fetus before conducting a secondary survey of the mother.

4 A search should be made for conditions unique to the injured pregnant patient, such as blunt or penetrating uterine trauma, abruptio placentae, amniotic fluid embolism, isoimmunization, and premature rupture of membranes.

5 Minor degrees of fetomaternal hemorrhage are capable of sensitizing the Rh-negative mother. All pregnant Rh-negative trauma patients should receive Rh immunoglobulin therapy unless the injury is remote from the uterus.

6 Presence of indicators that suggest domestic violence should serve to initiate further investigation and protection of the victim.

BIBLIOGRAPHY

1. ACEP Clinical Policies Committee and Clinical Policies Subcommittee on Early Pregnancy. American College of Emergency Physicians. Clinical Policy: critical issues in the initial evaluation and management of patients presenting to the emergency department in early pregnancy. *Ann Emerg Med* 2003;41:122-133.

2. Berry MJ, McMurray RG, Katz VL. Pulmonary and ventilatory responses to pregnancy, immersion, and exercise. *J Appl Physiol* 1989;66(2):857-862.

3. Buchsbaum HG, Staples PP Jr. Self-inflicted gunshot wound to the pregnant uterus: report of two cases. *Obstet Gynecol* 1985;65(3):32S-35S.

4. Connolly AM, Katz VL, Bash KL, et al. Trauma and pregnancy. *Am J Perinatol* 1997;14:331-336.

5. Curet MJ, Schermer CR, Demarest GB, et al. Predictors of outcome in trauma during pregnancy: identification of patients who can be monitored for less than 6 h. *J Trauma* 2000;49:18-25.

6. Dahmus M, Sibai B. Blunt abdominal trauma: are there any predictive factors for abruption placentae or maternal-fetal distress? *Am J Obstet Gynecol* 1993;169:1054-1059.

7. Eisenstat SA, Sancroft L. Domestic violence. *N Engl J Med* 1999;341:886-892.

8. Esposito TJ. Trauma during pregnancy. *Emerg Med Clin North Am* 1994;12:167-199.

9. Esposito T, Gens D, Smith L, et al. Trauma during pregnancy. *Arch Surg* 1991;126:1073-1078.

10. Feldhaus KM, Koziol-McLain J, Amsbury HL, et al. Accuracy of 3 brief screening questions for detecting partner violence in the emergency department. *JAMA* 1997; 277:1357-1361.

11. George E, Vanderkwaak T, Scholten D. Factors influencing pregnancy outcome after trauma. *Am Surg* 1992;58:594-598.

12. Goodwin T, Breen M. Pregnancy outcome and fetomaternal hemorrhage after noncatastrophic trauma. *Am J Obstet Gynecol* 1990;162:665-671.

13. Grisso JA, Schwarz DF, Hirschinger N, et al. Violent injuries among women in an urban area. *N Engl J Med* 1999;341:1899-1905.

14. Hamburger KL, Saunders DG, Hovey M. Prevalence of domestic violence in community practice and rate of physician inquiry. *Fam Med* 1992;24:283-287.

15. Higgins SD, Garite TJ. Late abruptio placenta in trauma patients: implications for monitoring. *Obstet Gynecol* 1984;63:10S-12S.

16. Hoff W, D'Amelio L, Tinkoff G, et al. Maternal predictors of fetal demise in trauma during pregnancy. *Surg Gynecol Obstet* 1991;172:175-180.

17. Hyde LK, Cook LJ, Olson LM, et al. Effect of motor vehicle crashes on adverse fetal outcomes. *Obstet Gynecol* 2003;102:279-286.

18. Ikossi DG, Lazar AA, Morabito D, et al. Profile of mothers at risk: an analysis of injury and pregnancy loss in 1,195 trauma patients. *J Am Coll Surg* 2005;200:49-56.

19. Kissinger DP, Rozycki GS, Morris JA, et al. Trauma in pregnancy—predicting pregnancy outcome. *Arch Surg* 1991;125:1079-1086.

20. Klinich KD, Schneider LW, Moore JL, Pearlman MD. Investigations of crashes involving pregnant occupants. *Annu Proc Assoc Adv Automot Med* 2000;44:37-55.

21. Kyriacou DN, Anglin D, Taliaferro E, et al. Risk factors for injury to women from domestic violence. *N Engl J Med* 1999;341:1892-1898.

22. Lee D, Contreras M, Robson SC, et al. Recommendations for the use of anti-D immunoglobulin for Rh prophylaxis. British Blood Transfusion Society and Royal College of Obstetricians and Gynaecologists. *Transfus Med* 1999;9:93-97.

23. Mattox KL, Goetzl L. Trauma in pregnancy. *Crit Care Med* 2005;33:S385-S389.

24. Metz TD, Abbott JT. Uterine trauma in pregnancy after motor vehicle crashes with airbag deployment: a 30-case series. *J Trauma* 2006;61:658-661.

25. Minow M. Violence against women—a challenge to the supreme court. *N Engl J Med* 1999;341:1927-1929.

26. Mollison PL. Clinical aspects of Rh immunization. *Am J Clin Pathol* 1973;60:287.

27. Nicholson BE, ed. Family violence. *J South Carolina Med Assoc* 1995;91:409-446.

28. Pearlman MD, Tintinalli JE, Lorenz RP. Blunt trauma during pregnancy. *N Engl J Med* 1991;323:1606-1613.

29. Pearlman M, Tintinalli J, Lorenz R. A prospective controlled study of outcome after trauma during pregnancy. *Am J Obstet Gynecol* 1990;162:1502-1510.

30. Rose PG, Strohm PL, Zuspan FP. Fetomaternal hemorrhage following trauma. *Am J Obstet Gynecol* 1985;153:844-847.

31. Rothenberger D, Quattlebaum F, Perry J, et al. Blunt maternal trauma: a review of 103 cases. *J Trauma* 1978;18:173-179.

32. Schoenfeld A, Ziv E, Stein L, et al. Seat belts in pregnancy and the obstetrician. *Obstet Gynecol Surv* 1987;42:275-282.

33. Scorpio R, Esposito T, Smith G, et al. Blunt trauma during pregnancy: factors affecting fetal outcome. *J Trauma* 1992;32:213-216.

34. Shah AJ, Kilcline BA. Trauma in pregnancy. *Emerg Med Clin North Am* 2003;21:615-629.

35. Sims CJ, Boardman CH, Fuller SJ. Airbag deployment following a motor vehicle accident in pregnancy. *Obstet Gynecol* 1996;88:726.

36. Sisley A, Jacobs LM, Poole G, et al. Violence in America: a public health crisis—domestic violence. *J Trauma* 1999;46:1105-1113.

37. Statement on Domestic Violence. *Bull Am Coll Surg* 2000;85:26.

38. Timberlake GA, McSwain NE. Trauma in pregnancy, a ten-year perspective. *Am Surg* 1989;55:151-153.

39. Towery RA, English TP, Wisner DW. Evaluation of pregnant women after blunt injury. *J Trauma* 1992; 35:731-736.

40. Tsuei BJ. Assessment of the pregnant trauma patient. *Injury* 2006;37:367-373.

41. Weinberg L, Steele RG, Pugh R, et al. The pregnant trauma patient. *Anaesth Int Care* 2005;33:167-180.

42. Wolf ME, Alexander BH, Rivara FP, et al. A retrospective cohort study of seatbelt use and pregnancy outcome after a motor vehicle crash. *J Trauma* 1993; 34:116-119.

RESOURCE

National Coalition Against Domestic Violence, PO Box 18749, Denver, CO 80218-0749; 303-839-1852; 303-831-9251 (fax).

CHAPTER **13** **Transfer to Definitive Care**

Upon completion of this topic, the student will demonstrate the ability to explain and apply general principles for the safe transfer of injured patients to definitive care. Specifically, the doctor will be able to:

OBJECTIVES

1 Identify injured patients who require transfer from a primary care institution to a facility capable of providing the necessary level of trauma care.

2 Initiate procedures to optimally prepare trauma patients for safe transfer to a higher-level trauma care facility via the appropriate mode of transportation.

Introduction

The Advanced Trauma Life Support course is designed to train doctors to be more proficient in assessing, stabilizing, and preparing trauma patients for definitive care. Definitive care, whether support and monitoring in an intensive care unit (ICU) or operative intervention, requires the presence and active involvement of a surgeon and the trauma team. If definitive care cannot be rendered at a local hospital, the patient requires transfer to a hospital that has the resources and capabilities to care for the patient. Ideally, this facility should be a verified trauma center, the level of which depends on the patient's needs.

The decision to transfer a patient to another facility depends on the patient's injuries and the local resources. Decisions as to which patients should be transferred and when transfer should occur are matters of medical judgment. Evidence supports the view that trauma outcome is enhanced if critically injured patients are cared for in trauma centers. **Therefore, trauma patients should be transferred to the closest appropriate hospital, preferably a verified trauma center.** See American College of Surgeons (ACS) Committee on Trauma, *Resources for Optimal Care of the Injured Patient;* Guidelines for Trauma System Development and Trauma Center Verification Processes and Standards.

A major principle of trauma management is to *do no further harm*. Indeed, the level of care of trauma patients should consistently improve with each step, from the scene of the incident to the facility that can provide the patient with the necessary, proper treatment. All providers who care for trauma patients must ensure that the level of care never declines from one step to the next.

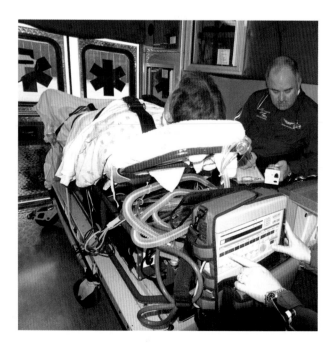

Determining the Need for Patient Transfer

The vast majority of patients receive their total care in a local hospital, and movement beyond that point is not necessary. **It is essential that doctors assess their own capabilities and limitations, as well as those of their institution, to allow for early recognition of patients who may be safely cared for in the local hospital and those who require transfer for definitive care.** Once the need for transfer is recognized, arrangements should be expedited and not delayed for diagnostic procedures (eg, diagnostic peritoneal lavage [DPL] or computed tomographic [CT] scan) that do not change the immediate plan of care.

TIMELINESS OF TRANSFER

❓ *When should I transport the patient?*

Patient outcome is directly related to the time elapsed between injury and properly delivered definitive care. In institutions in which there is no full-time, in-house emergency department (ED) coverage, the timeliness of transfer is partly dependent on the how quickly the doctor on call can reach the ED. Consequently, effective communication with the prehospital system should be developed to identify patients who require the presence of a doctor in the ED at the time of arrival. In addition, the attending doctor must be committed to respond to the ED prior to the arrival of critically injured patients. Identification of patients who require prompt attention can be based on physiologic measurements, specific identifiable injuries, and mechanism of injury.

The timing of interhospital transfer varies based on the distance of transfer, the available skill levels for transfer, circumstances of the local institution, and intervention that is necessary before the patient can be transferred safely. If the resources are available and the necessary procedures can be performed expeditiously, life-threatening injuries should be treated before patient transport. This treatment may require operative intervention to ensure that the patient is in the best possible condition for transfer. **Intervention prior to transfer is a surgical decision.**

TRANSFER FACTORS

❓ *Whom do I transport?*

To assist doctors in determining which patients may require care at a higher-level facility, the ACS Committee on Trauma recommends using certain physiologic indices, injury mechanisms and patterns, and historical information. These factors also help doctors decide which stable patients might benefit from transfer. Criteria for interhospital transfer when a patient's needs exceed available resources are out-

PITFALL

Patients frequently spend more time than necessary at the initial hospital after the necessity for transfer has been determined (eg, additional diagnostic tests for "completeness"). Once the decision to transfer the patient is made, little is gained by performing procedures other than those necessary to restore normal hemodynamic function. Delaying the transfer to wait for test results is not appropriate. In a patient with an obvious brain injury and focal neurologic findings, waiting for a CT scan of the brain before transferring the patient to the care of a neurosurgeon delays the patient's access to necessary specialty care. There are occasions when a patient cannot be hemodynamically normalized prior to transport. Direct consultation with the receiving doctor may be helpful in determining the most appropriate time to begin the transfer of a patient with hemodynamic abnormalities.

lined in Table 13-1. It is important to note that these criteria are flexible and must take into account local circumstances.

Certain clinical measurements of physiologic status are useful in determining the need for transfer to an institution that provides a higher level of care. Patients who exhibit evidence of shock, significant physiologic deterioration, or progressive deterioration in neurologic status require the highest level of care and will likely benefit from timely transfer.

Stable patients with blunt abdominal trauma and documented liver or spleen injuries may be candidates for nonoperative management. Implicit in such practice is the immediate availability of an operating room and a qualified surgical team. A general or trauma surgeon should supervise nonoperative management, regardless of the patient's age. Such patients should not be treated expectantly at facilities that are not prepared for urgent operative intervention; they should be transferred to a trauma center.

Patients with specific injuries, combinations of injuries (particularly those involving the brain), or historical findings that indicate high-energy-transfer injury may be at risk for death and are candidates for early transfer to a trauma center. High-risk criteria suggesting the necessity for early transfer are also outlined in Table 13-1.

Treatment of combative and uncooperative patients with an altered level of consciousness is difficult and fraught with hazards. These patients are often immobilized in the supine position with wrist/leg restraints. If sedation is required, the patient should be intubated. Therefore, before administering any sedation, the treating doctor must:

1. Ensure that the patient's ABCDEs are appropriately managed.

2. Relieve the patient's pain if possible (eg, apply splint fractures and administer small doses of narcotics intravenously).

3. Attempt to calm and reassure the patient.

Remember, benzodiazepines, fentanyl, propofol, and ketamine are all hazardous in patients with hypovolemia, patients who are intoxicated, and patients with head injuries. **When in doubt, pain management, sedation, and intubation should be accomplished by the individual most skilled in these procedures.** See Chapter 2: Airway and Ventilatory Management.

Abuse of alcohol and/or other drugs is common to all forms of trauma and is particularly important to identify. Doctors should recognize that alcohol and drugs can alter pain perception and mask significant physical findings. Alterations in the patient's responsiveness can be related to al-

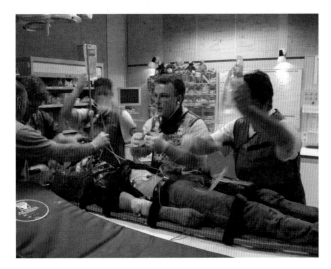

PITFALL

The process of transporting patients to other medical facilities is not, in and of itself, a treatment or cure for any disease or injury. The very process of transportation holds great potential for the level of care to deteriorate. The environment into which the patient is placed can be unpredictable and not well controlled. Careful planning can minimize the impact that these unintentional events may produce.

TABLE 13-1   ■   Criteria for Interhospital Transfer

CLINICAL CIRCUMSTANCES THAT WARRANT INTERHOSPITAL TRANSPORT WHEN THE PATIENT'S NEEDS EXCEED AVAILABLE RESOURCES:

Central Nervous System	Head injury: • Penetrating injury or depressed skull fracture • Open injury with or without CSF leak • GCS score <15 or neurologically abnormal • Lateralizing signs Spinal cord injury or major vertebral injury
Chest	Widened mediastinum or signs suggesting great-vessel injury Major chest wall injury or pulmonary contusion Cardiac injury Patients who may require prolonged ventilation
Pelvis/Abdomen	Unstable pelvic-ring disruption Pelvic-ring disruption with shock and evidence of continuing hemorrhage Open pelvic injury Solid organ injury
Extremities	Severe open fractures Traumatic amputation with potential for replantation Complex articular fractures Major crush injury Ischemia
Multisystem Injuries	Head injury with face, chest, abdominal, or pelvic injury Injury to more than two body regions Major burns or burns with associated injuries Multiple, proximal long-bone fractures
Comorbid Factors	Age >55 years Age <5 years Cardiac or respiratory disease Insulin-dependent diabetes Morbid obesity Pregnancy Immunosuppression
Secondary Deterioration (Late Sequelae)	Mechanical ventilation required Sepsis Single or multiple organ system failure (deterioration in central nervous, cardiac, pulmonary, hepatic, renal, or coagulation systems) Major tissue necrosis

Adapted with permission from ACS Committee on Trauma. *Resources for Optimal Care of the Injured Patient 2006.* Chicago: ACS; 2006.

cohol and/or drugs, but the absence of cerebral injury should never be assumed in the presence of alcohol or drugs. If the examining doctor is unsure, transfer to a higher-level facility may be appropriate.

Death of another individual involved in the incident suggests the possibility of severe, occult injury in survivors. **A thorough and careful evaluation of the patient, even in the absence of obvious signs of severe injury, is mandatory.**

Transfer Responsibilities

Specific transfer responsibilities are held by both the referring doctor and the receiving doctor.

REFERRING DOCTOR

❓ Where should I send the patient?

The referring doctor is responsible for initiating transfer of the patient to the receiving institution and selecting the appropriate mode of transportation and level of care required for optimal treatment of the patient en route. The referring doctor should consult with the receiving doctor and should be thoroughly familiar with the transporting agencies, their capabilities, and the arrangements for patient treatment during transport.

Stabilizing the patient's condition before transfer to another facility is the responsibility of the referring doctor, within the capabilities of his or her institution. Initiation of the transfer process should begin while resuscitative efforts are in progress.

Transfer agreements must be established to provide for the consistent and efficient movement of patients between institutions. These agreements allow for feedback to the referring hospital and enhance the efficiency and quality of the patient's treatment during transfer.

RECEIVING DOCTOR

The receiving doctor must be consulted with regard to the transfer of a trauma patient. He or she must ensure that the proposed receiving institution is qualified, able, and willing to accept the patient, and is in agreement with the intent to transfer. The receiving doctor should assist the referring doctor in making arrangements for the appropriate mode and level of care during transport. If the proposed receiving doctor and facility are unable to accept the patient, they should assist in finding an alternative placement for the patient.

The quality of care rendered en route is of vital importance to the patient's outcome. Only by direct communication between the referring and receiving doctors can the details of patient transfer be clearly delineated. If adequately trained ambulance personnel are not available, a nurse or doctor should accompany the patient. All monitoring and management rendered en route should be documented.

Modes of Transportation

❓ How should I transport the patient?

Do no further harm is the most important principle when choosing the mode of patient transportation. Ground, water, and air transportation can be safe and effective in fulfilling this principle, and no one form is intrinsically superior to the others. Local factors such as availability, geography, cost, and weather are the main determining factors as to which to use in a given circumstance. Interhospital transfer of critically injured patients is potentially hazardous unless the patient's condition is optimally stabilized before transport, transfer personnel are properly trained, and provision has been made for managing unexpected crises during transport. To ensure safe transfers, trauma surgeons must be involved in training, continuing education, and quality improvement programs designed for transfer personnel and procedures. Surgeons also should be actively involved in the development and maintenance of systems of trauma care.

PITFALL

Moving a patient from one location to another, regardless of the distance involved, is hazardous. The process must be approached with the same attention to detail as the resuscitation of the patient's vital functions. Problems during transportation must be anticipated so that their impact may be minimized should they occur. Anticipation of deterioration in the patient's neurologic condition or hemodynamic status allows for planning for such a contingency if it occurs before the patient arrives at the referral center.

PITFALL

The prudent doctor must review steps that ensure the safest possible transfer to another level of care. Remember, the doctor who begins the care of the injured patient must be committed to ensuring that the level of care does not deteriorate. This includes the care delivered during transfer to definitive care.

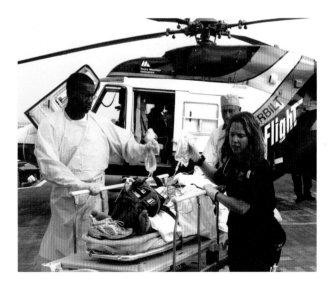

Transfer Protocols

Where protocols for patient transfer do not exist, the following guidelines are suggested.

INFORMATION FROM REFERRING DOCTOR

The local doctor who has determined that patient transfer is necessary should speak directly to the surgeon accepting the patient at the receiving hospital. The following information must be provided:

- Patient identification

- Brief history of the incident, including pertinent prehospital data

- Initial findings in the ED

- Patient's response to the therapy administered

INFORMATION TO TRANSFERRING PERSONNEL

Information regarding the patient's condition and needs during transfer should be communicated to the transporting personnel. This information includes, but is not limited to:

- Airway maintenance

- Fluid volume replacement

- Special procedures that may be necessary

- Revised Trauma Score, resuscitation procedures, and any changes that may occur en route

DOCUMENTATION

A written record of the problem, treatment given, and patient status at the time of transfer, as well as certain physical items, must accompany the patient (Figure 13-1). A facsimile transmission may be used to avoid delay in transfer.

TREATMENT PRIOR TO TRANSFER

Patients should be resuscitated and attempts made to stabilize their conditions as completely as possible based on the following suggested outline:

1. Airway
   a. Insert an airway or endotracheal tube, if needed.
   b. Provide suction.
   c. Insert a gastric tube to reduce the risk of aspiration.

2. Breathing
   a. Determine rate and administer supplementary oxygen.
   b. Provide mechanical ventilation when needed.
   c. Insert a chest tube if needed.

3. Circulation
   a. Control external bleeding.
   b. Establish two large-caliber intravenous tubes and begin crystalloid solution infusion.
   c. Restore blood volume losses with crystalloid fluids or blood and continue replacement during transfer.
   d. Insert an indwelling catheter to monitor urinary output.
   e. Monitor the patient's cardiac rhythm and rate.

4. Central nervous system
   a. Assist respiration in unconscious patients.
   b. Administer mannitol or diuretics, if needed.
   c. Immobilize any head, neck, thoracic, and lumbar spine injuries.

5. Diagnostic studies (When indicated, obtaining these studies should not delay transfer.)
   a. Obtain x-rays of cervical spine, chest, pelvis, and extremities.
   b. Sophisticated diagnostic studies, such as CT and aortography, are usually not indicated.
   c. Order hemoglobin or hematocrit, type and cross-match, and arterial blood gas determinations for all patients; also order pregnancy tests for females of childbearing age.
   d. Determine cardiac rhythm and hemoglobin saturation (ECG and pulse oximetry).

6. Wounds (Performing these procedures should not delay transfer.)
   a. Clean and dress wounds after controlling external hemorrhage.
   b. Administer tetanus prophylaxis.
   c. Administer antibiotics, when indicated.

7. Fractures
   a. Apply appropriate splinting and traction.

The flurry of activity surrounding the initial evaluation, resuscitation, and preparations for transfer of trauma patients often takes precedence over other logistic details. This may result in the failure to include certain items in the information that is sent with the patient, such as x-ray films, laboratory reports, or narrative descriptions of the evaluation process and treatment rendered at the local hospital. A checklist is helpful in this regard to make sure that all important components of care have been addressed (see Figure 13-1). Checklists can be printed or stamped on an x-ray jacket or the patient's medical record to remind the referring doctor to include all pertinent information.

TRANSFER FORM

County General Hospital

Patient Information

Name _____ Next of kin _____

Address _____ Address _____

City _____ State _____ Zip _____ City _____ State _____ Zip _____

Age _____ Sex _____ Weight _____ Phone # _____ / _____ – _____

Phone # _____ / _____ – _____ Relationship to patient _____

Date and Time

Date _____ / _____ / _____

Time of injury _____ AM/PM

Time admitted to ED _____ AM/PM

Time admitted to OR _____ AM/PM

Time transferred _____ AM/PM

Ample History

_____

_____

_____

_____

_____

Condition on Admission

HR _____ Rhythm _____

BP _____ / _____ RR _____ Temp _____

Probable diagnoses _____

_____

_____

_____

_____

Management During Transport

_____

Information in transfer materials

_____ MIST _____ AMPLE

Checklist

Airway: ___ Endotracheal tube ___ C-spine protection

Breathing: ___ Oxygen ___ SAO_2 ___ $EtCO_2$ ___ Chest tubes

Diagnostic: ___ X-Rays (chest, C-spine, pelvis) ___ Laboratory

Equipment: ___ ECG ___ BP ___ SAO_2 ___ IV ___ T°
___ Indwelling catheter ___ Splints ___ Gastric tube

Circulation: ___ Volume ___ Blood ___ Drugs

Family notification: ___

Referral Information:

Doctor _____

Hospital _____

Phone # _____ / _____ – _____

Receiving Information:

Doctor _____

Hospital _____

Phone # _____ / _____ – _____

■ **Figure 13.1 Sample Transfer Form.** This form includes all of the information that should be sent with the patient to the receiving doctor and facility.

(Adapted with permission from Schoettker P, D'Amours S, Nocera N, Caldwell E, Sugrue M. Reduction of time to definitive care in trauma patients: effectiveness of a new checklist system. Injury 34 (2003), 187-190.)

PITFALL

Endotracheal tubes may become dislodged or mal-positioned during transport. The necessary equipment for reintubation must accompany the patient and the attendants must be capable of performing the procedure.

TREATMENT DURING TRANSPORT

The appropriate personnel should transfer the patient, based on the patient's condition and potential problems.

Treatment during transport typically includes:

- Monitoring vital signs and pulse oximetry
- Continued support of cardiorespiratory system
- Continued blood-volume replacement
- Use of appropriate medications as ordered by a doctor or as allowed by written protocol
- Maintenance of communication with a doctor or institution during transfer
- Maintenance of accurate records during transfer

While preparing for transport and while it is underway, remember that, if air transport is used, changes in altitude lead to changes in air pressure, which may result in increases in the size of pneumothoraces and gastric distention. Hence, placement of a chest tube or gastric tube should be carefully considered. Similar cautions pertain to any air-filled device. For example, during prolonged flights, it may be necessary to decrease the pressure in air splints, endotracheal tube balloons, and pneumatic antishock garments.

Transfer Data

The information accompanying the patient should include both demographic and historical information pertinent to the patient's injury. Uniform transmission of information is enhanced by the use of an established transfer form, such as the example shown in Figure 13-1. Other data that should accompany the patient are outlined in Appendix C: Trauma Scores: Revised and Pediatric. In addition to the information already outlined, space should be provided for recording data in an organized, sequential fashion—vital signs, central nervous system (CNS) function, and urinary output—during the initial resuscitation and transport period. See Appendix D: Sample Trauma Flow Sheet.

CHAPTER SUMMARY

1 Patients whose injuries exceed an institution's capabilities for definitive care should be identified early during assessment and resuscitation. Individual capabilities of the treating doctor, institutional capabilities, and indications for transfer should be known. Transfer agreements and protocols should be in place to support definitive care.

2 Optimal preparation for transfer includes attention to ATLS principles and clear documentation. The referring doctor and receiving doctor should communicate directly. Transfer personnel should be adequately skilled to administer the required patient care en route.

BIBLIOGRAPHY

1. American College of Surgeons Committee on Trauma. *Resources for Optimal Care of the Injured Patient: 2006.* Chicago: ACS.

2. Champion HR, Sacco WJ, Copes WS, et al. A revision of the trauma score. *J Trauma* 1989;29:623-629.

3. Mullins PJ, Veum-Stone J, Helfand M, et al. Outcome of hospitalized injured patients after institution of a trauma system in an urban area. *JAMA* 1994;271:1919-1924.

4. Scarpio RJ, Wesson DE. Splenic trauma. In: Eichelberger MR, ed. *Pediatric Trauma: Prevention, Acute Care, Rehabilitation.* St. Louis: Mosby Yearbook; 1993:456-463.

5. Schoettker P, D'Amours S, Nocera N, Caldwell E, Sugrue M. Reduction of time to definitive care in trauma patients: effectiveness of a new checklist system. *Injury* 2003;34:187-190.

6. Sharar SR, Luna GK, Rice CL, et al. Air transport following surgical stabilization: an extension of regionalized trauma care. *J Trauma* 1988;28:794-798.

APPENDICES

APPENDIX A Injury Prevention

Injury should not be considered an "accident" which is a term that implies a random circumstance resulting in harm. In fact, injuries occur in patterns that are predictable and preventable. The expression "an accident waiting to happen" is both paradoxical and premonitory. There are high-risk individuals and high-risk environments. In combination, they provide a chain of events that can result in trauma. With the changing perspective in today's health care from managing illness to promoting wellness, injury prevention moves beyond promoting good health to take on the added dimension of reducing health care costs.

Prevention is timely. Doctors who care for injured individuals have a unique opportunity to practice effective, preventive medicine. Although the true risk takers may be recalcitrant about any and all prevention messages, many people who are injured through ignorance, carelessness, or temporary loss of self-control may be receptive to information that is likely to reduce their future vulnerability. Each doctor–patient encounter is an opportunity to reduce trauma recidivism. This is especially true for surgeons who are involved daily during the period immediately after injury, when there may be opportunities to truly change behavior. The basic concepts of injury prevention and strategies for implementation through traditional public health methods are included in this appendix.

Classification of Injury Prevention

Prevention can be considered as primary, secondary, or tertiary. *Primary prevention* refers to elimination of the trauma incident completely. Examples of primary prevention measures include stoplights at intersections, window guards to prevent toddlers from falling, swimming pool fences to keep out nonswimmers and prevent drowning, DUI laws, and safety caps on medicines to prevent ingestions.

Secondary prevention accepts the fact that an injury may occur, but serves to reduce the severity of the injury sustained. Examples of secondary prevention include safety belts, airbags, motorcycle and bicycle helmets, and playground safety surfaces.

Tertiary prevention involves reducing the consequences of the injury after it has occurred. Trauma systems, including the coordination of emergency medical services, identification of trauma centers, and the integration of rehabilitation services to reduce impairment, constitute efforts at tertiary prevention.

Haddon's Matrix

In the early 1970s, Haddon described a useful approach to primary and secondary injury prevention that is now known as the Haddon matrix. According to Haddon's conceptual framework, there are three principal factors in injury occurrence: the injured person (host), the injury mechanism (eg, vehicle, gun), and the environment in which the injury occurs. There are also three phases during which injury and its severity can be modified: the pre-event phase, the event phase (injury), and the post-event phase. Table A-1 outlines how the matrix serves to identify opportunities for injury prevention and can be extrapolated to address other injury causes. The adoption of this structured design by the National Highway Traffic Safety Administration resulted in a sustained reduction in the fatality rate per vehicle mile driven over the past two decades.

The Four Es of Injury Prevention

Injury prevention can be directed at human factors (behavioral issues), vectors of injury, and/or environmental factors and implemented according to the four Es of injury prevention:

- Education
- Enforcement
- Engineering
- Economics (incentives)

Education is the cornerstone of injury prevention. Educational efforts are relatively simple to implement; they promote the development of constituencies and serve to bring the issue before the public. Without an informed and activist public, subsequent legislative efforts (enforcement) are likely to fail. Education is based on the premise that

279

TABLE A-1 ■ Haddon's Factor-Phase Matrix for Motor Vehicle Crash Prevention			
	PRE-EVENT	**EVENT**	**POST-EVENT**
Host	Avoidance of alcohol use	Use of safety belts	Care delivered by bystander
Vehicle	Antilock brakes	Deployment of air bag	Assessment of vehicle characteristics that may have contributed to event
Environment	Speed limits	Impact-absorbing barriers	Access to trauma system

knowledge supports a change in behavior. Although attractive in theory, education in injury prevention has been disappointing in practice. Yet it provides the underpinning for implementation of subsequent strategies, such as that to reduce alcohol-related crash deaths. Mothers Against Drunk Driving is an organization that exemplifies the effective use of a primary education strategy to reduce alcohol-related crash deaths. Through their efforts, an informed and aroused public facilitated the enactment of stricter drunk-driving laws, resulting in a decade of reduced alcohol-related vehicle fatalities. For education to work, it must be directed at the appropriate target group, it must be persistent, and it must be linked to other approaches.

Enforcement is a useful part of any effective injury-prevention strategy because, regardless of the type of trauma, there always are individuals who resist the changes needed to improve outcome—even if the improved outcome is their own. Where compliance with injury prevention efforts lags, legislation that mandates certain behavior or declares certain behaviors illegal often results in dramatic differences. For example, safety belt and helmet laws resulted in measurable increases in usage when educational programs alone had minimal effect.

Engineering, often more expensive at first, clearly has the greatest long-term benefits. Despite proven effectiveness, engineering advances may require concomitant legislative and enforcement initiatives, enabling implementation on a larger scale. Adoption of air bags is a recent example of the application of advances in technology combined with features of enforcement. Other advances in highway design and safety have added tremendously to the margin of safety while driving.

Economic incentives, when used for the correct purposes, are quite effective. For example, the linking of federal highway funds to the passage of motorcycle helmet laws motivated the states to pass such laws and enforce the wearing of helmets. This resulted in a 30% reduction in fatalities from head injuries. Although this economic incentive is no longer in effect, and rates of deaths from head injuries have returned to their previous levels in states that have reversed their helmet statutes, the association between helmet laws and reduced fatalities confirmed the utility of economic incentives in injury prevention. Insurance companies have clear data on risk-taking behavior patterns, and the payments from insurance trusts, consequently, provide related discount premiums.

Developing an Injury Prevention Program—The Public Approach

There are five basic steps to developing an injury prevention program: define the problem, define the causes and risk factors, develop and test interventions, implement injury-prevention strategies, and evaluate the impact.

DEFINE THE PROBLEM

The first step is a basic one: define the problem. This may appear self-evident, but both the magnitude and community impact of trauma can be elusive unless reliable data are available. Population-based data on injury incidence are essential to identify the problem and provide a baseline for determining the impact of subsequent efforts at injury prevention. Information from death certificates, hospital and/or emergency department discharge statistics, and trauma registry printouts are, collectively, good places to start. Whereas sentinel events in a community may identify an individual trauma problem and raise public concern, high-profile problems do not lend themselves to effective injury prevention unless they are part of a larger documented injury-control issue.

DEFINE CAUSES AND RISK FACTORS

After a trauma problem is identified, its causes and risk factors must be defined. The problem may need to be studied to determine what kinds of injuries are involved and where, when, and why they occur. Injury-prevention strategies may begin to emerge with this additional information. Some trauma problems vary from community to community;

however, there are certain risk factors that are likely to remain constant across situations and socioeconomic boundaries. Abuse of alcohol and other drugs is an example of a contributing factor that is likely to be pervasive regardless of whether the trauma is blunt or penetrating, the location is the inner city or the suburbs, and whether fatality or disability occurs. Data are most meaningful when the injury problem is compared between populations with and without defined risk factors. In many instances, the injured people may have multiple risk factors, and clearly defined populations may be difficult to sort out. In such cases, it is necessary to control for the confounding variables.

DEVELOP AND TEST INTERVENTIONS

The next step is to develop and test interventions. This is the time for pilot programs to test intervention effectiveness. Rarely is an intervention tested without some indication that it will work. It is important to consider the views and values of the community if an injury prevention program is to be accepted. End points must be defined up front, and outcomes reviewed without bias. It is sometimes not possible to determine the effectiveness of a test program, especially if it is a small-scale trial intervention. For example, a public information program on safety-belt use conducted at a school

can be assessed by monitoring the incoming and outgoing school traffic and showing a difference, whereas the usage rates in the community as a whole may not change. Nonetheless, the implication is clear—broad implementation of public education regarding safety-belt use can have a beneficial effect within a controlled community population. Telephone surveys are not reliable measures to confirm behavioral change, but they can confirm that the intervention reached the target group.

IMPLEMENT INJURY-PREVENTION STRATEGIES

With confirmation that a given intervention can effect favorable change, the next step is implementation of injury-prevention strategies. From this point, the possibilities are vast.

EVALUATE IMPACT

With implementation comes the need to monitor the impact of the program or evaluation. An effective injury-prevention program linked with an objective means to define its effectiveness can be a powerful message to the public, the press, and legislators, and ultimately may bring about a permanent change in behavior.

APPENDIX A SUMMARY

Injury prevention seems like an immense task, and in many ways it is. Yet, it is important to remember that a pediatrician in Tennessee was able to validate the need for infant safety seats that led to the first infant-safety-seat law. A New York orthopedic surgeon gave testimony that played an important role in achieving the first safety-belt law in the United States. Although not all doctors are destined to make as significant an impact, all doctors can have an impact on their patients' behaviors. Injury-prevention measures do not have to be implemented on a grand scale to make a difference. Although doctors may not be able to prove a difference in their own patient population, if everyone made injury prevention a part of their practice, the results could be significant. As preparations for hospital or emergency department discharge are being made, consideration should be given to patient education to prevent injury recurrence. Whether it is alcohol abuse, returning to an unchanged hostile home environment, riding a motorcycle without wearing head protection, or smoking while refueling the car, there are many opportunities for doctors to make a difference in their patients' future trauma vulnerability.

Bibliography

1. American College of Surgeons Committee on Trauma. *Resources for Optimal Care of the Injured Patient.* Chicago: American College of Surgeons; 2006.

2. Cooper A, Barlow B, Davidson L, et al. Epidemiology of pediatric trauma: importance of population-based statistics. *J Pediatr Surg* 1992;27:149-154.

3. Haddon W, Baker SP. Injury control. In: Clark DW, MacMahon B, eds. *Prevention and Community Medicine.* 2nd ed. Boston: Little Brown; 1981:109-140.

4. Knudson MM, Vassar MJ, Straus EM, et al. Surgeons and injury prevention: what you don't know can hurt you! *J Am Coll Surg* 2001;193:119-124.

5. Laraque D, Barlow B. Prevention of pediatric injury. In: Ivatory R, Cayten G, eds. *The Textbook of Penetrating Trauma.* Baltimore: Williams & Wilkins; 1996.

6. National Committee for Injury Prevention and Control. *Injury Prevention: Meeting the Challenge.* New York: Education Development Center; 1989.

7. Rivera FP. Traumatic deaths of children in United States: currently available prevention strategies. *Pediatrics* 1985;85:456-462.

8. Schermer CR. Alcohol and injury prevention. *J Trauma* 2006;60:447-451.

Resources

1. British Columbia Injury Research and Prevention Unit, Centre for Community Health and Health Research, L408-4480 Oak St., Vancouver, BC V6H 3V4, Canada; 604-875-3776; *www.injuryresearch.bc.ca.*

2. Harborview Injury Prevention and Research Center, University of Washington, Box 359960, 325 Ninth Ave., Seattle, WA 98104-2499; 206-521-1520; *http://depts.washington.edu/hiprc.*

3. Harvard Injury Control Research Center, Harvard School of Public Health, 677 Huntington Ave., 2nd Floor, Boston, MA 02115; 617-432-3420; *www.hsph.harvard.edu/hicrc.*

4. Injury Control Research Center, University of Alabama-Birmingham, CH19 UAB Station, Birmingham, AL 35294; 205-934-1643; *www.uab.edu/icrc.*

5. Injury Free Coalition for Kids, Columbia University, Mailman School of Public Health, 722 W. 168th St., Rm. 1711, New York, NY 10032; 212-342-0517; *www.injuryfree.org.*

6. Injury Prevention and Research Center, University of North Carolina, 137 E, Franklin St., CB#7505 CTP, Chapel Hill, NC 27599-7505; 919-966-2251; *www.iprc.unc.edu.*

7. Johns Hopkins Center for Injury Research and Policy, Hampton House, 624 N. Broadway, 5th Floor, Baltimore, MD 21205-1996; 410-614-4026; *www.jhsph.edu/Research/Centers/CIRP.*

8. National Center for Injury Prevention and Control, Centers for Disease Control, Program Development and Implementation, Mailstop K65, 4770 Buford Hwy. NE, Atlanta, GA 30341-3724; 770-488-1506; *www.cdc.gov*

9. San Francisco Center for Injury Research and Prevention, San Francisco General Hospital, 1001 Potrero Ave., Department of Surgery, Ward 3A, Box 0807, San Francisco, CA 94110; 415-206-4623; *www.surgery.ucsf.edu/sfic.*

10. Slide Prevention Programs (Alcohol and Injury, Bicycle Helmet Safety), available from American College of Surgeons, Customer Service/Publications, 633 N. Saint Clair St., Chicago, IL 60611-3211; 312/202-5474; *https://secure.facs.org/commerce/2003/trauma.html.*

11. State and Local Departments of Health, Injury Control Divisions.

12. The Children's Safety Network, National Injury and Violence Prevention Resource Center, Education Development Center, Inc., 55 Chapel St., Newton, MA 02458-1060; 617/969-7100; *www.childrensafetynetwork.org.*

13. TIPP Sheets, available from American Academy of Pediatrics, 141 Northwest Point Blvd., Elk Grove Village, IL 60007; 800-433-9016; *www.aap.org.*

APPENDIX B Biomechanics of Injury

Introduction

Biomechanics plays an important role in injury mechanisms, especially in motor vehicle crashes. Impact biomechanics includes four principle areas of study: (1) understanding the mechanism of injury; (2) establishing levels of human tolerance to impact; (3) soliciting the mechanical response to injury; and (4) designing more humanlike test dummies and other surrogates. The details of the injury event can provide clues to identifying 90% of a patient's injuries. Specific information for doctors to elicit regarding the biomechanics and mechanism of injury includes:

- The type of traumatic event (eg, vehicular collision, fall, or penetrating injury)

- An estimate of the amount of energy exchange that occurred (eg, speed of the vehicle at impact, distance of the fall, and caliber and size of the weapon)

- The collision or impact of the patient with the object (eg, car, tree, knife, baseball bat, or bullet)

Mechanisms of injury can be classified as blunt, penetrating, thermal, and blast. In all cases, there is a transfer of energy to tissue—or, in the case of freezing, a transfer of energy (heat) from tissue. Energy laws help us understand how tissues sustain injury. These include:

1. Energy is neither created nor destroyed; however, its form can be changed.

2. A body in motion or a body at rest tends to remain in that state until acted on by an outside force.

3. Kinetic energy (KE) is equal to the mass (m) of the object in motion multiplied by the square of the velocity (v) and divided by two.

$$KE = \frac{(m)(v^2)}{2}$$

4. Force (F) is equal to the mass times deceleration (acceleration).

5. Injury is dependent on the amount and speed of energy transmission, the surface area over which the energy is applied, and the elastic properties of the tissues to which the energy transfer is applied.

Blunt Trauma

The common injury patterns and types of injuries identified with blunt trauma include:

- Vehicular impact when the patient is inside the vehicle

- Pedestrian injury

- Injury to cyclists

- Assaults (intentional injury)

- Falls

- Blast injury

VEHICULAR IMPACT

Vehicular collisions can be subdivided further into: (1) collision between the patient and the vehicle, or between patient and some stationary object outside the vehicle if the patient is ejected (eg, tree, earth), and (2) the collision between the patient's organ(s) and the external framework of the body (organ compression).

The interactions between the patient and the vehicle depend on the type of crash. Five crashes depict the possible scenarios—frontal, lateral, rear, angular (front quarter or rear quarter), and rollover.

Occupant Collision

Types of occupant collisions include frontal impact, lateral impact, rear impact, quarter-panel impact, rollover, and ejection.

Frontal Impact A frontal impact is defined as a collision with an object in front of the vehicle that suddenly reduces its speed. Consider two identical vehicles traveling at the same speed. Each vehicle possesses the same kinetic energy [KE = (m)(v²)/2]. One vehicle strikes a concrete bridge abutment, whereas the other brakes to a stop. The braking vehicle loses the same amount of energy as the crashing vehicle, but over a longer time. The first energy law states that energy cannot be created or destroyed. Therefore, this energy must be transferred to another form and is absorbed by the crashing vehicle and its occupants. The individual in the braking vehicle has the same *total* amount of energy applied, but the energy is distributed over a broad range of surfaces (eg, seat friction, foot to floorboard, tire braking, tire to road surface, and hand to steering wheel) and over a longer time.

Lateral Impact   A lateral impact is a collision against the side of a vehicle that accelerates the occupant away from the point of impact (acceleration as opposed to deceleration). A left-sided driver who is struck on the driver's side is at greater risk for left-sided injuries, including left rib fractures, left-sided pulmonary injury, splenic injury, and left-sided skeletal fractures, including pelvic compression fractures. A passenger struck on the passenger side of the vehicle may experience similar right-sided skeletal and thoracic injuries, with liver injuries being common.

In lateral impact collisions, the head acts as a large mass that rotates and laterally bends the neck as the torso is accelerated away from the side of the collision. Injury mechanisms, therefore, involve a variety of specific forces, including shear, torque, and lateral compression and distraction.

Rear Impact   Most commonly, rear impact occurs when a vehicle is at a complete stop and is struck from behind by another vehicle. The stopped vehicle, including its occupants, is accelerated forward from the energy transfer from impact. Because of the apposition of the seat back and torso, the torso is accelerated along with the car. In the absence of a functional headrest, the occupant's head may not be accelerated with the rest of the body. As a result, hyperextension of the neck occurs. Fractures of the posterior elements of the cervical spine—for example, laminar fractures, pedicle fractures, and spinous process fractures, may result and are equally distributed through the cervical vertebrae. Fractures at multiple levels are common and are usually due to direct bony contact.

Quarter-Panel Impact   A quarter-panel impact, front or rear, produces a variation of the injury patterns seen in lateral and frontal impacts or lateral and rear impacts.

Rollover   During a rollover, the unrestrained occupant can impact any part of the interior of the passenger compartment. Injuries may be predicted from the impact points on the patient's skin. As a general rule, this type of mechanism produces more severe injuries because of the violent, multiple motions that occur during the rollover. This is especially true for unbelted occupants.

Ejection   The injuries sustained by the occupant during the process of ejection may be greater than when the indi-

vidual hits the ground. The likelihood of serious injury is increased by more than 300% if the patient is ejected from the vehicle.

Organ Collision

Types of organ collision injuries include compression injury and deceleration injury. Restraint use is a key factor in reducing injury.

Compression Injury   Compression injuries occur when the anterior portion of the torso ceases to move forward, but the posterior portion and internal organs continue their motion. The organs are eventually compressed from behind by the advancing posterior thoracoabdominal wall and the vertebral column, and in front by the impacted anterior structures. Blunt myocardial injury is a typical example of this type of injury mechanism.

Similar injury may occur in lung parenchyma and abdominal organs. In a collision, it is instinctive for the patient to take a deep breath and hold it, closing the glottis. Compression of the thorax produces alveolar rupture with a resultant pneumothorax and/or tension pneumothorax. The increase in intraabdominal pressure may produce diaphragmatic rupture and translocation of abdominal organs into the thoracic cavity. Compression injuries to the brain may also occur. Movement of the head associated with the application of a force through impact can be associated with rapid acceleration forces applied to the brain. Compression injuries also may occur as a result of depressed skull fractures.

Deceleration Injury   Deceleration injuries occur as the stabilizing portion of an organ (eg, renal pedicle, ligamentum teres, or descending thoracic aorta) ceases forward motion with the torso, while the movable body part (eg, spleen, kidney, or heart and aortic arch) continues to move forward. In the case of the heart, shear force is developed in the aorta by the continued forward motion of the aortic arch with respect to the stationary descending aorta. The distal aorta, which is anchored to the spine, decelerates more rapidly with the torso. The shear forces are greatest where the arch and the stable descending aorta join at the ligamentum arteriosum.

This mechanism of injury also may be operative with the spleen and kidney at their pedicle junctions; with the liver as the right and left lobes decelerate around the ligamentum teres, producing a central hepatic laceration; and in the skull when the posterior part of the brain separates from the skull, tearing vessels and producing space-occupying lesions. The numerous attachments of the dura, arachnoid, and pia inside the cranial vault effectively separate the brain into multiple compartments. These compartments are subjected to shear stress by both acceleration and deceleration forces. Another example is the flexible cervical spine, which is attached to the relatively immobile thoracic spine, accounting for the frequent injury identified at the C7-T1 junction.

Restraint Use   The value of passenger restraints in reducing injury has been so well established that it is no longer a debatable issue. When used properly, current three-point restraints have been shown to reduce fatalities by 65% to 70% and to produce a 10-fold reduction in serious injury. At present, the greatest failure of the device is the occupant's refusal to use the system.

The value of occupant restraint devices can be illustrated as follows: A restrained driver and the vehicle travel at the same speed and brake to a stop with a deceleration of $0.5 \times g$ (16 ft/sec^2, or 4.8 m/sec^2). During the 0.01 second it takes for the inertial mechanism to lock the safety belt and couple the driver to the vehicle, the driver moves an additional 6.1 inches (15.25 cm) inside the passenger compartment.

The increasing availability of air bags in vehicles may significantly reduce the injuries sustained in frontal impacts. However, air bags are beneficial only in approximately 70% of collisions. These devices are *not* replacements for the safety belt and must be considered *supplemental* protective devices. Occupants in head-on collisions may benefit from the deployment of an air bag, but only on the first impact. If there is a second impact into another object, the bag is already deployed and deflated, and is no longer available for protection. Air bags provide no protection in rollovers, second crashes, or lateral or rear impacts. The three-point restraint system must be used. Side air bag systems offer promise for safer passenger compartments. **Currently, maximum protection is provided only with the simultaneous use of both seat belts and air bags.**

When worn *correctly*, safety belts can reduce injuries. When worn *incorrectly*—for example, above the anterior/superior iliac spines—the forward motion of the posterior abdominal wall and vertebral column traps the pancreas, liver, spleen, small bowel, duodenum, and kidney against the belt in front. Burst injuries and lacerations of these organs can occur. Hyperflexion over an incorrectly applied belt can produce anterior compression fractures of the lumbar spine (Chance fractures). (See Figure B-1.)

PEDESTRIAN INJURY

It is estimated that nearly 90% of all pedestrian-auto collisions occur at speeds of less than 30 mph (48 kph). Children constitute an exceptionally high percentage of those injured by collision with a vehicle. Thoracic, head, and lower-extremity injuries (in that order) account for the majority of injuries sustained by pedestrians.

There are three impact phases to the injuries sustained by a pedestrian: impact with the vehicle bumper, impact with the vehicle hood and windshield, and final impact with the ground. Lower-extremity injury occurs when the vehicle bumper is impacted; the head and torso are injured by impact with the hood and windshield; and the head, spine, and extremities are injured by impact with the ground.

INJURY TO CYCLISTS

Cyclists and/or their passengers also can sustain compression, acceleration/deceleration, and shearing-type injuries. Cyclists are not protected by the vehicle's structure or restraining devices, as are the occupants of an automobile. Cyclists are protected only by clothing and safety devices worn on their bodies—for example, helmets, boots, and protective clothing. Only the helmet has the ability to redistribute the energy transmission and reduce its intensity, and even this capability is limited. Obviously, the less protection worn by the cyclist, the greater the risk for injury. The concern that the use of bicycle and motorcycle helmets increases the risk of injury below the head, especially cervical spine injury, has *not* been substantiated.

FALLS

Similar to motor vehicle crashes, falls produce injury by means of a relatively abrupt change in velocity (deceleration). The extent of injury to a falling body is related to the ability of the stationary surface to arrest the forward mo-

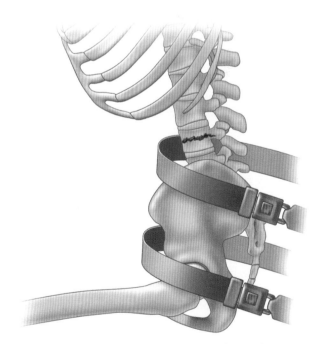

■ **Figure B-1** When worn *correctly,* safety belts can reduce injuries. When worn *incorrectly* burst injuries and organ lacerations can occur. Hyperflexion over an incorrectly applied belt can produce anterior compression fractures of the lumbar spine.

tion of the body. At impact, differential motion of tissues within the organism causes tissue disruption. Decreasing the rate of the deceleration and enlarging the surface area to which the energy is dissipated increase the tolerance to deceleration by promoting more uniform motion of the tissues. The characteristics of the contact surface that arrests the fall are important as well. Concrete, asphalt, and other hard surfaces increase the rate of deceleration and are therefore associated with more severe injuries.

Another factor that should be considered in determining the extent of injury after a fall is the position of the body relative to the impact surface. Consider the following examples:

- A man falls 15 feet (4.5 m) from the roof of a house, landing on his feet

- A man falls 15 feet (4.5 m) from the roof of a house, landing on his back

- A man falls 15 feet (4.5 m) from the roof of a house, landing on the back of his head with his neck in 15 degrees of flexion

In the first example, the entire energy transfer occurs over a surface area equivalent to the area of the man's feet; energy is transferred via the bones of the lower extremity to the pelvis and then the spine. The soft-tissue and visceral organs decelerate at a slower rate than that of the skeleton. In addition, the spine is more likely to flex than to extend because of the ventral position of the abdominal viscera. In the second example, the force is distributed over a much larger surface area. Although tissue damage may indeed occur, it is less severe. In the final example, the entire energy transfer is directed over a small area and focused on a point in the cervical spine where the apex of the angle of flexion occurs. It is easy to see how the injuries differ in each of these examples, even though the mechanism and total energy is identical.

BLAST INJURY

Explosions result from the extremely rapid chemical transformation of relatively small volumes of solid, semisolid, liquid, and gaseous materials into gaseous products that rapidly expand to occupy a greater volume than that occupied by the undetonated explosive. If unimpeded, these rapidly expanding gaseous products assume the shape of a sphere. Inside this sphere, the pressure greatly exceeds atmospheric pressure. The outward expansion of this sphere produces a thin, sharply defined shell of compressed gas that acts as a pressure wave at the periphery of the sphere. The pressure decreases rapidly as this pressure wave travels away from the site of detonation in proportion to the third power of the distance. Energy transfer occurs as the pressure wave induces oscillation in the media through which it travels. The positive-pressure phase of the oscillation may reach sev-

eral atmospheres in magnitude, but it is of extremely short duration, whereas the negative-pressure phase that follows is of longer duration. This latter fact accounts for the phenomenon of buildings falling inward.

Blast injuries may be classified into primary, secondary, tertiary, and quaternary. *Primary blast injuries* result from the direct effects of the pressure wave and are most injurious to gas-containing organs. The tympanic membrane is the most vulnerable to the effects of primary blast and can rupture if pressures exceed 2 atmospheres. Lung tissue can develop evidence of contusion, edema, and rupture, which may result in pneumothorax caused by primary blast injury. Rupture of the alveoli and pulmonary veins produces the potential for air embolism and sudden death. Intraocular hemorrhage and retinal detachments are common ocular manifestations of primary blast injury. Intestinal rupture also may occur. *Secondary blast injuries* result from flying objects striking an individual. *Tertiary blast injuries* occur when an individual becomes a missile and is thrown against a solid object or the ground. Secondary and tertiary blast injuries can cause trauma typical of penetrating and blunt mechanisms, respectively. *Quarternary blast injuries* include burn injury, crush injury, respiratory problems from inhaling dust, smoke, or toxic fumes, and exacerbations or complications of existing conditions such as angina, hypertension, and hyperglycemia.

Penetrating Trauma

Penetrating trauma refers to injury produced by foreign objects that penetrate tissue. Weapons are usually classified based on the amount of energy produced by the projectiles they launch:

- Low energy—knife or hand-energized missiles

- Medium energy—handguns

- High energy—military or hunting rifles

The velocity of a missile is the most significant determinant of its wounding potential. The importance of velocity is demonstrated by the formula relating mass and velocity to kinetic energy.

$$\text{Kinetic Energy} = \text{mass} \times (V_1^2 - V_2^2)/2$$
$$\text{where } V_1 \text{ is impact velocity and } V_2 \text{ is exit}$$
$$\text{or remaining velocity.}$$

VELOCITY

The wounding capability of a bullet increases markedly above the critical velocity of 2000 ft/sec (600 m/sec). At this speed a temporary cavity is created by tissue being compressed at the periphery of impact, which is caused by a shock wave initiated by impact of the bullet.

Cavitation is the result of energy exchange between the moving missile and body tissues. The amount of cavitation or energy exchange is proportional to the surface area of the point of impact, the density of the tissue, and the velocity of the projectile at the time of impact. (See Figure B-2.) Depending on the velocity of the missile, the diameter of this cavity can be up to 30 times that of the bullet. The maximum diameter of this temporary cavity occurs at the area of the greatest resistance to the bullet. This also is where the greatest degree of deceleration and energy transfer occur. A bullet fired from a handgun with a standard round can produce a temporary cavity of 5 to 6 times the diameter of the bullet. Knife injuries, on the other hand, result in little or no cavitation.

Tissue damage from a high-velocity missile can occur at some distance from the bullet track itself. Sharp missiles with small, cross-sectional fronts slow with tissue impact, resulting in little injury or cavitation. Missiles with large, cross-sectional fronts, such as hollow-point bullets that spread or mushroom on impact, cause more injury or cavitation.

BULLETS

Some bullets are specifically designed to increase the amount of damage they cause. Recall that it is the transfer of energy to the tissue, the time over which the energy transfer occurs, and the surface area over which the energy exchange is distributed that determine the degree of tissue damage. Bullets with hollow noses or semijacketed coverings are designed to flatten on impact, thereby increasing their cross-sectional area and resulting in more rapid deceleration and

consequentially a greater transfer of kinetic energy. Some bullets are specially designed to fragment on impact or even explode, which extends tissue damage. Magnum rounds, or cartridges with a greater amount of gunpowder than normal rounds, are designed to increase the muzzle velocity of the missile.

The wound at the point of bullet impact is determined by:

- The shape of the missile ("mushroom")
- The position of the missile relative to the impact site (tumble, yaw)
- Fragmentation (shotgun, bullet fragments, special bullets)

Yaw (the orientation of the longitudinal axis of the missile to its trajectory) and *tumble* increase the surface area of the bullet with respect to the tissue it contacts and, therefore, increase the amount of energy transferred (Figure B-3). In general, the later the bullet begins to yaw after penetrating tissue, the deeper the maximum injury. Bullet deformation and fragmentation of semijacketed ammunition increase surface area relative to the tissue and the dissipation of kinetic energy.

SHOTGUN WOUNDS

Wounds inflicted by shotguns require special considerations. The muzzle velocity of most of these weapons is generally 1200 ft/sec (360 m/sec). After firing, the shot radiates in a conical distribution from the muzzle. With a choked or narrowed muzzle, 70% of the pellets are deposited in a 30-inch (75-cm) diameter circle at 40 yards

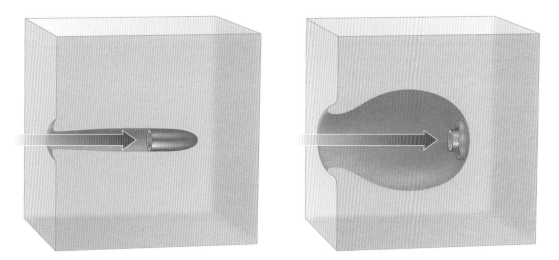

■ **Figure B-2** Sharp missiles with small cross-sectional fronts slow with tissue impact, resulting in little injury or cavitation. Missiles with large cross-sectional fronts, such as hollow-point bullets that spread or "mushroom" on impact, cause more injury and cavitation.

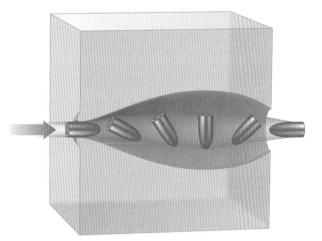

■ **Figure B-3** *Yaw* (the orientation of the longitudinal axis of the missile to its trajectory) and *tumble* increase the surface area of the bullet with respect to the tissue it contacts and, therefore, increase the amount of energy transferred. In general, the later the bullet begins to yaw after penetrating tissue, the deeper the maximum injury.

(36 m). However, the "shot" is spherical, and the coefficient of drag through air and tissue is quite high. As a result, the velocity of the spherical pellets declines rapidly after firing and further after impact. This weapon can be lethal at close range, but its destructive potential rapidly dissipates as distance increases. The area of maximal injury to tissue is relatively superficial unless the weapon is fired at close range. Shotgun blasts can carry clothing and deposit wadding (the paper or plastic that separates the powder and pellets in the shell) into the depths of the wound and become a source of infection if not removed.

ENTRANCE AND EXIT WOUNDS

For clinical reasons, it may be important to determine whether the wound is an entrance or exit wound. Two holes may indicate either two separate gunshot wounds or the entrance and exit of one bullet, suggesting the path the missile may have taken through the body. Missiles usually follow the path of least resistance once tissue has been entered, and the clinician should not assume that the trajectory of the bullet followed a linear path between the entrance and exit wound. The identification of the anatomic structures that may be damaged and even the type of surgical procedure that needs to be done may be influenced by such information.

Bibliography

1. Greensher J. Non-automotive vehicle injuries in the adolescent. *Pediatr Ann* 1988;17(2):114, 117-121.

2. Kraus JF, Fife D, Conroy C. Incidence, severity and outcomes of brain injuries involving bicycles. *Am J Public Health* 1987;77(1):76-78.

3. Leads from the MMWR. Bicycle-related injuries: Data from the National Electronic Injury Surveillance System. *JAMA* 1987;257:3334, 3337.

4. Mackay M. Kinetics of vehicle crashes. In: Maull KI, Cleveland HC, Strauch GO, et al., eds. *Advances in Trauma*, vol. 2. Chicago: Yearbook; 1987:21-24.

5. Maull KI, Whitley RE, Cardea JA. Vertical deceleration injuries. *Surg Gynecol Obstet* 1981;153:233-236.

6. National Highway Traffic Safety Administration. *The Effect of Helmet Law Repeal on Motorcycle Fatalities.* DOT Publication HS-807. Washington, DC: Government Printing Office; 1987:605.

7. Offner PJ, Rivara FP, Maier RV. The impact of motorcycle helmet use. *J Trauma* 1992;32:636-642.

8. Rozycki GS, Maull KI. Injuries sustained by falls. *Arch Emerg Med* 1991;8:245-252.

9. Wagle VG, Perkins C, Vallera A. Is helmet use beneficial to motorcyclists? *J Trauma* 1993;34:120-122.

10. Zador PL, Ciccone MA. Automobile driver fatalities in frontal impacts: air bags compared with manual belts. *Am J Public Health* 1993;83:661-666.

APPENDIX C Trauma Scores: Revised and Pediatric

Introduction

Correct triage is essential to the effective functioning of regional trauma systems. Overtriage can inundate trauma centers with minimally injured patients and delay care for severely injured patients. On the other hand, undertriage can produce inadequate initial care and cause preventable morbidity and mortality. Unfortunately, the perfect triage tool does not exist.

Revised Trauma Score

Experience with adult trauma scoring systems illustrates this problem by the multiplicity of scoring systems that have been proposed over the past decade. None of these scoring protocols is universally accepted as a completely effective triage tool. At present, most adult trauma surgeons utilize the Revised Trauma Score (RTS) as a triage tool and the weighted variation of this score as a predictor of potential mortality. This score is based totally on physiologic derangement on initial evaluation and entails a categorization of blood pressure, respiratory rate, and the Glasgow Coma Scale (See Table C-1).

Pediatric Trauma Score

Application of these three components to the pediatric population, however, is difficult and inconsistent. Respiratory rate is often inaccurately measured in the field and does not necessarily reflect respiratory insufficiency in the injured child. Although the Glasgow Coma Scale is an extremely effective neurologic assessment tool, it requires some revision for application to the preverbal child. These problems, in association with the lack of any identification of anatomic injury or quantification of patient size, undermine the applicability of the RTS to effective triage of injured children. For these reasons, the Pediatric Trauma Score (PTS) was developed. The PTS is the sum of the severity grade of each category and has been demonstrated to predict potential for death and severe disability reliably (Table C-2, page 291).

SIZE

Size is a major consideration for the infant-toddler group, in which mortality from injury is the highest. Airway is assessed — not just as a function, but as a descriptor of what care is required to provide adequate management. Systolic blood pressure assessment primarily identifies those children in whom evolving preventable shock may occur (50 to 90 mm Hg systolic blood pressure [+l]). Regardless of size, a child whose systolic blood pressure is below 50 mm Hg (-l) is in obvious jeopardy. On the other hand, a child whose systolic pressure exceeds 90 mm Hg (+2) probably falls into a better outcome category than a child with even a slight degree of hypotension.

LEVEL OF CONSCIOUSNESS

Level of consciousness is the most important factor in initially assessing the central nervous system. Because children frequently lose consciousness transiently during injury, the "obtunded" (+l) grade is given to any child who loses consciousness, no matter how fleeting the loss. This grade identifies a patient who may have sustained a head injury with potentially fatal—but often treatable—intracranial sequelae.

MUSCULOSKELETAL INJURY

Skeletal injury is a component of the PTS because of its high incidence in the pediatric population and its potential contribution to mortality. Finally, cutaneous injury, both as an adjunct to common pediatric injury patterns and as an injury category that includes penetrating wounds, is considered in the computed PTS.

USE OF THE PTS

The PTS serves as a simple checklist, ensuring that all components critical to the initial assessment of the injured child have been considered. It is useful for paramedics in the field, as well as for doctors in facilities other than pediatric trauma units. As a predictor of injury, the PTS has a statistically significant inverse relationship with the Injury Severity Score (ISS) and mortality. Analysis of this relationship has identified a threshold PTS of 8, above which injured children should have a mortality rate of 0%. All in-

TABLE C-1 ■ Revised Trauma Score

ASSESSMENT COMPONENT	VARIABLES	SCORE	START OF TRANSPORT	END OF TRANSPORT
A. Respiratory Rate (breaths/minute)	10–29 >29 6–9 1–5 0	4 3 2 1 0	_____	_____
B. Systolic Blood Pressure (mm Hg)	>89 76–89 50–75 1–49 0	4 3 2 1 0	_____	_____
C. Glasgow Coma Scale Score Conversion $C = D + E^1 + F$ (adult) $C = D + E^2 + F$ (pediatric)	13–15 9–12 6–8 4–5 <4	4 3 2 1 0	_____	_____
D. Eye Opening	Spontaneous To voice To pain None	4 3 2 1	_____	_____
E^1 Verbal Response, Adult	Oriented Confused Inappropriate words Incomprehensible words None	5 4 3 2 1	_____	_____
E^2 Verbal Response, Pediatric	Appropriate Cries, consolable Persistently irritable Restless, agitated None	5 4 3 2 1	_____	_____
F. Motor Response	Obeys commands Localizes pain Withdraws (pain) Flexion (pain) Extension (pain None	6 5 4 3 2 1	_____	_____
Glasgow Coma Scale Score (Total = $D + E^1$ or $E^2 + F$)			_____	_____
Revised Trauma Score (Total = A + B + C)				

Adapted with permission from Champion HR, Sacco WJ, Copes WS, et al: A revision of the Trauma Score. *Journal of Trauma*. 1989; 29(5):624.

jured children with a PTS of less than 8 should be triaged to an appropriate pediatric trauma center, because they have the highest potential for preventable mortality, morbidity, and disability. According to the National Pediatric Trauma Registry statistics, this group represents approximately 25% of all pediatric trauma victims, clearly requiring the most aggressive monitoring and observation.

Studies comparing the PTS with the RTS have identified similar performances of both scores in predicting po-

tential for mortality. Unfortunately, the RTS produces unacceptable levels of undertriage, which is an inadequate trade-off for its greater simplicity. Perhaps more importantly, however, the PTS's function as an initial assessment checklist requires that each of the factors that may contribute to death or disability is considered during initial evaluation and becomes a source of concern for those individuals responsible for the initial assessment and management of the injured child.

TABLE C-2 ■ Pediatric Trauma Score

ASSESSMENT COMPONENT	SCORE		
	+2	+1	−1
Weight	> 20 kg (> 44 lb)	10-20 kg (22–44 lb)	<10 kg (<22 lb)
Airway	Normal	Oral or nasal airway, oxygen	Intubated, cricothyroidotomy, or tracheostomy
Systolic Blood Pressure	> 90 mm Hg; good peripheral pulses and perfusion	50-90 mm Hg; carotid/ femoral pulses palpable	<50 mm Hg; weak or no pulses
Level of Consciousness	Awake	Obtunded or any loss of consciousness	Coma, unresponsive
Fracture	None seen or suspected	Single, closed	Open or multiple
Cutaneous	None visible	Contusion, abrasion, laceration <7 cm not through fascia	Tissue loss, any gunshot wound or stab wound through fascia
Totals:			

Adapted with permission from Tepas JJ, Mollitt DL, Talbert JL, et al: The pediatric trauma score as a predictor of injury severity in the injured child. *Journal of Pediatric Surgery*. 1987; 22(1)15.

TRAUMA RESUSCITATION RECORD

TRAUMA REGISTRY # _____

DATE: _____ / _____ / _____ TIME ARRIVED: _____ : _____

NAME: _____

EST. WGT.: _____ EST. AGE: _____ ☐ MALE ☐ FEMALE

TRAUMA I.D. BAND #: _____ WA / OR

TRAUMA TEAM
☐ ACTIVATED I
☐ ACTIVATED II
☐ MULTIPLES
☐ UPGRADED
☐ ED ROOM _____
☐ OR ROOM _____

	TR SURG	ED MD	ANEST	SR RES	JR RES	NEURO	ORTHO	PEDS		
NAME										
CALLED			$			$	$	$	$	$
RESPOND										
ARRIVE										

CIRCLE "S" FOR STAT CALL

TIME OF INJURY: _____ : _____ LOCATION: _____

XPORT: ☐ AMBU _____ ☐ HELI/FIXED _____ ☐ PRIV CAR ☐ WALK-IN OTHER _____

TRAUMA SYSTEM ENTRY BY: ☐ FIELD TRIAGE ☐ ED ☐ TRAUMA CONSULT ☐ TRANSFER

PRE-HOSPITAL EVENTS: _____

MEDICATION PTA: _____

CHILDREN / ADULT GLASGOW COMA SCALE

EYE OPENING	SPONTANEOUS	4
	TO VOICE	3
	TO PAIN	2
	NONE	1
VERBAL RESPONSE	ORIENTED	5
	CONFUSED	4
	INAPPROPRIATE WORDS	3
	INCOMPREHENSIBLE WORDS	2
	NONE	1
MOTOR RESPONSE	OBEYS COMMANDS	6
	LOCALIZES PAIN	5
	WITHDRAWS (PAIN)	4
	FLEXION (PAIN)	3
	EXTENSION (PAIN)	2
	NONE	1

☐ CHEMICALLY PARALYZED ON ARRIVAL

PUPIL CHART
2 3 4 5 6 7

KEY
A Abrasion
B Burn
C Contusion
D Amputation
E Paralysis
F Fracture
G Gunshot Wound
H Open Fracture
I Stab Wound
J Pain
K Paresthesia
L Laceration

R L   L R

INITIAL ASSESSMENT

TREATMENT PTA

☐ AIRWAY / BVM
☐ OET / NET / PEAD / CRICO
☐ O₂ _____
☐ C COLLAR
☐ SPINE STABILIZATION

☐ MAST PANTS (INFLATED)
☐ EXTREMITY SPLINT / TRACTION
☐ HEIMLICH VALVE R / L
☐ CPR/DEFIBRILLATE
☐ IV

HEALTH HISTORY: _____
_____
PREVIOUS SURGERIES: _____
CURRENT MEDS: _____
_____
ALLERGIES: _____
PREGNANT: ☐ YES ☐ NO LMP: _____
TETANUS STATUS: CURRENT ☐ YES ☐ NO
PCP: _____

	WNL	PRIMARY SURVEY
BEHAVIOR		☐ UNCOOPERATIVE ☐ COMBATIVE ☐ SEDATED ☐ RESTRAINTS ☐ PHARMACOLOGICAL PARALYSIS
AIRWAY		☐ UNOBSTRUCTED ☐ OTHER
BREATHING		☐ LABORED ☐ PANTING ☐ SPLINTING ☐ NOT BREATHING ☐ ASSISTED BREATHING ☐ NECKVEIN DISTENTION ☐ CREPITUS ☐ DEVIATED TRACH ☐ CYANOSIS ☐ OPEN PTX ☐ FLAIL CHEST ☐ HEMOPTYSIS
BREATH SOUNDS		L ☐ ABSENT ☐ DECREASED ☐ RALES ☐ WHEEZES R ☐ ABSENT ☐ DECREASED ☐ RALES ☐ WHEEZES
EXTERNAL HEMORRHAGE		LOCATION: _____
CARDIAC		RHYTHM: _____ HEART SOUNDS: ☐ MUFFLED ☐ MURMUR
PULSES		L ☐ RADIAL ☐ FEMORAL ☐ PEDAL ☐ THREADY R ☐ RADIAL ☐ FEMORAL ☐ PEDAL ☐ THREADY
SKIN		CYANOSIS: ☐ PERIPHERAL ☐ CENTRAL ☐ CLAMMY ☐ DELAYED CAP. REFILL

	WNL	SECONDARY SURVEY
NEURO-CRANIAL		☐ LETHARGY ☐ STUPOR ☐ DECEREBRATE ☐ DECORTICATE
NEURO SPINAL CORD		QUAD/PARAPLEGIC LEVEL: _____ MONOPLEGIA EXTREMITY: _____
SCALP		☐ LACERATIONS: _____ ☐ OPEN FRACTURE: _____ ☐ HEMATOMA: _____

	WNL	SECONDARY SURVEY CONT'D
PUPILS		L ☐ NON-REACTIVE ☐ CONSTRICTED ☐ DILATED SIZE: _____ R ☐ NON-REACTIVE ☐ CONSTRICTED ☐ DILATED SIZE: _____
FACE		☐ PALPABLE FACIAL FRACTURES ☐ MALOCCLUSION ☐ ABRASIONS ☐ LACERATIONS ☐ CONTUSIONS
EARS		OTORRHAGIA OTORRHEA T.M. L ☐ ☐ L: _____ R ☐ ☐ R: _____
NECK		☐ ABRASIONS ☐ LACERATIONS ☐ CONTUSIONS ☐ C-SPINE CLEARED CLINICALLY
CHEST		☐ LACERATIONS ☐ CONTUSIONS ☐ HEMATOMA ☐ BELT ABRASIONS ☐ PENETRATING WOUND
ABDOMEN		☐ PREV. SURG. ☐ PENETRATING WOUND ☐ BELT ABRASIONS ☐ DISTENTION ☐ SCAPHOID
PELVIS		☐ UNSTABLE ☐ GENITAL INJURY ☐ PROSTATE ☐ RECTAL TONE ☐ GUAIAC + − ☐ HEMATURIA
BACK (log roll)		☐ DEFORMED ☐ PENETRATION
UPPER EXTREMITIES		L ☐ LAC ☐ FX ☐ OPEN R ☐ LAC ☐ FX ☐ OPEN
LOWER EXTREMITIES		L ☐ LAC ☐ FX ☐ OPEN R ☐ LAC ☐ FX ☐ OPEN

147029 (2/07)   WHITE - ORIGINAL   YELLOW - TRAUMA REGISTRY   PINK - ED COPY

Used with permission from Legacy Trauma Services, Legacy Emanuel Hospital & Health Care Center, Portland, Oregon.

TIME	BP	P / Rhythm	RESP	T / SaO2	G E	C V	S M	PUPIL L/R	PAIN 1-10	ASSESSMENT / INTERVENTIONS / RESPONSE	I.V. SOLUTIONS	BLOOD	AMT INFUSED	OUTPUT
PTA														
	R													
	L													

DISPOSITION TOTALS

IV NO. _____ _____ cc Remaining
IV NO. _____ _____ cc Remaining
IV NO. _____ _____ cc Remaining
IV NO. _____ _____ cc Remaining

FLUID SUMMARY

INTAKE (cc)	OUTPUT (cc)
Crystalloids/Colloids _____	Urine _____
Blood _____	Gastric/Emesis _____
Other _____	Chest (L) _____ (R) _____
Total	Total

LABORATORY   ☐ LEVEL I   ☐ LEVEL II   ☐ PEDS   TIME DRAWN ▨▨▨▨

TIME	PH	PO₂	PCO₂	HCO₃	BE	TIME	HGB	HCT	PLTS	PT	PTT	INR	FIB	NA+	CL-	K+	BUN	CR	GLU	CA+
:						:														
:						:														
:						:														
:						:														

ETOH 0 •   HCG ±   TO LAB ☐   :   URINE TOX SCREEN   BLOOD BANK   CLOT   TYPE & SCREEN   TYPE & CROSS   UNITS   MTP   TIME INITIATED ____ : ____

AIRWAY / BREATHING

☐ INTUBATED   TIME _____ : _____
☐ NASAL   ☐ ORAL   ☐ CRICO/TRACH _____
SIZE _____   DEPTH OF TUBE _____
FiO2 _____   TIDAL VOLUME _____
MODE _____ RATE _____
END TIDAL CO₂ _____

TIME
L __:__ R __:__ NEEDLE THORACENTESIS
L __:__ R __:__ TUBE THORACOSTOMY(S)
__:__ ☐ NGT (NO MIDFACE TRAUMA)
__:__ ☐ OGT (MIDFACE TRAUMA)
__:__ ☐ FOLEY/SUPRAPUBIC
__:__ ☐ PERITONEAL LAVAGE
__:__ ☐ CERVICAL TRACTION DEVICE
__:__ ☐ ORTHO REDUCTION
__:__ ☐ SPLINT Type: _____ L+R
__:__ ☐ OTHER _____
_____
_____
_____
_____
_____

FAMILY NOTIFICATION

☐ HERE   ☐ CONTACTED
NAME _____
_____
TELEPHONE NUMBER _____
☐ UNABLE TO REACH
       TIME
____ : ____
____ : ____
____ : ____
____ : ____

CIRCULATION

TIME
__:__ ☐ INT/EXT JUGULAR VEIN   L   R
__:__ ☐ SUBCLAVIAN VEIN   L   R
__:__ ☐ PERIPHERAL SIZE _____   L   R
__:__ ☐ PERIPHERAL SIZE _____   L   R
__:__ ☐ FEMORAL   SIZE _____   L   R
__:__ ☐ INTRAOSSEOUS   SITE _____
__:__ ☐ SWAN GANZ   SITE _____
__:__ ☐ ART LINE   SITE _____
__:__ ☐ OTHER   SITE _____
__:__ ☐ EKG 12 LEAD

BELONGINGS: (SEE ITEMIZED LIST)
☐ HOME   ☐ ROOM
☐ POLICE   ☐ DISCARD

SEQUENCE OF EVENTS

▨▨▨ : ▨▨▨   TIME LEFT RESUSCITATION ROOM

RADIOLOGICAL STUDIES	
IN TIME	STUDY X-RAYS
:	C-SPINE LATERAL
:	C-SPINE COMPLETE SERIES
:	CHEST SUPINE
:	CHEST ERECT
:	PELVIS
:	EXTREMITIES
:	ABDOMEN
:	CAT SCAN - HEAD
:	CAT SCAN - SPINES - C T L
:	CAT SCAN - CHEST
:	CAT SCAN - ABDOMEN
:	THORACIC SPINE
:	LUMBAR SPINE
:	ULTRASOUND - ABDOMEN
:	ULTRASOUND
:	IVP/CYSTOGRAM
:	ANGIOGRAM
:	ECHO-CARD
:	
:	

▨▨▨ : ▨▨▨   TIME RADIOLOGICAL STUDIES COMPLETED
▨▨▨ : ▨▨▨   READY FOR DISPOSITION

DISPOSITION   TIME ▨▨▨ : ▨▨▨

ADMIT   ☐ I/P   ☐ OBSERVATION   ADMIT TIME: ▨▨▨ : ▨▨▨
☐ HOME   ☐ AMA
☐ TRANSFERRED TO: _____
VIA: ☐ GROUND ☐ AIR AGENCY: _____
☐ EXPIRED
    REMAINS TO: _____
    ORGAN DONOR: ☐ YES ☐ NO
C-SPINE CLEARED: ☐ YES ☐ NO   BY: _____ M.D.
C-COLLAR REMOVED: ☐ TIME: ____ : ____   BY: _____
THORACIC/LUMBAR CLEARED: ☐ YES ☐ NO   BY: _____

ADMITTING DIAGNOSIS: _____
_____
_____

_____
TRN

_____
RECORDER

_____
CIRCULATOR

_____
PHYSICIAN SIGNATURE

*NOTE: This flow sheet is only an example of information that may be required. All institutions that receive trauma patients should develop a form that meets the needs of the institution.

APPENDIX E Tetanus Immunization

Introduction

Adequate tetanus prophylaxis is important in patients with multiple injuries, particularly when open-extremity trauma is present. The average incubation period for tetanus is 10 days; most often it is 4 to 21 days. In severe trauma cases, tetanus can appear as early as 1 to 2 days after injury. All medical professionals must be cognizant of this important fact when providing care to injured patients. Recent studies conclude that it is not possible to determine clinically which wounds are prone to tetanus; tetanus can occur after minor, seemingly innocuous injuries, yet it is rare after severely contaminated wounds. Thus, all traumatic wounds should be considered at risk for the development of tetanus infection.

Tetanus immunization depends on the patient's previous immunization status and the tetanus-prone nature of the wound. The following guidelines are adapted from the literature, and information is available from the Centers for Disease Control and Prevention (CDC). Because this information is continuously reviewed and updated as new data become available, the American College of Surgeons Committee on Trauma recommends contacting the CDC for the most current information and detailed guidelines related to tetanus prophylaxis and immunization for injured patients.

General Principles

The following general principles for doctors who treat trauma patients concern surgical wound care and passive immunization.

SURGICAL WOUND CARE

Regardless of the active immunization status of the patient, meticulous surgical care—including removal of all devitalized tissue and foreign bodies—should be provided immediately for all wounds. If the adequacy of wound debridement is in question or a puncture injury is present, the wound should be left open and not closed by sutures. Such care is essential as part of the prophylaxis against tetanus. Traditional clinical features that influence the risk for tetanus infection in soft tissue wounds are listed in Table E-1. However, all wounds should be considered at risk for the development of tetanus.

TABLE E-1 ■ Wound Features and Tetanus Risk		
CLINICAL FEATURES OF WOUND	**NON–TETANUS-PRONE WOUNDS**	**TETANUS-PRONE WOUNDS**
Age of wound	< 6 hours	>6 hours
Configuration	Linear wound, abrasion	Stellate wound, avulsion
Depth	≤ 1 cm	>1 cm
Mechanism of injury	Sharp surface (eg, knife, glass)	Missile, crush, burn, frostbite
Signs of infection	Absent	Present
Devitalized tissue	Absent	Present
Contaminants (eg, dirt, feces, soil, saliva)	Absent	Present
Denervated and/or ischemic tissue	Absent	Present

Adapted with permission from the Centers for Disease Control and Prevention, Atlanta, GA, www.cdc.gov/mmwr/preview/mmwrhtml/00041645.htm. (Last updated 2007.)

PASSIVE IMMUNIZATION

Passive immunization with 250 units of human tetanus immune globulin (TIG) administered intramuscularly must be considered for each patient. TIG provides longer protection than antitoxin of animal origin and causes few adverse reactions. The characteristics of the wound, conditions under which it occurred, wound age, TIG treatment, and the previous active immunization status of the patient must all be considered (Table E-2). When tetanus toxoid and TIG are given concurrently, separate syringes and separate sites should be used. If the patient has ever received a series of three injections of toxoid, TIG is not indicated, unless the wound is judged to be tetanus-prone and is more than 24 hours old.

Bibliography

1. American College of Surgeons Committee on Trauma. Prophylaxis against tetanus in wound management. Poster, 1995.

2. Rhee P, Nunley MK, Demetriades D, Velmahos G, Doucet JJ. Tetanus and trauma: a review and recommendation. *J Trauma* 2005;58:1082-1088.

3. U.S. Department of Health and Human Services, Centers for Disease Control and Prevention. Tetanus. http://www.cdc.gov/vaccines/pubs/pinkbook/downloads/tetanus.pdf. Accessed October 22, 2007.

TABLE E-2   ■   Summary of Tetanus Prophylaxis for Injured Patients

HISTORY OF ADSORBED TETANUS TOXOID (DOSES)	NON–TETANUS-PRONE WOUNDS		TETANUS-PRONE WOUNDS	
	TD[a]	TIG	TD[a]	TIG
Unknown or < 3	Yes	No	Yes	Yes
≥ 3[b]	No[c]	No	No[d]	No

Adapted with permission from the Centers for Disease Control and Prevention, Atlanta, GA, www.cdc.gov/mmwr/preview/mmwrhtml/00041645.htm. (Last updated 2007.)

[a] For children younger than 7 years old, diphtheria-tetanus-pertussis (DPT) vaccine (DT, if pertussis vaccine is contraindicated) is preferred to tetanus toxoid alone. For patients 7 years old and older, tetanus and diphtheria toxoids are preferred to tetanus toxoid alone.

[b] If only three doses of fluid toxoid have been received, a fourth dose of toxoid, preferably an adsorbed toxoid, should be given.

[c] Yes, if more than 10 years since last dose.

[d] Yes, if more than 5 years since last dose. (More frequent boosters are not needed and can accentuate side effects.)

APPENDIX F **Ocular Trauma**
(Optional Lecture)

Introduction

The initial assessment of a patient with an ocular injury requires a systematic approach. The physical examination should proceed in an organized, step-by-step manner. It does not require extensive, complicated instrumentation in the multiple-trauma setting. Rather, simple therapeutic measures often can save the patient's vision and prevent serious sequelae before an ophthalmologist is available. This appendix provides pertinent information regarding the early identification and treatment of ocular injuries that will enhance doctors' basic knowledge and may save their patients' vision.

Assessment

Key factors in the assessment of patients with ocular trauma include patient history, history of the injury incident, initial symptoms, and results of physical examination.

PATIENT HISTORY

Obtain a history of any preexisting ocular disease. Key questions include:

1. Does the patient wear corrective lenses?

2. Is there a history of glaucoma or previous eye surgery?

3. What medications does the patient use (eg, pilocarpine)?

HISTORY OF INJURY INCIDENT

Obtain a detailed description of the circumstances surrounding the injury. This information often raises the index of suspicion for certain potential injuries and their sequelae, such as the higher risk of infection from certain foreign bodies (eg, wood vs. metallic). Key questions include:

Upon completion of this topic, the student will be able to assess and manage sight-threatening eye injuries. Specifically, the doctor will be able to:

OBJECTIVES

1. Obtain patient and event histories.

2. Perform a systematic examination of the orbit and its contents.

3. Identify eyelid injuries that can be treated by the primary care doctor, as well as those that must be referred to an ophthalmologist for treatment.

4. Explain how to examine the eye for a foreign body, and how to remove superficial foreign bodies to prevent further injury.

5. Identify corneal abrasion and describe its proper management.

6. Identify hyphema and describe its initial management and the necessity for referral to an ophthalmologist.

7. Identify eye injuries that require referral to an ophthalmologist.

8. Identify ruptured-globe injury and describe its initial management prior to referral to an ophthalmologist.

9. Evaluate and treat eye injuries that result from chemicals.

10. Evaluate a patient with an orbital fracture and describe its initial management and the necessity for referral.

11. Identify retrobulbar hematoma and explain the necessity for immediate referral.

1. Was there blunt trauma?

2. Was there penetrating injury? (In motor vehicular crashes there is potential for glass and metallic foreign bodies.)

3. Was there a missile injury?

4. Was there a possible thermal, chemical, or flash burn?

INITIAL SYMPTOMS

Key questions regarding the patient's initial symptoms include:

1. What were the initial symptoms?

2. Did the patient report pain or photophobia?

3. Was there an immediate decrease in vision that has remained stable, or is it progressive?

PHYSICAL EXAMINATION

The physical examination must be systematic so that function and anatomic structures are evaluated. As with injuries to other organ systems, the pathology also may evolve with time, and the patient must be reevaluated periodically. A directed approach to the ocular examination, beginning with the most external structures in an "outside-to-inside" manner, ensures that injuries are not missed.

Visual Acuity

Visual acuity is evaluated first by any means possible and recorded (eg, patient counting fingers at 3 ft [0.9 m]).

Eyelids

The most external structures to be examined are the eyelids. The eyelids should be assessed for: (1) edema; (2) ecchymosis; (3) evidence of burns or chemical injury; (4) laceration(s)—medial, lateral, lid margin, canaliculi; (5) ptosis; (6) foreign bodies that contact the globe; and (7) avulsion of the canthal tendon.

Orbital Rim

Gently palpate the orbital rim for any step-off deformity or crepitus. Subcutaneous emphysema can result from a fracture of the medial orbit into the ethmoids or a fracture of the orbital floor into the maxillary antrum.

Globe

The eyelids should be retracted to examine the globe without applying pressure to the globe. Specially designed retractors are available for this purpose. Cotton-tipped applicators can also be used; they should be placed gently against the superior and inferior orbital rims, enabling the eyelids to be rolled open. Then assess the globe anteriorly for any displacement from a retrobulbar hematoma and for any posterior or inferior displacement due to an orbit fracture. Also assess the globes for normal ocular movement, diplopia, and evidence of entrapment.

Pupil

Assess the pupils for roundness, with regular shape, equality, and reaction to light stimulus. It is important to test for an afferent pupil defect. Optic nerve trauma usually results in the failure of both pupils to constrict when a light is directed at the affected eye.

Cornea

Assess the cornea for opacity, ulceration, and foreign bodies. Fluorescein and a blue light can facilitate this assessment.

Conjunctiva

Assess the conjunctivae for chemosis, subconjunctival emphysema (indicating probable fracture of the orbit into the ethmoid or maxillary sinus), subconjunctival hemorrhage, and foreign bodies.

Anterior Chamber

Examine the anterior chamber for hyphema (blood in the anterior chamber). The depth of the anterior chamber can be assessed by shining a light into the eye from the lateral aspect of the eye. If the light does not illuminate the entire surface of the iris, a shallow anterior chamber should be suspected. This condition can result from an anterior penetrating wound. A deep anterior chamber can result from a posterior penetrating wound of the globe.

Iris

The iris should be reactive and regular in shape. Assess the iris for iridodialysis (a tear of the iris) or iridodonesis (a floppy or tremulous iris).

Lens

The lens should be transparent. Assess the lens for possible anterior displacement into the anterior chamber, partial dislocation with displacement into the posterior chamber, and dislocation into the vitreous.

Vitreous

The vitreous should be transparent, allowing for easy visualization of the fundus. Visualization may be difficult if vitreous hemorrhage has occurred. In this situation, a black rather than red reflex is seen on ophthalmoscopy. Vitreous bleeding usually indicates a significant underlying ocular injury. The vitreous also should be assessed for an intraocular foreign body.

Retina

The retina is examined for hemorrhage, possible tears, or detachment. A detached retina is opalescent, and the blood columns are darker.

Specific Injuries

Common traumatic ocular injuries include eyelid injury, corneal injury, anterior chamber injury, injury to the iris, injury to the lens, vitreous injuries, injury to the retina, globe injury, chemical injury, fractures, retrobulbar hematoma, and fat emboli.

EYELID INJURY

Eyelid injuries often result in marked ecchymosis, making examination of injuries to the globe and lid difficult. However, a more serious injury to the underlying structures must be excluded. Look beneath the lid as well to exclude damage to the globe. Lid retractors or cotton-tipped applicators can be used if necessary to forcibly open the eye to inspect the globe. Ptosis may result from edema, damage to the levator palpebrae, or oculomotor nerve injury.

Lacerations of the upper and lower lids that are horizontal, superficial, and do not involve the levator in the upper lid may be closed by the examining doctor using interrupted 6-0 (silk, nylon) skin sutures. The doctor also should examine the eye beneath the lid to rule out damage to the globe.

Lid injuries that require treatment by an ophthalmologist include: (1) wounds involving the medial canthus that may have damaged the medial canaliculus; (2) injuries to the lacrimal sac and nasal lacrimal duct, which can lead to obstruction if not properly repaired; (3) deep horizontal lacerations of the upper lid that may involve the levator and result in ptosis if not repaired correctly; and (4) lacerations of the lid margin that are difficult to close and can lead to notching, entropion, or ectropion. These wounds may be covered with a saline dressing pending emergency ophthalmologic consultation.

Foreign bodies of the lid result in profuse tearing, pain, and a foreign-body sensation that increases with lid movement. The conjunctiva should be inspected, and the upper and lower lids should be everted to examine the inner surface. Topical anesthetic drops may be used, but only for initial examination and removal of the foreign body.

Penetrating foreign bodies should not be disturbed and are removed only in the operating room by an ophthalmologist or appropriate specialist. If the patient requires transport to another facility for treatment of this injury or others, consult an ophthalmologist regarding management of the eye during transport.

CORNEAL INJURY

Corneal abrasions result in pain, foreign-body sensation, photophobia, decreased visual acuity, and chemosis. The injured epithelium stains with fluorescein.

Corneal foreign bodies sometimes can be removed with irrigation. However, if the foreign body is embedded, the patient should be referred to an ophthalmologist. Corneal abrasions are treated with antibiotic drops or ointment to prevent ulcers. Clinical studies have demonstrated no advantage to patching in terms of patient comfort or time required for the abrasion to heal. The patient should be instructed to instill the drops or ointment and should be followed up within 24 to 48 hours.

ANTERIOR CHAMBER INJURY

Hyphema is blood in the anterior chamber, which may be difficult to see if there is only a small amount. In extreme cases, the entire anterior chamber is filled. The hyphema can often be seen with a penlight. Hyphema usually indicates severe intraocular trauma.

Glaucoma develops in 7% of patients with hyphema. Corneal staining also may occur. Remember, hyphema can be the result of serious underlying ocular injury. Even in the case of a small bleed, spontaneous rebleeding often occurs within the first 5 days, which may lead to total hyphema. Therefore, the patient must be referred to an ophthalmologist. The affected eye will be patched, and the patient usually is hospitalized, placed on bed rest, and reevaluated frequently. Pain after hyphema usually indicates rebleeding and/or acute glaucoma.

INJURY TO THE IRIS

Contusion injuries of the iris can cause traumatic mydriasis or miosis. There may be disruption of the iris from the ciliary body, causing an irregular pupil and hyphema.

INJURY TO THE LENS

Contusion of the lens can lead to later opacification or cataract formation. Blunt trauma can cause a break of the zonular fibers that encircle the lens and anchor it to the ciliary body. This results in subluxation of the lens, possibly into the anterior chamber, causing shallowing of the chamber. In cases of posterior subluxation, the anterior chamber deepens. Patients with these injuries should be referred to an ophthalmologist.

VITREOUS INJURY

Blunt trauma may also lead to vitreous hemorrhage. This usually is secondary to retinal vessel damage and bleeding into the vitreous, resulting in sudden, profound loss of vision. Funduscopic examination may be impossible, and the red reflex, seen with an ophthalmoscope light, is lost. A patient with this injury should be placed on bed rest with the eye shielded and referred to an ophthalmologist.

INJURY TO THE RETINA

Blunt trauma also can cause retinal hemorrhage. The patient may or may not have decreased visual acuity, depending on involvement of the macula. Superficial retinal hemorrhages appear cherry red in color, whereas deeper lesions appear gray.

Retinal edema and detachment can occur with head trauma. In such cases, a white, cloudy discoloration is observed. Retinal detachments appear "curtain-like." If the macula is involved, visual acuity is affected. An acute retinal tear usually occurs in conjunction with blunt trauma to an eye with preexisting vitreoretinal pathology. Retinal detachment most often occurs as a late sequela of blunt trauma, with the patient describing light flashes and a curtain-like defect in peripheral vision.

A rupture of the choroid initially appears as a beige area at the posterior pole. Later it becomes a yellow-white scar. If it transects the macula, vision is seriously and permanently impaired.

GLOBE INJURY

A patient with a ruptured globe has marked visual impairment. The eye is soft because of decreased intraocular pressure, and the anterior chamber may be flattened or shallow. If the rupture is anterior, ocular contents may be seen extruding from the eye.

The goal of initial management of the ruptured globe is to protect the eye from any additional damage. As soon as a ruptured globe is suspected, the eye should not be manipulated any further. A sterile dressing and eye shield should be applied carefully to prevent any pressure to the eye that may cause further extrusion of the ocular contents. The patient should be instructed not to squeeze the injured eye shut. If not contraindicated by other injuries, the patient may be sedated while awaiting transport or treatment. Do not remove foreign objects, tissue, or clots before placing the dressing. Do not use topical analgesics—only oral or parenteral, if not contraindicated by any other injuries.

An *intraocular foreign body* should be suspected if the patient reports sudden, sharp pain with a decrease in visual acuity, particularly if the eye might have been struck by a small fragment of metal, glass, or wood. Inspect the surface of the globe carefully for any small lacerations and possible sites of entry. These may be difficult to find. In the anterior chamber, tiny foreign bodies may be hidden by blood or in the crypt of the iris. A tiny iris perforation may be impossible to see directly, but with a pen light the red reflex may be detected through the defect (if the lens and vitreous are not opaque).

CHEMICAL INJURY

Chemical injuries require immediate intervention in order to preserve sight. Acid precipitates proteins in the tissue and sets up somewhat of a natural barrier against extensive tissue penetration. However, alkali combines with lipids in the cell membrane, leading to disruption of the cell membranes, rapid penetration of the caustic agent, and extensive tissue destruction. Chemical injury to the cornea causes disruption of stromal mucopolysaccharides, leading to opacification.

The treatment for chemical injuries to the eyes involves copious and continuous irrigation. Attempts should not be made to neutralize the agent. Intravenous solutions (eg, crystalloid solution) and tubing can be used to improvise continuous irrigation. Blepharospasm is extensive, and the lids must be manually opened during irrigation. Analgesics and sedation should be used, if not contraindicated by coexisting injuries. Thermal injuries usually occur to the lids only and rarely involve the cornea. However, burns of the globe occasionally occur. A sterile dressing should be applied and the patient referred to an ophthalmologist. Exposure of the cornea must be prevented or it may perforate, and the eye may be lost.

FRACTURES

Blunt trauma to the orbit may cause rapid compression of the tissues and increased pressure within the orbit. One of the weakest points is the orbital floor, which may fracture, allowing orbital contents to herniate into the antrum—leading to the use of the term "blowout."

Clinically, the patient presents with pain, swelling, and ecchymosis of the lids and periorbital tissues. There may be subconjunctival hemorrhage. Facial asymmetry and possible enophthalmos can be evident or masked by surrounding edema. Limitation of ocular motion and diplopia secondary to edema or entrapment of the orbital contents may be noted. Palpation of the rims may reveal a fracture step-off deformity.

Subcutaneous and/or subconjunctival emphysema may occur when the fracture is into the ethmoid or maxillary sinuses. Hypesthesia of the cheek occurs secondary to injury of the infraorbital nerve. The Waters view and Caldwell view (straight on) are useful for evaluating orbital fractures. Examine the orbital floor and look for soft-tissue density in the maxillary sinus or an air fluid level (blood). Computed tomographic scans also are helpful, and may be considered mandatory.

Treatment of fractures may be delayed up to 2 weeks. Watchful waiting may help to avoid unnecessary surgery by allowing the edema to decrease. Indications for orbital blowout repair include persistent diplopia in a functional field of gaze, enophthalmos greater than 2 mm, and fracture involving more than 50% of the orbital floor.

RETROBULBAR HEMATOMA

A retrobulbar hematoma requires immediate treatment by an ophthalmologist. The resulting increased pressure within the orbit compromises the blood supply to the retina and optic nerve, resulting in blindness if not treated. If possible, the head should be elevated, with no direct pressure placed on the eye.

FAT EMBOLI

Patients with long-bone fractures are at risk for fat emboli. Remember, this is a possible cause of a sudden change in vision for a patient who has sustained multiple injuries.

APPENDIX F SUMMARY

Thorough, systematic evaluation of the injured eye results in few significant injuries being missed. Once the injuries have been identified, treat the eye injury using simple, systematic measures; prevent further damage; and help preserve sight until the patient is in the ophthalmologist's care.

Bibliography

1. Arbour JD, Brunette I, Boisjoly HM, et al. Should we patch corneal erosions? *Arch Ophthalmol* 1997;115:313-317.

2. Campanile TM, St Clair DA, Benaim M. The evaluation of eye patching in the treatment of traumatic corneal epithelial defects. *J Emerg Med* 1997;15:769-774.

3. Flynn CA, D'Amico F, Smith G. Should we patch corneal abrasions? A meta-analysis. *J Fam Pract* 1998;47:264-270.

4. Hart A, White S, Conboy P, et al. The management of corneal abrasions in accident and emergency. *Injury* 1997;28:527-529.

5. Patterson J, Fetzer D, Krall J, et al. Eye patch treatment for the pain of corneal abrasion. *South Med J* 1996;89:227-229.

6. Poon A, McCluskey PJ, Hill DA. Eye injuries in patients with major trauma. *J Trauma* 1999;46:494-499.

7. Sastry SM, Paul BK, Bain L, Champion HR: Ocular trauma among major trauma victims in a regional trauma center. *J Trauma* 1993;34:223-226.

8. Tasman WS. Posterior vitreous detachment and peripheral retinal breaks. *Trans Am Acad Ophthalmol Otolaryngol* 1968;72:217.

Austere Environments: Military Casualty Care and Trauma Care in Underdeveloped Areas and Following Catastrophes (Optional Lecture)

Introduction

Even the largest hospital or medical center can become an austere environment after a natural or human-made disaster. During a war or after a terrorist attack with explosives, and chemical, biologic, or nuclear weapons, the environment may be both austere and hostile. In a hostile environment, the safety of the patients, medical care providers, and even the medical facility is threatened, and provisions must be made to protect them. How do doctors support the ABCDEs of patient care in such situations? The goal of this chapter is to explain how to apply the principles of Advanced Trauma Life Support (ATLS) when standard equipment and supplies are not available or advisable in an austere or hostile environment.

Background

Many countries of the world are able to commit significant resources to health care, including the care of injured patients. The ATLS course is written with such well-equipped and well-staffed hospital facilities in mind. However, not all the equipment and supplies for diagnostic testing and treatment mentioned within the course are available to all doctors. Some countries and regions have few resources to devote to health care. The doctors who practice in these countries include local nationals, missionaries, military personnel, and members of charitable and relief organizations, such as the International Red Cross and Red Crescent Societies. Remote and wilderness areas in any country are austere medical environments.

Hostile environments are defined by ongoing risks to the patients and rescuers. These risks may be from things such as climate, collapsing buildings, explosions, and toxins, but are most commonly associated with enemy action in some advanced police situations and the military. Those who know that they will practice in such environments or who wish to be prepared for such events should seek additional training in the care of massive wounds from explosive weapons. Although the number of survivors with such wounds is small, they offer challenges in hemorrhage control and management that are not seen in most civilian

Upon completion of this topic, the doctor will be able to:

OBJECTIVES

1. Define austere and hostile environments.

2. In a given situation, describe patient treatment priorities in the context of environment and relative risk.

3. In a given situation, identify available resources and treatment options.

4. In a given situation, adapt available resources to meet the ABCDE goals of Advanced Trauma Life Support.

practices. ▪ Further description of such wounds is included in Appendix B: Biomechanics of Injury.

Some areas are thrust into austerity or become hostile environments because of the destruction of their infrastructures by disasters, either natural or human-made (eg, terrorist actions or war). These situations are particularly challenging because of their unpredictability. Citizens of large countries with strong militaries should not fail to prepare, believing themselves to be immune.

Doctors in disaster situations will be more prepared to care for injured patients when they recognize that ATLS is not comprised of the equipment and supplies that can be used for patient care. Rather, ATLS is an organized approach to the care of injured patients with the goal of treating the most life-threatening conditions first to decrease morbidity and mortality. This appendix is not an exhaustive manual for care in these environments. It describes some substitutions or adaptations to meet the goals of ATLS in this context.

Austere and Hostile Environments: Context

The ATLS course focuses on treatment priorities for trauma patients in a robust hospital environment. Austere and hostile environments are different for several reasons, including personnel and their safety, communication and transportation, and equipment and supplies.

PERSONNEL AND THEIR SAFETY

Personnel limitations are a key factor in austere and hostile environments. Available care providers may not have been trained to deal with injured patients, and specialty and surgical care may not be available. In addition, there may be blurring of specialty boundaries; a surgeon or nonsurgeon may be called upon to perform procedures that are typically performed by other specialists. There may be too few or no doctors or other health care providers. The abilities of the most highly trained specialist can be neutralized by the lack of equipment in a hostile environment, such as an environment under enemy fire. Such providers must evaluate what should be done, balancing what they are capable of doing with what can be done with the available resources.

COMMUNICATION AND TRANSPORTATION

Disrupted or nonexistent communication can prevent specialty consultation, provision of supplies, and arrangement for removal of casualties. Disrupted communication is the most commonly cited "lesson learned" in disasters. Plans must be in place for alternative means of communication prior to an event. Transportation to bring in resources and personnel or to transport patients to definitive care may be infrequent or nonexistent.

EQUIPMENT AND SUPPLIES

An austere environment is defined by limited equipment and supply resources. A typical community hospital emergency department is very well supplied when compared with most out-of-hospital settings. Doctors need to understand that even equipment that is outdated, suboptimal, or intended for other uses can be used to save lives. Triage decisions that change the treatment of ABC priorities may be necessary to balance the needs of the patients with the available resources. For example, a paucity of supplies relative to the number of casualties may make it inadvisable to start an intravenous line on many injured patients. Limiting fluid use to patients who are sufficiently hypovolemic to sustain cellular damage helps to extend fluid resources.

Definitive care is not usually possible in austere and hostile environments. Diagnostic challenges include management of possible fractures without radiology support and blood pressure determination in the absence of blood pressure cuffs. Operative considerations in these environments include deciding which operating room procedures can be performed outside the operating room under less than ideal circumstances versus which operative procedures should *never* be performed outside the operating room.

Pharmacologic support may be minimal or nonexistent, so clinicians must know how to make optimal use of a limited number of medications. Some treatments should not be started unless they can be completed appropriately or treatment regimens may need to be delayed or temporized until resources and definitive care are available. For example, frostbite should not be rewarmed if the individual cannot subsequently be kept warm, because the risk of re-freezing can cause more injury than simply leaving the part frozen for a longer period.

MILITARY COMBAT CASUALTY CARE

To some, the term *military combat casualty care* implies a single homogeneous entity. In fact, military combat casualty care is conducted over a continuum of that can progress from austere and hostile to robust and protected. Large military field hospitals may offer more resources than are available to the surrounding populace. Some have enough resources to use the tools described in the ATLS course, such as specialty care, CT scanners and interventional radiology. However, the various sized hospitals at sequential echelons of care may all become austere environments, depending on the number of casualties received within a certain period or on enemy action.

Military combat casualty care occurs in phases that are best described in Tactical Combat Casualty Care (TCCC or TC[3]), a program that was developed by the U.S. military and has been adopted by a number of other countries. The earlier phases of TCCC are the most austere and hostile and overlap greatly with prehospital care; in fact, the earliest levels of care are provided primarily by medics or fellow soldiers. This recognition has lead to the inclusion of the TCCC concepts in a military version of the Prehospital Trauma Life Support Course (PHTLS), which is a useful reference for doctors who are likely to practice in this environment. Review of TCCC and PHTLS is key for the doctors at the higher echelons who will receive the patients so they understand what the medics have done and why.

Care Under Fire

Care Under Fire, the first phase of TCCC, is the most austere and hostile. At this level, the main obligation of the provider is to prevent further injury by removing the casualty from the area of danger or by suppressing enemy fire. This concept also applies to some advanced special weapons police units in larger cities. Only a small percent of these casualties have airway or breathing injuries as their primary life-threatening injury; rather, the casualty frequently demonstrates a patent airway by requesting aid. In addition, the medic does not have the safety, time, or equipment for advanced airway management.

The most common life-threatening injury is external hemorrhage, usually from the extremities. In this context (risk of a specific injury and the de facto clearing of airway and breathing by use of the voice), the concept of "CAB" (circulation or hemorrhage control, followed by airway and breathing) has been proposed. This mantra, the inversion of the "ABC" of ATLS is proposed to be different from ATLS. In fact, CAB does not deny the importance of airway and breathing, but addresses the most likely danger and the only one that can be addressed rapidly in the situation. This suggests that ABC is not a linear mandate, but is instead important life-saving priorities in a circle; in many research-rich environments, they are addressed simultaneously. The context will decide which of the three may take treatment priority in a resource-constrained environment when only one can be addressed at a time. In Care Under Fire, hemorrhage control assumes the highest priority. Tourniquets are useful to save lives during this phase, as the medic cannot maintain pressure while under fire. Advanced hemostatic dressings may also be used, but they require some period of pressure to achieve benefit.

Tactical Field Care

After the casualty is removed from under fire to a relatively safe place, a more thorough evaluation of ABC is accomplished and treated if need be with the tools and skills available. This phase is termed Tactical Field Care.

Care During Evacuation

The evacuation phase may involve very austere vehicles and helicopters, implying basic care, and is often called "CASEVAC" for Casualty Evacuation care. Evacuation from larger hospitals may also involve worldwide air transport with ICU level care. This may also be referred to as Air Evac.

Medical Units

Along the way, depending on the countries involved and the situation, the casualty may be treated in medical units with various levels of capability—from aid stations with doctors and no surgeons to small surgical teams with limited postoperative care performing hemorrhage control with "damage control" procedures to very robust field hospitals. Care in each setting is applied according to the context.

Most tactical care must be accomplished with the resources that soldiers can carry with them. There is a premium for lightweight items that can perform more than one use, as well as items that are likely enough to be used as to justify the weight. Since resuscitation fluids are heavy, decisions on fluid types, volumes, and use are strongly impacted by their weight.

Some special military units function covertly in hostile areas, complicating trauma care, with prolonged times to definitive care and the need to avoid detection. Such units bring into sharp relief the understanding that a successful mission is likely to save more lives than any medical care, thus the care provided may also need to balance the context of the tactical situation with the medical needs.

OTHER CHALLENGING ENVIRONMENTS

Remote areas have problems that are unique, such as identification of the occurrence of injury, which is a significant problem in remote areas. For this reason, highway call boxes are in place in many developed countries, and some vehicles have been fitted with emergency locator transmitters similar to those in airplanes. In addition, the burden of rural and remote areas includes the problems generated by time and distance.

Wilderness activities such as hiking/biking, spelunking, and water sports create a special challenge for the medical care provider, as the bulk and weight of medical supplies becomes a tremendous issue. When supplies must be carried by backpack, medications and provisions must be thoughtfully selected. These also are the activities that can result in the most challenging evacuation because of the difficulty of contacting help.

Natural disasters (eg, hurricanes, tornados, and floods) and human-made disasters (eg, terrorism, war/armed conflicts, and industrial accidents/chemical spills) can rapidly turn a nonaustere environment into an austere one. Even doctors working in tertiary-care centers should have training and knowledge of trauma care under these circumstances. The hospital and the community should develop and practice plans for such situations.

Preparation and Planning

Successful trauma care in austere and hostile environments comes from careful preparation and planning.

TRAVEL TO AN AUSTERE OR HOSTILE ENVIRONMENT

Doctors traveling to austere or hostile environments must first prepare for self-protection and survival; otherwise, they can become a burden rather than a help in the situation. Good physical health and fitness are prerequisites. Appropriate shelter, clothing, food, and water must be planned for, and in many cases, brought with the individual. It cannot be assumed that such supplies are available. Before traveling, careful communication with the local authorities and an advance party must be accomplished.

Communication between members of the party, with local and international authorities, and with the home base must be planned. Planning for the care of loved ones and the medical practice left behind includes wills, powers of attorney, and access to funds to pay bills.

Administrative preparations include passports, visas, local currency, and transportation. It is important to have an invitation by local authorities to enter either the country or austere/hostile environment—unwanted and unprepared volunteers only place a burden on the local system.

Personal health protection includes vaccinations, appropriate personal prescriptions, and over-the-counter medications.

Further preparation for military physicians varies by country.

PREPARATION OF A HOSPITAL FOR BECOMING AN AUSTERE OR HOSTILE ENVIRONMENT

Preparation of a hospital for disaster requires a city- or region-wide plan that includes communications with fire and rescue personnel, police, and civil and military authorities. Such a plan includes how and when to involve each of these authorities and clearly delineates a chain of command, including who is in charge. These plans determine how patients are sorted and routed to the appropriate hospital to avoid overwhelming any one institution.

An assessment of the threats is important. Health care providers in the tropics may need to consider typhoons and volcanoes, whereas those in other regions may need to prepare for earthquakes. Terrorist threats are not predictable. Hospitals need to have a plan to recall key personnel and a personnel rotation plan to allow those personnel to rest if the situation is prolonged.

Spare equipment and supplies need to be stored in protected areas in the event regular equipment and supplies are destroyed or contaminated. Plans must include options for loss of electric power, water, steam sterilization ventilators, intensive care unit(s), etc.

Terrorist activities, industrial accidents, and war can contaminate the patients and facilities with toxic chemical or biologic agents. Although a detailed discussion of these agents and specific protections and treatments is outside the scope of this chapter, the doctor must become familiar with the symptoms, signs, and treatment of these conditions.

Plans must include decontamination of patients prior to their being brought into the health care facility so that the health care workers do not become secondary casualties who are unable to help. Protective clothing and respiratory protection must be available. Detection equipment for various threat agents must be available, and caregivers must be familiar with the use of these items. Finally, the plan must be exercised as a "full-dress" rehearsal on a regular basis.

Management of Airway and Breathing

The procedures needed to treat problems in "A" and "B" may vary substantially in an austere environment. The problems facing treatment in this type of environment center prima-

rily on the environment itself, the limited equipment that is usually available, and the evacuation constraints. If the patient is threatened with further injury because of environmental concerns (eg, rough terrain), preventing further injury to the patient and to the health care provider takes priority. Once the site is secure or the patient is moved to a safe location, then the doctor can attempt to aid the victim. ◼ See Chapter 2: Airway and Ventilatory Management.

AIRWAY

Discerning the patient's true airway status may be difficult in an austere or hostile environment. The "look, listen, and feel" approach remains important. However, under conditions of low light, high noise levels, etc., the recognition of airway problems may be challenging. It requires close attention, patience, and ingenuity to fully evaluate the patient. Feeling chest or abdominal movements may become the primary means of assessing airway patency and breathing efforts.

Airway Maintenance Techniques

Management of a compromised airway is usually performed in a standard fashion in the austere environment. However, because of limited equipment or personnel, other issues or mechanisms may become important. Foremost is the decision to initiate treatment. If a patient with a compromised airway can be treated rapidly and maintaining that airway does not risk the safety of others in the group, then the standard techniques remain unchanged.

Associated with initial airway management is protection of the cervical spine. Cervical collars and other devices normally used to protect the cervical spine during transport and evaluation are sometimes not available, so ingenuity is essential to protecting the neck. Common examples of equipment used in stabilizing the neck include blankets, pillows, shoes, sandbags, malleable splints, and padded hip belts. Cervical spine injuries are uncommon in penetrating trauma, particularly in the military, so complex methods to protect the C-spine in this situation are rarely necessary. During care under fire, such efforts are unlikely to be needed, and put the rescuer and victim at increased risk. If there is evidence of a fall, blunt injury, or motor vehicle crash associated with the penetrating injury, then C-spine protection should be considered. Even with these other mechanisms, efforts at cervical spine protection should not delay removing the victim from the line of fire.

Chin Lift/Jaw Thrust   Performance of chin-lift/jaw-thrust maneuvers remains unchanged in the austere environment. Placing the patient on his or her side in the "rescue position" may also be helpful. A temporary means of lifting the tongue off the posterior pharynx can be performed by attaching the anterior tongue to the lower lip or chin with safety pins or sutures. Alternatively, the pins can be held forward with string attached to the patient's clothing. Placing the pins transversely through the tongue will keep them from pulling through.

Oropharyngeal and Nasopharyngeal Airways
The use of oropharyngeal and nasopharyngeal airways remains important. If placement of one of these airways relieves the airway obstruction, then it must be well secured prior to evacuation. If ventilation must be assisted with a face mask, then the patient ties up additional valuable personnel resources prior to and during evacuation. When the proper equipment is not available, a nasal airway can be made with a urinary catheter, radiator hose, or other small tube.

Laryngeal Mask Airway
The laryngeal mask airway (LMA) is designed to be placed blindly into the posterior pharynx, with its final position resting over the epiglottis. It should be viewed as an interim airway between the oropharyngeal and nasopharyngeal airways and the endotracheal tube (ET). In addition, the modified LMA can be used as a conduit through which an ET can be placed.

The LMA is viewed as an alternative to the face mask to establish and maintain control of the patient's airway, but it is not a substitute for an ET. It establishes an airway in unconscious patients without a gag reflex, but because it does not completely occlude the tracheal inlet, it cannot reliably prevent aspiration. It can be inserted from virtually any position using one hand. As it is inserted blindly, the patient's head and neck are maintained in a neutral position.

Multilumen Esophageal Airway Devices
Multilumen esophageal airway devices contain two cuffs and two airway ports. They differ from the esophageal obturator airway in that lung insufflation does not require the use of a face mask, with all of its inherent problems and difficulties. Use of these tubes requires minimal skill and equipment; as with the LMA, they can be inserted rapidly and blindly with minimal cervical spine manipulation. Ventilation does not require the face mask to be sealed. Their design allows adequate ventilation regardless of whether the distal tube and cuff are in the esophagus or the trachea.

Definitive Airway

The definition of a definitive airway remains unchanged in the austere environment—a cuffed tube in the trachea. Endotracheal intubation with an ET and laryngoscope remain the standard against which all other airways' effectiveness is compared. However, under austere conditions, the environment or lack of required equipment may prevent the performance of standard endotracheal intubation.

Tactile/Digital Orotracheal Intubation
Tactile/digital orotracheal intubation is potentially useful in a difficult environment; it requires minimal equipment, is not hindered by the presence of blood or secretions, is performed blindly, and does not require manipulation of the cervical spine. Once learned, it can be performed rapidly to obtain a secure, definitive airway. However, it does not provide visualization of the laryngeal cords and exposes the doctor to bodily fluids. In addition, precautions must be taken to protect the operator's hand from the patient's teeth. To perform this procedure, the patient must be unconscious. Facing the patient from the front, hook the first and second fingers of one hand over the tongue and into the vallecula or grasp the epiglottis with the fingertips. The ET is guided along the groove between the fingers into the trachea.

Surgical Airway

The inability to obtain an airway using any of the previously mentioned techniques is the main indication for a surgical airway. Lack of training in performing the procedure and unavailability of necessary equipment may preclude this technique from being performed rapidly and safely.

Needle Cricothyroidotomy
Entering the cricothyroid membrane with a large-caliber intravenous catheter and insufflating the lung with pressurized oxygen is quick and easy. However, it requires an oxygen source. If the equipment is available, this technique can provide up to 45 minutes of oxygenation until a more stable airway can be established. See Chapter 2: Airway and Ventilatory Management, and Skill III-A: Needle Cricothyroidotomy.

Surgical Cricothyroidotomy
Surgical cricothyroidotomy and its advantages and disadvantages are outlined in Chapter 2: Airway and Ventilatory Management, and Skill III-B: Surgical Cricothyroidotomy. In the absence of an ET tube, an airway can be made from a syringe barrel, a flashlight or pen casing, or another small-diameter tube.

Percutaneous Puncture/Dilation Techniques
Percutaneous puncture/dilation uses one of several products on the market to penetrate the cricothyroid membrane. The opening in the cricothyroid membrane is dilated in a manner similar to that of the Seldinger technique to allow placement of the ET tube. Performance of the technique is similar to that of needle cricothyroidotomy for jet insufflation, yet permits a standard cuffed tube to be placed in the trachea. It does require special equipment and more time to perform, and has all of the inherent complications of other surgical airways.

VENTILATION AND OXYGENATION

After an airway is established, sufficient oxygenation and ventilation must be supported. The challenges in the austere environment focus on the equipment needed to support the failing respiratory system and the number of personnel required to assist the patient. Because supplemental oxygen usually is not available, the ability to support a patient with oxygen remains very difficult in an austere environment.

When oxygen is available in only limited amounts, it should be reserved for patients with evidence of hypoxia on physical examination (cyanosis), by pulse oximetry readings, or by blood gas analysis. The patients most likely to require the additional oxygen in the short term are those with chest injuries associated with lung contusion.

Initiating ventilation in the austere environment commits personnel and resources to the patient. Maintaining the airway in these environments and during transport requires close vigilance because of the risk of the airway device becoming dislodged. Monitoring includes ensuring a secure, patent airway and adequate ventilation. Ideally, monitoring also includes pulse oximetry and end-tidal CO_2 monitoring, if available.

CHEST INJURIES

Chest injury in an austere environment should be handled as discussed in ◾ Chapter 4: Thoracic Trauma. However, not all materials necessary to manage a chest wound may be available. Open chest wounds must be covered, but in the absence of a chest tube, an occlusive dressing using plastic bags, IV fluid bags, or something similar can be used. Such ancillary devices are taped on three sides to prevent a tension pneumothorax; however, three-sided taping may not be effective in dirty, sweaty casualties. In this case, complete occlusion with petroleum jelly gauze is used. The patient is then monitored for or prophylactically treated for a tension pneumothorax.

Needle decompression of a tension pneumothorax is performed as described previously. ◾ See Chapter 4: Thoracic Trauma, and Skill VII-A: Needle Thoracentesis. However, a tube other than a large-caliber IV catheter may have to be improvised. The decompression ideally is performed with an over-the-needle catheter with the catheter left in place to prevent recurrence. A Heimlich valve can be attached to the catheter. If a Heimlich valve is not available, one can be improvised with a finger from a rubber glove attached to the tube with a hole at the fingertip. This simulates the flutter valve of a Heimlich valve. Of course a simple small stab wound, such as would precede the placement of a chest tube, will decompress a tension pneumothorax and should be considered when other options are unavailable.

If air evacuation is planned, the effects of altitude, temperature, and other factors associated with flight must be considered. For airway management, endotracheal cuff pressures increase. If a manometer is not available for the flight, then the cuffs are filled with a nonexpanding liquid (water or saline) rather than air. Similarly, a pneumothorax also expands at high altitudes, with the potential for unexpected respiratory compromise. Ideally, supplemental oxygen should be made available because of the decreased partial pressure of oxygen at high altitudes. Finally, because gastric distention can easily occur, gastric tube placement should be considered.

Management of Circulation

The tools and supplies used to treat injured patients become less plentiful as the environment becomes more austere. Nowhere is this more obvious than in management of hypovolemic shock. Fluids (crystalloid, colloid, and blood) that are the mainstay of restoring circulating volume are very bulky and heavy. They are usually found in only minimal amounts in most field kits, and are quickly used up in disasters.

Although the presence of shock in an injured patient demands the immediate involvement of a surgeon, one may not be available, or the surgeon's skills may be negated without appropriate surgical equipment, anesthesia, and support personnel. The goal under such circumstances is to maintain life until a higher level of care can be delivered.

Successful treatment of hypovolemic shock under these conditions requires a thorough understanding of the compensatory mechanisms of the body. ◾ See Chapter 3: Shock. Although the goals of resuscitation are unchanged, the emphasis may shift in the austere environment. Less than ideal organ perfusion may have to be accepted. "Life-over-limb" and triage decisions assume a central role in saving as many lives as possible.

HEMOSTASIS

Control of bleeding is of utmost importance when there is minimal or no fluid with which to replace the lost blood. Direct pressure remains important and may be augmented with the compression of the artery above the bleeding site at a pressure point—points where arteries pass superficially and are felt as pulses. These pressure points are the radial, brachial, and axillary arteries in the arm, and the femoral, popliteal, and ankle arteries in the leg. Compression of the artery for 20 minutes can stop or decrease the bleeding sufficiently to allow a dressing to be placed.

Elevation of the bleeding area above the level of the heart reduces the pressure to the bleeding area and aids hemostasis for arterial bleeding. Elevation and a dressing may be all that are necessary for venous bleeding. The patient or another individual may be enlisted to hold pressure, while the doctor treats someone else.

In the worst cases, tourniquets are used. Although there is a real risk of limb loss with a tourniquet, blood loss must be stopped to save the life of the patient. Commercially available simple small windlass tourniquets that can be applied with one hand are used by many military services. Those venturing into austere environments of combat should ensure their availability. Any flexible material of enough length (rope, wire, cloth strips) can be used to encircle the limb and be tied in place. A rigid device (eg, a rod or stick) is placed through the loop and twisted to tighten it until bleeding ceases. Arterial flow to, as well as venous flow from, the extremity must be stopped to prevent paradoxically increased bleeding from venous injuries. The time of tourniquet application should be recorded, and this written record should accompany the patient. When the time to care is short, there is little risk to the limb, and a life can be saved. The risk to the limb increases with the duration of use of the tourniquet. Life over limb is a time-honored choice that should not be made lightly. Especially in combat, the receiving doctor should remember that the decision was made under fire.

A technique that stops vigorous scalp bleeding from a large flap is to fold the flap outward onto itself. This crimps the vessels and stops the bleeding. After 20 minutes the bleeding should be stopped or slowed enough to return the flap to its normal position and apply direct pressure and dressings. Prior to surgical management, endogenous hemostatic mechanisms must be relied on to control unseen bleeding.

With the possibility of ongoing or barely clotted bleeding sites, rapid restoration of normal blood pressure with a vigorous fluid bolus should be avoided. Smaller amounts of fluid given more slowly and stopped when the blood pressure rises to an acceptable, yet less than normal, level may allow the clot to be maintained and still provide adequate organ perfusion.

Advanced topical hemostatic dressings are increasingly available. All function as "pressure adjuncts" and require some period of pressure over them with a bandage after application to affect hemorrhage control. Some have the side effect of exothermia, which can damage normal tissue. A stepwise algorithm has been proposed in military care in several countries. It emphasizes the use of normal pressure techniques or tourniquets to control hemorrhage first. If these fail or an analysis of a large wound suggests that they will not be effective because of the wound's location, then the hemostatic agents that have no side effects should be used first. If ineffective, they can be followed by those with potential side effects if needed. This balances the potential risk of the exothermic reaction with the benefit of hemostasis.

RESUSCITATION

Fluid resuscitation in the austere environment may be challenging. Both difficulties in establishing access and having sufficient fluids are likely obstacles.

Venous Access

Central venous access kits, intravenous needles, and intraosseous needles may be unavailable in an austere or hostile environment, so performing venous cutdown assumes a more important role in these situations. Fluid administration tubing, with the connectors cut off, nasogastric tubes, and urinary catheters may be used for venous access with a cutdown. ◾ See Chapter 3: Shock, and Skill V-A: Venous Cutdown.

Alternative Fluid Routes

Although oral fluids are avoided in the usual clinical arena because of the possibility of aspiration, fluids may be administered orally to the awake patient, or via a gastric tube in the unconscious patient. Absorption may be decreased after injury, but it does occur. Similarly, rectal clysis allows excellent fluid absorption, as demonstrated during World War I. Only about 250 mL/hr can be absorbed safely by either of these routes, so they are most useful as substitutes for massive resuscitation in dehydrated patients and those who have had mild to moderate hemorrhage that is now controlled.

Patients who do not have partial stabilization on their own or who do not respond to some fluid using these alternative methods are unlikely to respond to large amounts of fluid. This might be used as a triage consideration, placing such patients in the expectant category

Fluid Choices

The fluids used are those that are available. Usually this is crystalloid or colloid fluid. In military situations, fluid choices are usually based on weight considerations; colloids and hypertonic fluids weigh less for equivalent intravascular volume than do crystalloids. The initial effect of increased blood pressure may dissipate over time as the body water equilibrates with the osmotic load. Blood transfusion from noninjured members of the group can be considered. Typing can be done by the patient's report of his or her own blood type. Quick "crossing" of drops of blood from the patient and the donor on a smooth white surface, which was the method used in the earliest days of blood transfusion, may reveal major incompatibilities by clumping. Of course, this is an unusual choice for difficult circumstances, and it carries some risk. Such fresh whole blood does bear the additional benefit of clotting factors useful in severe hemorrhage.

Careful consideration of the goals of fluid therapy is necessary in planning the use of a limited quantity of fluids. Patients who appear to be compensating for their fluid losses and maintaining organ perfusion may require no fluids. This can be judged by level of consciousness. The conscious cooperative patient can be observed. Units of fluid (bags, bottles, etc.) can be split among several patients, giving each only the amount absolutely necessary to maintain life. Fluids such as commercial beverages may be used as oral rehydration fluids. When balancing rebleeding with organ perfusion, careful reevaluation is key to determining whether further small amounts of fluid should be given to maintain the low level of perfusion necessary to maintain life until definitive care is possible. A less than normal blood pressure is acceptable with this technique. If the patient is unconscious, fluid is titrated on and off according to the presence or absence of the radial pulse. Care must be taken when titrating hypertonic or colloid fluids in this manner, as they may overshoot the target blood pressure as they recruit extravascular fluid.

Pain Management

Control of pain and alleviation of suffering is a primary goal of all doctors. This is important not only as a kindness, but also to minimize the adverse physiologic consequences of pain, such as increases in levels of catecholamines and cortisol, metabolic rate, and total body oxygen consumption. Management of pain in hospitals is facilitated not only by the availability of many different analgesic agents and cardiovascular monitoring, but also by the availability of anesthesiologists who are knowledgeable and helpful regarding pain management. Austere circumstances require alternatives to hospital-based pain management protocols.

Pain management is a challenge in austere military circumstances because of limitations in the numbers and types of personnel and equipment and drugs and the potential for even a few casualties to overwhelm existing resources. The doctors in these locations should be familiar with all uses of the agents they have available. Civilian remote and wilderness situations provide similar challenges to relieving a patient's pain. A wide spectrum of therapeutic agents is not always available to the doctor in these venues. Agents must be carefully selected, not only for their ability to relieve pain but also with consideration for safety.

Principles of pain management in the austere environment include: (1) type of environment; (2) available options; (3) anatomic location and severity of injury; (4) possibility of complications; (5) allergies; (6) associated injuries; and (7) availability of, timing of, and plan for evacuation. The choice of a drug or multiple drugs depends on many factors. Many agents are available to relieve pain or act as adjuncts.

Patients in a low-flow state secondary to hypovolemic shock should not be given intramuscular injections of narcotics, as these drugs can remain in the muscle until flow is restored. With restoration of flow, a bolus of drug is released, putting the patient at risk for respiratory depression. However, in the austere environment, with an inadequate supply of IV catheters, it may be necessary to consider the intramuscular use of narcotics. Oral use is reasonable in the absence of abdominal and head injury.

Local anesthetics are considered for hematoma blocks associated with fractures and regional blocks if the doctor is knowledgeable about the sites of injection and allowable doses. Remember, local anesthetics can cause seizures if too high a dosage is used. Epinephrine can be added to slow ab-

sorption and thereby decrease the likelihood of toxicity. A caveat is to not add epinephrine if the injection is used in fingers, toes, penis, or nose because of the risk of ischemia in these areas with arteriolae. Another point to remember is that the nonsteroidal antiinflammatory medications may inhibit platelet function, so they must be avoided if there is hemorrhage or an injury with significant risk of severe hemorrhage.

Ketamine, a dissociative anesthetic, can be used safely either intramuscularly or intravenously. It has an effect similar to that of general anesthetics in that the patient is unaware of his or her surroundings. Attention must be directed to keeping the airway free of secretions. Although ketamine is useful for suture repair of lacerations and setting of fractures with angulation or arterial compromise, the individual will not be able to function without assistance for 1 to 2 hours, making it necessary to carry the patient if evacuation is imminent. Other agents allow the patient to assist in his or her own transportation, if his or her injuries allow.

Management of Specific Injuries

ABDOMINAL INJURIES

The evaluation and management of abdominal injuries in austere settings is very different from what is practiced in well-equipped modern hospitals.   See Chapter 5: Abdominal and Pelvic Trauma. Mortality from untreated intraabdominal injury is high: patients either die quickly from uncontrolled hemorrhage or they die later from intraabdominal sepsis. For this reason, a high index of suspicion must be maintained in these patients. Those with suspected injury must be referred early for surgical consultation or evacuation. Sophisticated diagnostic techniques such as ultrasound and computed tomography (CT) are not available in the austere setting. Diagnostic peritoneal lavage (DPL), while potentially available, has very different indications and implications in this setting.

The actual mechanism of injury becomes paramount in establishing priorities in settings with limited resources. Gunshot wounds to the abdomen, unless clearly tangential, are associated with visceral injury in 90% of patients. These patients all require rapid surgical referral and celiotomy. In the civilian setting, stab wounds to the abdomen are associated with visceral injury in only 30% to 40% of patients. Unless there is clear evidence of intraabdominal injury (eg, evisceration, pneumoperitoneum, peritoneal findings, shock, or blood in the nasogastric tube or rectum), these patients are treated based on symptoms and wound exploration. Stab wounds usually can be explored under local anesthesia without much difficulty to determine whether the abdominal wall fascia is penetrated. If no fascial penetrations or abdominal symptoms are present, the wound can be managed primarily.

Blunt injury to the abdomen is associated with a variety of solid and hollow organ injuries and may be less dramatic in appearance than penetrating injury. Abdominal pain, tenderness, distention, shock, or blood in the nasogastric tube or urinary catheter are all suggestive of blunt intraabdominal injury. Although CT and ultrasound are not available in the austere setting, DPL can serve as a expedient substitute in the field.

DPL is accomplished with a minimum of resources and time, and is a reliable means to determine whether a significant hemoperitoneum exists. If gross blood is not encountered and newsprint-sized writing can be read through IV tubing containing the lavage fluid, the DPL is negative for significant intraperitoneal bleeding. DPL is limited in that it provides no information about extraperitoneal organs and structures. It is contraindicated in patients with obvious intraabdominal injury and is indicated only in patients with a high probability of intraabdominal injury. Many of these patients eventually require celiotomy because of continued bleeding or peritonitis. DPL might help to identify these patients earlier and assist in triage if evacuation is possible. ◾ See Chapter 5: Abdominal and Pelvic Trauma, and Skill Station VIII: Diagnostic Peritoneal Lavage.

In situations in which evacuation is impossible or significantly delayed, DPL has no role. If a major intraabdominal injury exists, it becomes quite apparent with time. In this setting, DPL adds nothing to physical examination or treatment.

Patients with a definite abdominal injury (as demonstrated by evisceration, shock, peritoneal findings, and pneumoperitoneum) are expeditiously referred for surgical treatment. They should receive a broad-spectrum antibiotic and intravenous fluids sufficient to maintain urinary output. Open wounds should be cleaned of gross contamination and dressed. Eviscerations should be covered with moist gauze or dressings, and the patient must be kept warm. If wounds are massive, resources are minimal, and evacuation unlikely, these patients are given comfort measures only and treated expectantly.

Every patient with a significant history of injury should be considered to have an intraabdominal injury until clinical examination, diagnostic test, or celiotomy proves otherwise.

EXTREMITY INJURIES

Extremity injuries are common in trauma patients. ◾ See Chapter 8: Musculoskeletal Trauma. Although these injuries are not usually immediately life-threatening, they are often dramatic in appearance and can divert attention from other injuries. Elicitation of a brief history of the injury and a pertinent medical history should be followed by a complete examination of the extremity.

The management of extremity injuries depends to a great extent on the available resources and the length of time it takes to transfer the patient to a definitive care facility. Vas-

cular injuries, if the patient does not exsanguinate, must be definitively repaired early, within 6 hours of injury, to preserve limb function. Likewise, because of the risk of arterial injury and osteonecrosis, major dislocations should be reduced early. Finally, traumatic amputations usually require early surgical debridement.

The immediate treatment of extremity injury should include, at a minimum, control of active bleeding by applying direct pressure, cleaning grossly contaminated wounds, and immobilizing the injured extremity until the patient is evacuated. Use tourniquets sparingly, if ever, since they place the entire limb at risk. Dislocations and major angulation deformities should be carefully reduced, while monitoring the limb's neurovascular status before and after reduction.

If definitive treatment is delayed, administer antibiotics, perform limited irrigation and debridement of open wounds, and keep the extremity immobilized with some type of splint or cast. The use of antibiotics in poorly debrided or nondebrided wounds does not prevent infections; rather, the goal is to shift the spectrum of infection from gram-positive synergistic gangrene or clostridial infections that can be fatal in a few hours to more indolent infections. However, the doctor must consider the risk of encouraging resistant organisms when choosing too broad a coverage. Patients with femur fractures should be put into some sort of traction to minimize further blood loss into the thigh.

Splints and traction devices can be improvised from equipment and resources at the scene. Any rigid item, if properly padded, can be used as a splint. Likewise, a makeshift frame can be constructed to provide traction for femur fractures, sometimes using the patient's own boot or shoe as the ankle hitch. These patients also should receive analgesics and sufficient hydration to prevent shock, if available. ◾ See Chapter 8: Musculoskeletal Trauma, and Skill Station XII: Musculoskeletal Trauma: Assessment and Management.

Compartment syndrome, a late complication of extremity injury, can present insidiously in injured patients, especially after a crush injury in which no fracture is present. If compartment pressures cannot be measured, early fasciotomy may be indicated, especially in the presence of any vascular injury.

Other late complications of extremity injuries include fat embolus syndrome, deep venous thrombosis, and osteomyelitis. These complications must be considered if transfer to definitive care is markedly delayed.

The management of pelvic fractures in the austere setting deserves some comment. Since the force required to fracture the pelvic ring is so great, pelvic fractures usually occur in association with intraabdominal or other injuries. Patients with these injuries may go into shock because of bleeding from the pelvic fracture itself and from both arterial and venous vessels in the pelvis. Patients also may have significant neurologic injury, as well as genitourinary or rectal injuries.

Very little can be done for such patients in austere environments, with the exception of immobilization of the lower extremities and pelvis. The patient should be kept immobilized and the pelvis stabilized as well as possible with sheets, sandbags, etc. If available, external fixation can be performed to reduce open-book pelvic fractures and help minimize bleeding. Although it is out of favor for use in trauma, a pneumatic antishock garment, if available, can function as an "air splint" for the pelvis or lower extremities. Care must be taken to prevent compartment syndromes by overinflation and prolonged use.

Patients with musculoskeletal injuries are classified according to the severity of their injury and the need for orthopedic evaluation and treatment. Patients with vascular injury and dislocations require urgent referral or evacuation, as do patients with significant pelvic fractures or suspected cervical or thoracolumbar spinal injuries. Patients with stable open or closed fractures also require referral or evacuation, though less urgently. If referral or evacuation is delayed for more than 6 hours, these patients should receive antibiotics, analgesia, hydration, immobilization, and wound management as resources allow. Patients with sprains and minor injuries can either be treated primarily or referred to an orthopedist in a more routine fashion.

BURN INJURIES

The mortality from major burn injuries is significant, even with unlimited resources. Patients with burn injuries often require airway support, mechanical ventilation, and massive fluid resuscitation, in addition to management of their burn wounds. ◼ See Chapter 9: Thermal Injuries. The initial evaluation and treatment of these patients follows closely the ABCDE algorithm. Remember, these patients often have other injuries in addition to their burn injury (eg, blast injury or injury from jumping in an attempt to get away from the fire).

Inhalation injury, either from breathing heated air or breathing toxic gases emitted during combustion, essentially doubles the mortality from burn injury. Patients with significant facial burns and smoke or steam inhalation, as well as those with toxic gas inhalation from burning plastics, require a definitive airway (ie, endotracheal intubation or tracheostomy) and mechanical ventilation.

Probably the most significant aspect of the care of burn patients is the massive fluid replacement they require. These patients also require urgent evacuation to a burn center; otherwise, the care necessitated by their injuries can quickly overwhelm even a well-equipped hospital. Under austere conditions, patients with severe burns may need to be treated expectantly.

The initial treatment of patients with smaller burns can be initiated in the austere setting by preventing further injury, limiting debridement to ruptured blisters only, initiating fluid resuscitation (orally if necessary), preventing hypothermia, and applying topical antibiotics and sterile dressings. If circumferential burns are present, distal circulation and the need for escharotomy should be assessed. If local resources are limited but evacuation is possible, even if delayed, the patient with a significant burn should be stabilized as much as possible prior to transport. If possible, the airway should be secured and fluid resuscitation begun. If resources are limited and evacuation is difficult or impossible, small (<5% of body-surface area) burns often heal with nonoperative care, although sometimes with significant scarring or loss of function, especially over joints.

Preparation for Transport

The following discussion highlights the major principles of preparing injured patients for evacuation from isolated circumstances in which resources are limited, including military operations, wilderness environments, and civil disasters with delayed rescue. It may be necessary to provide care for hours to days in proximity to dangers—for example, fire from hostile weapons, persistently threatening weather, and imminent flood.

Under these circumstances, the first priority is to protect the caregivers and the patients from further injury. In general, a minimum of medical care is attempted while the injured patients and caregivers are exposed to danger. Once the danger has been mitigated, care of injured patients may commence to the fullest extent possible, given limitations inherent in the circumstances, while applying ATLS principles with some modifications. The skills required are similar to those used by a military medic or corpsman in the field once the caregiver and the patient are no longer under hostile fire.

The odds of successful rescue/evacuation, if needed, increase dramatically when plans are made in advance for such contingencies. Initiating rescue and communicating with rescuers is beyond the scope of this appendix; however, it is essential that provisions be considered for establishing communications with or signaling rescuers. This requires a plan for rescue, which includes notification of individuals not involved in the movement or plan of action. A flight, float, or expedition plan should be filed with individuals who can initiate rescue, automatically and autonomously under certain conditions. It is easy to understand why emergency extraction and rescue plans are an essential part of any military operation.

Flexibility and improvisation while waiting for evacuation from isolation are important to a successful outcome. Seeking appropriate shelter until evacuation is possible is an early priority. Shelter should be sought as soon as the patients and caregivers are out of immediate danger. High ground is generally preferable if the patient can be moved. Simple shelters of various types can be constructed from available materials with a minimum number of simple tools.

Use the following principles while waiting to transport patients:

- Move patients as little as possible after shelter is obtained.

- Initiate appropriate medical interventions as soon as feasible, based on the available resources and the injuries.

- Arrange for a stretcher or litter for severely injured or unconscious patients while providing extra padding to pressure points.

- In general, place patients in a supine position.

- Place patients with thoracic injuries in a lateral decubitus position with the injured side down or in a semi-elevated position (head and chest elevated at approximately 45 degrees).

- Splint fractures with available materials or splint them to another extremity.

- Keep patients as dry as possible and prevent hypothermia.

- Shield patients from prolonged exposure to intense, direct sunlight.

- Do not leave unattended patients close to campfires.

If helicopter evacuation is a possibility, scout a landing site to facilitate rescue. The landing site should ideally be on level, flat terrain that is clear of obstructions. It may be necessary to mark the site with smoke, reflectors, or other devices that can be seen from the air (branch or stone pointer). Helicopter extraction (while hovering) is also a possibility, but it is much more difficult and riskier to the patient.

Environmental Extremes of Heat and Cold

Preventing heat and cold injuries is preferable to treating them. Understanding the effects of environmental extremes on the human body helps to avoid these injuries. Unfortunately, accidental heat and cold injuries still occur despite adequate precautions.

COLD INJURY AND HYPOTHERMIA

A high index of suspicion is essential to making the diagnosis of hypothermia. Patients suffering overwhelming environmental exposures (eg, cold-water drowning and cold exposure) are readily identified. Preventing hypothermia involves two strategies: reducing heat loss and increasing heat production. Heat is lost from the skin in four ways: radiation, convection, conduction, and evaporation. In a normal environment, an individual loses 50% to 60% of body heat because of radiation. In contrast, convection is the major source of heat loss in a cold environment, particularly with strong winds. Conduction is a major route of heat loss during cold-water immersion. Heat losses from convection and conduction can be effectively reduced with whatever clothing materials are available. Evaporative heat loss occurs through both respiration and perspiration. This route is most important during exposure to cool dry environments.

Also, keep in mind that:

- Clothing must provide adequate insulation.

- Adequate shelter must be sought for adequate protection from the environment.

- Food consumption must be adequate for the increased caloric energy requirements.

- Activity must be at an adequate level to produce the heat required to keep warm.

The amount of heat lost by convection is determined by the temperature difference between the air and the body surface with which it is in contact and by the speed with which the air is moving. A wind of 8 mph (12.8 kph) removes four times as much heat as a wind of 4 mph (6.4 kph). Wind-chill charts detail the relationship between the ambient temperature and the effective temperature based on the prevailing wind speed.

Many different materials are used for cold weather clothing. The oldest is wool, which is still one of the best because it contains innumerable small air pockets that provide excellent insulation. One of the greatest values of wool is its ability to provide insulation even when wet. Its major disadvantage is its weight. Down provides excellent insulation when dry, but provides little protection when it is wet.

Heat production by the body can be increased significantly only by muscular exercise, either by shivering or performing voluntary work. Large muscles (eg, leg muscles) produce more heat than small muscles. Vigorous exercising can produce more heat than shivering. If a threatening situation cannot be avoided, deliberate exercise that uses large muscles, such as repeatedly stepping on and off rocks or logs, produces more heat than just standing and shivering. No drugs or other behavior can substitute for exercise as a means of generating body heat.

When cold injury does occur in the austere environment, an important principle is to avoid rewarming until a sustained warm environment can be ensured. Clearly, as with systemic cold injury, the best management of local cold injury is prevention.

HEAT-RELATED ILLNESS OR INJURY

Heat illness is due to exposure to increased ambient temperature under conditions in which the body is unable to maintain appropriate homeostasis. The milder syndromes are exertional; the most severe may occur without exercise.

The three common heat-related conditions are heat cramps, heat exhaustion, and heat stroke.

Heat Cramps

Painful muscles after exertion in a hot environment are often attributed to a salt deficit. However, it is likely that many cases represent exertional rhabdomyolysis. Acute muscle injury due to severe exertional effort beyond the limits for which the individual is trained can result in myoglobinuria, but this rarely affects kidney function unless heat stroke is present. Treatment includes rest in a cool environment and salt replacement with a 650-mg sodium chloride tablet in 500 mL of water or a commercially available balanced electrolyte replacement solution.

Heat Exhaustion

Fatigue, muscular weakness, tachycardia, postural syncope, nausea, vomiting, and an urge to defecate can result from dehydration and heat stress. This occurs in unacclimatized individuals who exercise in the heat and results from loss of both salt and water. Body temperature is normal. There may be a continuum from heat exhaustion to heat stroke. Treatment consists of rest in a cool environment, acceleration of heat loss by fan evaporation, and fluid repletion with salt-containing solutions. After the patient recovers, exercise in a hot environment should be avoided for 2 to 3 days to avoid recurrence.

Heat Stroke

Core body temperature exceeds 40° C (104° F) with heat stroke and severe central nervous system dysfunction and anhidrosis occur. The two types of heat stroke are classic and exertional.

Classic heat stroke occurs after several days of extreme heat exposure in individuals who are not acclimated. Risk factors include chronic illness, advanced age, high humidity, obesity, chronic cardiovascular disease, poverty, alcohol abuse, dehydration, and use of sedatives. Sedentary heat stroke is a disease of the elderly or infirm whose cardiovascular systems are unable to adapt to the hot environmental stress.

Exertional heat stroke occurs rapidly in unacclimatized individuals who exercise in conditions of high ambient temperature and humidity. In the United States each year, about 4000 people die from heat stroke. Exercise-induced heat stroke most often affects young people (eg, athletes, military recruits, and laborers). Individuals with this type of heat stroke are more likely to have disseminated intravascular coagulopathy, lactic acidosis, and rhabdomyolysis.

The treatment for heat stroke is rapid cooling. The most efficient method is to induce evaporative heat loss by misting and fan cooling. Immersion in an ice-water bath or the use of ice packs also is effective but can cause vasoconstriction and shivering, which limits cooling and monitoring.

Resuscitation with approximately 20 mL/kg of balanced salt solution is often required within the first 4 hours. Vigorous cooling should be stopped when the patient's temperature reaches 38.9° C (102° F). If myoglobinuria is present, hydration must be maintained to ensure a good urine output. Intravenous mannitol (25 g, or 300-400 mg/Kg) may be given after ensuring adequate intravascular volume.

Poor prognostic signs are body temperatures of 42.2° C (108° F) or more, coma lasting longer than 2 hours, shock, and hyperkalemia. Mortality rates are about 10%.

As with all thermal environmental injuries, the best treatment for heat stress is prevention. Acclimation to extreme heat requires about 3 to 5 days. Best strategies for activity involve alternating work and rest cycles and emphasizing fluid intake. Work in a desert environment at 49° C (120° F) requires 2 liters of water per hour. Availability of shelter with shading from the sun is important.

Communications and Signaling

The principles of effective communications in the austere environment include:

- Having a working plan in place beforehand.
- Knowing what your communications system can and cannot do.
- Having a backup communications plan.

Doctor-to-doctor contact with at least a minimum of patient information for referral is the safest way to coordinate patient transfers. Unfortunately, the austere environment may not afford either a doctor or a reliable means of communication. Effective communications rely on a preestablished and tested means of communication, with contingencies for a backup system when the primary means of communication fail. Available technologies include hand-held radios, cellular phones, and newer technologies, such as telemedicine.

Limitations of a telephone system in a disaster setting include destruction of the phone lines, power loss, inclement weather, and an increase in phone calls that frequently result in system saturation and overload. Cellular phones should ideally serve as a backup to a VHF radio communication system, which emits a directional signal that could be pinpointed. In addition, Global positioning systems (GPS) are becoming relatively inexpensive and afford the medical care provider the opportunity to identify his or her location in the austere setting with extreme accuracy.

Oral reporting should be efficient and clear, particularly in disaster settings in which radio traffic is high. Information relayed should include scene safety, number of patients, and the patients' conditions. Use of a standardized phonetic alphabet and phonetic numerals is preferred. When no direct contact is made with the receiving facility or medical care providers, every effort must be made to provide an accurate record that survives with at least a minimum amount of transfer data, including patient identification, medical problem, treatment provided, and patient status at transfer. Online medical care protocols for nondoctor providers are critically important when direct medical control is not available.

Communications at a disaster site are frequently and severely disrupted. Effective means of communication in this setting may include handheld radios, messengers, and megaphones. Disaster management is a multidisciplinary community activity, and effective communication among disaster responders is best addressed through the Incident Command System (ICS). Military organizations can bring to these sites well-developed communication systems with the ability to communicate worldwide through a secure network. Hospitals are expected to report to their local emergency communications center about their bed availability, number of casualties they have received and are prepared to accept, and items in short supply. In a disaster situation, most patients are not likely to have accessed the emergency medical services (EMS) system prior to arrival at medical facilities. Communication backup systems may address unique situations such as communication by medical staff while operating in hazardous material suits or a chemical or biologic "protective posture." See also Appendix H.

In the austere environment, available communications equipment is frequently limited to that which is carried into the field by the participants. In the event that electronic equipment is unavailable, the best signaling devices are either audio or visual. A universally recognized distress signal is essentially considered three of anything—for example, three whistle blasts, three gun shots, or three columns of smoke. An effective ground-to-air device is a mirror reflecting sunlight, which may be seen up to 10 miles (16 km) away. Ground signals should be as large as possible and contain straight lines and square corners. An "X" on the ground is the symbol internationally recognized as needing medical assistance. Both day-and night-signaling devices are readily available; these include mirrors, smoke, dyes, flashlights, flares, search and rescue transponders (SARTs), and other pyrotechnic and nonpyrotechnic devices.

Triage

Mass-casualty triage is the process of sorting or prioritizing patients into specific care categories depending on the number and severity of casualties and the resources available at that time. By definition, *triage* means there are inadequate resources to care for this number of patients in the usual manner. Triage is the process of prioritizing injured patients to determine which need medical care immediately, which can wait for care, and which are so severely injured that attempts at care are futile given the existing circumstances. The philosophy behind triage is to do the greatest good for the greatest number. Triage in the austere environment may be required when there are as few as two injured patients, which may easily overwhelm the resources available to a single doctor. A decision must be made regarding which patient should first receive the benefit of the doctor's full attention and application of available resources.

Even large, well-organized medical teams, such as disaster-response teams or military hospitals, may face overwhelming numbers of casualties. Preplanning and practice must occur prior to team deployment. Typically, the most experienced surgeon acts as the triage officer. In the event the surgeons are all needed to perform operations, another experienced doctor can act as the triage officer. This individual should have prior training in triage.

In wilderness austere environments, the doctor may not have the benefits of preplanning and must rely on experience. In these circumstances, it is particularly important for care providers to be very familiar with their equipment and supplies in order to do the most good for the largest number of patients. Only with knowledge of available resources and the possible ways to make the best use of them can a doctor save the most lives.

Remember, the entire concept of triage is predicated on the fact that not every patient gets immediate attention for his or her most significant injury. In order to do the most good for the largest number of patients, it is critically important to have a basic understanding of triage methods and categories. The first step in a mass casualty event is to "sift" the patients rapidly. This may consist of an order for all patients who are able to move to gather at a single, clearly visible site in the immediate area—for example, "Everyone who can, please move to the base of the large tree." This enables the medical care providers to pay immediate attention to the remaining patients.

Next, a careful "sieve" of the more severely injured patients occurs. Patients with life-threatening injuries are treated first, using the ABCDEs. The next priority is patients with limb-threatening or other injuries that are not immediately life-threatening—for example, abdominal injuries without hypotension.

In order to do the most good using existing supplies in an austere environment, it may be necessary to categorize some patients as expectant (expected to die). Patients in this category are given pain medication, if available, so they do not suffer. Supplies in limited quantity, such as intravenous fluids, should not be used in the care of expectant patients.

Many mass casualty triage classification schemes exist. A simple and useful method of triage involves four categories:

1. Immediate (needs treatment of life-threatening injuries)

2. Delayed (can wait 1 to 2 hours or more before treatment)

3. Minimal or ambulatory (can wait many hours for treatment)

4. Expectant or expected to die (given current patient load and resources)

The names and number of triage categories are not as important as the fact that all care providers have an understanding of the system being used. Color-coded triage tags are useful in identifying the category into which a patient is placed (eg, red for immediate, yellow for delayed, green for minimal, and gray for expectant). Patients who are dead should be transported to the morgue or another designated area.

Triage of mass-casualty victims is not a one-time exercise. Triage can occur at several levels, and needs to be both accurate and repetitive. Disaster-scene triage may be performed by experienced paramedics initially and then later by an on-site doctor if evacuation of victims is prolonged because of the sheer number of victims or difficulties in extrication or transport to definitive care. It is extremely important to understand the need for repeated triage. Patients who are placed into the expectant category because of lack of resources in a mass-casualty scenario may become immediate-category patients once operating room resources become available and no additional patients are expected to arrive. This is only one of many possible scenarios that serves to underscore the need for triage to be continuous rather than discrete.

APPENDIX G SUMMARY

ATLS provides an organized approach to the care of injured patients and is taught in the context of a resource-rich environment. However, there are many circumstances that can result in a doctor needing to work outside the normal environment. These include both military and civilian austere and/or hostile environments. These may be either planned (wilderness or military) or unplanned (natural disaster or terrorist attack) austere and hostile environments. Preparation and familiarity with the principles of the care of injured patients under austere and hostile circumstances optimize the care provided using limited resources.

Bibliography

1. Adkisson GA, Butler FK, et al. In: *Manual for Prehospital Trauma Life Support*, 5th ed. St. Louis, MO: Mosby; 2006.

2. Alam HB, Burris D, DaCorta JA, Rhee P. Hemorrhage control in the battlefield: role of new hemostatic agents. *Milit Med* 2005;170(1):63-69.

3. Alam HB, Rhee P. New developments in fluid resuscitation. *Surg Clin North Am* 2007;87(1):55-72.

4. American College of Surgeons. *Advanced Trauma Life Support Program for Doctors.* Chicago, IL: ACS; 1997, 2002, 2003.

5. Arishita GI, Vayer JS, Bellamy RF. Cervical spine immobilization of penetrating neck wounds in a hostile environment. *J Trauma* 1989; 29:332-337.

6. Barkana Y, Stein M, Maor R, Lynn M, Eldad A. Prehospital blood transfusion in prolonged evacuation. *J Trauma* 1999;46:176-180.

7. Bellamy RF. The causes of death in conventional land warfare: implications for combat casualty care research. *Milit Med* 1984;149:55-62.

8. Bickell WH, Wall MJ, Pepe PE, et al. Immediate versus delayed fluid resuscitation for hypotensive patients with penetrating torso injuries. *N Engl J Med* 1994;331:1105-1109.

9. Bledsoe BE, et al. *Paramedic Emergency Care.* 2nd ed. Englewood Cliffs, NJ: Prentice-Hall; 1994.

10. Bowman WD. Basic patient assessment and life support techniques (Chapter 4), Oxygen and other types of respiratory system support (Chapter 5), and Environmental emergencies (Chapter 18). In: *Outdoor Emergency Care.* National Ski Patrol System; 1993.

11. Bowman WD. Wilderness survival. In: Auerbach P, ed. *Wilderness Medicine*, 5th ed. St. Louis, MO: Mosby-Yearbook; 2007.

12. Burris D, Rhee P, Kaufmann C, Pikoulis M, Austin B, Leppäniemi AK. Controlled resuscitation in uncontrolled hemorrhagic shock. *J Trauma* 1998;46:216-223.

13. Butler FK Jr, Hagmann J, Butler EG. Tactical combat casualty care in special operations. *Milit Med* 1996;161:Suppl:3-16.

14. Calkins MD, Robinson TD. Alternative airway use in the special operations environment: a comparison of laryngeal mask airway and esophageal tracheal combitube to endotracheal tube. *J Trauma* 1999;46:927-932.

15. DeHart RL. *Fundamentals of Aerospace Medicine.* 3rd ed. Philadelphia: Lea & Febiger; 2002.

16. Farmer CJ. Temperature-related injuries. In: Civetta JM, Taylor RW, Kirby RR, eds. *Critical Care.* 3rd ed. Philadelphia: Lippincott; 1997.

17. Fortune JB, Judkins DG, Scanzaroli D, McLeod KB, Johnson SB. Efficacy of prehospital surgical cricothyrotomy in trauma patients. *J Trauma* 1997;42:832-836.

18. Gentile DA, Morris JA, Schimelpfenig T, et al. Wilderness injuries and illnesses. *Ann Emerg Med* 1992;21:853-861.

19. *Instructor's Manual for Prehospital Trauma Life Support (PHTLS)*, Military Edition. St. Louis, MO: Mosby; 2006.

20. Kauvar DS, Holcomb JB, Norris GC, Hess JR. Fresh whole blood transfusion: a controversial military practice. *J Trauma* 2006:61:181-184.

21. Kaweski SM, Sise MJ, Virgilio RW. The effect of prehospital fluids on survival in trauma patients. *J Trauma* 1990;30:1215-1218.

22. Lakstein D, Blumenfeld A, Sokolov T, Lin G, Bssorai R, Lynn M, Ben Abraham R. Tourniquets for hemorrhage control in the battlefield—a four year accumulated experience. *J Trauma* 2003:54:S221-S225.

23. Lounsbury D, Bellamy RF, eds. *Emergency War Surgery, Third United States Revision.* Washington, DC: Government Printing Office; 2004.

24. Martin RR, Bickell WH, Pepe PE, et al. Prospective evaluation of preoperative fluid resuscitation in hypotensive patients with penetrating truncal injury: a preliminary report. *J Trauma* 1992;33:354-361.

25. Moss JF, Haklin M, Southwick HW, et al. A model for treatment of accidental severe hypothermia. *J Trauma* 1986;26:68-74.

26. Rosemurgy AS, Norris PA, Olson SM, et al. Prehospital traumatic cardiac arrest: the cost of futility. *J Trauma* 1993;35:468-474.

27. Salvino CK, Dries D, Gamelli R, et al. Emergency cricothyroidotomy in trauma victims. *J Trauma* 1993; 34: 503-505.

28. Wedmore I, McManus JG, Puateri AE, Holcomb JB. A special report on the citosan-based hemostatic dressing experience in current combat operations. *J Trauma* 2006;60:655-658.

29. Woodhouse P, Keatinage WR, Coleshaw SR. Factors associated with hypothermia in patients admitted to a group of inner city hospitals. *Lancet* 1989;2:1201.

30. Yeskey KS, Llewellyn CH, Vayer JS. Operational medicine in disasters. *Emerg Med Clin North Am* 1996;14:429-438.

Disaster Management and Emergency Preparedness (Optional Lecture)

Introduction

Disasters may be defined, from a medical perspective, as incidents or events in which the needs of patients overextend or overwhelm the resources needed to care for them. Although disasters usually strike without warning, **emergency preparedness**—the readiness for and anticipation of the contingencies that follow in the aftermath of disasters—enhances the ability of the health care system to respond to the challenges imposed. Such preparedness is the institutional and personal responsibility of every health care facility and professional. Adherence to the highest standards of quality medical practice that are consistent with the available medical resources serves as the best guideline for developing disaster plans. Commonly, the ability to respond to disaster situations is compromised by the excessive demands placed on resources, capabilities, and organizational structures.

Multiple casualty incidents (MCIs), or disasters in which patient care resources are overextended but are not overwhelmed, such as automobile crashes that involve 5 or more patients, can stress local resources such that triage focuses on identifying the patients with the most life-threatening injuries.

Mass casualty events (MCEs) are disasters in which patient care resources are overwhelmed and cannot be immediately supplemented, such as natural or human-made disasters that involve 20 or more patients, can exhaust local resources such that triage focuses on identifying those patients with the greatest probability of survival.

Note that MCIs and MCEs are both called MCIs by many experts. The ATLS course distinguishes between the terms because their different circumstances mandate alternative strategies for triage and treatment, based on illness and injury acuity and severity, versus availability and accessibility of existing and supplemental resources. It must also be emphasized that the numerical guidelines cited (eg, 5 or more patients for an MCI, and 20 or more for an MCE) are arbitrary and based on the capabilities of trauma hospitals and trauma systems that routinely care for trauma patients. Many hospitals would be overwhelmed by 5 or more disaster patients, whereas some could manage 20 or more without a significant disruption of daily routines. **Thus, each hospital must determine its**

Upon completion of this topic, the student will be able to explain the application of ATLS principles to patients injured in natural or human-made disasters. Specifically, the doctor will be able to:

OBJECTIVES

1 Define the terms *multiple casualty incident (MCI)* and *mass casualty event (MCE)* and describe the differences between them.

2 Describe the "all hazards" approach to disaster management and emergency preparedness, including its application to acute injury care.

3 Identify the four phases of disaster management and describe the key elements of each phase with respect to acute injury care.

4 Describe the incident command system that has been adopted in his or her specific practice area.

own thresholds, recognizing that the hospital disaster plan must address both MCIs and MCEs.

Like most disciplines, disaster management and emergency preparedness experts have developed a nomenclature unique to their field. Box H-1 is a glossary of all key terms (ie, those appearing in boldface type) in this appendix.

The Need

Disaster management and emergency preparedness constitute key knowledge areas that prepare ATLS providers to apply ATLS principles during natural and human-made disasters. Successful application of these principles during the chaos that typically comes in the aftermath of such catastrophes requires both familiarity with the disaster

Box H-1
Key Disaster Management and Emergency Preparedness Terminology

Acute Care—The early care of victims of disasters that is provided in the field and in the hospital (ie, emergency department, operating room, intensive care unit, acute care unit inpatient units) prior to recovery and rehabilitation.

Acute Care Specialists—Physicians who provide acute care to victims of disasters, including, but not limited to, emergency medicine physicians, trauma surgeons, critical care medicine physicians, anesthesiologists, and hospitalists—both adult and pediatric.

Area of Operations ("Warm Zone")—The geographic subdivision established around a disaster site into which only qualified personnel—for example, hazardous material (HAZMAT) technicians and emergency medical services (EMS) providers—are permitted.

Casualty Collection Point (CCP)—A sector within the external perimeter of an area of operations ("warm zone") where casualties who exit the Search and Rescue (SAR) area ("hot zone") via a decontamination chute are gathered prior to transport off site.

Chemical, Biological, Radiological, Nuclear, and Explosive (CBRNE), including incendiary, agents—human-made hazardous materials (HAZMATs) that may be the cause of human-made disasters, whether unintentional or intentional.

Decontamination Chute—A fixed or deployable facility where hazardous materials (HAZMATs) are removed from a patient, and through which the patient must pass before transport, either out of a Search and Rescue (SAR) area ("hot zone"), or into a hospital.

Disaster—A **natural** or **human-made** incident or event, whether **internal** (originating inside the hospital) or **external** (originating outside the hospital) in which the needs of patients overextend or overwhelm the resources needed to care for them.

Emergency Medical Services (EMS)—Emergency medical responders (EMRs), including emergency medical technicians (EMTs) and paramedics, who provide prehospital care under medical direction as part of an organized response to medical emergencies.

Emergency Operations Center (EOC)—The headquarters of Unified Incident Command (UIC) for a region or system, established in a safe location outside the area of operations ("warm zone"), usually at a fixed site, and staffed by emergency managers.

Emergency Preparedness—The readiness for and anticipation of the contingencies that can follow in the aftermath of natural or human-made disasters. Preparedness is the institutional and personal responsibility of every health care facility and professional.

Emergo Train System (ETS)—An organizational structure used chiefly in Europe and Australasia to help coordinate an in-field or in-hospital disaster response. (*Note:* Nations and hospitals typically adopt their own versions of this system.)

External Perimeter—The outer boundary of an Area of Operations ("warm zone") that is established around a disaster site to separate geographic subdivisions that are safe for the general public ("cold zones") from those that are safe only for qualified personnel.

Hazardous Materials (HAZMATs)—Chemical, biological, radiological, nuclear, and explosive (CBRNE), including incendiary, agents that pose potential risks to human life, health, welfare, and safety.

Hospital Incident Command System (HICS)—An organizational structure used chiefly in the Americas to help coordinate an in-hospital disaster response. (*Note:* Nations and hospitals typically adopt their own versions of this system.)

Hazard Vulnerability Analysis (HVA)—An analysis of the probability and severity of the risks of various hazardous materials (HAZMATs), industrial mishaps, natural disasters, and weather systems that pose potential risks to community health and safety.

Incident Command or **Incident Commander (IC)**—The final authority and overall coordinator or supervisor for the management of any disaster response.

Incident Command Post (ICP)—The headquarters for Incident Command (IC), established in a safe location within the area of operations ("warm zone"), but at a safe distance from the Search and Rescue (SAR) area ("hot zone"), for any disaster.

Incident Command System (ICS)—An organizational structure that provides overall direction for the management of the disaster response.

Internal Perimeter—The outer boundary of a Search and Rescue (SAR) area ("hot zone") that isolates this area from the surrounding Area of Operations ("warm zone").

Mass Casualty Event (MCE)—A disaster in which patient care resources are overwhelmed and cannot immediately be supplemented.

Mitigation—Activities that health care facilities and professionals undertake in an attempt to lessen the severity and impact of a potential disaster.

Medical Response Team—A team of 1 to 4 health care professionals, led by an acute care specialist, that provides emergency medical care to an individual patient.

Minimum Acceptable Care—The lowest appropriate level of medical and surgical treatment required to sustain life and limb until additional assets can be mobilized.

Multiple Casualty Incident (MCI)—A disaster in which patient care resources are overextended but not overwhelmed

Personal Protective Equipment (PPE)—Special clothing worn by disaster response personnel to avoid self-contamination by hazardous materials (HAZMATs).

Preparation—Activities that health care facilities and providers undertake to build capacity and identify resources that may be used if a disaster occurs.

Recovery—Activities that are designed to assist health care facilities and professionals resume normal operations after a disaster situation is resolved.

Response—Activities that health care facilities and professionals undertake in evaluating and treating victims of an actual disaster.

Search and Rescue (SAR) Area ("Hot Zone")—A sector within the internal perimeter of an area of operations for a disaster in which humans are directly affected by the hazard.

Surge Capability—The extra assets that can actually be deployed—for example, beds that can actually be staffed and ventilators and monitors that can actually be used—in a disaster.

Unified Incident Command (UIC)—The locus of incident command for an entire region or system, where incident commanders from all involved public safety and public health disciplines meet to direct the overall strategy of the incident response to mass casualty events (MCEs).

Weapons of Mass Destruction (WMDs)—Hazardous materials (HAZMATs) used, or intended to be used, for the explicit purpose of harming or destroying human life.

response and knowledge of the medical conditions likely to be encountered. Terror events constitute a minority of all disasters, but nearly all terror events cause physical injury, three-fourths of which are due to blast trauma and most of the rest to gunshot wounds. As such, the understanding and application of ATLS principles are essential in the evaluation and treatment of all disaster victims.

The Approach

Disasters are unpredictable because of their nature, location, and timing. An "all hazards" approach is used in contemporary disaster management. This approach is based on a single, common, initial emergency response protocol, with branch points that lead to specific actions depending on the type of disaster encountered. **The fundamental principle of disaster management is to do the greatest good for the greatest number.**

Phases of Disaster Management

The public health approach to disaster and mass casualty management consists of four distinct phases:

1. Preparation
2. Mitigation
3. Response
4. Recovery

In most nations, local and regional disaster response plans are developed in accordance with national response plans. Emergency medicine, trauma care, public health, and disaster medicine experts must be involved in all four phases of management with respect to the medical components of the operational plan. The elements that must be addressed during each of these four phases are described below.

PREPARATION

Preparation involves the activities a hospital undertakes to build capacity and identify resources that may be used if a disaster occurs. These activities include the development of a simple, yet flexible, disaster plan that is regularly reviewed and revised as necessary, and provision of disaster training that is necessary to allow these plans to be implemented when indicated.

Simple Disaster Plans

A basic and readily understood approach to MCIs and MCEs is the key to effective disaster and emergency man-

agement. Plans that are too complex or cumbersome to remember or implement are destined to fail. All plans must include training in disaster management and emergency preparedness appropriate to the educational preparation of the individuals being trained.

Community Planning Disaster planning, whether at the local, regional, or national level, involves a wide range of individuals and resources. All plans:

- Should involve **acute care specialists** (eg, emergency medicine physicians, trauma surgeons, critical care medicine physicians, anesthesiologists, and hospitalists, both adult and pediatric) and local hospitals, as well as officials of the local police, fire, **emergency medical services (EMS)**, homeland security, emergency management, public health, and governmental agencies charged with **hazardous material (HAZMAT)** management and disaster preparation.

- Should be frequently tested and reevaluated.

- Must provide for a means of communication considering all contingencies, such as loss of telephone land lines and cellular circuits.

- Must provide for storage of equipment, supplies, and any special resources that may be necessary based on local **hazard vulnerability analysis (HVA).**

- Must provide for all levels of assistance—from first aid through definitive care to rehabilitation.

- Must prepare for the transportation of casualties to other facilities by prior agreement should the local facility become saturated or unusable.

- Must consider the urgent needs of patients already hospitalized for conditions unrelated to the disaster.

Hospital Planning Although a regional approach to planning is ideal for the management of mass casualties, circumstances may require each hospital to function with little or no outside support. Earthquakes, floods, riots, or nuclear contamination may require the individual hospital to operate in isolation. The crisis may be instantaneous or it may develop slowly. Situations may exist that disrupt the infrastructure of society and prevent access to the medical facility. For this reason, it is vital that each hospital develop a disaster plan that accurately reflects its HVA. Once a state of disaster has been declared, the hospital disaster plan should be put into effect. Specific procedures should be automatic and include:

- Establishment of an **incident command post (ICP).**

- Notification of on-duty and off-duty personnel.

- Preparation of decontamination, triage, and treatment areas.

- Classification of in-hospital patients to determine whether additional resources can be acquired to care for them or whether they must be discharged or transferred.

- Checking of supplies (eg, blood, fluids, medication) and other materials (eg, food, water, power, communications) essential to sustain hospital operations.

- Activation of decontamination facilities and staff and application of decontamination procedures if necessary.

- Institution of security precautions, including hospital lockdown if necessary, to avoid potential contamination and subsequent hospital closure.

- Establishment of a public information center and provision of regular briefings to inform family, friends, the media, and the government.

Departmental Planning   Effective disaster planning builds on existing strengths to address identified weaknesses. Since patient care can best be delivered to individual patients by providers working in small teams, every hospital department with responsibility for the care of injured patients must identify its **medical response teams** in advance. These teams must be provided with specific instructions as to where to go and what to do in the event of an internal or external disaster. Such instructions should not be overly complex. They should also be readily accessible in the event of a disaster—for example, printed on the back of hospital identification cards or posted on wall charts. They should also be very specific in terms of the job action to be performed, as follows:

- Emergency department plans must identify who will be responsible for notifying the incident commander; deploying the decontamination team; organizing the available physicians, nurses, allied health personnel, patient care technicians, orderlies, and housekeepers into individual teams to care for individual patients; directing emergency department triage of disaster victims; and mobilizing additional staff as needed.

- Surgical department plans must identify who will be responsible for organizing the available surgeons into resuscitation and operating teams and where these teams will assemble, or "muster"; identifying the leaders of such teams; and determining which patients will receive priority if operating rooms or perioperative staff are in short supply.

- Operating room plans must identify who will be responsible for organizing perioperative staff, both

anesthesiology and nursing; mobilizing needed additional staff; retrieving and deploying appropriate equipment; and identifying additional resources, such as obstetric operating rooms and nursing staff, that are not typically used to care for injured patients.

- Critical care plans must identify who will be responsible for organizing critical care unit staff, both medical and nursing; mobilizing needed additional staff; retrieving and deploying additional ventilators and monitors; and preparing additional isolation rooms, suites, or units that are not typically used to care for contaminated or contagious patients.

Personal Planning   Since the hospital disaster response, of necessity, is built on the personal and family disaster response, personal and family disaster planning constitutes a vital part of pre-event hospital disaster preparation for both the hospital and its employees. Most health care providers have family responsibilities, and will be at best uncomfortable, and at worst unable, to meet their employment responsibilities in the event of a disaster if the health and safety of their families is uncertain. Hospitals can assist health care providers in meeting their responsibilities to the hospital and to their families in a number of ways, and it is obviously to the advantage of both for hospitals to ensure that employees' family needs are met. Among these needs are assistance in identifying alternative resources for the care of dependent children and adults and ensuring that all employees develop family disaster plans, since all hospital-specific response plans depend on mobilization of additional staff, whose first duty in any disaster will be to ensure their own and their families' health and safety.

Hospital Disaster Training

All health care providers must be trained in the principles of disaster management and emergency preparedness commensurate with their level of patient contact. Training in disaster management includes both operational and medical components. The ATLS provider should be well versed in the fundamental elements of the local, regional, and national disaster plans, as appropriate, and understand the role of medical care in the overall management plan. It is essential to realize that, although the purpose of all disaster management is to ensure the safety and security of the maximum number of human lives and the greatest mass of public and private property, the medical component is but one element of the operational plan, at both the hospital and the community level. This is because the provision of medical care requires a complex infrastructure of logistical support before medical professionals can safely and securely apply their skills.

Beyond this basic understanding, it is also vital that the ATLS provider have a working understanding of the application of ATLS principles in disaster situations. It is important to recognize that the approach to the patient injured in a disaster is no different from the approach to the patient injured in the course of everyday activities: **A**irway, **B**reathing, **C**irculation, **D**isability, and **E**xposure. Rather, it is the application of this basic approach that may be altered, which is best summarized by the phrase, "Care ordinary, circumstances extraordinary." For example, the fact that the ATLS provider may need to care for multiple victims more or less simultaneously, and may not have sufficient equipment or assistance to carry out all needed tasks in a timely manner, requires that routine standards of care may need to be altered such that disaster medicine must focus on the **minimum acceptable** care required for salvage of life and limb, not the highest possible standard of care normally offered to severely injured patients.

As such, it is vital that the ATLS provider obtain sufficient basic education to initiate the medical care of multiple victims not only of natural disasters, but also of human-made disasters, including those caused by HAZMATS—including **weapons of mass destruction (WMDs)** such as **CBRNE (chemical, biological, radiological, nuclear, and explosive)** and incendiary agents—in the potentially austere environment of an emergency department overwhelmed by panicked patients and staff shortages. Although brief outlines of such treatment are provided in this appendix, additional training in disaster medical care is currently beyond the scope of the ATLS provider course, but can be obtained through participation in the appropriate national disaster management courses.

MITIGATION

Mitigation involves the activities a hospital undertakes in attempting to lessen the severity and impact of a potential disaster. These include adoption of an incident command system for managing internal (originating inside the hospital) and external (originating outside the hospital) disasters, and the exercises and drills necessary to successfully implement, test, and refine the hospital disaster plan.

Incident Command System

An **incident command system (ICS)** is vital to operational success during disasters and must be known to all personnel within every health care facility and agency. The ICS establishes clear lines of responsibility, authority, reporting, and communication for all health care personnel, thereby maximizing collaboration and minimizing conflicts during the disaster response. It is also important that the hospital ICS follow normal lines of hospital authority as closely as possible to avoid confusion about who is in charge, provided that all hospital officials within the chain of command understand the ICS and their roles and responsibilities within the ICS

The effective ICS includes both vertical and horizontal reporting relationships, to ensure that urgent decisions can

be made without the need for prior confirmation by incident commanders, which consumes valuable time. In MCEs that affect an entire region or system, the effective ICS must be fully integrated with the **unified incident command (UIC)** serving the entire region or system, which is comprised of all involved public health and safety agencies.

A hierarchical approach to incident command, such as the **Hospital Incident Command System (HICS)** developed under the auspices of the California EMS Authority (http://www.emsa.ca.gov/hics/hics.asp), is favored in the Americas. A more collaborative and medically centered approach to incident command, such as the **Emergo Train System (ETS)** promulgated by the Linköping University Trauma Center in Sweden (http://www.emergotrain.com), is favored in Europe and Australasia. Most nations adopt one of the two approaches for **incident command (IC)** in developing their response plans, adapting them to fit local needs and resources. The models used by these two systems are shown in Table H-1.

Regardless of the ICS system used, incident command (IC) is responsible for all aspects of the disaster response under its jurisdiction—operational, medical, or both. The initial responsibility of IC is to declare an internal disaster or an external disaster. All operational and medical section heads report directly to, and must be in constant communication with, the IC, either in person or by telecommunications, for unified incident command to be effective and efficient.

As soon as possible after an internal or external disaster is declared by IC, an **incident command post (ICP),** also known as the **hospital command center (HCC)**, must be established, with reliable communication links to all functional units—operational/logistic or medical. The ICP must

TABLE H-1 ■ Commonly Used Models for Incident Command Systems[a]

HICS FUNCTIONAL JOB ACTIONS[b]	ETS FUNCTIONAL JOB ACTIONS[c]

Incident command (hospital)
• Command staff
  Public information
  Liaison
  Safety
  Medical/technical
• Finance and administration
• Logistics
• Operations
• Planning and intelligence
	Field
	• Ambulance incident command
	• Medical incident command
	Hospital
	• Logistics command
	• Medical command

[a]Regardless of the system being used, like structures are used in-field and in-hospital.
[b]http://www.emsa.ca.gov/hics/hics.asp
[c]http://www.emergotrain.com

be established in a secure location, distant from, but with ready access to, the site of primary patient care activity, whether field or hospital. In the field, it should be located within the **area of operations**, or **"warm zone,"** uphill, up-wind and upstream of the **search and rescue (SAR)** area, or **"hot zone," decontamination chutes**, and **casualty collection points (CCPs)**. In the hospital, it should be located at a safe distance from decontamination areas, patient care areas family support areas, and potential hazards, such as contaminated ventilation and drainage, but close enough to patient care and family support areas so that messages can be transmitted in person if electronic communications fail.

Frequent Disaster Drills

As in trauma resuscitation, medical management of mass casualties can be provided to individual patients only by in-dividual providers, working in small **medical response teams,** led by a senior acute care specialist. It is crucial to an effective disaster medical response that such teams have been drilled, not simply trained, in disaster medical care, under circumstances that are as realistic as possible. Disas-ter drills should always emphasize the disasters expected on the basis of the hospital's HVA. The purpose of disaster drills and exercises is not only to train emergency medical responders to provide care to disaster victims, but also to identify gaps in the hospital disaster plan so they can be closed prior to the occurrence of an actual internal or ex-ternal disaster. In addition, they should involve scenarios that emphasize the needs of special populations, such as burn patients, pediatric patients, geriatric patients, and dis-abled patients, which may require the mobilization and de-ployment of population-specific resources. The types of disaster drills and exercises hospitals should hold are de-scribed in Box H-2. It is wise to proceed from simple drills to complex exercises as staff members gain familiarity with the ICS and experience with the problems likely to arise during a disaster.

RESPONSE

Response involves activities a hospital undertakes in treating victims of an actual disaster. These include activation of the hospital disaster plan, including the ICS, and management of the disaster as it unfolds, implementing schemes for pa-tient decontamination, disaster triage, surge capacity (mo-bilization and deployment of the necessary staff, equipment, resources, and facilities to treat increased numbers of pa-tients, better termed **surge capability**), and alternative care (provision of the **minimum acceptable care** needed to save life and limb). Given the increased level of activity in disas-ter events, traffic control is needed to ensure an uninter-rupted forward flow of communications, patients, supplies, and personnel. The medical disaster response must also ad-dress the needs of special populations, including children, elders, the disabled, and the dispossessed.

Prehospital Care

The prehospital (EMS) response to natural and human-made disasters typically occurs in four stages:

1. Chaos phase, typically lasting 15 to 20 minutes
2. Organizational phase, usually lasting 1 to 2 hours
3. Site-clearing and evacuation stage of variable length, depending on disaster type, complexity of SAR ef-forts, and number of evacuees
4. Gradual recovery

All SAR efforts at the scene should be the responsibil-ity of HAZMAT technicians specifically trained for this pur-pose, and must proceed as rapidly and safely as possible, due to the potential for a "second hit" designed to injure first re-sponding personnel, including volunteers. Since the first re-sponsibility of field providers is to protect themselves, first-response personnel, including EMS professionals,

Box H-2
Types of Disaster Drills and Exercises

- **Disaster Drill** Supervised activity with a limited focus to test a procedure that is a limited compo-nent of a facility's overall disaster plan.
- **Tabletop Exercise** Written and verbal scenarios that evaluate the effectiveness of a facility's overall disaster plan and coordination.
- **Functional Exercise** Simulation of a disaster in the most realistic manner possible without moving real people or real equipment to a real site.
- **Field Exercise** Culmination of previous drills and exercises that tests the mobilization of as many of the response components as possible in real time, using real people and real equipment.

should not enter the disaster scene until it has been declared safe and secure by the appropriate authorities. Appropriate **personal protective equipment** (**PPE**) is mandatory for all health care personnel in direct contact with patients.

In-Hospital Care

Once the hospital disaster plan is activated, the first priority of IC is to ensure sufficient resources to mount an effective disaster response. This includes mobilization and deployment of adequate patient care staff, facilities, and equipment to meet anticipated needs, as well as early discharge of eligible patients from hospital inpatient and fast track units; cancellation of elective operations and outpatient clinics; selective withholding of "elective" blood component therapy; and accurate determination of each unit's surge capability, not merely its capacity, including identification and mobilization of alternative care sites. The next priority is to sustain the disaster response, through adjustment of shifts and schedules, provision of room and board for in-house hospital staff, and assistance in activating family disaster plans, including child and elder care as needed. Preprinted job action sheets should be made available to appropriate facility staff for each functional job description within the ICS, to serve as a tangible reminder of the tasks each staff member is expected to undertake.

Patient Decontamination   Hospital disaster care begins with decontamination, the principles and methods for which are shown in Box H-3. Ninety percent of hazardous materials to which disaster victims may have been exposed can be eliminated simply by removal of outer garments contaminated with hazardous materials. However, it may not be pos-

sible for HAZMAT teams or first responders to perform decontamination under all circumstances. Moreover, many patients are likely to transport themselves to the closest hospital, and will arrive at the emergency department before being decontaminated, demanding urgent care.

For this reason, hospitals must rapidly and conscientiously determine the likelihood of contamination and proceed accordingly. Although the safest course might be to consider all disaster patients contaminated until public safety officials determine otherwise, this approach slows patient throughput and can result in further deterioration of high-risk patients. Another approach is to segregate patients who transport themselves to the hospital in a holding area outside the hospital until HAZMAT teams determine the nature of the event, recognizing that such patients are far less likely to deteriorate than patients transported by ambulance. Either way, hospitals must plan for decontamination of potentially contaminated patients before they can enter the emergency department. Failure to do so can result in contamination and subsequent quarantine of the entire facility. Involvement of hospital security, and local police, may be necessary if lockdown is required to prevent presumptively contaminated patients from entering the emergency department or hospital before they can be effectively decontaminated.

Disaster Triage Scheme   Whether the disaster is an MCI that overextends or an MCE that overwhelms the resources of an institution, a method for rapid identification of victims requiring priority treatment is essential. Most triage schemes use color-coded tags to indicate acuity and severity of needed treatment (red = immediate, yellow = delayed,

Box H-3
Principles and Methods of Decontamination

Remember, "Dilution is the solution to pollution."

Gross (primary) decontamination

- Performed in the field or outside the hospital after removal of clothing
- Patient is hosed with a fine mist spray under moderate pressure
- Washes away most remaining contaminants

Technical (secondary) decontamination

Self-decontamination with soap and water under a warm shower bath

OR

Assisted decontamination with soap and water via a warm sponge bath

- Eradicates almost all residual contaminants, suffices for radioactive agents
- Additional cleansing with dilute chlorine bleach may be recommended if susceptible biologic agents or chemical agents are suspected

green = minor, blue = expectant, black = dead). The goal of treatment in MCIs is to treat the sickest patients first, whereas the goal in MCEs is to save the greatest number of lives. As such, triage schemes in MCEs should adopt an approach that separates patients with minor injuries from those with more serious injuries, before proceeding with evaluation and sustentative treatment of patients with major injuries. Unsalvageable patients receive terminal or comfort care only after other patients have been treated.

Overtriage and undertriage can substantially affect the medical disaster response in the emergency department and after admission to the hospital. Overtriage slows system throughput, and undertriage delays medically necessary care. Both increase the fatality rate among potentially salvageable patients. Therefore, triage should be performed by an experienced clinician with specific knowledge of the conditions affecting most patients. In addition, all injured patients should be continually reevaluated and reassessed.

Effective Surge Capability   The initial disaster response is invariably a local response, as regional or national assets cannot typically be mobilized for 24 to 72 hours. Thus, local, regional, and national disaster plans must presume that hospitals will be able to deploy sufficient staff, equipment, and resources to care for an increase, or "surge," in patient volume that is approximately 20% higher than its baseline, an estimate that reflects recent worldwide experience with limited MCEs.

The term *surge capacity* is more often used in disaster plans than *surge capability,* but the ATLS course uses the latter term, as it is more inclusive than the former term. This is because *surge capacity* too often is used to refer only to the number of additional beds or assets, such as ventilators or monitors, that might be pressed into service on the occasion of an MCE. By contrast, *surge capability* refers to the number of additional beds that can actually be staffed or ventilators and monitors that can actually be operated. In large urban areas, many staff may work multiple jobs, and may unknowingly be part of more than one hospital's disaster plan. In addition, most hospital staff are working parents, who must consider the needs of their families and relatives, in addition to those of their workplaces.

Alternative Care Standards   In MCEs, it can be expected that during the first 24 to 72 hours of the disaster there will be insufficient local assets to provide a level of care comparable to that routinely provided in local hospital emergency departments or intensive care units. If scarce resources, particularly intensive resources, are devoted to the first several critically ill or injured patients who require them, it will be difficult, if not impossible, to later redirect them to others in greater need.

To achieve this goal, hospital disaster plans must strive to provide the largest possible number of patients with the **minimum acceptable care**, defined as the lowest appropriate level of medical and surgical treatment required to sus-

tain life and limb until additional assets can be mobilized. Since each disaster response presents health care providers with a different mix of patient needs and available resources, no single description of a minimum acceptable standard of care is applicable to every facility or every disaster circumstance. However, because the selection of patients to receive scarce or intensive resources will present the trauma specialist with an ethical dilemma and potentially a later legal problem, general criteria should be developed *before* the disaster event, based on demographic and geographic circumstances as well as the community HVA. It is wise to develop such criteria in collaboration with the hospital's legal counsel, bioethics committee, and pastoral care department to ensure consistency with the community standard of legal, ethical, and moral values. They should then be included as part of the facility's disaster plan.

Traffic Control System   Controlling the flow of information (communications), equipment (supplies), patients (transport), and personnel (providers, relatives, the public, and the press) is of paramount importance in a medical disaster response. These are the issues most often cited in after-action reports as causes of disaster *mis*management. The unidirectional flow of patients from the emergency department to inpatient units must be ensured, since emergency department beds will be made available for later-arriving patients as they are emptied.

Redundant communications systems, reliable supply chains, and redoubtable security measures are also vital components of an effective disaster medical and operational response. These assets must be tested on a regular basis through drills and exercises that realistically reflect the disaster scenarios that are most likely to be encountered by a particular facility, whatever its location.

Special Needs Populations   Special needs populations include tribal nations; children, especially those who are technology-dependent; elders, especially those who are bedridden, including the nursing home population; the disabled, both physically and emotionally, for whom assistance will be illness- or injury-specific; and the dispossessed, including the poor and the homeless, who will be difficult to reach by traditional means for purposes of disaster education and treatment. Specific response plans are needed to ensure that their special needs are met.

Pathophysiology and Patterns of Injury

As with all trauma, natural and human-made disasters result in recognizable patterns of injury that are based on the properties of the particular wounding agent and the unique pathophysiology that results from each such agent. Although detailed descriptions of the pathophysiology and patterns of injury encountered in the acute disaster response are beyond the scope of this appendix, 100% of all natural disasters and 98% of all terror events worldwide involve physical trauma.

Thus, the principles of ATLS are ideally suited to the early care of patients with blunt and penetrating injuries observed in natural or human-made disasters, provided that the mechanisms and patterns of physical injury that are typically observed in natural and human-made disasters are distinctly understood. However, certain additional factors must also be considered in the early and later care of seriously injured disaster patients, including the very real possibility that chemical, radiologic, and biologic injuries may coexist with blast injuries—specifically, that the blast device may be a "dirty bomb" that is contaminated with deadly agents.

WMDs are HAZMATs—particularly CBRNE agents—that are used, or intended to be used, for the express purpose of harming or destroying human life, or causing fear of the same. Members of the medical team should be familiar with the basics of decontamination and initial treatment of all patients injured by WMDs, not only those injured by bomb blasts and gunshot wounds. WMDs may be the sole agent used, or may be added as adulterants to explosive devices to construct a "dirty bomb." If present, WMDs can complicate the care of individuals who have suffered blast trauma, although their effectiveness in such scenarios may be limited by the effects of the blast. Descriptions of WMD agents and care of WMD injuries other than contagious illnesses are summarized in Boxes H-4 through H-10. **Remember, the emergency care of these patients becomes even more complex in the face of MCEs, with their associated needs for disaster triage, additional staff, and adequate supplies.** The treatment of contagious illnesses, which typically present days after exposure with fever and rash, or influenza-like symptoms is microbe-dependent.

RECOVERY

Recovery involves activities designed to help facilities resume operations after an emergency. The local public

Box H-4
Special Considerations in the Care of Blast Injury

Early Care

Airway

- Lateral recovery position (field care of facial trauma without cervical spine injury)
- Modified HAINES* position (field care of facial trauma with cervical spine injury)

Breathing

- Supplemental oxygen (blast lung)
- Needle decompression (tension pneumothorax)

Circulation

- Tourniquets (field care of bleeding from traumatic amputations)
- HemCon™ (chitosan), QuikClot™ (zeolite) (field care of bleeding from soft tissues)
- Hypotensive resuscitation (field care of patients in shock)
- Damage control laparotomy/thoracotomy
- Completion amputations for unsalvageable mangled extremities
- Liberal use of fasciotomies and escharotomies (to avoid compartment syndromes)

- Active and passive rewarming (to avoid hypothermic coagulopathies)
- Preferential use of fresh whole blood, if available (for treatment of coagulopathies)
- Administration of recombinant factor VIIa (rVIIa) (for treatment of coagulopathies)
- Judicious crystalloid fluid resuscitation (for combined blast lung and blast burn)

Later Care

- Compartment syndrome despite fasciotomy (especially during aeromedical transport)
- Early recognition and repair of vascular injury (intimal tears caused by shock wave)
- Wound management (reopening, irrigation, debridement, reclosure of dirty wounds)
- Tertiary survey (should be performed by different team of examiners)
- Documentation (essential for providers in subsequent echelons of care)
- Feedback (all providers must learn of outcome for care to improve)

***High Arm IN Endangered S**pine (lateral recovery position + head on outstretched arm)

Box H-5
Chemical Agents Commonly Associated with Human-Made Disasters

Nerve (cholinergic) agents

- Tabun (GA)
- Sarin (GB)
- Soman (GD)
- VX (an oily, brown liquid ; all other nerve agents are gases)

Blood (asphyxiant and hemolytic) agents

- Hydrogen cyanide (AC)
- Cyanogen chloride (CK)
- Arsine (SA)

Choking (pulmonary) agents

- Chlorine (CL)
- Phosgene (CG)

- Diphosgene (DP)
- Ammonia

Blister (vesicant) agents

- Mustards (HD, HN, HT)
- Lewisite (L)
- Phosgene oxime (CX)

Incapacitating (psychogenic) agents

- Agent 15
- BZ

---

health system plays a major role in this phase of disaster management, although health professionals will provide routine health care to the affected community consistent with available resources, in terms of operable facilities, usable equipment, and credentialed personnel. Acute care physicians who provide care for neglected injuries and chronic illnesses may find both the medical and organizational skills required for the early care of the trauma patient useful in the days after the response phase subsides. The principles of ATLS—that is, treatment of the greatest threat to life first, without waiting for a definitive diagnosis, and causing the patient no harm, are no less useful in the austere environments that may follow natural or human-made disasters.

Pitfalls

The four common pitfalls in the disaster medical response are always the same—communications, supplies, security, and volunteers—leading many disaster experts to ask why humans seem incapable of learning from the mistakes made in past disaster events. The answer lies in the very nature of

the disaster event, the word *disaster* being derived from the Latin words for *evil* and *star.* Falling stars are seldom seen, and when they are, they vanish from view almost immediately, and do not reenter the collective consciousness until the next star falls. While the exact dates, times, and places of future disasters are unknown, the lessons learned from previous disasters are invaluable in teaching us how to better prepare for them.

It can be expected, not merely anticipated, that land and mobile telecommunications systems will be overwhelmed. Communications systems must be fully interoperable and overly redundant, both in terms of duplicate equipment and disparate modes. Capability for both vertical and horizontal communications must be ensured. Supplies needed for disasters must be sequestered and stored in high, dry, safe, and secure areas. Security must be ensured for providers, patients, supplies, and systems needed for disaster care, such as communications and transport. Volunteers, well meaning as they may be, must be properly trained and credentialed to participate in a disaster response, and must participate only as part of a properly planned and organized disaster response, since they otherwise place both themselves, and the intended recipients of their aid, in danger.

Box H-6
Special Considerations in the Care of Chemical Injuries

Nerve (cholinergic) agents (GA, GB, GD, VX)

- Pathophysiology: form complexes with $AChE \rightarrow \uparrow$ ACh; victim drowns in secretions
- Sx: cholinergic crisis (both muscarinic and nicotinic effects; see Box H-7)
- Rx: atropine (dries secretions); pralidoxime* [2-PAM] (inactivates complexes)
- *Note: A bendodiazapene should also be given if seizure activity is evident.*

Blood (asphyxiant and hemolytic) agents (AC, CK and SA)

- Pathophysiology:
  - AC, CK: CN- replaces O_2 in Cya_3
  - SA: acute hemolysis ± renal failure
- Sx: telltale odor in association with cardinal signs
  - AC, CK: almonds, in association with LOC
  - SA: garlic, in association with hematuria, jaundice
- Rx:
  - AC, CK: OHCbl ($\rightarrow$CNCbl) [or $NaNO_2$ (Hb$\rightarrow$MetHb)] + $Na_2S_2O_3$
  - SA: supportive
- *Note: OHCbl has largely replaced $NaNO_2$ in treatment of AC, CK exposure.*

Choking (pulmonary) agents

- Pathophysiology: chemical pneumonia, severe tracheobronchitis and alveolitis†
- Sx: telltale odor in association with shortness of breath
  - CL: bleach
  - CG, DP: green corn, mown hay
  - NH_3: ammonia
- Rx: supportive
- *Note: Dry oxygen in CL exposure avoids HCl damage to tracheobronchial tree.*

Blister (vesicant) agents

- Pathophysiology: severe/painful/blistering cutaneous/pulmonary/mucous burns
- Sx: telltale odor in association with epithelial damage
  - HD,HN,HT: garlic, mustard, onions
  - L: geraniums
  - CX: pepper
- Rx: aggressive decontamination, wound care
- *Note: Administer British anti-Lewisite (BAL) in L exposure.*

Incapacitating (psychogenic) agents (Agent 15, BZ)

- Pathophysiology: agent specific
- Sx: bizarre behavior
- Rx: await recovery

*GD-AChE complexes age rapidly; pralidoxime must be given as soon as possible
†Phosgene is fatal if pulmonary edema develops in 2-4 hr

Box H-7
Classic Toxidromes Associated with Cholingeric Crisis due to Nerve Agents

SLUDGEM*

Salivation
Lacrimation
Urination
Defecation
Gastrointestinal
Emesis
Miosis

DUMBELS*

Diarrhea, **D**yspnea, **D**iaphoresis
Urination
Miosis
Bradycardia, **B**ronchorrhea, **B**ronchospasm
Emesis
Lacrimation
Salivation, **S**ecretions, **S**weating

MTW(t)HF†

Mydriasis
Tachycardia
Weakness
(t)**H**ypertension
Fasciculations

*Muscarinic effects (treated with atropine)
†Nicotinic effects

Box H-8
Radioactive Agents Commonly Associated with Human-Made Disasters

Ionizing radiation

- Particles:
  - Alpha (a) [He^{++} nucleus]
  - Beta (b) [energized e$^-$]
- Rays:
  - x [high energy photon waves]
  - Gamma (g) [high energy photon waves]

Likely agents

- "Dirty bomb":
  - Low level radioactive waste (^{137}Cs, ^{192}Ir) of medical or industrial origin
- Nuclear accident:
  - Pressure water reactor: ^{133}Xe, ^{135}Xe, ^{88}Kr (based on Three Mile Island experience)
  - Graphite reactor: ^{133}I, ^{131}I, ^{132}Te, ^{137}Cs, ^{90}Sr (based on Chernobyl experience)
  - Note: Pressure water reactors are most common; graphite reactors are now obsolete.

Radiation dosimetry

- For b, x, and g emitters, 1 R (Roentgen) = 1 rad (radiation absorbed dose) [or 0.01 Gy]
- For a or n emitters, 1 rad x Q* = # rem† (Roentgen equivalent man) [or 0.01 Sv]
- Note: In most circumstances, 1 R = 1 rad [or 0.01 Gy] = 1 rem [or 0.01 Sv].
- Note: "rad" and "rem" are preferred in the Americas, "Gy" and "Sv" elsewhere.

*Q = quality factor (b, x, g emitters: 1; inhaled/ingested a emitters: 20; n emitters: 3-20)
†It is this unit that denotes extent of biological damage (background dose = 360 mSv/yr)

Box H-9
Special Considerations in the Care of Radiation and Nuclear Injuries

Ionizing radiation

- Pathophysiology:
  - Strips electrons from atomic nuclei, damaging cellular DNA; rapidly dividing tissues (gastrointestinal, hematopoietic, epidermal) are most susceptible to ionizing radiation
  - *Note: Radioactive atoms emit particles (or rays) during decay; risk of exposure depends upon energy of emissions ("dirty bomb": low; nuclear accident: high).*
- Sx:
  - Specific to dose and type, distance to source, density of shielding; asymptomatic <50 rad (0.5 Sv), β burns >100 rad (1 Sv), acute radiation syndrome >200 rad (2 Sv)

- *Note: The more rapid the symptom onset, the higher the dose; patients who develop gastrointestinal symptoms within 4 hours of exposure rarely survive.*
- Rx:
  - α and β: external [± internal] decon + supportive care; x and γ: supportive care (treat external contamination as dirt; no risk to provider from patient x or γ exposure)
  - *Note: Do NOT delay resuscitation for decontamination, as risk to provider is nil; perform operations by day 3 to avoid wound complications 2° RES failure.*

Box H-10
Classic Toxidromes Associated with Acute Radiation Syndrome

Stage I: (chiefly gastrointestinal)

- Onset: minutes to hours*; duration: 48-72 hr
- Presentation: nausea, vomiting; also diarrhea, cramps

Stage II (chiefly hematopoietic[†])

- Onset: hours to days; duration: $1\frac{1}{2}$-2 wk
- Presentation: asymptomatic → bone marrow suppression

Stage III (multisystem involvement)

- Onset: 3-5 weeks; duration: variable
- Presentation[‡]: CNS/CVS (>15 Sv); CRS/GIT (>5 Sv); RES (>1 Sv)

Stage IV (gradual recovery)

- Onset: weeks; duration: weeks to months
- Presentation: leading cause of death before recovery is sepsis

*Acute radiation syndrome is fatal if gastrointestinal symptoms develop within 2-4 hours
[†]Hematopoietic (RES) derangements interfere with healing, may last weeks to months
[‡]CNS = central nervous system, CVS = cardiovascular system, CRS = cardiorespiratory system, GIT = gastrointestinal tract, RES = reticuloendothelial system

APPENDIX H SUMMARY

The medical disaster response occurs within the context of the public health disaster response—**preparation**, **mitigation**, **response**, and **recovery**.

Preparation requires both the conviction that a disaster will occur, and the commitment to be ready when it happens, and must ensure both that a simple plan is developed and that all are educated in its implementation.

Mitigation is the key to the success of the disaster response, since it provides the framework within which medical care must be rendered—for example, incident command systems and effective disaster drills and exercises.

Response is the essence of disaster management. It comprises both prehospital and in-patient care, and must embrace the minimal acceptable standard of care needed to provide the greatest good for the greatest number. It requires a sound understanding of pathophysiology and patterns of injury for care to be delivered expeditiously and deterioration anticipated and avoided.

Recovery is mainly the province of public health personnel, but it depends on support from acute care physicians for treatment of untreated injuries and chronic illnesses that may develop or become exacerbated in the aftermath of the acute response.

However, it is not enough to be competent in the medical aspects of disaster management, whether acute or chronic. Pitfalls must be foreseen and forestalled through redundant communication systems, reliable supply chains, situational awareness, and professional self-discipline.

Bibliography

1. American Academy of Pediatrics (Foltin GL, Schonfeld DJ, Shannon MW, eds.). *Pediatric Terrorism and Disaster Preparedness: A Resource for Pediatricians.* AHRQ Publication No. 06-0056-EF. Rockville, MD: Agency for Healthcare Research and Quality; 2006. http://www.ahrq.org/research/pedprep/resource.htm. Accessed February 26, 2008.

2. auf der Heide E. *Disaster Response: Principles of Preparation and Coordination.* Chicago, IL: CV Mosby; 1989.

3. Committee on Trauma, American College of Surgeons. Disaster Management and Emergency Preparedness Course Student Manual. Chicago: American College of Surgeons, 2007.

4. DiPalma RG, Burris DG, Champion HR, Hodgson MJ. Blast injuries. *N Engl J Med* 2005;352:1335-1342.

5. Frykberg ER, Tepas JJ. Terrorist bombings: lessons learned from Belfast to Beirut. *Ann Surg* 1988;208:569-576.

6. Gutierrez de Ceballos JP, Turegano-Fuentes F, Perez-Diaz D, Sanz-Sanchez M, Martin-Llorente C, Guerrero-Sanz JE. Casualties treated at the closest hospital in the Madrid, March 11, terrorist bombings. *Crit Care Med* 2005;33(1 Suppl);S107-S112.

7. Gutierrez de Ceballos JP, Turegano-Fuentes F, Perez-Diaz D, Sanz-Sanchez M, Martin-Llorente C, Guerrero-Sanz JE. 11 March 2004: the terrorist bomb explosions in Madrid, Spain–an analysis of the logistics, injuries sustained and clinical management of casualties treated at the closest hospital. *Crit Care* 2005;9:104-111.

8. Hirshberg A, Scott BG, Granchi T, Wall MJ, Mattox KL, Stein M. How does casualty load affect trauma care in urban bombing incidents? A quantitative analysis. *J Trauma* 2005;58(4):686-693; discussion 694-695.

9. Holden PJ. The London attacks—a chronicle: Improvising in an emergency. *N Engl J Med* 2005;353(6):541-543.

10. Jacobs LM, Burns KJ, Gross RI. Terrorism: a public health threat with a trauma system response. *J Trauma* 2003;55(6):1014-1021.

11. Kales SN, Christiani DC. Acute chemical emergencies. *N Engl J Med* 2004;350(8):800-808.

12. Klein JS, Weigelt JA. Disaster management: lessons learned. *Surg Clin North Am* 1991;71:257-266.

13. Mettler FA, Voelz GL. Major radiation exposure—what to expect and how to respond. *N Engl J Med* 2002;346(20):1554-1561.

14. Multiple authors. Perspective: The London attacks-a chronicle. *N Engl J Med* 2005;353:541-550.

15. Musolino SV, Harper FT. Emergency response guidance for the first 48 hours after the outdoor detonation of an explosive radiological dispersal device. *Health Phys* 2006;90(4):377-385.

16. National Disaster Life Support Executive Committee, National Disaster Life Support Foundation and American Medical Association. *Advanced, Basic, Core, and Decontamination Life Support Provider Manuals.* Chicago, IL: American Medical Association, 2007.

17. Pediatric Task Force, Centers for Bioterrorism Preparedness Planning, New York City Department of Health and Mental Hygiene (Arquilla B, Foltin G, Uraneck K, eds.). *Pediatric Disaster Toolkit: Hospital Guidelines for Pediatrics in Disasters.* 2nd ed. New York: New York City Department of Health and Mental Hygiene, 2006. http://www.nyc.gov/html/doh/html/bhpp/bhpp-focus-ped-toolkit.shtml. Accessed November 17, 2007.

18. Roccaforte JD, Cushman JG. Disaster preparation and management for the intensive care unit. *Curr Opin Crit Care* 2002;8(6):607-615.

19. Sever MS, Vanholder R, Lameire N. Management of crush-related injuries after disasters. *N Engl J Med* 2006;354(10):1052-1063.

APPENDIX | Triage Scenarios

Introduction

This is a self-assessment exercise, to be completed *before* you arrive for the course. Please read through the introductory information on the following pages before reading the individual scenarios and answering the related questions. This skill station is conducted in a group discussion format in which your participation is expected. Upon completion of this session, your instructor will review the answers.

The goal of this station is to apply trauma triage principles in multiple patient scenarios.

Definition of Triage

Triage is the process of prioritizing patient treatment during mass-casualty events.

Principles of Triage

DO THE MOST GOOD FOR THE MOST PATIENTS USING AVAILABLE RESOURCES

This is the central guiding principle that underlies all other triage principles, rules, and strategies. Multiple-casualty events, by definition, do not exceed the resources available. Mass-casualty events, however, do exceed available medical resources and require triage; the care provider, site, system, and/or facility is unable to manage the number of casualties using standard methods. Standard of care interventions, evacuations, and procedures cannot be completed (for each injury) for every patient within the usual time frame. The principles of triage are applied when the number of casualties exceeds the medical capabilities that are immediately available to provide usual and customary care.

MAKE A DECISION

Time is of the essence during triage. The most difficult aspect of this process is making medical decisions without

Upon completion of this session, the doctor will be able to:

OBJECTIVES

1 Define triage.

2 Explain the principles involved and the factors that must be considered during the triage process.

3 Apply the principles of triage to actual scenarios.

complete data. The triage decision maker (or triage officer) must be able to rapidly assess the scene and the numbers of casualties, focus on individual patients for short periods, and make immediate triage determinations for each patient. Triage decisions are typically made by deciding which patients' injuries constitute the greatest immediate threat to life. As such, the airway, breathing, circulation, and disability priorities of ATLS are the same priorities used to make triage decisions. That is, in general, airway problems are more rapidly lethal than breathing problems, which are more rapidly lethal than circulation problems, which are more rapidly lethal than neurologic injuries. All available information, including vital signs, when available, should be used to make each triage decision.

TRIAGE OCCURS AT MULTIPLE LEVELS

Triage is not a one-time, one-place event or decision. Triage first occurs at the scene or site of the event as decisions are made regarding which patients to treat first and the sequence in which patients will be evacuated. Next, triage typically occurs just outside the hospital to determine where patients will be transported within the facility (emergency department, operating room, intensive care unit, ward, or clinic). Triage then occurs in the preoperative area as decisions are made regarding the sequence in which patients are taken for operation.

KNOW AND UNDERSTAND THE RESOURCES AVAILABLE

Optimal triage decisions are made with knowledge and understanding of the available resources at each level or stage of patient care. The triage officer must also be immediately aware of changes in resources, whether additional or fewer.

A surgeon is the ideal triage officer for hospital triage positions because he or she understands all components of hospital function, including the operating rooms. This arrangement will not work in situations with limited numbers of surgeons and does not apply to the incident site. The medical incident commander (who may or may not elect to serve as the triage officer) should be the highest-ranking medical professional on the scene who is trained in disaster management.

PLANNING AND REHEARSAL

Triage must be planned and rehearsed, as possible. Events that are likely to occur in the local area are a good starting point for mass-casualty planning and rehearsal. For example, simulate a mass-casualty event from an airplane crash if the facility is near a major airport, a chemical spill if near a busy railroad, or an earthquake if in an earthquake zone. Specific rehearsal for each type of possible disaster is not possible, but broad planning and fine tuning of facility responses based on practice drills is possible and necessary.

DETERMINE TRIAGE CATEGORY TYPES

The title and color markings for each triage category should be determined at a systemwide level as part of planning and rehearsal. Many options are used around the world. One common, simple method is to use tags the colors of a stoplight: red, yellow, and green. Red implies life-threatening injury that requires immediate intervention and/or operation. Yellow implies injuries that may become life- or limb-threatening if care is delayed beyond several hours. Green patients are the walking wounded who have suffered only minor injuries. These patients can sometimes be used to assist with their own care and the care of others. Black is frequently used to mark dead patients. Many systems add another color, such as blue, for "expectant" patients—those who are so severely injured that, given the current number of casualties requiring care, the decision is made to simply give palliative treatment while first caring for red (and perhaps some yellow) patients. Patients who are classified as expectant because of the severity of their injuries would typically be the first priority in situations in which there are only two or three casualties requiring immediate care. However, the rules, protocols, and standards of care change in the face of a mass-casualty event. Remember: "Do the most good for the most patients using available resources."

TRIAGE IS CONTINUOUS (RETRIAGE)

Triage should be continuous and repetitive at each level or site where it is required. Constant vigilance and reassessment will identify patients whose circumstances have changed—either because of a change in physiologic status or because of a change in resource availability. As the mass-casualty event continues to unfold, the need for retriage becomes apparent. The physiology of injured patients is not constant or predictable, especially considering the limited rapid assessment required during triage. Some patients will unexpectedly deteriorate and require an "upgrade" in their triage category, perhaps from yellow to red. In others, an open fracture may be discovered after initial triage has been completed, mandating an "upgrade" in triage category from green to yellow. An important group requiring retriage is the expectant category. Although an initial triage categorization decision may label a patient as having nonsurvivable injuries, this may change after all red (or perhaps red and some yellow) patients have been cared for or evacuated (eg, a young patient with 90% burns may survive if burn center care becomes available).

Triage Scenario I
Gas Explosion in the Gymnasium

SCENARIO: You are summoned to a triage area at a construction site where 5 workers are injured in a gas explosion during the renovation of a gymnasium ceiling. You quickly survey the situation and determine that the patients' conditions are as follows:

    PATIENT A—A young man is screaming, "Please help me, my leg is killing me!"

    PATIENT B—A young woman has cyanosis and tachypnea and is breathing very noisily.

    PATIENT C—A 50-year-old man is lying in a pool of blood with his left trouser leg soaked in blood.

    PATIENT D—A young man is lying face down on a stretcher and not moving.

    PATIENT E—A young man is swearing and shouting that someone should help him or he will call his lawyer.

Questions for Response

1 *For each patient, what is the primary problem requiring treatment?*

    PATIENT A—is a young man screaming, "Please help me, my leg is killing me!"

    Possible Injury/Problem: _____

    _____

    PATIENT B—appears to have cyanosis and tachypnea and is breathing very noisily.

    Possible Injury/Problem: _____

    _____

    PATIENT C—is a 50-year-old man lying in a pool of blood with his left trouser leg soaked in blood.

    Possible Injury/Problem: _____

    _____

    PATIENT D—is lying face down on a stretcher and not moving.

    Possible Injury/Problem: _____

    _____

    PATIENT E—is swearing and shouting that someone should help him or he will call his lawyer.

    Possible Injury/Problem:_____

    _____

2 *Establish your patient priorities for further evaluation by placing a number (1 through 5, with 1 being the highest priority and 5 being the lowest) in the space next to each patient letter.*

    _____ Patient A

    _____ Patient B

    _____ Patient C

    _____ Patient D

    _____ Patient E

3 *Briefly outline your rationale for prioritizing these patients in this manner.*

    Priority 1—Patient _____:

    Rationale: _____

    _____

    _____

    _____

(Continued)

Triage Scenario I (Continued)

Priority 2—Patient _____:
Rationale: _____
_____
_____
_____
_____
_____

Priority 3—Patient _____:
Rationale: _____
_____
_____
_____
_____
_____

Priority 4—Patient _____:
Rationale: _____
_____
_____
_____
_____
_____

Priority 5—Patient _____:
Rationale: _____
_____
_____
_____
_____
_____

4 *Briefly, describe the basic life support maneuvers or additional assessment techniques you would use to further evaluate the problem(s).*

Priority 1—Patient _____:
Basic life support maneuvers or additional assessment techniques: _____
_____
_____
_____
_____
_____

Priority 2—Patient _____:
Basic life support maneuvers or additional assessment techniques: _____

_____

_____

_____

_____

_____

Priority 3—Patient _____:
Basic life support maneuvers or additional assessment techniques: _____

_____

_____

_____

_____

_____

_____

Priority 4—Patient _____:
Basic life support maneuvers or additional assessment techniques: _____

_____

_____

_____

_____

_____

_____

Priority 4—Patient _____:

_____

_____

_____

_____

_____

_____

Priority 5—Patient _____:
Basic life support maneuvers or additional assessment techniques: _____

_____

_____

_____

_____

_____

Triage Scenario II
Gas Explosion in the Gymnasium

Continuation of Scenario I:

1 *Characterize the patients according to who receives basic life support (BLS) or advanced life support (ALS) care and describe what that care would be. (Patients are listed in priority order as identified in Scenario I.)*

PATIENT	BLS	ALS	DESCRIPTION OF CARE
_____	☐	☐	_____
_____	☐	☐	_____
_____	☐	☐	_____
_____	☐	☐	_____

2 *Prioritize patient transfers and identify destinations. Provide a brief rationale for your destination choice.*

PRIORITY	PATIENT	DESTINATION	RATIONALE
1	☐ Trauma center	☐ Nearest hospital	_____
2	☐ Trauma center	☐ Nearest hospital	_____
3	☐ Trauma center	☐ Nearest hospital	_____
4	☐ Trauma center	☐ Nearest hospital	_____
5	☐ Trauma center	☐ Nearest hospital	_____

3 *In situations involving multiple patients, what criteria would you use to identify and prioritize the treatment of these patients?*

_____
_____
_____
_____

4 *What cues can you elicit from any patient that could be of assistance in triage?*

_____
_____
_____
_____

5 *Which patient injuries or symptoms should receive treatment at the scene before prehospital personnel arrive?*

_____
_____
_____
_____

6 *After prehospital personnel arrive, what treatment should be instituted, and what principles govern the order of initiation of such treatment?*

_____
_____
_____
_____

7 *In multiple-patient situations, which patients should be transported? Which should be transported early?*

_____
_____
_____
_____

8 *Which patients may have treatment delayed and be transported later?*

_____
_____
_____
_____

Triage Scenario III
Trailer Home Explosion and Fire

SCENARIO: An explosion and fire, due to a faulty gas line, has involved one trailer home in a nearby trailer park. Because of the close proximity of the incident to the hospital, the prehospital personnel transport the patients directly to the hospital without prior notification. The five patients, all members of the same family, are immobilized on long spine boards when they arrive at your small hospital emergency department. The injured patients are:

PATIENT A—**A 45-year-old man** is coughing and expectorating carbonaceous material. Hairs on his face and head are singed. His voice is clear, and he reports pain in his hands, which have erythema and early blister formation. Vital signs are blood pressure, 120 mm Hg systolic; heart rate, 100 beats per minute, and respiratory rate, 30 breaths per minute.

PATIENT B—**A 6-year-old girl** appears frightened and is crying. She reports pain from burns (erythema/blisters) over her back, buttocks, and both legs posteriorly. Vital signs are blood pressure, 110/70 mm Hg; heart rate, 100 beats per minute, and respiratory rate, 25 breaths per minute.

PATIENT C—**A 70-year-old man** is coughing, wheezing, and expectorating carbonaceous material. His voice is hoarse, and he responds only to painful stimuli. There are erythema, blisters, and charred skin on the anterior chest and abdominal walls, and circumferential burns of both thighs. Vital signs are blood pressure, 80/40 mm Hg; heart rate, 140 beats per minute, and respiratory rate, 35 breaths per minute.

PATIENT D—**A 19-year-old woman** is obtunded but responds to pain when her right humerus and leg are moved. There is no obvious deformity of the arm, and the thigh is swollen while in a traction splint. Vital signs are blood pressure, 140/90 mm Hg; heart rate, 110 beats per minute, and respiratory rate, 32 breaths per minute.

PATIENT E—**A 45-year-old man** is pale and reports pain in his pelvis. There is clinical evidence of fracture with abdominal distention and tenderness to palpation. There is erythema and blistering of the anterior chest and abdominal walls and thighs. He also has a laceration to the forehead. Vital signs are blood pressure, 130/90 mm Hg; heart rate, 90 beats per minute, and respiratory rate, 25 breaths per minute.

Management priorities in this scenario can be based on information obtained by surveying the injured patients at a distance. Although there may be doubt as to which patient is more severely injured, based on the available information, a decision must be made to proceed with the best information available at the time.

1 *Identify which patient(s) has associated trauma and/or inhalation injury in addition to body-surface burns.*

☐ Patient A   ☐ Patient B   ☐ Patient C   ☐ Patient D   ☐ Patient E

2 *Using the table provided below:*

a. Establish priorities of care in your hospital emergency department by placing a number (1 through 5, with 1 being the highest priority and 5 being the lowest) in the space next to each patient letter in the column "Treatment Priority."

b. Identify which patient has associated trauma and/or an airway injury and place a mark in the appropriate column under "Associated."

c. Estimate the percent of body-surface-area (BSA) burn for each patient and enter the percent for each patient letter in the column "% BSA."

d. Identify which patient(s) should be transferred to a burn center and/or a trauma center and place a mark in the appropriate column under "Transfer."

e. Establish your priorities for transfer and enter the priority number under "Transfer Priority."

PATIENT	ASSOCIATED		TREATMENT PRIORITY	%BSA	TRANSFER		TRANSFER PRIORITY
	Trauma	Airway Injury			Burn	Trauma	
A							
B							
C							
D							
E							

Triage Scenario IV
Cold Injury

SCENARIO: You are in your hospital when you receive a call that five members of a doctor's family were snow-mobiling on a lake when the ice broke. Four family members fell into the lake water. The doctor was able to stop in time and left to seek help. The response time of basic and advanced life support assistance was 15 minutes. By the time prehospital care providers arrived, one individual had crawled out of the lake and removed another victim from the water. Two individuals remained submerged; they were found by rescue divers and removed from the lake. Rescuers from the scene provided the following information:

PATIENT A—**The doctor's 10-year-old grandson** was removed from the lake by rescuers. The ECG monitor shows asystole.

PATIENT B—**The doctor's 65-year-old wife** was removed from the lake by rescuers. The ECG monitor shows asystole.

PATIENT C—**The doctor's 35-year-old daughter,** who was removed from the water by her sister-in-law, has bruises to her anterior chest wall. Her blood pressure is 90 mm Hg systolic.

PATIENT D—**The doctor's 35-year-old daughter-in-law,** who had been submerged and crawled out of the lake, has no obvious signs of trauma. Her blood pressure is 110 mm Hg systolic.

PATIENT E—**The 76-year-old retired doctor,** who never went into the water, reports only cold hands and feet.

1 *Establish the priorities for transport from the scene to your emergency department, and explain your rationale.*

TRANSPORT PRIORITY	PATIENT (IDENTIFY BY LETTER)	RATIONALE
1		
2		
3		
4		
5		

2 *In the emergency department, all patients should have their core temperature measured. Core temperatures for these patients are:*

PATIENT A: 29° C (84.2° F)

PATIENT B: 34° C (93.2° F)

PATIENT C: 33° C (91.4° F)

PATIENT D: 35° C (95° F)

PATIENT E: 36° C (96.8° F)

Briefly outline your rationale for the remainder of the primary assessment, resuscitation, and secondary survey.

PATIENT A: Priority _____:

_____

_____

_____

_____

_____

PATIENT B: Priority _____:

_____

_____

_____

_____

_____

PATIENT C: Priority _____:

_____

_____

_____

_____

_____

PATIENT D: Priority _____:

_____

_____

_____

_____

_____

PATIENT E: Priority _____:

_____

_____

_____

_____

_____

Triage Scenario V
Car Crash

SCENARIO: You are the only doctor available in a 100-bed community emergency department. One nurse and a nurse assistant are available to assist you. Ten minutes ago you were notified by radio that ambulances would be arriving with patients from a single motor vehicle crash. No further report is received. Two ambulances arrive with five patients who were occupants in an automobile traveling at 60 mph (96 kph) before it crashed. The injured patients are:

PATIENT A—**A 45-year-old man** was the driver of the car. He apparently was not wearing a seat belt. Upon impact, he was thrown against the windshield. On admission, he is notably in severe respiratory distress. The prehospital personnel provide the following information to you after preliminary assessment: Injuries include (1) severe maxillofacial trauma with bleeding from the nose and mouth, (2) an angulated deformity of the left forearm, and (3) multiple abrasions over the anterior chest wall. The vital signs are blood pressure, 150/80 mm Hg; heart rate, 120 beats per minute; respiratory rate, 40 breaths per minute; and Glasgow Coma Scale (GCS) score, 8.

PATIENT B—**A 38-year-old female** passenger was apparently thrown from the front seat and found 30 feet (9 meters) from the car. On admission she is awake, alert, and reports abdominal and chest pain. The report you are given indicates that, on palpating her hips, she reports pain, and fracture-related crepitus is felt. The vital signs are blood pressure, 110/90 mm Hg; heart rate, 140 beats per minute; and respiratory rate, 25 breaths per minute.

PATIENT C—**A 48-year-old male** passenger was found under the car. You are told that on admission he was confused and responded slowly to verbal stimuli. Injuries include multiple abrasions to his face, chest, and abdomen. Breath sounds are absent on the left, and his abdomen is tender to palpation. The vital signs are blood pressure, 90/50 mm Hg; heart rate, 140 beats per minute; respiratory rate, 35 breaths per minute; and GCS score, 10.

PATIENT D—**A 25-year-old woman** was extricated from the back seat of the vehicle. She is 8 months pregnant, behaving hysterically, and reporting abdominal pain. Injuries include multiple abrasions to her face and anterior abdominal wall. You are told that her abdomen is tender to palpation. She is in active labor. The vital signs are blood pressure, 120/80 mm Hg; heart rate, 100 beats per minute; and respiratory rate, 25 breaths per minute

PATIENT E—**A 6-year-old boy** was extricated from the floor of the rear seat. At the scene, he was alert and talking. He now responds to painful stimuli only by crying out. Injuries include multiple abrasions and an angulated deformity of the right lower leg. There is dried blood around his nose and mouth. The vital signs are blood pressure, 110/70 mm Hg; heart rate, 180 beats per minute; respiratory rate, 35 breaths per minute.

Questions and Response Key for Students' Response

1 *Outline the steps you would take to triage these five patients.*

_____

_____

_____

_____

_____

_____

_____

_____

_____

2 *Establish your patient priorities by placing a number (1 through 5, with 1 being the highest priority and 5 being the lowest) in the space next to each lettered patient. Then, in the space provided, briefly outline your rationale for prioritizing these patients in this manner.*

Priority _____   **Patient A :** _____

Rationale: _____

_____

_____

_____

_____

Priority _____   **Patient B :** _____

Rationale: _____

_____

_____

_____

_____

_____

Priority _____   **Patient C:** _____

Rationale: _____

_____

_____

_____

_____

_____

Priority _____   **Patient D:** _____

Rationale: _____

_____

_____

_____

_____

_____

Priority _____   **Patient E:**

Rationale: _____

_____

_____

_____

_____

_____

Triage Scenario VI
Train Crash Disaster

SCENARIO: Two trains collide head-on at 1800 hours. One train is a commercial tanker carrying eight tanker cars and is driven by an engineer and fireman. No other personnel are on board. The tanks are filled with a highly flammable liquid. The other train is a passenger train traveling on the same track. Weather conditions are mild, and the ambient temperature is 20 C (72 F). Upon arrival at the scene, EMTs and paramedics find:

DECEASED—Two engineers and one fireman

Five passengers, including one infant with a fatal head injury

INJURED—The fireman from the commercial train, ejected 30 feet, with 40% BSA second- and third-degree burns

Forty-seven passengers from the passenger train:

- 12 category Red patients, 8 with extensive (20-50% BSA) second- and third-degree burns
- 8 category Yellow patients, 3 with focal (<10% BSA) second-degree burns
- 22 category Green patients, 10 with painful hand and forearm deformities
- 5 category Blue patients, 3 with catastrophic (>75% BSA) second- and third-degree burns

Two fire companies and two additional ambulances have been called. The local community hospital has 26 beds, 5 primary care providers, and 2 surgeons, 1 of whom is on vacation. The nearest trauma center is 75 miles (120 kilometers) away, and the nearest designated burn center is over 200 miles (320 kilometers) away.

1 *Should community disaster plans be invoked? Why, or why not?*

_____

_____

2 *If a mass-casualty event is declared, who should be the medical incident commander?*

_____

_____

3 *What is the first consideration of the medical incident commander at the scene?*

_____

_____

4 *What considerations should be taken into account in medical operations at the scene?*

_____

_____

5 *What is the second consideration of the medical incident commander at the scene?*

_____

_____

6 *What is the meaning of the red, yellow, green, blue, and black triage categories?*

_____

_____

7 *Given the categories in Question 6, which patients should be evacuated to the hospital, by what transport methods, and in what order?*

_____

_____

8 *What efforts should be taken by the medical incident commander to assist with response and recovery?*

_____

_____

INDEX